WOMEN'S HEALTH SOLUTIONS

WOMEN'S HEALTH SOLUTIONS

GARY NULL

SEVEN STORIES PRESS

New York | Toronto | London | Sydney

Parts of this book have been adapted from an earlier work by Dr. Null on this topic, *For Women Only!,* a Seven Stories Press book published in 1999.

This book is not intended to replace the services of a physician. Any application of the information set forth in the following pages is at the reader's discretion. The reader should consult with his or her physician before making any use of the information in this book.

Seven Stories Press
140 Watts Street
New York, NY 10013
http://www.sevenstories.com

In Canada:
Hushion House, 36 Northline Road, Toronto, Ontario M4B 3E2

In the U.K.:
Turnaround Publisher Services Ltd., Unit 3, Olympia Trading Estate, Coburg Road, Wood Green, London N22 6TZ

In Australia:
Tower Books, 2/17 Rodborough Road, Frenchs Forest NSW 2086

Library of Congress Cataloging-in-Publication Data
Null, Gary.
   Women's health solutions / Gary Null.—1st ed.
     p. cm.
Includes index.
   ISBN 1-58322-419-X
   1. Women—Health and hygiene. 2. Women—Diseases—Alternative treatment.
I. Title.
   RA778 .N885 2002
   613'.04244–dc21   2001006594

9 8 7 6 5 4 3 2 1

College professors may order examination copies of Seven Stories Press titles for a free six-month trial period. To order, visit www.sevenstories.com/textbook, or fax on school letterhead to (212) 226-1411.

Book design by Cindy LaBreacht

Printed in Canada.

CONTENTS

CHAPTER 1 **Aging** 11
Causes 12
Symptoms 14
Clinical Experience 14
Brain Aging 32

CHAPTER 2 **AIDS** 39
AIDS in Women 40
Causes 41
Clinical Experience 43
Specific Alternative Treatment Approaches 45

CHAPTER 3 **Anemia** 57
Causes 57
Symptoms 59
Clinical Experience 59

CHAPTER 4 **Arthritis** 63
What Is Arthritis? 63
Causes 65
Clinical Experience 65
Specific Alternative Treatment Approaches 73

CHAPTER 5 **Birth Control** 95
Fertility Awareness 95
Methods of Birth Control 97

CHAPTER 6 **Breast Cancer and Other Breast Diseases** 107
Causes 107
Symptoms 112
Clinical Experience 112
Patient Stories 121
Fibrocystic Breast Disease .122
Lymphedema 126

CHAPTER 7 **Cervical Dysplasia, Fibroids, and Reproductive System Cancers** 129

Cervical Dysplasia 129
Fibroids and Uterine Bleeding 132
Reproductive System Cancers 138
Patient Stories 145

CHAPTER 8 **Chronic Fatigue Syndrome** 147

Potential Causes 148
Symptoms 152
Clinical Experience 154

CHAPTER 9 **Diabetes** 163

Causes 163
Types of Diabetes 164
Symptoms 165
Clinical Experience 165
Gestational Diabetes 171

CHAPTER 10 **Digestive Disorders** 175

Causes 175
Symptoms 177
Clinical Experience 178
Food Allergy and Digestion 181
Lactose Intolerance 183
Gastritis 183
Pressure Diseases 184
Ulcers 187

CHAPTER 11 **Eating Disorders** 191

Causes 191
Clinical Experience 194
Why Popular Diets Don't Work 202

CHAPTER 12 **Endometriosis** 207

Causes 207
Symptoms 208
Clinical Experience 209
Patient Story 214

CHAPTER 13 **Environmental Illness** 215
    Causes 216
    Symptoms 218
    Clinical Experience 218
    Patient Story 231

CHAPTER 14 **Everyday Health** 237
    Diet and Nutrition 237
    A Home Detoxification Program 238
    Natural Medicine Cabinet 242
    Colds 246
    Headaches 249
    Hangovers 251
    Insomnia 252
    Aphrodisiacs 255
    Skin Care 257
    Dental Care 266
    Hair Care 270

CHAPTER 15 **Food Allergies** 273
    Types of Food Allergies 274
    Causes 275
    Clinical Experience 276

CHAPTER 16 **Heart Disease** 287
    Causes 287
    Symptoms 288
    Clinical Experience 289

CHAPTER 17 **Herpes** 307
    Causes 308
    Symptoms 309
    Clinical Experience 310

CHAPTER 18 **Hormonal Imbalance** 315
    Causes 315
    Symptoms 317
    Clinical Experience 318

CHAPTER 19 Infertility 321
    Causes 322
    Clinical Experience 323

CHAPTER 20 Lupus 333
    Causes 333
    Symptoms 333
    Clinical Experience 334

CHAPTER 21 Menopause 337
    Causes 337
    Symptoms 338
    Clinical Experience 339

CHAPTER 22 Menstrual Cramps and Irregular Menstruation 351
    Causes 351
    Clinical Experience 352
    Amenorrhea and Menorrhagia 355
    Toxic Shock Syndrome 359

CHAPTER 23 Mental Health Concerns 363
    Depression 363
    Anxiety Disorders 378
    Obsessive-Compulsive Disorders .384
    Addiction 386

CHAPTER 24 Migraines 399
    Causes 399
    Symptoms 401
    Clinical Experience 401

CHAPTER 25 Musculoskeletal Injuries 413
    Repetitive Strain Injuries 413
    Temporomandibular Joint (TMJ) Dysfunction 420
    Pain Management 423

CHAPTER 26 Nervous System Disorders 435
    Multiple Sclerosis 435
    Parkinson's Disease 440
    Alzheimer's Disease 444

CHAPTER 27 **Osteoporosis** 449

    Causes 449

    Diagnosis 450

    Clinical Experience 450

CHAPTER 28 **Pregnancy** 457

    Natural Childbirth 458

    What is Midwifery? 459

    Stages of Pregnancy 460

    Miscarriage 461

    Healthy Pregnancy the Natural Way 462

    Breast-feeding 474

    Corrective Vaginal Surgery (Episiotomy) 476

    Postpartum Depression 477

    Abortion Aftercare 479

    Is Circumcision Necessary? 481

CHAPTER 29 **Premenstrual Syndrome (PMS)** 483

    Causes 483

    Symptoms 483

    Clinical Experience 484

    A Final Note:

    Premenstrual Dysphoric Disorder (PMDD) 489

CHAPTER 30 **Sexual Dysfunction** 491

    Causes 491

    Clinical Experience 493

CHAPTER 31 **Sexually Transmitted Diseases** 495

    Gonorrhea 495

    Chlamydia 496

    Pelvic Inflammatory Disease (PID) 498

    Human Papilloma Virus (HPV) 499

    Genital Warts 501

CHAPTER 32 **Stroke** 503

    Causes 503

    Symptoms 503

    Clinical Experience 504

CHAPTER 33 **Thyroid Disease** 507

    Importance of the Thyroid 507
    Hypothyroidism 508
    Thyroiditis 512
    Patient Stories 516

CHAPTER 34 **Urinary Incontinence** 521

    Causes 521
    Symptoms 522
    Clinical Experience 522

CHAPTER 35 **Urinary Tract Infections and Inflammations** 525

    Causes 525
    Symptoms 528
    Clinical Experience 528
    Urinary Tract Inflammations 532
    Interstitial Cystitis 533

CHAPTER 36 **Vaginal Inflammation and Infection** 537

    Causes 537
    Symptoms 538
    Clinical Experience 538
    Vaginal Yeast (Candidiasis) 539
    Patient Story 548
    Trichomonas 549
    Patient Story 551
    Bacterial Vaginosis 551

CHAPTER 37 **Varicose Veins** 553

    Causes 553
    Symptoms 554
    Clinical Experience 554

CHAPTER 38 **Selecting an Alternative Health Practitioner** 557

    Your Rights As a Patient 557
    Your Role As a Patient 558
    The Importance of Commonplace Symptoms 559
    Types of Therapies 559

    Resource Guide 577

    Index 583

CHAPTER 1

AGING

I n the largely unread, fourth book of *Gulliver's Travels*, the hero comes to an island, near Japan, where a race has realized mankind's dream of living forever. The irony is that these immortals all wish they were dead because, though they have lived hundreds of years, these have been miserable years, since they have all the infirmities of the aged, such as blindness, deafness, arthritis, and senility. Jonathan Swift's satirical thrust can be applied today, when we consider the following facts: People are living longer than ever before, but many are unable to enjoy longevity because its potential pleasures are canceled out by the prematurely early encroachments of aging.

The idea that aging inevitably means gaining weight and having high blood pressure, high cholesterol, and arthritis is widely accepted. Since so many people have these problems, we think of them as normal. Even doctors are likely to say that when we get to be a certain age, these conditions are to be expected and, since they are irreversible, accepted.

Fortunately, research over the last decade has given us a better understanding of the causes of aging; in particular, several theories have led to new therapies offering women opportunities not only to improve their health but to actually slow down the aging process. We now know that it's possible to live to a hundred and beyond and to stay healthy throughout our life spans, thus "rectangularizing" the aging curve.

Dr. Martin Feldman, a traditionally trained physician who practices complementary medicine, supports this stand. "We need to have optimum energy as we grow old, not accept the diminishment many find encroaching as they grow older," he says.

Dr. Feldman cites joint disease as an example of a condition that medicine has accepted as inevitable, a condition that is reversible. There is now an epidemic of joint disease in the United States. Osteoarthritis, the most common form, afflicts 21 million people in the United States, more than 15 million of whom are women. Conventional doctors call osteoarthritis a "wear-and-tear disease," as if the joints wear out like the parts of a car. That sounds plausible, but it is nonsense. The disease is a product of deficiencies and occurs when the joint is not being nourished. A nourished joint will remain healthy. Dr. Feldman has seen marathon runners in their seventies and eighties who use their joints ten-fold or even fifty-fold more than a normal person does, yet their joints remain robust. (See chapter 4 for a full discussion of arthritis.)

CAUSES

Free Radical Damage

It is widely accepted that aging and degenerative diseases are the result of cellular damage brought on by free radicals, molecules that have become unstable after losing one of their orbiting electrons. The unpaired electrons make the molecules highly reactive, and in an attempt to restore balance, a free radical will steal electrons from other molecules, causing cellular damage and destruction.

Free radicals are produced through normal metabolism in the body, but increase with exposure to animal fat, alcohol, cigarettes, and other toxic chemicals. Dr. Christopher Calapai, a proponent of complementary medicine who has a medical practice in New York, gives an example of how this damage can occur: "Free radicals generated by cigarette smoke are huge in number. They steal healthy electrons from the lining of the lungs, thereby oxidizing lung tissue. When lung tissue is oxidized, cells break down and die. As hundreds of thousands of cells become oxidized and damaged, tissues and organs throughout the body are affected. Aging and disease are magnified."

Low Thyroid Function

Low thyroid function can prompt diseases associated with aging. Dr. Ray Peat, a distinguished research scientist from Eugene, Oregon, says that doctors in the first part of the twentieth century were better informed than today's doctors about the importance of correcting this condition: "Most of the basic research on the thyroid was done before World War II. Pharmaceutical companies came in after the war with what they thought was the latest word in understanding the thyroid. It turns out they were wrong. Until 1940 it was accepted that 40 percent of Americans benefited from taking thyroid supplements. After faulty tests were established, it was believed that only 5 percent of Americans needed or benefited from thyroid supplements. In the 1930s indications of hypothyroidism included such things as too much cholesterol in the blood, insomnia, emphysema, arthritis, and failure of the immune system. Many conditions now considered mysterious diseases were recognized as traits of low thyroid. Very often these conditions would simply disappear when thyroid supplements were given.

"When the thyroid is low we have to rely on emergency systems—such as the production of adrenaline and cortisone—to adapt to stress. Cortisone and adrenaline are now recognized as factors that cause damage, setting degenerative diseases in motion and causing damage to the lining of blood vessels and brain cells, but very often people don't realize that it is the thyroid that keeps us from relying excessively on these stress hormones." (See chapter 33 for more on thyroid dysfunction.)

Biological Clock

Another theory on aging holds that women have a built-in cellular "biological clock" that is set so that cells self-destruct after a certain amount of time. Dr. Lance Morris, a naturopathic physician from Tucson, Arizona, notes that since the theory was first propounded, the proposed upper limits for the clock's running time have increased. "At this time," he says, "there is a feeling that the top limit is pushing 140 years. Individuals have actually lived to that age, and even longer."

Shrinking Thymus Gland

Another theory relates aging to atrophy of the thymus gland, which plays a role in maintaining a healthy immune system and fighting infection. As Dr. Morris explains, "When we are born, this gland covers our entire chest. It's huge. As we grow older, it diminishes in size, a process known as thymic involution. One of the theories of aging is that if we could stop thymic shrinking we could stop the aging process altogether."

Mercury

Dr. Hal A. Huggins of Colorado Springs, Colorado, highlights another cause of premature aging, the mercury in silver amalgam fillings. According to Dr. Huggins, the mercury in your fillings does not just sit there—you inhale it and it goes into your lungs. Every time you eat and chew, minute amounts of mercury get into your stomach and digestive system and from there to cells in all parts of your body, where it can undergo oxidation, forming methyl mercury, a highly toxic substance. (In chapter 14 you will find more on mercury and other dental concerns.)

Other Theories

Dr. Elson Haas, an integrated medicine physician, is director of the Preventive Medical Center in San Rafael, California, and author of *The Staying Healthy Shopper's Guide,* among other best-selling books. In an article on the HealthWorld Online website (www.healthy.net), he summarizes a few other theories of aging: errors in DNA, possibly caused by free radicals; alterations in brain function; imbalance in the hormonal and nervous systems; a breakdown in immune system function; and stress. His own theory, he explains, is that all these processes combine in various ways in each person to result in aging, with the key factor being "stagnation of bioenergy circulation and stagnation of the digestive tract and bowels."

SYMPTOMS

A wide variety of gradual bodily changes are associated with aging, such as an increased susceptibility to weight gain and fatigue. But there is no physiological reason why women should become obese or get tired more easily as they grow older: these are society's, not nature's, norms. It can be just as natural, for example, for a woman to eat and sleep a little less as she grows older, compensating for any slowing down of metabolic processes and thus maintaining stable weight and energy levels.

The risk of contracting degenerative diseases such as cancer and heart disease, and suffering from thyroid dysfunction, musculoskeletal problems, and gastrointestinal disorders, also typically increases with age. As women age, they may suffer from elevated blood sugar, an increase in cholesterol and triglycerides, and other chemical imbalances. Decreases in memory, concentration, and sharpness may occur. Typical signs of aging also include changes in skin, hair, nails, and connective tissue. Again, it is not inevitable that these changes take place.

CLINICAL EXPERIENCE

Diagnosing Problems

Aging well means being healthy and balanced from within. To check that all systems are running optimally, Dr. Calapai recommends a full spectrum of diagnostic tests, with special attention to adrenal function, vitamin and mineral levels, blood chemistry, pancreatic enzymes, and stool. "The adrenal glands produce our antiaging hormones. With age, some people start producing less. This can be from free radical damage, excessive stress, injuries, and all sorts of reasons. As a result we see changes in memory, concentration, skin, hair, hormonal fluctuations, and energy levels. We start to see problems with immune response and increases in blood sugar, cholesterol, and abdominal deposition of body fat. So we need to look at adrenal function.

"Certainly, tests should look at vitamin and mineral levels to check our digestive and absorptive abilities. Looking at the basic blood chemistry tells us how well we are absorbing protein. We need to look at the fat-soluble vitamins and cholesterol, triglycerides, and the ratio of good HDL cholesterol to bad LDL cholesterol, which can provide information about our fat absorption. I also recommend looking at enzymes of the pancreas to assess function and having a comprehensive stool analysis done to see whether or not there are too many undigested particles in the stool. If parasites are present, this can decrease our absorptive ability. These are some of the main tests we need to perform to get a thorough picture of the individual."

Antiaging Diet

A basic healthy diet will vastly improve the quality of life and reduce the aging process in women of all ages. This diet should consist of high-quality organic foods, emphasizing complex carbohydrates such as beans and whole grains, fruits, and vegetables. Adolescents, who are still growing, may need more of certain nutrients, and people in specific age groups may have specific nutrient requirements that can be addressed through supplements.

Antiaging diets contain no animal proteins. Let me repeat that. Not a little bit, not a moderate amount, but zero animal products. What you do want are high-fiber foods. This means about 50 to 60 grams of fiber a day, soluble and nonsoluble. High-fiber diets help prevent common afflictions associated with aging, such as constipation, hemorrhoids, pressure in the intestines, ulcers, high blood pressure, colorectal cancer, and overall body toxemia.

One of the principles of longevity is eating to the point of being not quite full. As we get older, it is advisable to eat small servings more frequently. I'd rather see you eat three small servings a day than one big meal because your body requires energy throughout the day and if you only eat one meal, your body is not going to be able to sustain its energy. You'll think it's normal to be fatigued about four hours after you've eaten your meal when what's happening is your blood sugar level is simply low. It takes you twice as long to digest food when you're older because your whole metabolism is slowed down.

Many senior citizens suffer from dehydration because their intake of fluid is inadequate. Dehydration adversely affects the body's electrolytes, which carry electricity and are important for normal functioning of the nervous system. You should drink at least ten 8-ounce glasses of liquid daily. I don't want you drinking tap water. It's too polluted, no matter what your public health official says. I've done so much work showing what's in a glass that you can't even see. In addition to water, either filtered or distilled, you should be drinking juices. There is a proper way to take the juices so you don't overwhelm the system. Start with one glass of juice per day for the first month. Then add a glass a day per month until you reach six glasses a day at the end of six months. The juice floods the body with phytochemicals and chlorophyll, which are really important for healing.

Supplements

The first thing to look at as a means of reversing the symptoms of aging is supplements. Many people do not understand the effective use of vitamins and minerals as dietary supplements. Basically, you must follow the law of compensation. If you are a woman who smoked, used sugar, caffeine, or alcohol, if you were an angry person who held in your anger, if you have not honored the life force, if you have not exercised, if you have felt unfulfilled, you must work to compensate for these deficiencies.

One-a-day supplements are the easy way out. I have met people who say, "I eat meat. I eat sugar. But it's all right because I take my one-a-day vitamin." My friend, that does not work. The body cannot be lied to. After thirty or forty years of the body's being debilitated by an unhealthy lifestyle and environment, a little pill will not do the trick. You need to detoxify and cleanse the body.

You have to know what your bodily state is and plan accordingly. I would suggest one level of usage for healthy women who know they are healthy, and a very different level for those processing diseases. A person becoming conscious of her health will need to consult a nutritionist who can design a personalized supplement program to meet her individual needs.

The reason that supplements are even more crucial as we get older is that as we age, certain fatty acids, amino acids, and members of the main groups of nutrients are lost. Scientists looking into this issue already know that choline, tyrosine, glutathione, cysteine, vitamin E, zinc, and chromium are poorly absorbed and deficient in older people. Meanwhile, as these substances grow scarce, there is a buildup of heavy metals, such as aluminum and lead. These metals can be removed from the body through a process known as chelation. Vitamin C and zinc are also useful in flushing them out. Most importantly, all the nutrients that are lost, for whatever reason, must be restored for optimum physical and mental functioning.

At the same time, the free radicals in our bodies, which grow in number as we age, have to be fought. Remember, when you eat meat, drink alcohol, and are exposed to pollutants, the body creates free radicals. They cause the skin to wrinkle in the sun, and they foster cancer, arthritis, and heart disease. However, antioxidants, such as beta carotene and vitamin A, are able to neutralize the effect of the free radicals, slowing down the aging process.

Antioxidants

Dr. Morris calls aging a catch-22: "Oxygen is the great substance that sustains and gives life, but unfortunately it is also the substance that destroys us through oxidation." For this reason, antioxidants are essential. Here are the most important ones:

VITAMIN E—400–1,600 IU, taken at the largest meal. Women with herpes, chronic fatigue syndrome, hepatitis, and even AIDS have dramatically improved after taking large doses of this vitamin on a regular basis. Vitamin E is best in its natural form (as a mixed tocopherol or d-alphatocopherol). Synthetic vitamin E (dl-alpha) should be avoided.

BETA CAROTENE—25,000 IU per meal. Beta carotenes can be obtained in all the green, red, and orange fruits and vegetables. They help slow down aging and lessen cancer risk. They are nontoxic, since the body converts beta carotenes into vitamin A and will not convert more than it can use.

VITAMIN A— 5,000–10,000 IU per day. Vitamin A is a fat-soluble vitamin essential for healthy bones, skin, eyes, digestion, and immune function. Blood tests will determine whether or not a woman is getting too much vitamin A, which can be toxic.

SELENIUM—100 mcg once or twice a day. One cause of premature aging and even death, particularly in professional athletes, is cardiomyopathy, an enlargement of the heart. This is usually associated with selenium deficiency. Adequate amounts of this critical nutrient are needed to help the body produce the antioxidant enzyme glutathione peroxidase, which is on the front line of aging defense.

ZINC—30–90 mg daily. Zinc feeds more than one hundred enzyme systems in the brain, as well as various systems throughout the body. It is essential in the formation of stomach acid; without sufficient zinc, malabsorption syndrome occurs. Malabsorption is the failure of the body to absorb at the cellular level the nutrients that have been ingested. Most older people are zinc-deficient.

VITAMIN C—The single most important dietary supplement is vitamin C. I generally suggest people start at 1,000 mg a day. Then, in divided doses of 500 mg several times a day, you start to gradually take yourself up to 10,000–20,000 mg a day. This process takes several months. To really fight disease, you may have to take 200,000 mg daily via intravenous drips, under medical supervision of course. The benefits of this vitamin are multiple. Vitamin C is important for the skin, giving it youthful elasticity. This is because it produces collagen, a type of connective tissue that holds the muscles and skin together. It helps the body produce interferon and increases white blood cell disease-fighting activity. It aids the thymus gland, the liver, and the brain, and acts to prevent arthritis, cataracts, and heart disease.

At the Healing Center of New York City, drips of vitamin C and other nutrients are used to counteract the aging process. Dr. Howard Robins points out that toxins and free radicals are stressful to both the body and the mind. A body in pain, fatigued, and under attack from heavy metal and other pollutants is weakened, and the mind is adversely affected. Dr. Robins asserts that intravenously administered vitamin C cleanses the body. The Healing Center also uses drips with other nutrients, such as EDTA (ethylenediaminetetra-acetic acid) to cleanse the heavy metals from the body, and destroy viruses and keep them from replicating. These drips will also help boost energy levels.

GRAPESEED EXTRACT—50 mg per day and up to 200 mg per day for people in a disease state. This is a bioflavonoid, a water-soluble substance that ensures the strength and proper function of the capillaries, helps manufacture collagen, and protects the cells against attack and invasion by viruses and bacteria. It has the highest known antioxidant properties of any nutrient.

SUPEROXIDE DISMUTASE (SOD)—This important antienzyme nutrient is produced by the body. It is not effective when taken orally unless it is enteric-coated. According to Dr. Haas, manganese and copper, together with zinc, support the action of superoxide dismutase.

Hormones

Dr. Richard Ash has talked to his large New York City radio audience about the revivifying power of DHEA (dihydroepiandrosterone), which is a key ingredient underlying the normal functioning of the adrenal gland. He tells us that when the body is under stress, the adrenal gland requires higher amounts of cortisone and adrenaline. If these hormones are overused, they will become depleted, as will DHEA, their precursor.

An eighty-year-old woman may have only one-twentieth of the DHEA she had at age twenty. According to Dr. Ash, this can result in all sorts of negative consequences for the immune system, leading to a weakened capacity to fight diseases. One of the earliest signs of DHEA depletion is an inability to get REM sleep, which can lead to insomnia and chronic fatigue. An uninformed doctor may prescribe sleeping pills for a patient with insomnia, which will not get at the root of the problem. Other symptoms of low DHEA levels are hyperglycemia (an excess of glucose in the blood), palpitations, sweating, confusion, poor concentration, and the inability to cope with everyday stress.

Another effect of low DHEA is a reduction in salivary IgA, an antibody that fights infection in the gastrointestinal (GI) tract. When IgA is depleted or absent, there will be more antigen penetration in this area as well as increased sensitivity reactions to foods and chemicals. There may be inflammation of the GI tract, a condition called "leaky gut," in which certain foods and chemicals are not absorbed but pass out into the bloodstream. When the body tries to defend itself against these unexpected intruders, autoimmune disease may arise. Dr. Ash notes that by administering DHEA and building back up salivary IgA, we can diminish food sensitivity, lower toxic load, and repair the GI tract, restoring normal immune system functioning by treating the cause, not the symptoms.

Dr. Eric Braverman, founder of Princeton Associates for Total Health in Princeton, New Jersey, has found that counteracting the aging process has to be undertaken on an individual basis. His treatments are personalized on the basis of each patient's specific hormone balance, brain function, attention span, memory capacity, and cardiac and exercise capacities. Once these have been evaluated, the patient's nutritional needs are assessed. He recommends natural yam extract, which contains progesterone, estrogen, and testosterone (PET), the three hormones he considers essential. Progesterone has anticancer properties and helps calm the brain. Estrogen strengthens the bones, has anticancer effects, especially in the colon, aids memory, and gives cardiovascular protection.

Testosterone reduces the side effects of other hormones, and helps keep the sex drive vigorous through a person's fifties, sixties, and beyond. For a woman, the ovary produces all three of these substances, but, as Dr. Braverman puts it, "If the ovary dies, you must resurrect it. If you permit an organ to die, you allow yourself to die. We must stop this if we want abundant life. We replace depleted hormones with PET, and missing adrenal with DHEA."

Bioflavonoid Complex

Another invaluable supplement group is the citrus bioflavonoid complex, which can be obtained from lemons, plums, and oranges, among other fruits. With an orange, one can cut open the skin and right below is the nutrient, the bioflavonoid. Another good bioflavonoid is rutin, which comes from buckwheat. To take the bioflavonoid in pill form, I recommend 300 mg per day for a healthy woman, while someone in poor health should take 500 to 1,000 mg. As for the rutin, the proper dosage for a healthy person is 25 mg per day, while the ill person may take up to 50 mg.

BLUEBERRY AND RED CABBAGE EXTRACTS—Blueberry extract is good for the eyes. During World War II, the Royal Air Force gave this to its pilots to improve night vision and strengthen the immune system. Red cabbage extract is also important. There are cultures that lack a variety of foodstuffs, but those people eat cabbage and obtain its antibacterial, antiulcer properties. Cabbage, eaten juiced or steamed, is very healthful.

GREEN TEA—If you lived in China, you would probably be drinking green tea and taking green tea extract. We know it has anticancer properties. It is an immune system stimulator. Decaffeinated green tea is very beneficial.

GLUTATHIONE—Glutathione is good for the immune system, but it is not easily assimilated by the body, so it should be taken with something that produces it in the body, such as N-acetyl-cysteine (NAC). Generally you need 500 mg of NAC and 500 mg of reduced glutathione.

Other Supplements

CALCIUM—Calcium protects against osteoporosis and colon cancer, is important for strong teeth, and helps energy production as well as heart and nerve function.

CHROMIUM—Chromium supports glucose tolerance, decreasing the craving for sugar, and plays a role in preventing atherosclerosis by helping to lower blood cholesterol.

COENZYME Q10—Every cell in the body needs this coenzyme to create energy and build stamina.

L-CARNITINE—L-carnitine, a nonessential amino acid involved in fat metabolism, may help reduce fat and weight.

L-CYSTEINE—This amino acid, which scavenges free radicals, protects the tissues from chemicals and aids detoxification, partly by helping the liver produce and store glutathione. Most often it is taken with vitamin C to prevent the formation of kidney stones of cysteine, which is produced when cysteine is metabolized. Take 250 mg with a gram of vitamin C twice a day. When you take L-cysteine on a regular basis, you should also take a formula that contains the other amino acids the body needs.

DIGESTIVE AIDS—*Lactobacillus acidophilus,* along with other intestinal bacteria, may be needed occasionally to support the balance of bacteria in the colon. Similarly, supplements of hydrochloric acid and digestive enzymes aid digestion and metabolism of food, and thus prevent both nutritional deficiencies and free-radical formation due to food reactions.

ESSENTIAL FATTY ACIDS—Essential fatty acids, such as EPA (eicosapentaenoic acid) and DHA (docosahexaenoic acid), diminish the risk of cardiovascular disease. Omega-3 fatty acids, derived primarily from plant oils, help regulate blood cholesterol and promote the health of the immune, cardiovascular, and nervous systems. Flaxseed oil is a superb source of omega-3. Omega-6 fatty acids, which come from fish oils, are important for blood clotting and constriction of blood vessels.

FOLIC ACID—Folic acid also helps in RNA, DNA, and red blood cell synthesis.

MAGNESIUM—Magnesium supports the cardiovascular system and decreases nervous tension.

MOLYBDENUM—Molybdenum is a trace mineral that may help prevent cancer.

NIACIN—Niacin, a form of vitamin B3, decreases cholesterol and helps improve circulation.

NADH (NICOTINAMIDE ADENINE DINUCLEATIDE)—Also known as coenzyme 1, NADH is a naturally occurring substance in the body that supplies energy to the cells, allowing them to live longer.

RNA—RNA, taken in blue-green algae, spirulina, chlorella, and wheatgrass (all of which are also rich in chlorophyll), can decelerate the aging process.

SEA ALGAE—High in trace elements, antioxidant cofactors, flavonoids, and carotenoids.

THYMUS EXTRACT—Pure oral thymus extract enhances immune function and helps reverse the aging process.

TYROSINE—Strengthens the thyroid and adrenal glands, protecting against stress.

VITAMIN B12—Vitamin B12 boosts energy and protects the fatty sheaths that cover the nerves. It is involved in synthesis of red blood cells and DNA and RNA, which are needed for important rebuilding processes.

Herbs

Herbs are an important part of any antiaging nutritional protocol, and can be taken as capsules, powders, teas, or tinctures.

FO-TI—Fo-ti rejuvenates the endocrine system and is an excellent digestive tonic.

GINKGO BILOBA—The ginkgo tree has survived for hundreds of thousands of years due to its powerful immune system. An extract of the leaf of the tree improves circulation to the microcapillaries of the brain and heart so that needed nutrients and oxygen can get to all the tissues.

GINSENG—Ginseng is the best-known longevity herb. For centuries, the Chinese have revered ginseng for its rejuvenating effects. Research has shown that ginseng can stop the free radical damage associated with aging. It helps people focus better when under stress and increases overall energy levels.

GOTU KOLA—Gotu kola is useful for increasing vitality and endurance, and may lower blood pressure.

HAWTHORN BERRIES—Hawthorn berries support circulation and cardiac function.

MILK THISTLE—Milk thistle protects liver function. The liver releases toxins from the body, promoting health and youthfulness.

YAM—Wild yam supports adrenal gland production of DHEA, a building block for the development of estrogen, progesterone, testosterone, and cortisols, which decrease with age. As an adaptogen, wild yam balances the body's hormonal functions. It has been shown to ameliorate numerous chronic conditions, including heart disease, cancer, arthritis, and autoimmune diseases. DHEA is extremely safe, with no known side effects.

Dr. Haas mentions two other beneficial herbs: **CAPSICUM** stimulates elimination, and circulation, and its mild diuretic properties help cleanse the kidneys. **GARLIC** is antiviral, antibacterial, and antifungal. It boosts energy but—unlike coffee—helps lower cholesterol and blood pressure. Garlic also stimulates liver and colon detoxification and may have anticancer properties.

Detoxification Therapies

The more toxic we are, the faster we age. Cosmetic changes such as face-lifts and hair dye may temporarily make women appear younger, but they do not make a real difference. To keep youthful and healthy, we must address what is happening inside.

"Everyone needs detoxification," says Susana Lombardi, founder and president of the We Care Health Center in Palm Springs, California, and author of *Ten Easy Steps for Complete Wellness*. "I am vegetarian, and I take care of myself. Do I still need detoxification? Yes, because the air that we breathe is polluted, the water that we drink is full of chlorine, the clothing we wear is made of artificial fabrics and chemicals, the lotions and shampoos that we use all contain chemicals. Once these chemicals are inside us, we never fully eliminate them unless we go through a detoxification procedure."

Lombardi recommends rejuvenating the system from the inside out by, once a week, limiting food intake to fresh raw vegetable juices. She and many other practitioners also recommend the following simple, yet effective, detoxification therapies.

JUICE FASTING

Juice fasting gives the digestive system a rest and speeds up the growth of new cells, which promotes healing. (If you have any medical problems, do not fast without medical approval and supervision.)

On a juice fast, a person abstains from solid foods and drinks juice, water, and herbal teas throughout the day. "We should be drinking every half hour to an hour," advises Lombardi. "If we go for long periods of time without drinking anything, then a little glass of juice will not be able to sustain us. But if we are constantly drinking, the day will go by very smoothly."

Lombardi recommends a combination of the following:

CARROT JUICE—High in the antioxidant beta carotene and full of wonderful enzymes.

CELERY JUICE—High in sodium, not the artificial type poured from the saltshaker, which is bad for you, but the good, natural kind that promotes tissue flexibility.

BEET JUICE—Beets nourish the liver, one of the most important organs in the body, with hundreds of different functions. If your liver is functioning well, most likely everything else in your body will be too.

CABBAGE JUICE—Cabbage juice is high in vitamin C.

Mix the juice from each vegetable in equal proportion and drink this combination throughout the day. A little cayenne, which increases circulation, sending blood to every corner of the body to promote healing, can be added for flavor. Lemon juice in water and different herbal teas—some good ones are parsley and dandelion tea for the liver and kidneys and pau d'arco for blood purification—can be added for variety. "Any herbal tea free of caffeine will be good," Lombardi says. "Since you need to drink on an hourly basis, you don't want to drink the same thing over and over."

Other juices that I recommend, not necessarily as part of a fasting program but important to your daily health regimen, include tomato, watermelon, cherry, blueberry, and raspberry. These contain phytochemicals, such as lycopene and anthocyanin, the blockbuster antioxidants that protect against cancer, heart disease, and other ailments.

CHELATION THERAPY

Dr. Martin Dayton, who is board-certified in family medicine, chelation therapy, and clinical nutrition, says that chelation therapy has multiple benefits, and long life is one of them: "Dramatic increases in life span are found with chelation. While there are no longevity studies per se, this conclusion is implied indirectly by studies that show a lessening of killer degenerative diseases. In fact, chelation favorably impacts all four major causes of death in the United States [heart disease, cancer, cerebrovascular disease, and lung disease]."

During the chelation process, many beneficial changes occur at the cellular level. A synthetic amino acid called EDTA is administered to the patient via intravenous drip. Once in the bloodstream, EDTA attaches itself to heavy metals such as lead, cadmium, and mercury and holds onto those toxic substances until they exit the body through the urine. Dr. Dayton explains why removal of these substances is vital to good health: "The toxic material prevents normal function and repair. For example, lead prevents normal enzymatic processes so that the body cannot function properly and repair itself. This leads to premature aging and the premature development of disease. Removal of toxic material through chelation keeps the body functioning optimally."

Dr. Dayton notes that even an excess of iron, which is necessary for life, accelerates free radical production and causes harm: "Periodic purging of iron from the body via menstrual bleeding is thought to protect women from hardening of the arteries. However, this protection is lost at menopause with the cessation of menstruation. At this time, arterial clogging accelerates. Chelation removes this excess iron."

Since modern people are overwhelmed by pollutants, Dr. Dayton recommends chelation therapy for anyone over the age of thirty. "Lead is found everywhere, in the air we breathe, the water we drink, the food supply. It is even found at the North Pole. Lead and other toxic pollutants are hard to avoid in today's world. As a matter of fact, the concentration of lead found in the human skeleton now is several hundred times greater than that found in our preindustrial revolution ancestors. In one study, where lead was thought to be involved, eighteen years following chelation therapy a ten-fold decrease in cancer death rate was found for those who had the treatment versus those who had nothing."

Aside from its overall benefits, chelation therapy specifically helps aging individuals by improving brain function. Dr. Dayton cites the following evidence: "Research shows that circulation improves greatly in the brain and to the brain. One study of fifteen patients who had twenty infusions of chelation therapy found that fourteen out of fifteen demonstrated significant cerebral blood flow. Some showed dramatic improvement in cognitive abilities. In another study, thirty patients with carotid blockages were given thirty chelation treatments over a ten-month period. The carotid artery extends from the chest through the neck to the brain. It is the brain's main source of blood flow. Blockage decreased between twenty and forty percent.

"Unclogging carotid blockage is vitally important because the American College of Physicians states that patients with an obstruction of 70 percent or greater are at a high risk for stroke. They even recommend chelation therapy as a preferred treatment. I take that to heart and use chelation therapy on these individuals. People who have carotid artery disease improve as their arteries open up. I see this happen over and over again."

COLON CLEANSING

Colon cleansing is an ancient and time-honored health practice for rejuvenating the body; it was used in Egypt more than four thousand years ago. Later, Hippocrates taught these procedures in his health care system. The large intestine, or colon, is healed, rebuilt, and finally restored to its natural size, normal shape, and correct function.

Colon therapist Anita Lotson explains the procedure and some of its physical and psychological benefits: "There are several stages of therapy. The first segment involves cleansing, a thorough washing of the large intestine. The colon is irrigated by a technique whereby water is gently infused into the large bowel, flowing in and out at steady intervals. Through this method, water is allowed to travel the entire length of the colon, all the way around to the cecum area. The walls of the colon are washed and old encrustations and fecal material are loosened, dislodged, and swept away. This toxic waste material has often been attached to the bowel walls for many, many years. It is laden with bacteria, which set up the perfect environment for disease to take root and entrench itself in the system, wreaking havoc. As this body pollution is eliminated, many conditions—from severe skin disorders to breathing difficulties, depression, chronic fatigue, nervousness, severe constipation, and arthritis—are reduced in severity, providing great relief, especially when augmented with dietary changes and other treatment modalities.

"The next phases are healing, rebuilding, and finally restoration of a healthy colon, functioning at maximum efficiency for the final absorption of nutrients, and the total and timely elimination of all remaining waste materials. During the healing phase, we begin to infuse materials into the bowel that will cool inflamed areas and strengthen weak sections of the colon wall. Flaxseed tea, white oak bark, and slippery elm bark all soothe, lubricate, and introduce powerful healing agents directly into the large intestine. These herbal teas may be taken orally as well. Simple dietary changes have been made by now, such as the addition of water. This simple measure spells the difference between success and failure in alleviating many bowel conditions. I ask all my clients to double their intake of water.

"I love to see people's change in attitude from the time they come in to the time that they leave. Sometimes people are very irritable when their bowels are backed up. They're often depressed, and sometimes nasty. By the time they leave, you can see a smile and a bounce in their step. It's a different person altogether."

ENZYME THERAPY

Nina Anderson, author of *Over Fifty, Looking Thirty: The Secrets of Staying Young*, attributes slow aging to sufficient enzyme levels: "Many scientists say that people get old before their time due to enzyme exhaustion. Some people are old at forty because of the lack of enzymes, while others are young at eighty because of an abundance. Above all else, I would advise anybody who is trying to avoid looking and feeling older as they get older to take supplemental enzymes."

She goes on to explain that enzymes allow nutrients to be used. For example, you have enzymes in the heart that allow magnesium to be used. Without those enzymes, magnesium cannot get to the heart: "Enzymes are molecule catalysts found everywhere in your body. In fact, there are over thirteen hundred different ones. They make everything happen. In my book I use this analogy: minerals are building blocks of your body. They are the nose, eyes, ears, bones, all the things that hold you together. Something has to build this. Enzymes are the construction workers that facilitate everything in the body going together."

Anderson recommends that women eat more raw foods, mineral supplements, and digestive plant enzymes to increase enzyme levels. Raw foods are loaded with enzymes. Fruit and vegetable juices are filled with enzymes. When food is processed, the first things taken out are enzymes. Why? Because the enzymes are what allow the food to ripen. However, if the food becomes too ripe, it rots. To stop it from ripening and rotting so that it can be sold longer, these enzymes must be destroyed. But if you destroy the enzymes, you destroy the food's life force. It will have carbohydrates, vitamins, fats, and minerals, but not its life force.

"The mineral supplements to take," Anderson adds, "should be in crystalloid form, with electrolytes. The crystalloid form goes right into the cell walls. This fortifies your body.

"Plant enzymes assist in the digestion of food right on through the intestinal tract. You want to help the digestive process for the whole length of the digestive tract. With supplemental enzymes, you won't have an upset stomach anymore or feel bloated and exhausted after a big meal. The skin will start to improve too. The skin manifests everything that happens inside. If your inner organs start to degenerate, if they are not functioning properly, this kind of stress shows up on your face. The first thing people do when they start getting older is look in the mirror and go, 'Oh my God, I've got wrinkles.' They spend millions trying to get rid of them. But what they have to realize is that wrinkles start from inside. You have to work on the inside to get the outside to reflect that good health.

"Without the proper enzymes, none of the other good things you do matter. For example, the fat-soluble vitamins A, D, E, and K require fat for absorption. That fat has to be broken down by an enzyme, lipase. If lipase is not present in sufficient quantities, that fat will not be broken down. If the fat isn't broken down, the vitamins will not be released. Therefore, you can spend a fortune on vitamin pills, and if you don't have the proper enzymes to release those vitamins into your system, they are just going to be flushed out."

Enzymes can be used externally as well as internally for youthful effects. Anderson explains, "There are amazing enzyme treatments for the skin. Papaya enzymes are wonderful. Or you can mix a plant enzyme powder and put it on as a mask. Not only does it take the lines out of your face, but it fills them in and builds up collagen. It can also get rid of age spots and shrink moles. When you use enzymes as a mud pack when you come in from the sun, it fights free radicals that otherwise might foster melanoma."

EXERCISE AND OTHER PHYSICAL TECHNIQUES

When we exercise, we detoxify as we sweat through our skin and exhale from our lungs. Some good exercises include jogging or daily brisk walks, yoga stretches, and jumping on a minitrampoline, which exercises every cell in the body. Exercise slows down the aging process because it stimulates detoxification.

Chiropractor Mitch Proffman says that traditional cultures have appreciated the connection between physical fitness and longevity, making athletic activities a part of women's ritual ceremonies: "In traditional Navajo society women would run three times daily as a formal part of the four-day rites of passage after the onset of menstruation. The first run was at dawn, and each subsequent run would be for a longer distance. It was believed that the total distance a woman could run would determine her longevity."

He goes on to state that recent research supports the connection between exercise and a longer life: "The *Journal of the American Medical Association* has reported that exercise increases people's life spans. Women walking forty to fifty minutes, three to four times per week, live longer. The same article claims that exercise decreases the chance of dying from all known diseases. This can be attributed to the fact that most major diseases, such as cancer, diabetes, and heart disease, are stress-related, and exercise reduces stress.

"Another important function of exercising is that people's mental abilities improve. In a recent study at the University of Illinois, Dr. William Greenboro studied four different groups of rats. One group led a sedentary life. Another group played aimlessly on wood and plastic in their cages. A third group was on a special motorized wheel, and a fourth group walked through intricate mazes and ropes. The finding was that all rats that exercised in any manner had more capillaries in their brains and better brain function. This suggests that exercise fuels the brain with more oxygen and increases natural growth factors, in humans as well as in rats."

Dr. Joseph Pizzorno, past president of John Bastyr College of Naturopathic Medicine in Washington, says that strengthening exercises are the best defense against the increased frailty women face as they age: "It turns out that the majority of the debility of old age is simply due to people not using their muscles. The full strength of what one had at twenty and thirty is almost completely returned with weight-strengthening exercises. There are a lot of different weight-training programs out there. I have been doing some research. The one I find most effective, and am now using personally, is something called Super Slow. Weights are used in a very, very controlled, very, very intense way to get maximum effects from the exercise. I am quite impressed with what I have seen."

STRESS RELEASE

"In my personal opinion, the single most important factor influencing aging and disease is stress," says Dr. Morris. "We need to control emotional anxieties and tensions, and learn how to not let life get to us. It is important to learn to let go and enjoy life." Methods Dr. Morris and others suggest to overcome stress include deep breathing exercises, Reiki, skin brushing, saunas, and magnetic healing. Tai chi, yoga, meditation, qi gong, massage, biofeedback, and the Feldenkrais method are also recommended.

Since exercise increases oxygenation, it also has the potential to foster free radical damage. To prevent undesirable effects, women may want to combine exercise with sufficient amounts of antioxidants in the diet and/or as dietary supplements.

BREATHING EXERCISES

Breathing exercises combined with physical activity increase the action of lymphatic cleansing. Detoxification expert Susana Lombardi explains: "For lymphatic cleansing, you want to synchronize your breathing with the movement of your legs and arms. When you are walking or jumping on the trampoline, inhale four times and exhale four times. Move your arms and legs each time you take a little breath. Inhale through your nose and exhale through your nose or mouth.

"This breathing technique was learned from the Taromaro Indians, who live in the northern part of Mexico. They are famous for their fantastic health. They have no need of hospitals or homes for the elderly. They have no disease, no police force, no jails, and no mental institutions."

REIKI

Reiki is a type of massage therapy or bodywork in which pressure point techniques are used to move energy through the body, achieving balance and harmony. Reiki therapist Nilsa Vergara reports below on her clients' experiences with Reiki therapy.

"My first example is a fifty-nine-year-old woman who came to our healing circle feeling old and tired. She suffered from aches and severe pain in her neck and knee from car accidents. She was also going through job changes, and was estranged from her adult son.

"Each week she received a fifteen-minute session, and she quickly began feeling better. She released a lot of emotional toxins via crying and verbal expression of what she was feeling. She decided to take a Reiki class so that she could give herself daily treatments.

"Within a month, her changes were quite dramatic. She had a tremendous increase in energy and vigor. She told me she now feels like she is twenty-eight. With the Reiki, she now has very little pain. She feels emotional and vital. Her attitude has changed. She feels self-fulfilled and in control of her life. Her relationship with her son has greatly improved. To quote her, 'I feel like my whole life is as it should be.'

"My next client is a sixty-five-year-old woman. When she first came to see us, she was depressed. She had been in therapy for years, but nothing seemed to lift the depression. She felt tired all the time and would catch colds easily. Emotionally, she felt like a victim, and others treated her like one.

"After her first fifteen-minute session she felt immediately better. She knew that something powerful was happening. She returned and eventually studied Reiki. Today, she reports feeling much healthier. She has more energy and an optimistic outlook. She no longer feels like a victim, and if anyone tries to put her in that role, she is no longer afraid to set limits. In addition, she is much more able to tolerate cold weather, which indicates that her body has improved its oxygen intake.

"One of my students has an eighty-three-year-old mother who fell and broke her hip bone as well as bones in her wrist and arm. She decided to give her mother Reiki regularly, and her mother responded quite well. She began feeling stronger and stronger. Within four weeks she was out of her cast, walking with just the aid of a cane, not a walker. This is pretty remarkable for an eighty-three-year-old, because a broken hip does not always lead to a good outcome. So, as you can see, Reiki really enhances the body's ability to recuperate.

"Another client is a fifty-three-year-old woman who had some serious memory problems. Her thinking was scattered; emotionally, she was fearful and guilt-ridden; and she was estranged from her adult children.

"I recommended Reiki to her to see if we could work through some of these emotional blockages and change these negative patterns. She took a Reiki class, and within six months, her memory improved tremendously. She was much more focused in her thinking, and her job performance improved greatly. She became more insightful and much less fearful. Now she can speak with her adult children and set limits, and she no longer feels anxious and guilt-ridden. In addition to using Reiki, she uses herbal teas for detoxification, drinks vegetable juices, fasts, and gets colonics."

SKIN BRUSHING

Using a natural brush on dry skin removes dead cells and leaves pores open, so that more toxins can be expelled. Lombardi explains why this is so important: "We are supposed to eliminate toxins through the pores of the skin. Due to pollution, smog, the creams we use, the clothes we wear, and so forth, our pores are more closed than open. Always brush toward the heart."

SAUNAS

The sauna is a good follow-up to dry skin brushing because it pushes toxins out through the skin. The main thing to remember with saunas is to be prudent. You want to perspire but not remain there for too long. Nor do you want too much heat. "Follow the directions," says Lombardi. "And wear a cooling drape on your head. You don't want to heat up the brain area."

There are multiple benefits from sauna detoxification, explains Lombardi: "You will look and feel better. Your skin will be clear and you will not have constipation. Your nails will improve as well as your heart and digestive system. It will clear your mind and improve concentration. Nothing will destress your body like a sauna."

MAGNETIC HEALING

Susan Bucci is a holistically trained nurse who has spearheaded the development of magnetic healing products. "Magnets oxygenate tissues and allow cell walls to absorb more oxygen," she explains. "They promote mental acuity and normalize pH balance by increasing alkalinity. Restorative sleep is enhanced. Therapeutically, they stop pain, fight infection, and reduce inflammation and fluid retention. Over time, fatty and calcium deposits dissolve and the circulatory system opens up. Put that all together and you've got healing from A to Z. Take that a step further: If you achieve optimal well-being, you can actually live a long, productive life."

In addition, magnets can eliminate many specific signs and symptoms of old age. Bucci reports these antiaging benefits from her own use of magnetic healing techniques: "My energy level has increased. I used to have chronic fatigue in the worst way, but now that's gone. My immune system is functioning much better, so my susceptibility to viruses and colds has decreased dramatically. Allergies are basically gone, and there are no more killer sinus headaches. My circulation has improved so that I withstand weather a whole lot easier. Wounds heal quickly, and my spider veins have disappeared. Also, I was headed for an early menopause, but now my menstrual cycle is very much on track, very regular.

"Hair, skin, and nails have definitely improved. My hair grows faster and has a much better quality to it. Within two weeks of using magnets on a daily basis, I was able to see new, thick, dark hair growing. My grays started falling out and disappearing. I was going to color my hair about four years ago, and I still haven't touched it with an ounce of anything. My skin definitely looks and feels younger. And my nails grow so well that if I break one, it doesn't upset me. I know that it will grow right back."

How can magnets do so much? Simply stated, magnets confer a wide range of benefits because we are magnetic beings who derive energy from the earth's magnetic field. Bucci explains: "One reason we get sick is that the earth has lost a good deal of its magnetism, which leaves the body in an unbalanced state. Additionally, we are bombarded by unhealthy energies." Magnets create overall benefit by restoring internal harmony.

It is important to realize that not just any magnet will do. The negative pole restores health and good energy to the system, while exposure to the positive pole is detrimental. This has been proved repeatedly in studies where a variety of creatures, from earthworms, mice, and chickens to larger animals, live twice as long as untested control groups when exposed to negative field magnets, and half as long when exposed to positive fields. Bucci recommends unipolar magnets, marked by the Davis and Rawls system with an "N" or the word "negative" and a green label. "That's the healthy side, and that's the one we face toward the body." Negative field ions support biological systems, which help the body to heal itself. "The body is an amazing machine with a remarkable capacity to cure itself," Bucci says. "Give it a boost in the right direction and it does the rest on its own. The negative field is completely safe and risk-free."

Bucci finds that magnets work best when worn on a daily basis. During the day she wears a magnet over her heart to improve circulation and oxygenation. "It keeps the heart open and flowing and sends all that wonderful oxygen throughout my body," she says. At night, she takes the magnet off and sleeps with her head on a magnetic mattress pad. She does this because the most important benefit while sleeping is increased melatonin production from the brain's pineal gland: "People are running out to buy melatonin, but guess what? We can encourage our own melatonin production.

"People ask me how long magnets should be worn. Generally speaking, the longer you wear them, the more healing takes place. You can wear them all night and during the day. Generally, the body will tell you when it has had enough. It also will tell you when a condition has healed, although you should check with a physician just to make sure."

BRAIN AGING

One of the most disturbing symptoms of aging is diminished brain function, which can cause everything from forgetfulness and loss of concentration to Alzheimer's and other serious diseases. (Alzheimer's disease is discussed in chapter 26.) Fortunately, modern research reveals that much can be done to keep the brain in top form your entire life. Below, several experts in antiaging discuss new advances in the field.

Dr. Eric Braverman says that brain aging affects people differently and that brain health is a preventative process. "Even when you feel halfway decent in your fifties, sixties, and seventies, parts of your body may be breaking down," he cautions.

The part of the brain affected determines which symptoms manifest themselves. "Individuals age in all different shapes and forms, just as a face can have wrinkles on the brow or wrinkles under the eye," Dr. Braverman says. "The area of the brain that slows down can affect such things as general memory, concentration, and logic."

Another leading researcher in the field of antiaging, Dr. Ross Pelton of San Diego, author of *Mind, Food, and Smart Pills,* agrees that our brains do not have to deteriorate as we age: "It is simply poor nutrition and abuse that allows this condition to develop. Virtually everyone can enhance their memory, learning capabilities, and intelligence." Dr. Pelton helps his patients optimize brain functioning with two goals in mind: to slow down or stop the brain aging process and to optimize the function that they do have.

Dr. Dharma Singh Khalsa is a physician trained at Creighton University School of Medicine and Harvard Medical School, and the author of *Brain Longevity.* "There are many simple things that we can do right now to improve our memories, to forestall any degeneration, to be at our highest mental potential no matter what age or what stage of life we are in," Dr. Khalsa says. "We just have to look at the brain as a physical organ. We have to give it the oxygen it needs, the blood flow it needs, the nutrients it needs. We have to eat right, lower our fat intake, take supplements, meditate or do something to lower the stress in our lives, get physical exercise, think positively, and use our brain. If we do all of these things we can improve our brains. Combine this with a knowledgeable doctor in the field of antiaging medicine and look at hormone replacement therapy. I think hormone replacement therapy is coming into its own now and there is no question that it is definitely beneficial."

How the Brain Works

Dr. Khalsa explains how the brain works: "We have energy in the brain in the form of a power plant called the mitochondria. We have the synapse, a very important juncture where electrical-chemical energy is transferred from one cell to another to create memory or help us produce other memories, draw up old memories, or restore new memories."

The endocrine system affects our emotions and we see a decline in mood and sex drive that normally occur as people age. Dr. Khalsa highlights some of the changes in the endocrine system.

"The endocrine system is primarily the hypothalamus, which is the brain's brain that controls just about everything, including aging. It sends hormones called releasing hormones or factors down to the pituitary gland, which is the master gland of the brain. It orchestrates the secretions of all the glands in your body: the thyroid gland, the adrenal gland, the gonads (in men the testicles, in women the ovaries) and this causes the release of various hormones. When you are young it is responsible for growth and development and as we get older it is responsible for reproductive functions. Then after we reach a certain age, these hormones decline and that is when we start to devitalize. They peak at age thirty and start to decline at around forty and at about fifty they really start to plateau. Don't forget the pineal gland, which is so important in creating a healing environment in the body so we can regenerate ourselves daily and have more energy and vitality as we get older. And you have DHEA released by the adrenal gland. There is an exquisite intimate relationship between all these hormones. These hormones affect our emotions, our mood, the sex drive, our overall feeling of well-being, and our feeling of vitality as we get older. That is why it is so important to follow a brain longevity program."

Diet and Nutrition

Dr. Pelton recommends building total body health with a healthy diet. An organic vegetarian diet supplies the body with more protective nutrients and healthful fiber, and at the same time decreases toxins. Additionally, he believes that people should take a high-potency multivitamin and/or mineral supplement and extra antioxidants with each meal: "We are no longer looking at the Recommended Daily Allowance (RDA) as the level of nutrients appropriate for people. I say RDA stands for Really Dumb Allowance. It's more like the minimum wage, the minimal amount you can get by on. If we want to get into lifestyles of antiaging and life extension, we need to consider not only healthy diets but a program of optimal nutritional supplementation. Antioxidants are among the most important protectors against the aging process in general and against brain aging in particular. They will stop the onset of senility, Alzheimer's disease, and other brain injuries."

Dr. Khalsa elaborates: "What works for the heart works for the head. We know that high fat in the diet will contribute to hardening of the arteries in the heart, the large arteries in the neck, and the small arteries in the brain. Therefore it is critical to move away from these high fat diets and follow a more holistic type of diet. We construct a diet according to the patient's preferences that has about 15 to 20 percent fat so it is tasty. But it is not the 30 to 40 percent fat that you see in the standard American diet. Some of the high protein diets may be effective short-term for weight loss and I think in the long term they are not going to prove to be healthy."

SUPPLEMENTS

Dr. Khalsa goes on to talk about vitamin and mineral supplements that affect the brain. "An all-purpose insurance-policy multiple vitamin/mineral pill that has vitamin E, vitamin C, vitamin A in all its forms, the B vitamins, and the minerals is very useful day to day. Then we use brain-specific nutrients backed by strong scientific research. Vitamin E slows the progression of memory loss. Ginkgo is a good brain-specific nutrient. Coenzyme Q10 is a very energetic cofactor that works in the brain's power plant, the mitochondria. Phosphatidyl serine, or PS, from bovine brains has some excellent results even with patients with dementia. Newer types of phosphatidyl serine synthesized from soybeans is excellent in reversing memory loss and rejuvenating the brain. It is great for depression and mood and has even been shown to improve seasonal affective disorder. There are some other nutrients as well that I like, like fish oil or DHA. It is an algae or you can get it from salmon."

Flaxseed oil, an important brain nutrient, is the greatest source of the essential fatty acid omega-3 (EPA). Omega-3 is converted into another fatty acid, which nourishes the fat cells in the brain. Dr. Pelton says that 1 tablespoon of flaxseed oil is needed daily. It should be refrigerated, not cooked, and taken with the largest meal of the day.

DMAE (dimethylaminoethynol) is a naturally occurring but little-known B vitamin that enhances memory, boosts natural energy, and improves sleep. Additionally, it helps learning problems in children who have short attention spans. DMAE is safe, but if too much is taken, it can produce mild headaches, insomnia, and muscle tension.

Melatonin is a substance from the armamentarium of alternative medicine that has attracted attention in the mainstream media recently. This is a brain hormone produced by the pineal gland, and it diminishes with age. A dose of 3 milligrams once daily taken at bedtime can help normalize sleep cycles and support the pineal gland.

Dr. Khalsa describes two new compounds. "There are two compounds I use for sixty-year-olds who have early memory loss. I don't use them for everybody. The compounds I spoke of before are regenerating or protective, not stimulating like these two. Hypericin A in combination with vitamin E can be as effective as some of the drugs that are mildly effective or moderately effective. Hypericin has the same effect. It blocks the enzyme that destroys the memory compound. Hypericin A, from Chinese cub moss, can be taken in capsule form, 50 micrograms to 100 micrograms twice a day. Combine it with vitamin E and you have a very good reversal compound. I don't think hypericin should be taken by everybody because most normal people have enough of this memory compound. We must be much more scientific and much more specific about how we use these supplements.

"There is another one and that is vincristine. This is from the periwinkle plant. It increases metabolism in the brain and oxygenation. It can be over-stimulating so you have to be careful. Select a program, hopefully in concert with a holistic practitioner. See how to create your own brain longevity program because not each one of these supplements is right for everybody."

There are two minerals that also affect memory: zinc and boron. "Studies showed that those who had the right amounts of these minerals did better on short-term memory tests than those who had low amounts," Dr. Khalsa says. "However taking megadoses didn't result in any further improvement. A good source of zinc is oysters. Good sources of boron are apples, prunes, dates, raisins, and peanuts."

OTHER NUTRIENTS

Dr. Pelton utilizes some additional nutrients to enhance brain function. Hydergine (codergocrine mesylate) increases oxygen to brain cells and makes a person less susceptible to free radical damage and aging. Dr. Pelton says this is one of the most important substances for preventing brain aging because of its oxygenating capabilities. Hydergine is available in the United States, although as a prescription drug.

Lucidril (meclofenoxate hydrochloride), as its name suggests, makes you more lucid. This exciting drug can actually reverse brain aging. Dr. Pelton explains: "The primary yardstick in brain aging is the buildup of lipofuscin, the result of free radical damage over the years. This buildup is really cellular garbage that collects and coalesces inside the cells into a black, tarlike mass. In elderly people you can see this in the skin as liver spots or age pigment. It is theorized that when 60 to 70 percent of the brain cell is clogged, it breaks down and stops working. That's when the symptoms of senility kick in very quickly. Lucidril actually dissolves and flushes out these garbage deposits from brain cells and restores the brain cell to a much younger state." Lucidril has been shown to extend the life of laboratory animals and to enhance intelligence, learning, and recall.

Like Hydergine, piracetam prevents brain cell destruction caused by a lack of oxygen. Piracetam can also increase the flow of electrical information between the left and right hemispheres of the brain, a process known as superconnecting. It has proven effective in treating the learning disorder dyslexia. When used in conjunction with high-potency lecithin, piracetam is highly effective in helping some Alzheimer's patients improve cognition, memory, and recall.

Lucidril and piracetam must be ordered from overseas. Although classified as drugs by the FDA, Hydergine, Lucidril, and piracetam have few, if any, negative side effects, according to Dr. Pelton—only positive effects on memory and the prevention of brain aging. Overseas mail-order sources sell Hydergine in 4.5-milligram tablets, while in the United States it is available only in 1-milligram tablets. The higher dose, taken twice a day, is highly effective in helping people with early signs of memory loss.

Deprenyl (selegiline hydrochloride) has been shown in animal studies to prevent the destruction of a specific group of neurons in the substantia nigra, the area of the brain that goes bad when people develop Parkinson's disease. Moreover, it helps enhance intelligence and cognition when 5 milligrams is taken once daily.

Brain Electronic Activity Map (BEAM)

Dr. Eric Braverman has mapped brain aging and studied how nutrients influence this process. Using a test called the Brain Electronic Activity Map (or BEAM), a technique developed at Harvard Medical School and refined, strengthened, and expanded by Dr. Braverman, the brain's level of electric activity is studied. This is a crucial area of concern because such things as substance abuse, hormonal imbalance, chronic fatigue, anxiety, hypertension, and even Lyme disease may affect the brain and cause premature aging. Often electroencephalography (EEG) or magnetic resonance imaging (MRI) will show nothing wrong, while the BEAM test reveals that the brain has been suffering from stress. It gives a window on the brain and how it is aging. So, as Dr. Braverman says, he is using "the BEAM that lights the path to wellness."

He says that one thing this test registers is the speed of brain cycles, since slowing is a key marker of aging. The normal, healthy rhythm of the brain is 10 cycles per second of alpha waves, considerably faster than the heart's normal rate of 1 cycle per second. As people age, their brain rhythm decreases to 9, 8, or 7 beats per second. There is a decrease in alpha rhythms and an increase in theta waves.

This can occur prematurely for many reasons, including head trauma, Alzheimer's disease, and abuse of substances such as cocaine, marijuana, and alcohol. Any one of these conditions can cause the frontal and temporal lobes to age in an accelerated manner. Aging is also accelerated by whiplash, metabolic disorders, loss of circulation, and "toxic home syndrome," which refers to the damage that can be done to the body by substances, such as cleansers, that vaporize; pesticides; and herbicides found around the house or garden. Add to that possible harm from fluorescent lights and electromagnetic pollution. The latter is that which may be caused by the electromagnetic grid that characterizes our environment, surrounded as we all are by digital clocks, VCRs, CD players, computers, electric blankets, cellular phones and beepers, and microwave ovens.

Dr. Braverman notes that a computerized spectral analysis will pick up how these factors have affected the brain. A PET (positron emission tomography) scan, which provides data about the metabolism of the brain, can be correlated with a BEAM test, which may record not only weaker brain electrical activity but a loss of metabolism of the neurotransmitters.

Exercise

Research shows that the whole neurotransmitter system of the brain can be improved through exercise. Exercise boosts your ability to think because it increases the blood circulation to the brain. This brings more oxygen to the brain. It also increases the production of brain chemicals that are needed for information processing. It may also promote nerve synapses—the bridges between the brain cells—and make information coding faster and more efficient.

Mental Stimulation and Stress Management

"Combine physical exercise with some type of mental stimulation," Dr. Khalsa says. "Mental stimulation includes activities like reading a book, listening to a book on tape, or listening to an informational show and then discussing it with someone else. Also, reading a newspaper and doing headline discussion or what I call column discussion, where you first read the headline and then read the column to the right of it and then talk about it to somebody. Combine this with some physical exercise, sometimes at the same time, for example riding on a stationary bike and reading the newspapers or listening to a book on tape, and you can actually make new connections. Our brains are hungry for connections, hungry to communicate, hungry to reach out and make new neuronal connections so that we can maintain our intelligence. The greatest way to do that is to keep using your brain, doing mental exercise, and to combine that with physical exercise."

Depression slows the brain processing. Relaxation and destressing helps memory. There are lots of ways to reduce stress. Something as easy as taking a deep, long breath and holding it for a moment will not only relax you but bring some oxygen to the brain and make it easier to think and concentrate. Yoga and meditation do the same thing. Listening to music can also be very relaxing.

A good night's sleep allows the entire body to recharge. If you get some quality sleep, you are better able to concentrate. Research shows that people who are awakened during dream sleep fail to process memories from the day before and thus forget more. Dr. Khalsa points out that "recent studies have shown that you don't need to sleep as much as you think because in the last two hours you have very weird dreams and the rapid eye movement sleep is very intense. This raises cortisol levels and can actually cause some problems. In fact, people who have heart attacks have them most often in the morning. High amounts of REM sleep produce high levels of cortisol, which is why many people awaken with morning stress and anxiety. This particular feeling has been found to lead to memory loss specifically and other illnesses perhaps as well."

Dr. Khalsa emphasizes the need for a stress management program. "Anyone who does not have a regular stress management program that is proactive, like a daily or almost daily practice of meditation, won't enjoy good health. It is also important to have stress management tools that reduce the stress in your life and reduce the nasty chemicals such as cortisol. Cortisol attacks the memory center of the brain. It is like battery acid there.

"Start your day in a positive way, what I call 'Wake Up to Wellness'. There have been so many studies lately talking about prayer or meditation. Just take ten, fifteen, twenty minutes in the morning before you rush headlong into your day."

Other Alternative Therapies

Dr. Braverman believes that each person must be individually tested to determine weak areas of brain function and to devise a program that addresses specific needs. For overall general improvement, he endorses exercise and the following important therapies: chelation, electrostimulation, and Reiki.

CHELATION THERAPY

As described earlier, chelation therapy pulls out aluminum and other heavy metals from the bloodstream, resulting in improved memory.

ELECTROSTIMULATION

Amino acids and neurotransmitter precursors are more effective when accompanied by electrostimulation of the brain. A transcutaneous electrical nerve stimulation (TENS) unit, worn on the forehead and left wrist, helps drive these substances along a good pathway. A cranioelectrical stimulation (CES) device also helps electrical fields and enhances the entire neurotransmitter system.

REIKI

In this bodywork technique, described earlier, pressure points are used to move energy through the body, achieving balance and harmony.

CHAPTER 2

AIDS

P robably the most popular new musical on Broadway in the 1990s was *Rent*. Although it suffered from a saccharine quality, it was a crowd pleaser because it mirrored something in the times. The central characters were a pair of couples—one straight, one gay—and all four members of the group were HIV positive. One dies of AIDS in the course of the drama but even more important for the theme of this chapter is the fate of the straight male's former girlfriend. When she finds out she is positive, she commits suicide.

In some ways this death may be more tragic than the AIDS death, insofar as it's partly driven by an establishment-induced myopia. The plain fact is: It has not yet been proven that HIV (human immunodeficiency virus) causes AIDS, though there is clearly an association between the two. Moreover, the woman's despair may have been so overwhelming partly because she only knew about AZT and the other drastic treatments touted by conventional doctors. She was probably unaware of the less toxic, more natural treatments we will explore in this chapter.

In 1984 at a conference in Maryland, Dr. Robert Gallo claimed to have isolated the HIV retrovirus, which he conjectured was the active agent causing AIDS. The press front-paged the story, not only lauding Dr. Gallo and his fellow researchers but also predicting a cure was just a short distance down the road.

Well, nearly twenty years have passed and we find that in relation to AIDS, we are not on the high road of hope but slogging through a quagmire of failed studies that provide little sense or information about how the disease progresses; confusing, unworkable, and expensive treatments; and toxic drugs that often do more harm than good. That's the bad news coming from the medical establishment. The good news is where the establishment failed, that is, in the accuracy of their doomsday predictions about the inevitable, plaguelike spread of AIDS. AIDS has not spread with either the speed or decimating broadness that was foreseen. On the other hand, if there is to be any good news on the treatment front, it will have to come from the alternative doctors who concentrate on such healing remedies as the use of nutritional and lifestyle changes as well as oxygen and ozone therapies.

AIDS IN WOMEN

While men represent a greater proportion of the 34 million people worldwide with HIV or AIDS, women are increasingly bearing the burden of this disease. The number of new AIDS cases among American women has tripled over the last fifteen years. In 2001, women comprised 25 percent of the nearly 1 million total HIV/AIDS cases in the United States. African-American and Latina women, while accounting for less than one-quarter of U.S. women, represented more than three-quarters of the female AIDS cases. Women also comprise the majority of AIDS cases among teens.

CAUSES

Does HIV = AIDS?

In 1984, Dr. Gallo found the presence of human immunodeficiency virus (HIV) in the majority of the AIDS sufferers whose blood he tested. From this he concluded that HIV causes AIDS. So far this is still the best evidence that HIV equals AIDS, but it relies on a peculiarly strained logic.

Even if HIV were found in every AIDS patient, this alone does not settle the question of what causes the syndrome. HIV could simply be a cofactor, an agent that is necessary but not sufficient to create AIDS. Prominent AIDS researcher Dr. Root-Bernstein writes in *The Scientist*, "We also thought we knew that HIV alone is sufficient to cause AIDS. But such researchers as Luc Montagnier...and many others...now believe that cofactors are necessary and, therefore, that HIV by itself cannot cause AIDS."

The case for labeling HIV as partially, not wholly, the cause of AIDS is summed up well by Dr. Root-Bernstein. He notes, "All AIDS patients do have multiple, well established causes of immunosuppression prior to, concomitant with, subsequent to, and sometimes in the absence of, HIV infection." If HIV infection in AIDS patients is always found with other debilitating conditions—"chronic or repeated infectious diseases caused by immunosuppressive microorganisms; recreational and addictive drugs; anesthetics; antibiotics; semen components; blood; and malnutrition"—then it seems reasonable to conclude that these factors are as necessary as the presence of HIV to bring on the disease.

The Nature of the Retrovirus

HIV is a retrovirus, and part of the debate around it is whether a retrovirus could be powerful enough to play a determinative role in creating the AIDS disease.

First, we need to describe a virus. A virus is an extremely simple organism that contains genes (strands of DNA or RNA holding the information needed by the virus to copy itself) within a shell with, possibly, an outer membrane around that. The virus is so absolutely simple it cannot reproduce, feed itself, or carry out any other functions on its own. To survive, it has to get into a living cell and use that cell's machinery. It can only survive as a parasite, though; and perhaps surprisingly, these viruses are not always detrimental to their host. A virus may move from cell to cell, leaving its own genetic material behind as it travels. In the best of cases, this new material may be valuable and, if nothing else, will account for increased genetic diversity.

A retrovirus is a particular, only recently discovered, subtype of virus. To understand its action, we need to step back a minute and look at how genes operate. Until 1970, it was believed the DNA in a cell's nucleus was the sole possessor of the genetic code. When it was necessary to direct cell operation, RNA (a messenger version of the code, created on the DNA template) would be manufactured and sent to carry out the DNA's orders. This seemed to be an adequate explanation, except for viruses. They were so simple they could only contain either RNA or DNA, not both. However, while a DNA-carrying virus could be easily understood—it entered a host cell and used its DNA to form RNA out of materials from the host cell—the operation of RNA-carrying viruses seemed inexplicable.

In 1970, biochemists Howard Temin and David Baltimore overthrew accepted thinking by showing that certain types of RNA could themselves manufacture DNA. They deservedly won a Nobel Prize for their findings. This is relevant to our study because it led to an explanation of how RNA-carrying virus operated successfully. Once it entered a likely host, it used the host's machinery to manufacture its own DNA, which then took over operation of the host cell. A virus that functions in this manner, as does HIV, is called a retrovirus.

Where this causes a problem for AIDS researchers is that it adds yet another puzzling element to the disease, since the retrovirus, in general, is not actually threatening and tends to leave its host unaffected by its presence.

Harvey Bialy, editor of the science journal *Bio/Technology*, rounds out this point by mentioning, "HIV is an ordinary retrovirus. There is nothing about this virus that is unique. It does not differ substantially from all the benign retroviruses.... It contains no gene different enough from the genes of other retroviruses to be a possible AIDS gene."

He also remarks that HIV uses all of its genetic information when it first infects a cell. "It doesn't hoard any for later use, so there is no conceivable reason HIV should cause AIDS ten years after infection, rather than early on when it is unchecked by the immune system."

Why AIDS Hasn't Spread As Predicted

For the moment we can leave these problems to be sorted out by the scientists, since we want to turn to the less speculative question of what inroads AIDS has made into the world's populations.

Predictions based on the HIV theory have failed spectacularly. Here are the bare facts. AIDS in the United States and Europe has not spread through the general population. The number of HIV-infected Americans has remained relatively constant for years instead of increasing rapidly as predicted.

These statements may seem bold to the point of being outrageous to anyone who keeps up with the AIDS story by following it in the mass media. However, there is one thing that escalating predictions of the ravages of AIDS conveniently tend to leave out of their reports. That, in many cases, when a report of a sudden increase of AIDS patients is made, it is accompanied by a redefinition of what the disease is.

Recall that people only die indirectly of AIDS. AIDS weakens the immune system and then they die of another disease, such as tuberculosis. Now suppose—and this is not a theoretical case—a fatal disease that was not classified as AIDS-related is reclassified as AIDS-related. Obviously, you would be adding the people who had died of that disease previously to the AIDS death list and driving up the figures.

As I said, this is not hypothetical. In January 1993, the Centers for Disease Control (CDC) changed the definition of AIDS so that anyone who had a low CD4 blood cell count was defined as an AIDS statistic. According to the previous definition, a person did not have AIDS until he or she came down with an AIDS-related disease. Is it any surprise, then, after this redefinition, that the CDC said the disease was exploding? The reported cases had doubled from about 48,000 to about 107,000. However, a task force for the Society of Actuaries didn't fall for this explosion. Robert Maver, speaking for the task force, said the increase was artificially produced, created by widening the net of people who were considered to be suffering from the disease. He commented, "Under this new category [low CD4 level] alone, more than 50,000 cases were added to the 1993 total."

There is a similar numbers game being played with the statistics of African AIDS victims. At this point, the reader might wonder why projections have been and continue to be so flawed. In the book *Rethinking AIDS*, P. Plumley lists three reasons why public health officials tend to vastly exaggerate the number of people who will get AIDS in the future: "(1) No one wants to appear complacent; (2) the worse the epidemic is projected to be, the more money will be available for public health work; and (3) when the numbers turn out to be lower, the officials can take credit for having done a good job of AIDS education."

Of course the downside of this is that the money the public health officials have accrued by pumping up the number is largely wasted, because it is not properly targeted. David Mertz points out, "Only 5 percent of all U.S. AIDS educational materials are directed at gay men. Instead, a sizable majority of safe-sex material is targeted to young, white heterosexuals. Injecting drug use receives similar short shift in these materials." This results in a dangerous squandering of resources.

CLINICAL EXPERIENCE

Conventional Treatments

Among the difficulties I have with conventional programs is that they are restricted in purview almost exclusively to drugs. Various drugs are used to treat the opportunistic infections and illnesses, and to prevent HIV from reproducing and attacking the body's immune system. Since 1995, the number of medications used to treat AIDS has more than tripled. Among the types of drugs available are reverse transcriptase inhibitors, including abacavir, didanosine (ddI), nevirapine, and zidovudine (AZT), and protease inhibitors, such as amprenavir, indinavir, nelfinavir, and saquinavir. Many people take several of these drugs in antiretroviral combinations, or "cocktails."

If one brings up measures to help the AIDS patient that go beyond ingesting pharmaceuticals, according to Dr. Dean Black, "This opens up the door to all the lifestyle measures that medicine has so long discounted, the idea that it could be in the behavior of the AIDS victim, in the diet, in the lifestyle in some fashion."

Researcher Bill McCreary points to the absurdity of doctors' ignoring their own intuitions about the people they are treating in order to await orders from on high: "Doctors say it's not approved by the FDA so we can't touch it…. Doctors usually do a better job because they're there, they know the patient…. Today, the doctor works from a cookbook that is issued out of the federal government. They have to abide by that cookbook or they may be found guilty of malpractice."

A CASE IN POINT: AZT

AZT was developed as a chemotherapy agent in the late 1960s for the treatment of leukemia, but was never patented by its creator, Dr. Richard Beltz, after he established that his chemotherapy compound was "too toxic for even short-term use" and "caused cancer at any dose." Because of this, AZT was never used for its intended purpose as a cancer chemotherapy. Laboratory studies revealed some of its side effects to be hair loss, weight loss, muscle loss, anemia, and the very same pneumonia associated with AIDS. The drug was then shelved.

The drug's antileukemic mechanism of action is to kill growing lymphocytes by termination of DNA synthesis. The rationale of AZT therapy is simple, if not naive: the retrovirus HIV depends on DNA synthesis for multiplication, and AZT terminates DNA synthesis. Thus AZT should stop AIDS.

It should—but there's one catch. As Huw Christie explains, "Cancer cells, which AZT was designed to kill, grow faster than normal tissue cells, the idea therefore being that, when incorporating AZT, they die more quickly than normally replicating cells too. When the treatment is finished and the chemotherapy stopped, the normal tissue cells can set about making up for their own lower rate of loss." Studies show, on the other hand, that no more than one in a thousand lymphocytes are ever infected by HIV—even in people dying from AIDS. Since AZT cannot distinguish between an infected and an uninfected cell, 999 uninfected cells must be killed in order to kill just one HIV-infected cell.

In 1984, the U.S. Department of Health granted a contract for AZT to Burroughs-Wellcome, which remarketed AZT to AIDS doctors as an "antiviral." AZT was first given to human beings in the initial AIDS treatment trials.

A campaign was then waged to get every HIV-positive person on AZT. Researcher John Lauritsen explains: HIV-positive patients "were told that they should go for what was called early medical intervention. There were slogans put out, 'Put time on your side.' The early intervention meant purely and simply AZT. And rather than putting time on the side of these people, what the drug did and is doing is to terminate their lives."

Here's another difference from cancer treatment. In cancer, you begin to take chemotherapy after you contract the disease. AZT, which, as we saw, was originally developed for chemotherapy, has become the first "chemotherapy" prescribed as a preventative before a person shows any symptoms.

Activist G. Hazlehurst put it like this: AIDS "is the only disease I know of where treatment with powerful drugs is begun several to many years prior to the actual onset of any illness, when there is still the possibility it may not even develop."

HOW AZT AFFECTS THE IMMUNE SYSTEM

Dr. Martin Feldman told me, "The current drugs on the market, primarily AZT, tend to severely weaken the immunity and make the body have to work harder to have immune strength. The body uses up its basic nutrients in the process. Really, the body is fighting against the AZT."

Another commentator notes that if you give AZT indefinitely, so that every six hours the patients take 250 milligrams of AZT, they are going to "lose weight, they become anemic, they lose their white cells, they have nausea, they lose their muscles…. That is what you call AIDS by prescription."

AZT challengers agree that it can only weaken the immune system further. Dr. Dean Black castigates the developers of the drug for the whole rationale of the treatment. "By virtue of determining to substitute for the immune system, by attacking this alien agent with a drug, medicine has literally replaced the body's immune system. What can it do but become weak?"

Advocates of alternative treatment tell us that we need to change the focus of treatment toward "stimulating, activating, and increasing" the body's antibody system. "Since it is the evolutionary responsibility of the cytotoxic T-lymphocytes to destroy infected and abnormal self-cells, increasing their numbers would be beneficial." The best direction of treatment, according to this perspective, would be to help the body to use the immune system it already has instead of forcing it to tolerate an artificial one.

Alternative Treatments

A number of alternative treatments are having some success with AIDS. In this chapter we will highlight three of the newer approaches, pairing each description with a brief mention of a doctor who has pioneered the approach as well as the histories of some of the patients he has worked with. It is important to discuss with a medical professional any alternative therapies you are considering or already using. The three approaches are: (1) supporting the body's own methods of healing and defense by bringing nutrient levels up to optimal levels; (2) working on improving the body's metabolism using a special fatty acid preparation; and (3) elevating the level of oxygen in the blood to boost the immune system and cell activity.

SPECIFIC ALTERNATIVE TREATMENT APPROACHES

Optimizing Nutrient Levels: Dr. Christopher Calapai

In an article published in a scientific journal, Cohen and Kutler note that evaluations of the health conditions of HIV-infected persons before they showed any disease symptoms showed that most had poor nutrition. They had decreased body mass, fat, and protein, resulting from malabsorption. They would be eating but their bodies were not adequately breaking down the food and assimilating its nutrients. A further study, "Influence of HIV Infection on Vitamin Status and Requirement," points out that a vicious circle will result from this malabsorption. "Once occurring, malnutrition leads to immunosuppression, infection, and mucosal damage...resulting in further malnutrition."

Dr. Christopher Calapai sees the body's inability to profit from food nutrients as stemming not only from absorption problems but also from anorexia and high resting energy expenditure (REE). REE means that the body is overstimulated. While it should have slowed during rest, the metabolism is still using up nutrients at an accelerated pace. In any case, the HIV-infected person is either not getting or using too quickly the nutrients he or she needs to support bodily functions.

There is no question that certain vitamins are needed to maintain immune response. These include E, B6, C, and beta carotene. Studies of the elderly, who generally have impaired immune systems, have long shown that these vitamins, taken as supplements, will improve immune response.

In fact, there is evidence that certain vitamins as well as herbs can counter the progress of AIDS as they bolster the immune system. Let's highlight some of the more notable successes that have been seen with these types of therapies, many of which are used by Dr. Calapai.

In my book *AIDS: A Second Opinion*, I detail the vitamins and herbs that have been used for treating people with AIDS with positive results. In this briefer space, I will touch upon some of the substances that have recorded good results.

GLUTATHIONE —Glutathione is an antioxidant that protects against cellular damage. It stimulates lymphocytes that help defend the body against viral illnesses, such as AIDS. When N-acetyl-cysteine (NAC) is given to a patient, the body will convert it to glutathione.

A study in *Nutrition Review* indicates that HIV-positive individuals are deficient in glutathione. On the other hand, results have been reported from a number of studies that indicate HIV activity is reduced by glutathione's presence.

Dr. Joan Priestley gives her HIV-infected and AIDS patients intravenous glutathione, because, she says, "Glutathione specifically attacks the AIDS virus in about four different steps."

At an AIDS symposium, Dr. Calapi stated, "When we add glutathione intravenously with vitamin C, we see a significant turnaround in the patient's comfort, attitude, and well being…. NAC taken intravenously can inhibit reverse transcriptase [HIV replication] activity better than 90 percent. There is no drug available for any treatment or disease that can do better than 90 percent with minimal or no side effects."

BETA CAROTENE—Beta carotene is a safe form of vitamin A, which stops damage from bodily pollution, bolsters the immune system, inhibits viruses, and prevents premature aging.

A study done by Dr. Semba of Johns Hopkins showed that a vitamin A deficiency found in HIV-positive and AIDS patients was a serious risk factor for the disease. In a different study, Dr. Semba's team found that a lack of vitamin A was positively correlated with death from AIDS.

On the other hand, a number of studies chart improvements when beta carotene is administered. In one, eleven HIV-positive patients received 60 milligrams of the vitamin per day for four months. They recorded an increase in natural killer cells and other vital parts of the immune system, which HIV infection tends to diminish. Another study was done on ten patients who had just gotten off AZT and began taking 120 milligrams a day of beta carotene. Although one died a few months into the treatment, the other nine experienced an HIV-burden diminution, clinically measured improvements in health, and evaluated themselves as having a better quality of life.

VITAMIN C—Vitamin C is one of the stars among the vitamins in treating AIDS. Basing his opinion on numerous clinical studies, Dr. Robert Cathcart confidently states, "Vitamin C can double the life expectancy of AIDS patients." He says that his treatment, which involves using massive doses of buffered ascorbate of 50 to 200 grams every twenty-four hours (in combination with other treatments for secondary infections), will produce a clinical remission of the disease that shows every evidence of being prolonged if the treatment goes on.

Other doctors report similar results. Dr. Raxit Jariwalla, a virologist from the Linus Pauling Institute, says, "In laboratory cultures of HIV-infected cells...vitamin C can significantly suppress both the activity and the replication of the AIDS virus."

Joy DeVincenxo, who is HIV positive and has used massive doses of vitamin C, explains, "A lot of doctors...do not believe in giving me vitamin C...[but] without it, I know I wouldn't have stayed stable for so long."

These statements are supported by a host of studies, such as the one that appeared in the volume *Nutrition and AIDS*, which summarized the results of various examinations of C's value. The authors point out, "A striking property of ascorbic acid is its ability to inactivate viruses and inhibit viral growth in their host cells." Experimental studies reported in the same volume show that vitamin C will directly interfere with HIV replication, carrying the assault on the disease into the enemy's camp.

VITAMIN E—Vitamin E is an antioxidant that seems to prevent many diseases caused by environmental stressors. It is found in fish and vegetable oil, nuts, and whole grains. However, most Americans do not get enough of this vitamin in their foods and need supplementation.

Studies are piling up showing that vitamin E is a warrior against AIDS. One study showed that the administration of 50 milligrams per kilogram per day over five days already began to inhibit the replication of HIV. Another study showed that if the dosage of E was increased fifteen-fold (to 160 IU/liter), immune system functions that had been suppressed by HIV presence were restored.

HERBAL TREATMENTS

Again, we can only skim the surface in mentioning some herbal treatments that have shown themselves to be powerful agents in working against AIDS.

The Institute for Traditional Medicine in Portland, Oregon, has done some vital work in looking at how Chinese herbs can be used in treating AIDS. The founder of the institute has developed a specific herbal combination that combines strong tonic herbs with those that fight inflammation and infection. Of 150 patients who have undergone therapy with this herbal formula over three months, 76 percent experienced an increase of energy, and 62 percent of the patients who suffered from diarrhea saw a cessation of the problem. Other symptoms were similarly improved.

Dr. Chang of the Sun Yat Sen Medical Center also found a mix of Chinese herbs to work strenuously against AIDS. He found that extracts from eleven different herbs inhibit the activity of HIV. Dr. Quingcai Zhang notes these Chinese herb treatments are effective because they work with the body to fight infection, rather than by trying to override the body's own creative functioning, the way drugs such as AZT do.

Following are some of the herbs that have a good reputation for working against HIV:

ASTRAGALUS—Astragalus root has been used for centuries in China because it was thought to strengthen the immune system. Current research shows the truth of this belief, since astragalus is now known to correct T-cell (part of the immune system) deficiency and to promote antiviral action.

A study at the University of Texas showed that taking astragalus extract stimulates T-cell production in healthy animals and restores it in cancer patients who have seen their T-cell production impaired. In another study involving nineteen cancer patients with weakened immune systems, an extract of astragalus induced such a complete recovery that it was noted, "People whose immune systems were devastated by cancer experienced full restoration of immune function."

Of course, studies need to be conducted on AIDS sufferers, but astralagus's aid to the immune system is evident.

GARLIC—Garlic has a number of antitumor and antiviral mechanisms. It stimulates the immune system's production of phagocytosis, which eliminates abnormal cells from the body. It is toxic to some abnormal cells and inhibits the implantation of others. It has even proven effective against some bacteria that do not respond to antibiotics.

In fighting AIDS, it is especially good in eliminating the opportunistic infections that set in once immune systems have been weakened. A German study of seven AIDS patients who were given 5 g of garlic daily found that five of them showed significant improvements in their T cells, along with other improvements in health and fewer outbreaks of opportunistic infections.

GINSENG—Numerous studies of ginseng's benefits were conducted in Russia in the 1960s and 1970s. Norman Farnsworth collected and translated many of these studies, which indicated that various types of ginseng acted to normalize body temperature, enhance the body's ability to resist infection, improve cells' ability to dispose of the by-products of metabolism, and counter the effects of environmental pollution.

Its effects in treating AIDS patients have also been shown. In a study by Y. K. Cho and others, Korean red ginseng improved weakened immune response in subjects infected with HIV.

LICORICE ROOT—Licorice root has also been effective in stopping the HIV virus from replicating. A study, done at the World Life Research Institute, recorded no toxicity to normal cells.

The plant is known to strengthen the immune system by increasing macrophage activity and that of interferon-gamma, both vital actors in combating infections and viruses. Licorice is a detoxifying agent and has anti-inflammatory, antiallergic, and antispasmodic properties.

ST. JOHN'S WORT—Studies at New York University have shown that St. John's wort contains two potent chemicals that are highly effective in preventing the spread of retroviruses, such as HIV, both in laboratory samples and in patients.

One of the researchers found that one of these chemicals would stop the spread of AIDS, even crossing the barrier into the brain, which serves as a reservoir of HIV cells, to combat the disease there. This researcher comments that St. John's wort's "antiviral activity is remarkable both in its mechanism…and in the potency of one administration of a relatively small dose of the compounds."

PHYTOCHEMICALS

Before moving on to the lifestyle components that form part of Dr. Calapai's program, I want to mention a newer area of research in supplementation that I believe will have a lot to offer toward helping AIDS patients in years to come. This is the area of phytochemicals.

Phytochemicals are disease-preventing or healing substances found in edible plants, such as those found in licorice root, which are believed to account for the plant's valuable immune-system strengthening qualities that have already been outlined. These chemicals are found in frequently consumed foods such as fruits, vegetables, grains, legumes, and seeds as well as in less common foods such as soy and green tea. They have already been associated with the prevention and treatment of four of the leading causes of death in this country: cancer, diabetes, cardiovascular disease, and hypertension. Although not enough studies have been done on these substances, those that have been done hint that quite large benefits are to be expected.

Research on limonene, found in citrus fruits, shows that it increases the body's production of enzymes that help it dispose of potentially carcinogenic substances. It is well known that people whose diets are heavy in fruits have lower rates of most cancers than do those who don't have such diets. Many are attributing this low cancer rate to the effect of the phytochemicals.

LIFESTYLE CHANGES

Dr. Calapai's treatment program involves building up the body with proper nutrients and making lifestyle changes. Research supports the long-term efficacy of dietary counseling and use of nutritional supplementation for people with AIDS to increase or maintain weight, restore lean tissues, and lessen the effects of the disease.

Patrick Donnelly, program coordinator for the Whole Foods Project, says AIDS patients must be made aware of the need to eat nutritious foods. He advises working with "the new four food groups, which are grains, legumes, fruits, and vegetables." These foods are high in antioxidants and have nutrients like beta carotene, vitamin C, zinc, and selenium. Such nutrients are not found in the high-fat, high-protein standard American diet. Donnelly says, "We're trying to get people to look at a new way of eating that is not about providing calories so much as supporting the immune system."

Another member of the project staff, Richard Pierce, comments, "You only have to look at this food [we provide] to see that it's full of life…. The vitality of the food is what nurtures us."

Along with eating healthy foods, one must learn to avoid the foods that contribute to the growth or virulence of disease, counterproductive foods, particularly yeast and sugar. Yeast is a natural part of our makeup, but it can wreak havoc on the body when it gets out of control. Sugar is an immune suppressant. If one takes 100 grams of sugar, it will cut antibody production by 50 percent for 24 hours.

Studies have shown that regular exercise has long-term benefits on the biological condition of HIV and AIDS patients as well as on the course of the illness. Researchers have found that exercise will improve a patient's health at all stages of the disease. Moreover, it seems that complications of the disease will be delayed by exercise.

ACUPUNCTURE

Acupuncture has proven to be one of the most popular treatments for people with HIV. One study found that people with HIV who use the treatment have extended survival rates. In addition, they regularly report a substantial reduction in symptoms and side effects from HIV-related drugs. Acupuncture frequently provides relief from AIDS-related diseases, and most patients report a reduction in fatigue, abnormal sweating, diarrhea, and acute skin reactions after four to five treatments. Some patients have a fifteen- to twenty-pound weight gain and return to long hours of work.

Abigail Rist-Podrecca, a registered nurse, notes that acupuncture works by "dilating the blood vessels, so that the vessels can open. You get more circulation, more of the nutrients, more oxygen flowing through those meridians [the places where the acupuncture needles are stuck]."

She believes one of the reasons people with AIDS weaken is that they lose the ability to take up nutrition through the intestines. Acupuncture acts to reverse this digestive problem as well as working on the lungs and other bodily centers.

Studies conducted at the Lincoln Hospital Acupuncture Clinic in New York, the AIDS Alternative Health Project in Chicago, and the Quan Yin Herbal Support Program in San Francisco have reported symptomatic relief and overall physical improvement following acupuncture.

REFLEXOLOGY AND AROMATHERAPY

Reflexology is a form of relaxation treatment. It was used in an AIDS program in Uganda. Four months after the program began, 85 percent of those treated noted pain relief, better relaxation, and better sleep following the reflexology sessions.

Aromatherapy is the use of plant essences in healing. Pure oils are used, some of which have already proven to have antifungal and antiviral effects. One study looked at the effect of aromatherapy when used in conjunction with other therapies to see if it would lessen the need for toxic drugs. Using eighty randomly selected AIDS patients, the study concluded that the group that utilized aromatherapy, in contrast to the control group, reported fewer aches and pains, faster healing of wounds, greater physical strength, and a better ability to cope.

HOW DR. CALAPAI'S PROGRAM WORKS

As mentioned, Dr. Calapai's program centers on nutrition and lifestyle changes. When he first sees a patient, he asks her to bring in a week's worth of diet history, which he goes over very carefully. He immediately tells the patient how important it is to institute lifestyle changes that will provide strong benefits. These changes include immediately stopping smoking and drinking alcohol.

He orders a detailed diagnostic protocol that includes blood evaluations of cellular, mineral, vitamin, hormone, and viral and antigen levels. He also does aggressive testing for common infections, such as herpes and tuberculosis (TB), which can contribute to the progression of the disease. He allows a patient to take the antiretroviral drugs if she so desires. He also lets the patient consult other doctors.

Once Dr. Calapai has the test results, he uses them along with the patient's history to devise dietary recommendations.

Dr. Calapai reports good results with his program. "Many of the patients that I have put on the protocol after two weeks or so say they're feeling very good." He continues, "They have a lot of energy; they're sleeping better…. The overwhelming majority say they feel better in a number of ways." He has had patients who have followed his nutritional and lifestyle alteration program and, though they have very low T-cell counts, have been free of coughs, colds, and other opportunistic infections for a year.

Improving Metabolism: Dr. Emmanuel Revici

Dr. Emmanuel Revici's program is similar to Dr. Calapai's insofar as it also affirms that AIDS must be managed by addressing nutritional deficiencies. However, it is much narrower in locating the deficiency only in certain fats. At the same time, it is broader in that it is based on a well-worked-out philosophy.

This philosophy, though not based on Chinese medicine, does resemble the Asian system in viewing the body as driven by two crosscurrents, *yin* and *yang*, that create the body's vitality. The body's health depends on their balance. Similarly, Dr. Revici's program sees two basic processes in the body: the anabolic, which builds up, and the catabolic, which breaks down. When an organism is working normally, it maintains its characteristic rhythms and intensities by means of this oscillation. However, when there is a breakdown, it will be because the alternations are lopsided, and either catabolic or anabolic influences are unduly dominating. It is as if a pendulum's swing were being artificially pulled to one side.

In the case of AIDS, there is a deficiency in certain of the body's phospholipids (a type of fat), which normally play a role in disease prevention. The course of the disease is as follows: A primary viral infection occurs, which brings about the weakening of the body's line of lipidic defense. This is followed by secondary, opportunistic infections that are allowed to run wild due to the body's lowered defense threshold. Then comes an exaggerated catabolic imbalance whereby the body's breakdown of substances is outrunning its construction of others.

The treatment called for in such a case is a four-pronged one. To deal with the viral infections, antiviral agents should be introduced into the system. To deal with the lipid deficiency, these lipids have to be reintroduced by injection. For the secondary opportunistic infections, proper antibiotics are applied. And for the catabolic imbalance, balancing agents are prescribed.

I examined ten of Dr. Revici's cases and I can make these generalizations about them: Of these patients, only three seem not to have improved during therapy. Yet, of these three, one, though worsening in immunologic markers, nevertheless felt "well" at the end of 10 years of treatment. Another, though his T4 count also declined considerably over 4 years of treatment, was still "feeling fine" at the end of that period. Thus, of the ten patients, eight currently (or recently) report feeling well after an average period of 5.2 years of therapy. Five of the eight also report no remaining symptomatic complaints; and two of those have had a marked improvement in immune markers. All are currently continuing in therapy.

Oxygen and Ozone: Dr. John Pittman

Dr. John Pittman's treatment is based on the use of ozone and oxygen. Oxygen is an essential nutrient. It is, in fact, the most essential, as it is the only one which must be continuously available, at pain of quick death. As we all know, life ceases if the supply of oxygen is cut off for more than a few minutes. A number of studies indicate that ozone inactivates HIV at low and safe concentrations. It has been conjectured that ozone kills HIV cells. Ozone is also able to strengthen immune responses.

TREATMENT PROTOCOL

Ozone therapy is a prime component at Dr. John Pittman's Carolina Center for Alternative and Nutritional Medicine. Dr. Pittman believes that ozone can arrest the progression of AIDS' diseases and turn the syndrome into a manageable condition. He values ozone's ability to help alleviate chronic problems that plague patients, including dermatological conditions and low-level infections. He also notes a relationship between ozone and improved T-cell and CD4 counts. Best results occur when an intensive series of treatments is taken every four to six months.

Dr. Pittman uses ozone as an integral part of a wider treatment protocol: "The first ten days of their program entails a modified juice fast. Everyone drinks fresh-pressed vegetable juices and eats no solid food." Patients are then put on an intensive detoxification program. Nutritional supplements are given. The patient begins autohemotherapy. This involves the removal of blood from the body so that it can be filled with ozone and then reinfused.

After five days of autohemotherapy, Dr. Pittman says, "if the patient has tolerated that…we begin with the direct intravenous infusion of ozone gas…on a daily basis, gradually increasing concentrations and volume until we observe a healing crisis in the patient." The patient will experience fevers, chills, and sometimes flu symptoms. When the healing crisis passes, the doctor tapers off dosage and concentration, and goes into lower doses, "which have a more immune-stimulating effect."

Concurrent with ozone therapy are other intravenous therapies, which include intravenous vitamin C and mineral infusions as well as EDTA chelation therapy. The doctor also employs acupuncture and other dietary therapies throughout the program.

Although I was not able to obtain the same detailed case histories from Dr. Pittman that I had from the other practitioners mentioned here, I did gather very positive anecdotal evidence, including the story of a man who came to the clinic with a CD4 count of 42. In two weeks of intensive therapy, his count soared to 285.

As you can see, Dr. Pittman believes in a nontoxic multifactorial approach in the treatment of AIDS. He says, "I think the approach for AIDS has got to be one from a multimodality standpoint. There is no one single approach. It is only through the combination of appropriate antiviral therapy, immune-stimulating therapy, diet, and detoxification programs that a patient is really going to be maintained and have any hope of improvement."

Alternative Health Therapy Concepts

Theories and methods that seem very different can have broadly similar results. All three of the treatment approaches mentioned have, at the very least, reversed some of the symptoms of HIV infection in some patients and have improved the quality of life, according to the patients themselves, in many cases.

The three approaches are not mutually exclusive. Is there any reason why they should not be used together, complementing each other? For example, it was noteworthy that some of the reported actions of the vitamin C infusions used by Dr. Calapai were very similar to those of the ozone infusions used by Dr. Pittman. Both were found to be highly effective in inactivating many viruses, and HIV in particular; and both seemed to augment the effectiveness of the immune system. Perhaps if they were used together, the effects of each would potentiate the other, with results better than either alone.

One of the very important advantages of many of these "nonconventional" methods is that, whether or not they are effective (and there is evidence that some are), they are generally safe. Most nutritional and herbal methods cause far fewer side effects than the pharmaceutical and surgical methods now in favor. This is a major argument for permitting them to be used at the discretion of the individual.

That is a reason for not bringing these modalities under the regulatory authority of the state or organized medicine. It is a matter of constitutional freedoms. But there are also strong economic arguments. The costs of these alternative techniques are almost always far lower than the treatments now approved by organized medicine for the same disorders. Thus, encouraging the use of these other approaches can save the American public, both as taxpayer and as health-care consumer, vast amounts of money.

Yes, the physicians whose work with HIV infection we have examined approach health and illness from different perspectives. But they do share a basic worldview that separates them from the practitioners of conventional medicine.

According to the conventional view, my body consists of congeries of mechanisms, with subsystems that can be adequately understood separately, with little regard to the status of all the myriad other subsystems. The view of the body found in alternative health care is one that sees its level of interconnectedness as far higher. In a healthy organism all the subsystems are supporting each other in myriad ways (most of which are not yet observable or understood). In the first (allopathic) worldview, most disease originates through the breakdown of some one mechanism, or a few discrete mechanisms; disease, then, is to be treated by fixing (or bypassing) the defective mechanism(s). In the second (holistic) worldview, however, disease has to do not only with individual mechanisms but with weakening of many kinds of couplings between mechanisms, and with overstressing supporting systems through excessive demands for support.

Survivor Portraits

Literature on long-term survivors with AIDS is replete with anecdotal evidence linking survival to such things as holding a positive attitude toward the illness, taking control of one's health, participating in health-promoting behaviors, engaging in spiritual activities, and taking part in AIDS-related events.

Survivors are very pragmatic problem solvers who educate themselves about alternative treatments, nutrition, and exercise. If something isn't working for them, they change it.

While AIDS survivors generally do not follow mainstream treatments, they are not loners. They maintain good relationships with their friends, families, and doctors, and often belong to support groups. Another feature of long-term survivors is that they are passionately committed to life, believe in the possibility of survival, and surround themselves with people who will love and support them. They make major lifestyle changes. They have also dabbled with dietary changes. A writer who studied the lives of survivors says:

> They all talked about what they called "emotional house cleaning." Usually after they had survived their first major opportunistic infection, it represented a crisis to them and they did some soul-searching. They either repaired relationships or ended them. And all but two talked about a rebirth of spirituality. Half had returned to the religions of their childhood—although none in a fundamentalist, judgmental way—and half spoke more generally of there being a meaning to suffering…. This gave them a sense of purpose in the here and now. They were not done with life yet. They had a reason to stick around.

CHAPTER 3

ANEMIA

A nemia is a health condition characterized by red blood cells deficient in hemoglobin, the iron-containing portion of the blood. Hemoglobin enables the blood to transport oxygen from the lungs and circulate it throughout the body, and to carry away carbon dioxide. The listlessness, pallor, and shortness of breath experienced by a person with anemia reflect a lack of oxygen and buildup of carbon dioxide in the tissues.

CAUSES

Dr. Dahlia Abraham, a complementary physician from New York City, describes three major classifications of anemia, each of which is associated with a specific cause:

EXCESSIVE BLOOD LOSS—This can result from conditions such as hemorrhoids and a slowly bleeding peptic ulcer, or in association with menstruation.

EXCESSIVE RED BLOOD CELL DESTRUCTION—Dr. Abraham explains: "Normally, old and abnormal red blood cells are removed from the circulation. If the rate of destruction exceeds that of manufacture of new cells, anemia can result. A number of factors can cause excessive red blood cell destruction, such as defective hemoglobin synthesis, injury, and trauma within the arteries."

NUTRITIONAL DEFICIENCIES OF IRON, VITAMIN B12, AND FOLIC ACID—This is the most common type of anemia, with iron deficiency the most frequent.

Dr. Abraham further explains: "People require extra iron during growth spurts in infancy and adolescence. Pregnancy and lactation are other times when women need iron supplementation. During the childbearing years, many women experience anemia caused by an iron deficiency."

Do supplements help? "Supplementation may not solve the problem because many people have difficulty absorbing iron," Dr. Abraham says. "They lack enough hydrochloric acid, the stomach acid that helps the body assimilate iron. This is common among the elderly, who generally produce less hydrochloric acid." Chronic diarrhea also may cause decreased iron absorption.

A defect in absorption is the most common cause of a vitamin B12 deficiency. Dr. Abraham remarks, "Vitamin B12 must be liberated from food by hydrochloric acid and bound to a substance called intrinsic factor, which is also secreted in the stomach. For B12 to be absorbed, then, an individual must secrete enough hydrochloric acid and enough intrinsic factor." For this type of anemia, supplements of vitamin B12, hydrochloric acid, and intrinsic factor may help.

A deficiency in folic acid may also cause anemia. Alcoholics and pregnant women are particularly at risk. "Folic acid is vital for cell production in the growing fetus and prevents birth defects, such as neural tube imperfections," Dr. Abraham says. "This is why prenatal vitamins must contain this nutrient. In addition, a number of pharmaceutical drugs, such as anticancer drugs and oral contraceptives, can drain the body of folic acid."

Dr. Pat Gorman, an acupuncturist and educator in New York City, explains anemia and other blood disorders in women from an Asian perspective: "In women, blood has an actual cycle that rises and falls every month. There is a building phase that occurs for about a week after the menstrual period. Then there is a peak phase where the blood reaches its richest moment; that's the moment you ovulate. This is followed by a storage phase. (If you are pregnant, the blood is stored.) A week before the period, you go through a cleansing phase where your organs release toxins into the blood. That's the week before your period, when you can go through a PMS hell if the toxins are not being properly released. Next is the purging of the actual period."

Using this philosophy as her framework, Dr. Gorman holds that women become anemic when they are out of touch with their monthly cycles. In a fast-paced society, one of the major reasons for this condition is that women do not rest at the appropriate times. "Women work all the time. They show no vulnerability and just keep on going no matter what. There is no respect for the actual rhythm of the cycle. I believe that we need to bring back the menstrual hut. When you are bleeding, you need to stop working for a day or two. I know I am saying things that sound impossible, but if you have anemia—and 60 to 70 percent of the women I see do—you need to face the fact and work with it."

Another major reason women become anemic is that they approach pregnancy incorrectly: "There is a law called the one-month, one-year law," Dr. Gorman says. After a pregnancy is terminated, whether by abortion, miscarriage, or birth, one month of absolute rest is needed. Women say, 'That's not possible. I just gave birth, but I have other children. I have to take care of things.' The Chinese say this is a straight road to a severe problem with anemia.

"The one-year aspect is the avoidance of pregnancy for at least another year. Women who try to conceive and who then miscarry often frantically begin again. They need to build up the blood for an entire year's cycle before trying to conceive again. It is very difficult for me to help anxious patients relax and understand that this is the way to overcome anemia and to have a really healthy baby." (See chapter 28, "Pregnancy.")

Additionally, Dr. Gorman warns that birth control pills disturb the integrity of the blood's cycle. They trick the body into believing that it is continuously pregnant by locking blood into its storage phase. By eliminating the cycle of building, peaking, storing, cleansing, and purging, oral contraceptives may create many problems. (For more on birth control, see chapter 5.)

SYMPTOMS

The general symptoms of anemia are weakness and a tendency to tire easily. When there is a vitamin B12 deficiency, the symptoms may also include paleness; shortness of breath; a sore, red, swollen tongue; diarrhea; heart palpitations; and nervous disturbances.

CLINICAL EXPERIENCE

Diagnosis

According to Dr. Abraham, the treatment of anemia is dependent on proper clinical evaluation by a physician. Too often, physicians assume that anemia is caused by an iron deficiency, but this is just one possible reason. "It is absolutely imperative that a comprehensive laboratory analysis of the blood be performed. Do not be satisfied when your physician offers a simple diagnosis of anemia," she warns. "Insist that your doctor investigate the underlying causes."

While Dr. Gorman agrees that clinical studies help confirm the diagnosis, she adds that Asian physicians are trained to detect anemia and other blood disorders through observation: "In Chinese medicine, you examine the body. Look at your tongue. Is it pale? Look at your lips. Are they pale? See if the mucous membranes under the eyes are pale. These signs indicate whether you are anemic."

Dietary Remedies

Green, leafy vegetables are high in iron and folic acid. It is best to purchase organic vegetables, since pesticides interfere with absorption. Eating vegetables raw or lightly cooked preserves their folic acid content. Soy or shoyu sauce, miso (a fermented soybean paste), and tempeh (another soybean preparation) are rich sources of vitamin B12.

Proteins should be eaten every day, preferably vegetarian proteins such as those from grains and legumes such as rice and beans or oatmeal with soy milk. When animal protein is eaten, it should be from fish. Caffeine and alcohol are detrimental to healthy blood and should be eliminated.

Supplements

According to Dr. Abraham, iron, vitamin B12, and folic acid should be prescribed as needed. Additionally, hydrochloric acid and intrinsic factor are often required to aid the absorption of these nutrients.

Naturopath Dr. Tori Hudson, in a column in *Prevention* magazine, advises that iron citrate and iron aspartate are forms of iron supplementation that are less likely to cause constipation. She suggests taking 1,000 to 3,000 milligrams of vitamin C with the iron to enhance absorption.

Herbs

Dr. Janet Zand, a naturopathic physician, acupuncturist, and doctor of Oriental medicine in Los Angeles, in an article posted on the HealthWorld Online website (www.healthy.net), suggests an herbal program that anemic women can use to build the blood. It is meant to accompany iron and iron-synergistic nutrient supplementation as directed by a health care practitioner. Dr. Zand bases her herbal regimes for women on the shifting hormonal balance over the four weeks of the menstrual cycle.

During all four weeks of the cycle, red raspberry leaf and dong quai are used to build blood and balance hormones. These herbs can be taken as a tea, tincture, capsule, or tablet three times a day. Then, during the specified weeks, one also takes the herbs listed below:

FIRST WEEK—Take yellow dock leaf (*Rumex crispus*) and chlorophyll as a tea or tincture three times a day.

SECOND WEEK—Take American ginseng (*Panax quinquefolius* root), a blood builder, as a tea or tincture three times a day.

THIRD WEEK—Take nettle (*Urtica dioica* leaf) and chlorophyll as a tea or tincture three times a day.

FOURTH WEEK—Take alfalfa (*Medicago sativa* leaf), with chlorophyll as a tea or tincture three times a day.

Ayurveda

According to Swami Sada Shiva Tirtha, founder of the Ayurveda Holistic Center in Bayville, New York, in an article on the center's website (ayurvedahc.com), practitioners of Ayurvedic medicine consider anemia an imbalance of the blood that can have a number of causes. Too many sour, salty, or hot foods; drinking alcohol; poor nutrition; injury; excessive menstruation or bleeding; liver disorders; pregnancy; excessive sexual activity; and fevers are all factors that can cause a disorder in the kidneys, blood, and *ojas* (life force) and lead to anemia.

Swami Sada Shiva recommends certain foods that help build blood. These foods include organic milk, pomegranate or black grape juice, boiled black sesame seeds, molasses, and Sucanat (whole cane sugar). Otherwise, people should follow the diet that is appropriate for their body type, according to Ayurvedic guidelines. Ayurveda uses meat as a medication only when anemia is extremely severe.

Women should use blood-building herbs after the menstrual period. To properly assimilate iron supplements, take them with ginger or cinnamon. You can take two or three teaspoonfuls of *chyavan prash* twice daily with warm milk as well as turmeric and ghee.

Aloe vera gel and triphala are very gentle laxatives that regulate the bowels and thus can help remove excess bile from the liver, a common reason for thinning of the blood. Other Ayurvedic herbs used to treat anemia are saffron, *shatavari, manjishtha,* and *punarnava.*

PATIENT STORY

I was born in Nicaragua, and I used to be a very healthy person. But in June 1993 I went to the emergency room. My hemoglobin was down to 2.8; the normal count for a woman is between 12 and 14. There I was with aplastic anemia, meaning that my bone marrow was not making any blood cells: no red cells, no white cells, no platelets. I almost had no blood.

The doctor said that my sickness was idiopathic, meaning that they didn't know what caused it. They said that one possible cause was the use of an antibiotic. But the only time I had ever taken one was fifteen years earlier. Another possible cause was exposure to chemicals or pesticides. A lot of towns in Nicaragua are surrounded by cotton plantations where cotton growers use a lot of pesticides to spray their crops.

In July 1993 I was referred to a bone marrow transplant unit and was put on a medication, a kind of chemotherapy. After one month of treatment, the medication failed to work. Then the doctors wanted to do a bone marrow transplant. I have seven siblings, so I had donors, and one of them was a perfect match. But I had reservations. A bone marrow transplant is very costly. Also, you get bone marrow that is working, but because of the chemotherapy or radiation, your liver, kidneys, pancreas, and so forth, pay a terrible toll.

Before my sickness I was following a macrobiotic diet. I was starting to use Oriental and alternative medicine, and I knew about the power of the body to heal itself. I decided to stay on my macrobiotic diet and was able to more or less clean myself of the chemotherapy. During this time I did not even get a cold. I didn't sneeze through all my sickness.

I was clean, but my blood counts were still very low. I needed a transfusion every ten days. The transfusions were very helpful, and I was grateful to be able to get them. But through transfusions I was also receiving a lot of genetic and other information completely foreign to my body. I could not control what the person who donated that blood was eating. So I was trying to clean my body of toxins, and I decided to look for help.

I went to a naturopath, who helped me a lot. Then I read an article on Ayurveda. It said that Ayurveda is very specific, even with the use of grains and vegetables. There are grains and vegetables that are not appropriate for your body type. In early February 1994 I went to an Ayurvedic doctor. He gave me a very gentle treatment consisting of diet, aromatherapy, massage, and meditation. After three weeks of following that treatment, my blood count went up for the first time.

I keep up with this treatment still. My last checkup at the hospital showed normal white cells. Red cells were a little bit low. They were 3.83, and the normal count is 4. But they are increasing day by day. My energy level is excellent. I went back to work 3 months ago and am now leading a completely normal life. I am very grateful to Ayurveda.

—Yolanda

CHAPTER 4

ARTHRITIS

M ore than 43 million Americans suffer from some form of arthritis, a large percentage of whom are women. By 2020, the number is expected to reach 60 million, or one-fifth of the population. We know the kind of discomfort this can mean: swollen joints and excruciating pain. It can be so bad it prevents a person from having a quality life.

With so many millions suffering from arthritis, maybe we should be thinking of something by way of treatment other than simply dulling the pain with drugs or performing dangerous and expensive operations. As you will see in reading this chapter, alternative practitioners have been thinking this way for years with quite astounding results.

There are signs that alternative therapies are starting to gain some of the recognition they so rightly deserve. A report published in March 2000 in the *Journal of the American Medical Association* concluded that two popular nutritional supplements, glucosamine and chondroitin compounds, are safe and "have some efficacy in treating osteoarthritis symptoms."

WHAT IS ARTHRITIS?

The word *arthritis* means pain and "swelling of the joints." A joint is the place where two bones meet. Cartilage covers the end of each bone and prevents the bones from rubbing together. The joint capsule surrounds and protects the joint, and special membranes cover it with a fluid that lubricates it. Muscles and ligaments around the joint provide support and make it move. When all these parts are working right, the joint moves smoothly and easily, but when something is wrong with the joint, arthritis may develop.

There are many types of arthritis. Some of the most common are described below.

Osteoarthritis

Osteoarthritis, also known as degenerative joint disease, is the most common form of chronic arthritis. It is estimated to affect more than twenty million Americans, three-quarters of whom are women. In osteoarthritis, the cartilage is worn away so that the bones rub against each other. When the cartilage breaks down, the joint may lose its shape. The ends of the bone may thicken and form spurs.

Adds Dr. Jason Theodosakis, whose treatment program is profiled later in this chapter, "At a biochemical level, the breakdown of cartilage is happening more rapidly than the buildup of cartilage. That brings up an important point. Cartilage on the end of the bones is not like a pencil eraser, which, once it is rubbed off, is gone. It is constantly breaking down and being replaced."

Osteoarthritis most often affects middle-aged and older women. Many people consider it a part of the aging process. The joints of the fingers, neck, low back, and legs are usually involved. Symptoms include joint pain, tenderness, stiffness, loss of function, and restricted mobility. Diagnosis is made by physical examination, X rays, and ruling out other types of arthritis.

Rheumatoid Arthritis

Rheumatoid arthritis, one of the most destructive forms of arthritis, is a severe inflammatory condition that affects the joints as well as other body organs. It is an autoimmune disease in which the body attacks its own tissue. More than 60 percent of the two million Americans with rheumatoid arthritis are middle-aged women. Symptoms include pain and swelling in many joints, morning stiffness, afternoon fatigue, and low-grade fevers. Significant joint deformity and disability may occur.

Rheumatoid arthritis can be difficult to diagnose. It often begins gradually and may resemble other types of arthritis. The condition is unpredictable, marked by episodes of remission and exacerbation.

Gout

Gout is a form of inflammatory arthritis caused by excess uric acid in the body. This excess can result from overproduction of the acid by the body itself, decreased elimination by the kidneys, or increased consumption of foods containing purines, which are metabolized into uric acid. Foods that are particularly high in purines include meats and seafood. Alcohol also increases uric acid levels. Acid crystals, which build up and congregate in the joints, are identified as invaders by the body's white blood cells. The cells attack the joints, creating painful episodes of inflammation.

Acute gouty arthritis is a sudden affliction that may last a few days to a few weeks and then disappear temporarily. Usually just one or a few joints are affected. In most cases, the big toe is the initial target. Often a person is awakened from sleep with intense pain. Gout tends to run in families, and more commonly affects overweight men in middle age. Gout may also result from blood disorders or cancers, or from the use of certain drugs. The symptoms of gout may appear following periods of excessive eating or drinking, or physical or mental stress.

CAUSES

A host of factors are triggers for people who are genetically susceptible to arthritis. Dr. Ray Wunderlich explains: "We talk about inadequate repairs, inadequate defenses for our body. As we go along with inadequate food, digestion, metabolism, and porosity of gut, we develop increasing levels of immune disturbance, and the joints are a major place where this manifests. That may be because of their movement or because of the tremendous amount of connective tissue around them."

Joint disorders are very common in our society. Connective tissue needs high amounts of vitamin C, glucosamine, and appropriate minerals such as silica, magnesium, zinc, and pantothenic acid. "Without these," says Dr. Wunderlich, "there will be a decline of the connective tissue, which is the glue that keeps our bodies together. As the body sails along through space in our journey through life, we get bombarded with more and more toxins. Rachel Carson was right. It's a toxic planet, and it's not getting any better."

Environmental stress is central to arthritis, as it is to so many other illnesses. There has been an intellectual blind spot on our medical, health, and legislative screens. We look out there and we see herbicides, pesticides, genetically engineered foods, pollution in our water—so much new pollution that government regulators cannot even abide by the old standards, so they keep raising the allowable amount of toxins in the body.

CLINICAL EXPERIENCE

Traditional Medicine

Typically, arthritis is diagnosed on the basis of a patient's symptoms, which most commonly include pain or swelling in the joint areas or some limitation of movement. Some diagnostic tests and X rays may show abnormalities in the joints, but often these tests are not accurate. Thus, the patient's symptoms are the central factor in determining the diagnosis.

Because medical students have been taught that there is no cure for arthritis, as doctors they do not look for the cause of the disease but instead focus on alleviating the symptoms. This approach can be very dangerous because many of the drugs used to counteract pain and swelling can have serious side effects. Even aspirin, which is ordinarily considered one of the least toxic medications and normally constitutes the first line of attack in the traditional treatment of arthritis, is not without side effects. In the treatment of arthritis, aspirin is given in large doses on a constant basis. Consequently, arthritis patients have consistently high levels of aspirin in their systems; this can result in dizziness, ringing in the ears, intestinal tract bleeding, and kidney damage.

When aspirin does not work or when an arthritis sufferer develops adverse reactions to it, other medications called nonsteroidal anti-inflammatory drugs (NSAIDs), such as the widely advertised Motrin, are used to control inflammation. Since these drugs are nonsteroidal (i.e., do not contain cortisone), they are less toxic than are some medications commonly used to combat inflammation, but they nevertheless do have side effects.

NSAIDs came onto the market as effective alternatives to aspirin, which had caused internal bleeding in many long-term users. Ironically, while the NSAIDs are less effective than aspirin as anti-inflammatories, they also have side effects that include gastrointestinal bleeding and peptic ulcers. Other side effects include dizziness, nervousness, nausea, vomiting, and ringing in the ears. If these drugs are unsuccessful, doctors often prescribe cortisone-derived drugs such as prednisone. These drugs are notorious for their severe toxicity. They interfere with the immune system, leaving the patient defenseless against infection and other diseases. Cortisone-type drugs also interfere with the body's healing ability, and it is not uncommon for a person taking these drugs to have bone fractures or wounds that do not heal for long periods.

Some rheumatologists (doctors who treat arthritis patients) use injections of gold. This method of treatment was abandoned years ago because it was considered too dangerous, but today gold treatments are finding their way back into medical practice. Another technique finding acceptance among arthritis doctors is the use of chemotherapy drugs. The theory behind this drastic measure is that when a patient's immune system is knocked out, the patient's body is no longer able to form the antibodies that may be causing the inflammation in her joints. Other techniques include radiation therapy in the area of the inflammation, again with the intent of destroying the patient's immune response, and plasmapheresis, a procedure by which a patient's blood is drained, filtered to remove antibodies, and then reinjected into the patient.

While the traditional medical approach to arthritis is undeniably becoming more sophisticated, it also appears to be missing the mark. Not only do these treatments fail to get at the cause of the disease, they are becoming more expensive, invasive, and toxic, leading to the inevitable question, Do the ends justify the means? When traditional medicine begins to turn to anticancer therapies to treat arthritis—therapies that are often cancer-causing themselves and result in side effects ranging from nausea and hair and weight loss to depletion of the immune system—this question becomes even more pressing.

Dr. Warren Levin of Physicians for Complementary Medicine recalls that a couple of years ago the American Medical Association (AMA) put out a series of videotapes to teach physicians how to take care of and diagnose rheumatoid arthritis. The lecturer on the tape was adamant that nutrition has nothing to do with arthritis: "His whole face filled the screen, and he said, 'Nutrition has no place in the treatment of arthritis. We can use drugs.' That is the AMA way. They have not come to Physicians for Complementary Medicine to see what success we have with our methods and how the vast majority of our patients dramatically improve without the use of the toxic drugs that characterize American medicine's treatment of arthritis."

Alternative Treatments

"The way I treat arthritis is probably quite different from the approach of most physicians," says Dr. Peter D'Adano. "As a naturopath, I was taught that we should not always think about treating a disease but about treating a person. Arthritis is a very good example of a disease that is highly individualized. Not only are there different types of arthritis, but people get it and express it in different manners."

It's a good idea to try to listen to the body and realize that it has an intelligence. In other words, if you are following a certain lifestyle and your problems are the result of that lifestyle, a change in lifestyle may change the illness.

People say that as the body gets older, the most natural thing in the world is for it to get decrepit. But give the body credit for the intelligence it has. When the body tells you something, if you listen and follow what it says, you will improve.

DIET AND NUTRITION

Dr. Peter Agho of the Healing Center says, "I do diet. Not just for arthritis. The thing about the whole diet is this. Change the diet, and the arthritis—along with obesity, high blood pressure, and other problems—will get better. The diet should include fresh fruit, including fresh fruit juice, and vegetables. You should eliminate animal fats and cut high-fat foods."

Dr. Howard Robins outlines his treatment: "We use a complete vegetarian diet, including a lot of green, leafy vegetables. These are important because of all the phytochemicals and phytoestrogens that help in all the chemical processes that are necessary to getting well again. We give them juices, six to eight fresh green juices a day—the best way to take in these chemicals."

Dr. Luke Bucci, author of *Pain Free: The Definitive Guide to Healing Arthritis*, notes that part of the reason people get arthritis is the lack of essential nutrients in a highly processed, refined diet. Sure, you get plenty of calories, protein, and fat—usually the wrong kind of fat. What you do not get is just as important—the minerals: magnesium, zinc, copper, manganese, boron. Many people are not aware of boron as a nutrient, but boron may turn out to be essential to our joints' health. These are what you do not get with the current, typical American diet. We lack the substances that enable the joints to repair themselves from the damage they sustain. That is why you want to start eating a whole-food diet that is rich in organic vegetables, fruits, and nuts.

Dr. Rich Ribner tells this story: "Recently, a woman came to the clinic with a terrible case of arthritis. She was in terrible pain and had been taking anti-inflammatory medication and tranquilizers. She was miserable. She said she thought about killing herself. I said, 'Stop this nonsense. I'm going to ask you to do something. You may not even want to do it.' She said, 'Anything.' I said, 'Between now and next week, I want you to drink six to eight glasses of water a day, but it has to be distilled or spring water. And eat nothing but brown rice, just brown rice.' 'But, but…' she began. 'Wait,' I said, 'You were talking about killing yourself. So listen, I'll add a few green vegetables to that.'

"You have to make sure there is a cleansing. Make sure they drink the water. Have a bowel movement daily.

"Well, this woman was so desperate that she stayed on the diet one week. When she came back, there was marked improvement. She still had a long way to go, but there was a change."

SUPPLEMENTS

Vitamins, minerals, and nutritive substances can play important roles in the treatment and prevention of arthritis. There is some evidence that the essential fatty acids furnished by substances such as cod liver oil, linoleic acid, and marine lipids, by replacing missing fatty substances in the joint-lubricating synovial fluid, can be important in treating arthritis. When the joint surfaces become irritated and undergo degeneration, some of the fat from the joint itself is lost. This fat acts as a lubricant and keeps the joint surfaces apart so that the cartilage-covered bone ends are protected and can move smoothly. When a person takes extra cod liver oil or other essential fatty acids, the oil goes to the joints and provides more lubrication.

Vitamin A, which is found in large quantities in cod liver oil, is also important for the maintenance of the mucous membranes, which manufacture mucus to cleanse the body of infectious bacteria and toxins. Without adequate supplies of vitamin A, infection and accumulation of toxic materials can set in around the joints. Furthermore, a vitamin A deficiency can lead to insufficient production of synovial fluid; when this occurs, the joints lack proper lubrication, the cartilage becomes subject to drying and cracking, and movement becomes difficult and painful.

Because lubrication is vital to the smooth functioning of the joints, vitamin E, whose primary role is to protect against the destruction of the essential fatty acids by oxidation, is also an important antiarthritic nutrient. Both vitamins E and C, which generally act as free radical scavengers within the body, can be especially important in the treatment as they can "clinch" the free radicals present at the site of inflamed or irritated joints, thereby decreasing pain, swelling, and inflammation.

Many symptoms of arthritis are alleviated by establishing a proper balance of calcium and phosphorus in the body, since these are the two minerals most responsible for bone formation and healing. This can be one of the most confusing aspects of arthritis, because X rays of arthritic joints often show excessive calcification. Afraid of further calcification, patients mistakenly believe that they must avoid calcium-rich foods. Actually, the calcification is due not to an excess of calcium but to malabsorption of existing supplies caused by an imbalance in the ratio of calcium to phosphorus. This imbalance is caused by two major factors: (1) excessive consumption of foods containing high levels of phosphorus, such as meat, dairy products, and soft drinks; and (2) the process of joint degeneration, which releases high levels of phosphates. This excess phosphorus at the joint site binds with calcium and results in calcification. Taking extra calcium orally does not contribute to this localized calcification. Rather, by increasing calcium levels in the blood, it draws the excess phosphorus away from the joints to bind with the blood calcium so that both are eliminated; this in turn inhibits calcification around the joints.

It should be noted here that soft drinks are the number-one source of phosphorus in the American diet today. These drinks contain more phosphorus than most other foods or beverages, and the typical American consumes nearly 500 gallons of them a year. According to Dr. David Steenblock, excess phosphorus is one of the major contributing factors to the development of osteoarthritis. He says, "We see this clinically in many people, who come with osteoarthritis in their early forties who are large consumers of soft drinks, who also consume excess quantities of meats and other high-phosphorus foods, and who do not eat enough of the green, leafy vegetables which contain calcium." The other problem associated with soft drinks is that most contain citric acids, which bind calcium and cause it to be excreted. "So," says Dr. Steenblock, "not only is there extra phosphorus in the soft drinks, they contain the material that takes calcium out of the body. If you want to develop osteoarthritis, that's a very good way of doing it."

Other useful supplements include glucosamine and chondroitin. According to Dr. Luke Bucci, these substances act to "convince" your joint tissues to repair the damage caused by arthritis. (See "Specific Alternative Treatment Approaches" later in this chapter for more information on glucosamine and chondroitin.)

Several studies have shown that a small supplemental dose of boron, about 3 to 6 milligrams a day, can reverse the symptoms of osteoarthritis. Magnesium is also helpful.

AVOIDING CERTAIN FOODS AND CHEMICALS

Arthritis may be caused or exacerbated by allergies to foods and chemicals. Dr. Warren Levin says that removing offending substances from the patient's environment can produce dramatic changes.

Some doctors believe that arthritis is caused by the foods a person eats most often. Dr. Morton Teich stresses that the food the patient wants the most may be the problem. Studies have shown that milk, for example, can cause severe allergies and arthritis.

Dr. Teich also warns us about the glycoproteins in milk, wheat, corn, and cinnamon, as well as inhalants such as dust, mold, and pollen. Chemicals and food additives are also potential contributors to allergies and arthritis.

HERBS

Letha Hadady, an herbalist, tries to eliminate the toxins that result from poor digestion and poor circulation. She shares some of her herbal remedies.

In dealing with arthritis, one thing you must have every day is alfalfa. You could chew ten tablets a day with a little water to eliminate much of the uric acid that can build up to create joint pain. Rhubarb also eliminates acid. It is a laxative, but it also breaks apart the painful crystals that form around your joints.

Dandelion greens are full of vitamins and minerals. Dandelions break down pain-giving acid, too.

Star fruit is a sweet, delicious fruit you can find in the grocery store or at the vegetable stand. Juice it. Add a cup and a half of cold water per serving of six star fruits. Taken three times a day, it can eliminate inflammatory joint pain, bleeding hemorrhoids, and burning urine. It is cooling and cleansing.

It is important to realize that not everyone's arthritic pain is the same. Do you wake up in the morning with your joints feeling stiff and sore? Do they feel better after you move them around and after you exercise? If so, you need to take warming, tonic herbs that build vitality, increase circulation, and warm joints. Add a pinch of turmeric to your stews. Turmeric and cinnamon are a good combination for achy shoulders. If you have rheumatism that gets worse in cold weather, add 1/4 teaspoon of turmeric and cinnamon to a little water and drink it as a tea.

Asafetida is a spice that is available in Indian stores. A little asafetida added to cooking beans or other hard-to-digest foods will help cleanse the body and warm the joints.

Also useful is the resin myrrh; a few drops added to your tea will make your joints feel warm and your blood move, thus improving the circulation.

Hadady says that Asian medicine uses many herbs that can be added in cooking. For example, dong quai increases circulation and warms joints. Another classic Chinese remedy, one that Chinese doctors have used for generations, is du huo jisheng wan. Hadady's favorite—guan jie yan wan—is translated as "walk as smoothly as a tiger." Other Asian remedies include raw Tienchi ginseng, Efficacious Corydalis, tien ma, Three Snakes Formula, Mobility 3, Clematis 19, du zhong, leigong ten pian, and rinchen dragjor-rilnag chenmo.

CHIROPRACTIC

Many arthritis sufferers interviewed for this chapter said that of all the things they tried in their efforts to eliminate the pain, going to a chiropractor helped the most.

Dr. Mitchell Proffman, a chiropractor at the Healing Center, showed me two X rays. The first showed bones that were nice and clean and square in shape; the second showed degeneration of the bones.

He showed what arthritis looks like in the human body: thinned disks and a little lip or spur, the body's defense mechanism to heal or shore up the area so that it does not totally disintegrate. He said a woman might have a pinched nerve somewhere in the body, in the neck, for example. He administers a gentle push with his hand, which is not painful, to move the bone back into position. The nerve energy comes through, and the joint can start to heal.

RECONSTRUCTIVE THERAPY

The noted physician Dr. Arnold Blank has used reconstructive therapy to treat arthritis. Reconstructive therapy, created in the 1920s by the osteopathic physicians Gedney and Schumann, works by stimulating the body's ability to heal itself. The doctors found that by injecting substances that caused a slight irritation to tissues, they could help blood vessels grow into a region, thus bringing more oxygen, vitamins, and minerals into the cartilage and promoting tissue growth.

Dr. Blank says this therapy is most effective in patients who are in an optimal nutritional state. "Vitamin and mineral levels are important in our healing response and ability. The injection consists of a variety of different liquids. Primary liquids I use are calcium, lidocaine, and saline. They take a moment and really aren't painful. The majority of patients feel improvement after the first three or four treatments, developing some strength and feeling less pain, even increasing the range of movement.

"The nutrients we may use, natural ones, include substances that have an anti-inflammatory effect, such as vitamin C, shark cartilage, sea cucumber, glutathione, and glucosamine sulfate. All these substances are used once reconstructive therapy has begun because the new blood vessels going to the tissues will enhance healing. These nutrients may not work well when there are no blood vessels going into the area, so they should be administered after the therapy has begun its work."

ACUPUNCTURE

Acupuncture has been used by countless people throughout the world to help alleviate the pain and suffering of arthritis. Dr. Yuan Yang of the Healing Center explains briefly how this works. "We put the needle around the joint to create circulation, taking the pain away. There may be cold, blocked blood and low energy, so I apply the needle for smooth blood flow. Moving blocked energy takes the pain out."

PHYSICAL THERAPY

Shmuel Tatz typically works with people who have arthritic problems from overuse syndromes or accidents. He works directly on the joints. For example, for a pianist who has problems with the hands, he will try to move the bones, separating the joints to make more space.

As Tatz explains, "Today in physical therapy we use many modalities. One of these is magnetic pulse therapy. We know of the positive effects of magnetism on the body. Scientists have developed a machine with different programs so that we can adjust for every different situation.

"We put electrodes on the body, for example, on the hip joint, and we leave them on for fifteen to twenty minutes. Usually patients report a very mild relaxing sensation, and the pain decreases.

"Many people with pain from osteoarthritis are afraid to be touched. People with a swollen knee, for instance, can do reflex therapy. For the knee we touch an acupuncture point on the ear, which gives relief."

Once this manipulation has had an effect, they start to exercise the knee by putting the legs in slings, relieving the pressure on the joint and making it easier for the patient to move the body. Trying to open the joint and make more space around the bones allows for better circulation. Movement is very important for people with arthritis.

One patient, Lori, speaks about her improvement: "Here at Medical Arts I was able to receive physical therapy, which has enabled me to avoid surgery and has greatly improved the quality of my life. I'm still dancing."

YOGA

Molly McBride, a yoga instructor, believes you do not have to stop working on your health simply because you may have some physical limitations. Even by working with something as simple as a chair, it is easy to stay fit and help yourself with the problems of arthritis.

The basis of yoga is breath and breathing practices, she says, which help circulation and also help flush the body out by collecting toxins so that they can be exhaled. Breath is the foundation of all the yoga stretches.

"We start with just taking a simple breath; the basic beginning exercise is a three-part breath. Let the air fill the abdomen, then the rib cage, then the upper chest. Exhale, letting the breath exit the upper chest, then the rib cage, and then abdomen. Inhale, exhale."

It is important to take time every day to do these breathing exercises. A really good time to do them is first thing in the morning, when your stomach is empty; if you have eaten, wait a few hours before you start. These breathing exercises can be combined with some simple joint lubrication exercises. To regenerate the body and increase the flow of oxygen through the system, to help release all the toxins that build up in the muscles and the protective cartilage around the joints, try simple yoga exercises.

SPECIFIC ALTERNATIVE TREATMENT APPROACHES

In the following pages, we discuss some specific alternative approaches to treating arthritis. Although there are many other approaches, these have had a consistently high success rate, are not toxic or expensive, and may get to the cause of the disease rather than merely masking its symptoms.

Treatment for Gout

Traditional medicine treats gout symptoms with drugs to relieve pain and decrease uric acid levels in the body. These drugs include colchicine, corticosteroids, analgesics, uricosuric agents, and allopurinol. They may be beneficial but they do have side effects. More important, they're reactive, not proactive.

An article on www.healthwell.com from Integrative Medicine Communications provides a good summary of the alternative and complementary ways to prevent and treat this painful condition. First, it's important to maintain a healthy weight, drink adequate amounts of water, avoid alcohol, and eliminate or limit foods that contain purines. Beef, goose, organ meats, mussels, herring, mackerel, and yeast contain high amounts of purine, Moderate amounts of purine are found in other meats and fish, as well as spinach, asparagus, lentils, mushrooms, and dried peas.

Helpful nutrients include berries, vitamin C, and folic acid. Cherries, hawthorn berries, and blueberries all contain anthocyanins, a class of natural dyes that have been found to reduce inflammation and enhance the quality of collagen. They also act as antioxidants. According to Dr. Muraleedharan Nair from Michigan State University, the anthocyanins in tart cherries are ten times more effective than aspirin in reducing inflammation. As an added benefit, they don't irritate the stomach like aspirin does. Half a pound of cherries per day for two weeks has been found to lower uric acid levels and prevent episodes of gout. Also beneficial is cherry juice, 8 to 16 ounces daily.

Eight grams of vitamin C per day have been found to reduce uric acid levels in the blood. Caution must be noted, however, as gout symptoms will get worse in some people with this amount of vitamin C. In terms of folic acid, 10 to 75 milligrams daily are recommended.

A good herbal remedy for gout is bromelain, 125 to 250 milligrams three times a day during an attack. Also recommended is devil's claw, which can be taken in the following dosages: 1 to 2 grams three times daily of dried powdered root, 4 to 5 milliliters three times daily of tincture, or 400 milligrams three times daily of dry solid extract. Both bromelain and devil's claw act as anti-inflammatories.

Among the homeopathic remedies used for gout are the following:

ACONITE, recommended for burning pain, anxiety, and restlessness that comes on suddenly.

BELLADONNA, recommended for intense, throbbing pain that increases with motion and decreases with pressure.

BRYONIA, indicated for pain exacerbated by motion and decreased by pressure and heat.

COLCHICUM, suggested for pain that increases with motion and weather changes.

LEDUM, for swollen, mottled joints that respond better to cold than to heat.

In addition, hot and cold compresses, and bed rest may help.

Dr. Jason Theodosakis: Maximizing the Arthritis Cure

Dr. Theodosakis is the author of *The Arthritis Cure* and *Maximizing the Arthritis Cure,* and·board-certified in preventive medicine. He is a lecturer on preventive medicine, an assistant clinical professor at the University of Arizona College of Medicine, and the former director of its Preventative Medicine Residency Training Program.

"I've come up with my arthritis program out of necessity, both to treat patients and for personal use," he says. "I see a lot of patients mainly with osteoarthritis but also with the other types of arthritis.

"My program is an integrated, comprehensive approach to creating a situation that optimizes the buildup of cartilage. I will basically use anything—diet, exercise, even medicine when it's called for. We hit it from all angles, including the psychological aspects."

Nonsteroidal anti-inflammatory drugs (NSAIDs), he remarks, are part of a $37 billion worldwide market that involves such huge corporations as Whitehall-Robins, which makes Advil and Motrin; other NSAIDs are Aleve, which is naproxen sodium, and aspirin. According to Dr. Theodosakis, these drugs may cause serious problems, such as bleeding ulcers, kidney dysfunction, and adverse drug interactions. "At a rheumatology conference I was at, it came out that none of these anti-inflammatories have been studied long term," he says. "Studies have suggested that they may even worsen the condition."

Dr. Theodosakis's program can be broken down into the following components: diagnosis, supplementation with glucosamine and chondroitin, a change in biomechanics, exercise, and medical approaches.

DIAGNOSIS

"The very first step is getting an accurate diagnosis and working with the physician," Dr. Theodosakis explains. "Be up front with your doctor. In my book, I lay out what you should be telling your doctor and what your doctor should be asking you, the tests you should be getting for a diagnosis, and so on. Even if you are in a managed-care setting where you get only five or ten minutes with your doctor, you have to know what information to get to use that time optimally. Getting an accurate diagnosis so that you'll know what you are treating is step one."

SUPPLEMENTS: GLUCOSAMINE AND CHONDROITIN

Glucosamine and chondroitin are natural supplements from seashells and cow's cartilage, respectively. When taken orally, they improve the balance between breakdown and buildup of cartilage. Several recent studies support their use. "These supplements are a part of the treatment," Dr. Theodosakis cautions. "Alone, these supplements are not the answer; they need to be part of a complete program.

Dr. Theodosakis has a website listing the studies on glucosamine and chondroitin (www.drtheo.com). Further, he states, "I also set up a national reporting center for drug side effects related to glucosamine and chondroitin to see if any negative effects have been noted. So far, although millions of people are using these supplements, I'm not aware of any side effects. And I would be the first person to be aware of them if they were occurring."

The one problem with these supplements is that there are about one hundred different brands on the market. In Dr. Theodosakis's opinion, "maybe as many as 30 percent do not meet the label claims. In other words, you are not getting what the bottle says. This is a very big concern of mine."

BIOMECHANICS

Biomechanics refers to the way the body absorbs shock from everyday movement. "You have different forces on your joint," Dr. Theodosakis says, "and if you learn to dissipate these forces throughout your body, there is likely to be less damage to your cartilage. People can learn to improve their biomechanics. They certainly do in the sports arena, which you will see if you look at athletes as well as performers in such disciplines as ballet. They have wonderful biomechanics and can absorb and dissipate tremendous shock. So my patients are taught how to alter their own biomechanics."

EXERCISE

Exercise is absolutely necessary for arthritis sufferers, but the wrong kind of exercise can worsen the condition. You need a specific program for whatever ails you, Dr. Theodosakis says. If you have a hip problem, for example, you will need to do the appropriate exercises for that.

DIET

Another component of Dr. Theodosakis's program is diet. He remarks, "The fasting in order to detoxify the body, the juicing, the vegetarian diet are all things I agree with 100 percent.

"Diet has a tremendous impact on arthritis for several reasons. One is weight control. A major risk factor for getting arthritis is being overweight. For example, women in the highest fifth of weight are eight times more likely to get arthritis of the knee than are women in the lowest fifth. Another factor is that different foods will either aggravate or alleviate arthritis. Some of the fish oils, omega-3 fatty acids, can help, while certain components of meat, such as arachidonic acid, can worsen the condition. You also need to eat a wide variety of fruits and vegetables, making sure you get a wide variety of nutrients and also taking supplements. With these nutritional elements, we are making sure your body has the optimal environment to win this cartilage battle."

MEDICAL APPROACHES

Dr. Theodosakis also incorporates medical approaches into his program. This may include prescription drugs, surgery, and treatment for depression associated with arthritis.

RESULTS

Dr. Theodosakis describes what he calls "one of my most remarkable cases," that of one of his nurses. "She is about forty years old. She had terrible arthritis, to the point where she was going to have her knee cartilage scraped off, she had so many crystals in it. She used my program for about four months and saw tremendous improvement. She was taking the supplements at that time, then she stopped taking the supplements—that was about two years ago. Now she's become a runner; she did a half marathon. But she would have been crippled if she had had the surgery.

"I have had a number of patients who were scheduled for joint replacement therapy and after going through this program were able to avoid the surgery. Many are pain-free. It won't reverse the bony changes that occurred in the joint, but it gives them the opportunity to exercise and do some of the things they want to do."

Dr. Robert Liefman: Holistic Balanced Treatment

Holistic Balanced Treatment (HBT) is derived from the work of the physician Dr. Robert Liefman (1920–1973). Dr. Liefman first used this treatment in 1961, after twenty years of research. Since that time more than thirty thousand arthritis sufferers have received the treatment, and many of them are living pain-free, normal lives.

HBT is based on the results of Dr. Liefman's research, which showed that many arthritis sufferers, especially those with rheumatoid arthritis, have specific hormonal imbalances. Within the body there are naturally occurring hormones called glucocorticoids whose role is to reduce inflammation and raise the level of simple sugars in the blood. One of the ways these hormones raise blood sugar levels is by converting nonglucose molecules such as protein into glucose. If unchecked, these glucocorticoids can be responsible for the collagen breakdown of cartilage in joints, which may be a contributing factor in the development of arthritis. The glucocorticoids are balanced within the body by other hormones, such as testosterone and the feminizing hormones, which include estradiol; these hormones induce tissue building and hence balance the tissue-wasting effects of the glucocorticoids. If the body is not regulating these hormones, there are therapies to correct these imbalances. Dr. Liefman developed formulas consisting of varying amounts of three basic ingredients: (1) prednisone, an anti-inflammatory steroid, (2) estradiol, an estrogenic hormone, and (3) testosterone.

According to the proponents of HBT, the anti-inflammatory property of the steroid prednisone and the healing properties of sex hormones can be used to treat arthritic conditions with minimal side effects because of the balancing action between the different components. The anabolic, or building, quality of the sex hormones acts to control the catabolic, or destructive, effects of the steroidal drug therapy (these effects include infection, decreased immunity, improper healing, suppression of pituitary and adrenal function, and fluid retention). The feminizing and androgenic activities of sex hormones are kept in check both by the catabolic nature of the glucocorticoids and by careful adjustment of the concentration of the sex hormones in accordance with the specific requirements of the individual patient during treatment.

THE SUCCESS OF HBT

In contrast to the symptom-suppressing approach taken by the traditional medical establishment, HBT is designed to address the causes of arthritis. It does this first by restoring a positive protein-building balance within the body through the administration of the trihormonal formulas, which works to stop pain and inflammation. Second, according to Dr. Henry Rothblatt, "HBT is never administered without considering the particular need of the individual patient. The medication is adjusted for every patient so that the proper tissue-building and healing response can be obtained. Respect for the uniqueness and the unique need of the individual patient is one of the essential principles of the holistic approach to medicine."

Dr. Liefman developed four basic formulas to account for the different requirements of each individual using HBT: (1) White Cap, which contains prednisone, testosterone, and estradiol, (2) Black Cap, which has only prednisone and estradiol, (3) Red Cap, which contains prednisone and testosterone, and (4) Green Cap, which contains only prednisone and is used only to allow women to shed the endometrium proliferation caused by the intake of the estrogen-containing preparations. In turn, the proportions of these different compounds may vary from individual to individual and may be altered for the same person during the course of treatment.

If, for example, a female patient begins to exhibit an adverse reaction to the treatment, such as the growth of excess body hair, the testosterone level in the medication will be reduced to eliminate those reactions. Patients who exhibit some of the typical side effects of cortisone-type drugs will have the amounts of prednisone in their medication decreased, or appropriate increases in one of the sex hormones will be made to counterbalance the negative effects of the steroids. Generally, the adverse reactions to any of the elements in the compounds disappear within a short time once the proper balance among the hormones has been attained.

HBT also incorporates principles of nutrition and stresses the importance of regular exercise. The diet recommended in HBT eliminates junk foods such as sugar and sugar products, and salty and processed foods such as luncheon meats and canned goods, fried foods, and refined foods. The diet is essentially moderate in protein and emphasizes high-fiber complex carbohydrates in the form of fresh fruits and vegetables, whole grains, and legumes. Vitamin and mineral supplements are used to bolster the patient's immune system and enhance the body's natural healing abilities. For instance, vitamin D is important for strong and healthy bones because it regulates the absorption of calcium from the stomach into the bloodstream, which carries it to bone tissue. Vitamins C and A are important for the maintenance and repair of collagen, the gluelike substance that holds the tissues together and is essential for joint and muscle stability. Vitamin E and the B-complex vitamins are important for bone growth. Among the minerals, adequate supply and absorption of calcium, phosphorous, and magnesium are essential for the formation of healthy bones, while zinc and selenium are important immune system nutrients.

Exercise is also an important adjunct to HBT and is recommended to restore joint and muscle mobility and function as well as muscle mass lost during periods of inactivity. However, patients generally are told not to exercise until they are free of pain, swelling, and stiffness and feel confident enough to engage in it. Walking may be the first exercise; then, as patients improve, they can be given specialized exercises for the hands, knees, fingers, shoulders, and other areas that may have been affected by arthritis.

The medical establishment has basically ignored, attacked, or criticized HBT therapy even though its basis is drugs already widely used by physicians. All Dr. Liefman did was combine certain commonly prescribed drugs to maximize the benefits and minimize the side effects of each component drug. The balanced hormonal approach to arthritis did, however, do one unorthodox thing: It challenged the rigidly held position of the medical establishment that arthritis is an incurable disease.

PATIENT STORIES

Here are some of the results arthritis patients have had over the years from using HBT:

CYNTHIA—At age nineteen, Cynthia began to experience the symptoms of rheumatoid arthritis. Initially the arthritis was confined to her jaw and elbows, but over a period of two and a half years, while she was undergoing treatment by a traditional physician, the arthritis spread to nearly every part of her body. Five years later Cynthia was so crippled with pain and stiffness that it took her a half hour to get out of bed in the morning. The morning after she started HBT, her pain had almost disappeared except for some stiffness and soreness, which also went away during the following three days. About her condition and her subsequent treatment at the Arthritis Medical Center in Fort Lauderdale, which administers HBT, Cynthia said,

"I was getting worse and worse. When I first went to my doctor, I had it just in my jaw and elbows. After two and a half years, I had it in just about every place except my hips and knees. l couldn't turn my head at all.

"The doctor actually told me once that he felt really bad, that he had tried everything and didn't know what else to do, and that I had better go to the crippled children's center in Palm Beach. To tell a young woman that.... I just wanted to drive off a bridge. But I thank him for saying it because if he hadn't, I don't think I ever would have tried this place. I did it in desperation."

At the time Cynthia started HBT she was taking thirty aspirin tablets a day, which were causing headaches, ringing in her ears, and ulcers. She was spending approximately a thousand dollars a month on painkillers alone. While Cynthia found that she bruised and bled more easily after starting HBT, she notes that she had the same symptoms while taking large doses of aspirin. However, while the aspirin and other treatments did nothing to arrest the progression of Cynthia's arthritis, a day after she started treatment with HBT, her pain virtually disappeared, and it returned only when she forgot to take her medication. At present Cynthia is pain-free and works out three times a week at a health spa. She continues on her medication, but in much smaller doses than when she started treatment with HBT.

JUNE —June suffered from severe crippling arthritis for two years before starting treatment with HBT. Over that two-year period June received almost every form of traditional arthritis treatment available: gold injections, penicillamine, Butazolidin (phenylbutazone), small doses of prednisone, and sixteen aspirins daily. June says that she was spending more than one hundred dollars a week for medication alone. In the meantime she kept getting worse, and when she started HBT, she says, "I was immobile in my hands and shoulders. It was at that point that I thought, What's the use of living? I couldn't even turn my head." Additionally, her liver, stomach, and kidneys were damaged by the large doses of medication. She was forced to give up her business because she was too weak and in too much pain to work. Her medical bills were ruining her financially. The second day after June received HBT, her pain disappeared. June says about her progress with HBT:

"I woke up and I could move my ankles, I could move my hands and my feet. When I stood up, the pain wasn't there. I said to [my husband], 'My God, there's been a miracle.' It got better and better, and I guess within two months I didn't even know I had rheumatoid arthritis. I got a bicycle, and I started dancing again and going to the beach again. It used to be if I lay on the sand, I couldn't get up again."

June continues to be pain-free, leading a normal life, and her medication has been reduced by more than half the initial amount.

Dr. Theron Randolph and Dr. Marshall Mandell: Environmental Allergies

Environmental medicine, also called clinical ecology, was developed by Dr. Theron Randolph in the 1940s and 1950s when he observed early in his medical career that food allergies and sensitivities to environmental chemicals were a major contributing factor in a wide range of diseases, including arthritis. Dr. Randolph also noted that the causal relationship of allergy to disease was a very individualized phenomenon: One person could eat beef every day and never have an adverse reaction, while another person could develop a food allergy to beef even when consuming it only on rare occasions. Similarly, people with an allergy to the same product did not necessarily manifest the same symptoms. One might break out with hives, while another developed depression, and still another became arthritic. Dr. Randolph also found that seemingly innocuous chemicals found in the home, workplace, or school could in certain individuals trigger symptoms ranging from mental problems to aching joints to chronic fatigue.

The work of Dr. Randolph was applied to arthritis by Dr. Marshall Mandell, a physician from Connecticut and one of the country's leading environmental medical specialists. He has found that a considerable number of patients who come to him with arthritis or arthritislike symptoms are in fact suffering from a form of environmental allergy such as the ones outlined by Dr. Randolph. According to Dr. Mandell, "The basic process that underlies many cases of arthritis is a completely unrecognized or unsuspected allergy or allergylike sensitivity to substances that are part of daily life, including the food we eat, the liquids we drink, including the water supply, the chemicals that are deliberately or accidentally introduced into a diet, and the various forms of chemical pollutants in the indoor and outdoor air that get into our bodies." From his clinical experience, Dr. Mandell has found that more than half the patients he treats who would be confirmed arthritics by standard medical diagnostic techniques can be helped by means of simple dietary or environmental changes.

THE TREATMENT

"My approach and that of my colleagues in the field of environmental medicine and clinical ecology, supplemented by the benefits of nutritional therapy, begins by looking at the person who is predisposed to having arthritis to see if there are identifiable substances in the diet and environment that can trigger or cause the episode of illness," says Dr. Mandell. "We deal with demonstrable cause-and-effect relationships. What we do is study the patient.

"First, we take a carefully formulated history that is designed to help identify people who have problems with foods, with various chemicals, with pollutants, and perhaps with seasonal airborne substances. From this, we are able to get a fairly good idea of what we're dealing with."

Before patients are tested for food or environmental allergies, Dr. Mandell often has them fast or go on a restricted diet for four to seven days to rid the body of any residue of substances suspected to be responsible for the symptoms.

"Next," says Dr. Mandell, "we test these people using a technique known as 'provocative testing' to determine their response to extracts prepared from all the foods in their diet. The most commonly ingested foods are often the culprits, so it shouldn't come as any surprise that wheat, corn products, milk, beef, tomatoes, and potatoes are leading offenders.

"The most common technique used for provocative testing is to place a few drops of the test substance under the tongue of the patient, where it is almost immediately absorbed. This is called 'sublingual' provocative testing. When we test in this manner, only small doses are used, so the effect is brief, but since the solution enters the bloodstream, the entire body is exposed. Symptoms can show up in the joints, muscles, brain, skin, or any other part of the body.

"If we are able to produce joint pain, stiffness or swelling, or redness within a few minutes after placing the solution under the tongue for absorption into the bloodstream, we know that we've found something that must be important, because we have flared up the patient's familiar symptoms—we have actually precipitated an attack of the patient's own illness.

"Many people will have what we call 'polysymptomatic illness,' meaning that many bodily structures, organs, or systems can be involved at the same time. The arthritic person's whole body may be sensitive, and this is why such patients may have a headache or fatigue or asthma or colitis, although they may not actually have any of the well-known allergies such as hay fever, eczema, or hives.

"We also find that many people react to chemicals. We have some people whose arthritis may be due in part or exclusively to the chlorine that is in the water supply, or perhaps to an artificial flavoring or coloring which is used very frequently, or perhaps to a preservative. We have people who have trouble because they are inhaling fumes such as tobacco smoke. We have people who in heavy traffic have trouble because the exhaust fumes will travel, along with the oxygen, through the walls of the lung into the circulation; once again, the whole body is exposed."

After Dr. Mandell determines the substances in the patient's overall environment that he suspects are responsible for arthritic symptoms, he double-checks with test meals of the specific substances.

He explains, "If we're able to reproduce that patient's specific symptoms, if we can actually turn the symptoms on and off like a switch, we know that we have nailed it down, because we have demonstrated a cause-and-effect relationship that can't be questioned. Should food be the primary causative factor, we will design a diet that eliminates all of those foods. Then, depending on how well they follow the diet, the patients will be either well or sick."

PATIENT STORIES

SARAH—Sarah was a rabbi's wife who began to have arthritis in her hands, but the flare-ups would take place only on Saturday mornings and then disappear during the course of the day. Using Saturday as a starting point, Dr. Mandell began to explore the possible sources of Sarah's "Saturday arthritis."

"Since she woke up with the arthritis in the morning," Dr. Mandell explains, "we knew it was not caused by something she was doing in the morning. So we went back twenty-four hours to explore Friday. What did she do on Friday? What did she eat? Drink? Breathe? What came into her system? Could it be, perhaps, the paraffin fumes from the candles on the table which were lit ceremonially every Friday night? Or could it be something they ate? Was it caused by something she was exposed to when she went to temple on Friday night, perhaps from clothing just taken out of the dry cleaners? Or was it hair spray, perfume, cologne, or men with aftershave lotion? Was it that the temple had had the rug shampooed the day before the services or that the furniture was polished? I had no way of knowing, but I retraced all her activities, and then I tested her systematically.

"This actually turned out to be an easy one, and it was humorous, because the great 'Jewish penicillin,' chicken soup, was the thing that was undoing her. When I placed a few drops of chicken extract under her tongue, within minutes the knuckles that were affected by arthritis swelled up and became painful and red. I did this on a few occasions, so we were able to demonstrate this. It is rare to find a patient in whom a single substance is the factor, but it does happen now and then. So here is a rabbi's wife with chicken-and-chicken-soup arthritis—Friday-night ingestion, Saturday-morning appearance of arthritis."

JANET—This example not only documents the dramatic effects that can be achieved by eliminating an offending food from an arthritic person's diet, it also shows the degree of resistance orthodox arthritis doctors have to accepting this even when it has been unequivocally demonstrated.

Back in the mid-1970s Dr. Mandell sent out a mailing to rheumatologists in the northeastern part of the country, indicating that he was studying the relationship between food allergies and arthritis and was interested in studying some of their patients free of charge. Out of ninety letters, he received six responses, of which three said yes and three said no. Through one of the doctors who agreed to send patients, Janet eventually saw Dr. Mandell. He discusses her testing and the results:

"I want to emphasize that we never tell the patient what the test material is, so we completely eliminate suggestion. When we tested her with pork, she had pain almost immediately in one finger on her right hand, and this was her arthritis joint. We caused the joint to swell up and become red and painful.

"This test was repeated three times, once a week, and after the last test I told her to stay off pork for at least a week and then have a large portion of it one morning as a feeding test. Once again the same thing happened. However, when she told her rheumatologist, the man who was willing to have her come to me, he said he didn't believe it because we didn't have any controls. This is…more than pathetic, it's almost a medical crime! Here the patient had her symptom reproduced…and the doctor says he doesn't believe what has happened to her."

The ironic thing about this skepticism on the part of the

orthodox medical establishment is that many of the treatments it prescribes for arthritis have never been proved either safe or effective. Gold injections are a good example. This treatment is extremely costly, has very high toxicity, and is only rarely of benefit to arthritis sufferers. Furthermore, in cases where gold does provide some relief, rheumatologists are unable to offer a scientific explanation of how it operates within the body. Nevertheless, gold continues to be endorsed by the arthritis establishment while something as simple as eliminating a food from a patient's diet, even if that food has been demonstrated to cause the patient's symptoms, is ignored or criticized as being unscientific.

Dana Ullman's Homeopathy for Arthritis and Fibromyalgia

Homeopathy is based on the idea that the cure for an illness is similar to its cause. As a result, treatment consists of administering small doses of a very diluted natural substance that would cause the symptoms of the condition being treated if it were taken in larger amounts.

Dana Ullman of the Foundation for Homeopathic Education and Research is the author of several books on homeopathy, including *The Consumer's Guide to Homeopathy: The Definitive Resource for Understanding Homeopathic Medicine and Making It Work for You* and *Discovering Homeopathy: Medicine for the 21st Century.* Ullman explains the homeopathic viewpoint:

"There are estimated to be two hundred types of arthritis. I'm glad that [the medical establishment has] increased that number from before. [In the past,] it's been...about ten or twenty. From the homeopathic point of view, every person with arthritis has his or her own species of arthritis. Homeopaths see disease as a syndrome.

"Before rushing into the practical stuff, I want to comment about the research behind homeopathy, specifically in light of arthritis. The *British Journal of Clinical Pharmacology,* a major pharmacology journal, published a double-blind, placebo-controlled study on the homeopathic treatment of rheumatoid arthritis; this was way back in 1980. This study showed that 82 percent of the patients given an individualized homeopathic medicine got some degree of relief, whereas among those given a placebo, only 21 percent got that similar degree of relief."

Ullman describes some of the homeopathic approaches: "One approach is the use of single remedies to treat the acute exacerbation of the problem. Acute exacerbation of the problem means an immediate problem of a short-term nature, like a flare-up of some sort. Homeopathy and homeopathic remedies can be used to allay and relieve some of the pain and discomfort that a person is having.

"A better approach, however, is using the single remedy prescribed by a professional homeopath. This provides what we call constitutional care. It's a more highly individualized remedy, not just for the acute flare-up but for the person's overall genetic health and entire health history. For the homeopath to do this, it requires a detailed interview, lasting at least one to sometimes two hours. And sometimes a homeopath doesn't prescribe on that first interview but needs more information. This type of care is probably, in my estimation, one of the more profound ways to augment the body's own immune defense system, to not just relieve a person's condition but to really initiate a healing and curative process."

FIBROMYALGIA

To explain in specific terms how homeopathy can be effectively utilized, Ullman uses the treatment of fibromyalgia as an example:

"Fibromyalgia is also called fibrositis. For those who aren't familiar with it, it's a somewhat newly defined disease. At first, there was controversy as to whether it existed or not, but now there's basic acceptance that it is a condition. It's not officially arthritis, although it is thought to be a type of rheumatism where the person experiences pain and discomfort in the joints. They can also experience fatigue and even emotional and mental changes such as poor concentration, anxiety, and irritability. There might also be an irritable bowel, headaches, and cramps. The syndrome comes on in exacerbations. The person may be fine at one point and then all of a sudden have all these symptoms.

"A study was published in the *British Medical Journal* on fibromyalgia. The researchers admitted into the study only those patients who fit the most popular homeopathic remedy used to treat the acute stages of fibromyalgia. It's a remedy called Rhus tox [*Rhus toxicodendron*], which is poison ivy, believe it or not. [With] actual poison ivy, not only [does] an overdose cause skin eruptions, but if taken internally, and I don't recommend it, at least in a crude dose, it can and will have effects upon connective tissue that make the person feel extremely stiff, re-creating many of the symptoms that people experience when they have not only fibromyalgia but even many types of arthritis.

"They found that 42 percent of the people they interviewed fit this remedy. So they admitted these people into this study. In the first half of the study, half the people got a placebo and half the people got the real remedy. Then halfway through the study they switched, and the people who got the placebo now got the real remedy, and the people who began with the remedy got the placebo. The researchers found that when people began the real remedy, the homeopathic medicine, that's when relief began. And in this type of study, which is not only a double-blind placebo study—'controlled and crossover' is what it's called—the researcher is comparing patients with themselves. It's the most sophisticated type of research currently being done. It cannot always be done because these crossover effects, which we notice in homeopathy, are problematic since often homeopathic remedies have effects even after the person stops taking the remedy. So, when they begin taking the placebo, they're still feeling better. That sort of muddies the water. But this study did show, very clearly, that whenever people started to take Rhus tox, they began experiencing relief."

SPECIFIC REMEDIES

Rhus tox is also used in many musculoskeletal problems. It is one of the leading remedies for arthritis, carpal tunnel syndrome, and lower back pain. Rhus tox is known for alleviating the type of pain syndrome in the joints that is worse on initial motion, in other words, when the person initiates movement of a particular part of the body. When the part has been moved for some time, it loosens up and doesn't hurt as much. The people who need Rhus tox also tend to have an exacerbation of their symptoms from cold and wet weather.

"One of the nice things about homeopathy is that you can talk about this broad field of musculoskeletal problems. Although initially I was talking about fibromyalgia, these remedies can be used for many of these conditions. Another remedy that comes to mind is Bryonia. Bryonia is an herb called wild hops. This is not the same hops that you drink in a beer. It's a different botanical substance entirely. This is for people with various types of musculoskeletal problems where any type of motion exacerbates the condition. By contrast, people who benefit from Rhus tox have this rusty-gate syndrome where they feel worse only on initial motion and then loosen up and limber up. People who need Bryonia, the more they move, the worse they are. Here is a really obvious difference. That's one of the unique and nice things about homeopathy. We can be quite precise in finding a remedy that fits each person because the bottom line is that we are all biologically individual. We don't have the same type of joint disease or headache or depression or fatigue. We all have our own unique constellation, our own pattern of symptoms, and homeopathy is an exclusively effective, individualized approach to using these substances from the plant, mineral, or animal kingdom to augment the body's own defenses."

Another remedy Ullman describes is honeybee venom (Apis mellifera). "For those of us who have ever been stung by a honeybee, or at least we know what it's like, it's a burning and stinging type of pain, somewhat sharp. If you've ever had a bee sting, you also know that if you put ice on the bee sting, it provides some relief. But if you get near heat or you apply heat to it, it worsens the pain. Likewise, people who will benefit from homeopathic doses of Apis will have joint pain with swelling, much like a bee might cause, because the bee not only causes that burning, stinging pain but also causes that inflammatory redness and heat. Thus, there will be swelling that will be increased by cold applications and aggravated by heat.

"One of the known parts of folklore is that beekeepers do not seem to get arthritis very often. Part of the reason for this is that they occasionally do get stung, though they don't react the way the rest of us do because they become more immune to it. Their body has developed more sophisticated histamine responses so that when there is any type of sting, the body just deals with it very rapidly and easily. And there's something about that sting that also provides protective effects. It's as if one were taking, if you will, a homeopathic medicine. You're taking something that will cause a similar syndrome to what the arthritis causes. I don't recommend bee venom therapy, usually. I don't recommend that a person with arthritis be stung multiple times by a bee. Not that I discourage it; I [just] think there are safer, easier ways, like taking homeopathic doses of bee venom."

DOSAGES AND STRENGTHS OF HOMEOPATHIC MEDICINES

Ullman feels that it is important to understand some basics about the dosages in homeopathy and the strength of homeopathic medicines. "Don't be fooled by these extremely small doses. Don't think that just because we use small doses, you need to take more frequent repetitions of the remedy. During acute exacerbations, you do need to repeat them approximately every two hours in intense types of syndromes and every four hours in less intense syndromes. However, the idea of homeopathy is to take as minimal a dose as possible but as often as necessary. It's a fine balance. In other words, at times you might take it more frequently, but then as pain and discomfort diminish, you reduce the frequency of taking the remedy.

"If you look in a health food store or pharmacy, it will list the name of the medicine, usually in Latin. Homeopathic manufacturers have to be really precise on the source and species of the plant, mineral, animal, or chemical that we're using. Next to the name will be a number such as 6x or 30c. Well, x and c refer to the number of times that particular substance has been diluted. X is a Roman numeral that stands for 10. So 6x means it was diluted 1 to 10 six times. That is, that 1 part of the original substance is diluted into 10 parts of the diluting substance, usually water. C is the Roman numeral for 100. [If it says 30c,] that means it was diluted 1 to 100 thirty times. Thus, the C potencies are a little more dilute because they're diluted 1 to 100. But both of these potencies are widely sold and widely effective, and generally we recommend that people who are not professionals in homeopathy should not use medicines higher than the thirtieth potency. The sixth potency, the twelfth, and the thirtieth are quite fine, quite effective. But even though the two hundredth and the thousandth are even more effective, you have to be highly knowledgeable about these remedies because the higher the potency used, the more precise the prescription must be.

"Another choice is not just the use of single remedies but various combination homeopathic remedies or formulas. These are mixtures of homeopathic medicines, usually two to eight of the most common remedies for a specific ailment, such as arthritic pain, back pain, PMS, allergies, sinusitis, and headaches. You see these in health food stores and pharmacies these days. Although these are not part of what would be called classical homeopathy and although they are not as precise as prescriptions, they are a user-friendly and quite effective means of providing help and relief to people, akin to using a single remedy for acute care.

"These formulas do not provide constitutional treatment. They do not really cure a person of their underlying problem. But they do provide wonderful relief. I do recommend that people consider using formulas when they cannot find the single remedy that they need or do not know how to find that remedy. Or they may know how to find the remedy but it is not immediately available, as is often the problem.

"There is a place for both single-remedy homeopathy, professional homeopathy, and formula homeopathy. In fact, in speaking of formula homeopathy, in terms of some injuries and trauma, I personally believe that people will experience—and I have observed this myself—even more rapid relief of an injury from using a formula of some sort. Because when you have an injury, you often need to give the person Arnica [wolfsbane]. But at some other point, you need to give the person another remedy for the specific ailment. If it's a nerve injury, you give Hypericum [St. John's wort]; if it's a connective tissue injury, you might give Rhus tox or Ruta [*Ruta graveolens*]. The bottom line here is that eventually anyone involved in homeopathy will need to give several remedies to the person. And I say, well, why not give several remedies together? A colleague of mine is a homeopath and a podiatrist. Every other day or so he conducts surgery on patients with various types of foot disorders, and he always gives a combination of homeopathic remedies, and he has systematically observed that people heal better from a combination rather than just a single medicine given sequentially. I do want to acknowledge that there is some controversy over these formulas, but as far as I'm concerned, the controversy should be null and void."

Dr. Laurie Aesoph's Six-Step Nutritional Approach

Dr. Laurie Aesoph is a naturopathic physician as well as a medical writer. She has authored more than two hundred articles on topics ranging from nutrition to herbs and homeopathy.

Dr. Aesoph describes her views on the relationship between food and arthritis prevention and treatment:

RESTORATIVE FOODS

"Many, many studies tell us that what I call restorative foods, which merely are the good foods we should be eating anyway, [such as] whole grains, fruits, and vegetables, are what we need to insert into our diet. The studies show not only that good diets help out with arthritis but that specific types of food seem to have healing qualities. For example, the oils from different fish have an anti-inflammatory and pain-relieving benefit for arthritis patients. Many fruits, vegetables, and even spices double as herbs. You can use those specifically for different arthritis symptoms.

"In an article printed in *The Lancet,* a British medical journal, in 1991, researchers put their patients on a cleansing diet. But eventually what they did is switch them over to a lacto-ovo-vegetarian diet in different stages, and they had a group that was their control, their placebo, that just ate as normal. They found that even on the lacto-ovo, where people are eating vegetarian diets but also eating eggs and dairy, the benefits continued throughout that year and at the end of the year. So here's evidence where we know that diet is helping.

"Even the Arthritis Foundation is admitting this. There are enough studies that they are taking notice. They have always said that of course, if you're overweight, there is stress on the joints, so if you have something like osteoarthritis or what we call degenerative joint disease, that's going to aggravate and wear out your joints. But they are also looking at studies involving food allergies and cleansing and fish oil, and of course the purines are involved with gout. And diet has always been a large part of treating gout."

STRESSOR FOODS

Dr. Aesoph asserts that it is equally important to minimize what she calls stressor foods from the diet: "Basically, the stressor foods are what set the stage for joint degeneration and breakdown to occur. And just to give you an example of what these foods are, look at the fat category. I want to remind [people] that fats per se are not bad. In fact they're essential, and there's something called essential fatty acids that we need to have—the fish oils fit into that category. But the trans-fatty acids—hydrogenated vegetable oils, for example, and margarine—[contain] too much saturated fat. Those are the sorts of things that are stressor foods and that we should be avoiding. Alcohol doesn't do us any good, nor does caffeine. Refined carbohydrates, such as sugars, flour, white rice, the different sweeteners, the artificial sweeteners such as aspartame and saccharine, processed foods, of course, and the additives and chemicals that are added to our foods are other things that we should also be avoiding.

"When you eat stressor foods, a lot of them really deplete the different nutrients: vitamins, minerals, and all the other phytochemicals and nutrients that we're discovering are in our foods. These, of course, are essential for general body function. Now, arthritis isn't just restricted to the joints. We've discovered that there is a link between the joints and different body systems, and so the immune system is involved. Rheumatoid arthritis is actually what we call an autoimmune disease, where the immune or defense system of your body is attacking yourself. So if you don't have the vitamins and minerals, your immune system isn't going to function as well as it can. Also, with regard to the intestinal tract, it's also vital that it function properly for all sorts of different conditions. When that isn't functioning right, it will aggravate an arthritic condition. I mentioned that if you are overweight, that will stress the joints. If you tend to eat stressor-type foods, that tends to play into or add to conditions of obesity. Also, we talk about stress in our lives, and I really believe that foods that are not complete in nutrition and aren't as whole as they should be are a stress on the body. So that doesn't help your body function any better.

"Also, if you are eating a lot of cooked or processed foods, they tend to be lower in the enzymes that help us digest our foods. There have been numerous studies done where when people eat a diet that is largely composed of cooked foods, their digestive systems, the pancreas, different organs that contribute digestive enzymes to the gut, have to work a little harder, which makes it harder to digest, and then that adds to your gut being a little thicker than it should be, and then that aggravates the arthritis down the road. So, you can see that there are direct and indirect effects that these stressor foods have.

"When you use natural medicine and conventional medicine, it doesn't need to be an either-or situation. You can also use nutrition to cut back on the medication that you're using. You can think of it as a compromise and perhaps gradually get away from the drugs. Also, if you happen to be on steroids, [such as] prednisone, if you plan to cut back and use nutrition, you need to work with your doctor on that. That's something you don't want to cut out cold turkey. The nonsteroidal anti-inflammatory drugs are not as much of a problem. But when going off any prescription drug or steroids, talk to your doctor first."

THE PROGRAM

Dr. Aesoph outlines her nutritional program:
1. Cut out all the stressor foods. You want to eliminate anything that is harming your body or undermining your body's functions and really setting the stage for joint problems to develop. These foods not only weaken the joints but impinge on their ability to repair themselves as well. These are also the foods that add to excess weight, which can overburden the joints. Some of these foods are also high in purines, which tend to aggravate gout.

2. Cleanse the body with a real whole-foods diet and start to add the restorative foods. This helps repair the gastrointestinal tract, which is an imperative part of healing arthritis. At this point you should be starting to learn how to incorporate healthy eating habits and what foods to choose.

3. Test for and then begin to cut out allergy foods.

4. Rebuild damaged joints and overall health by refining your choice of restorative foods. Sea cucumber at 1,000 milligrams may help, as can manganese at 25 milligrams and the bioflavonoid complex. Glucosamine sulfate

and chondroitin sulfate, both at 500 milligrams, can also produce phenomenal results. Flax at 1,000 milligrams from the omega-3 fatty acid group reestablishes normal fluid and osmotic pressure, the synovial fluid in those joints. Taking an alpha lipoic acid, the best all-around intracellular antioxidant, actually fights free radical damage inside the cell. Then you have a very powerful healing mechanism to get your joints circulating nutrients and oxygen and expelling carbon dioxide and waste products as they should. There are many supplements: minerals, vitamins, and herbs. Other ones that you can add are ginger, cumin, and cayenne. Cayenne cream can be rubbed on arthritic joints because it depletes substance p, which in turn decreases pain.

5. Decrease weight, if that's a problem, because it is a stress on the joints.

6. Eliminate any stress by learning to eat properly, such as by chewing your food properly and eating in a relaxed way.

Dr. David Steenblock: Arthritis and Atherosclerosis

Because of the susceptibility of the joints to the accumulation of toxic material that can scratch and irritate the inner linings, leading to the pain and inflammation that characterize arthritis, an analogy has been made between arthritis and atherosclerosis (degeneration of the arteries). In both diseases corrosive substances scratch the inner linings of the body part involved, causing irritation that can lead to degeneration. These substances can come from toxic material in the bowel that gets into the bloodstream. They can also come from food. In the case of atherosclerosis, these foods include cholesterol, fats, and fried foods, which, when they get into the blood, scratch and irritate the very sensitive inner linings of the blood vessels. The same substances can also pass from the blood into the joint space and irritate the inner linings of the joints.

According to Dr. David Steenblock, this correlation between arthritis and atherosclerosis is one of the reasons why a low-fat, low-cholesterol, high-fiber diet has been useful in treating arthritis. "Many patients on this type of diet," he says, "show substantial improvement because the fiber cleanses the colon and removes many of the toxic bacterial waste products, which frees up the blood system and makes it more pure. This in turn allows the toxic materials to be eliminated from the joints, and so the joints themselves can begin to heal."

HIGH-FIBER DIET

Dr. Steenblock also explains how a diet that eliminates processed foods and focuses on the consumption of high-fiber natural grains, fruits, and vegetables works specifically in the treatment of arthritis:

"We want to eliminate white sugar and white flour products and processed foods and foods which contain food additives because these processed foods cause abnormalities in the state of health of the intestine. When you eat processed foods with little fiber, the bacterial content of the colon changes from the so-called good bacteria, which are *Lactobacillus bifidus* and *L. acidophilus,* to organisms that are anaerobic such as anerococci and streptococci and organisms that generally are not healthy and produce many toxic substances themselves. When these toxic substances are present as a result of eating a diet high in refined food and lacking fiber, these toxins pass through the bowel into the blood. Also, refined foods, because they are so easily digestible and do not require work by the intestine, cause the muscle wall of the intestine to atrophy, or become thinner. This thinness of the wall allows more toxic material to pass through the bowel into the blood. Once it is in the blood, it can pass easily into the joints and cause more problems.

"The use of the high-fiber natural diet counteracts this trend because the fiber changes the bacterial content of the colon back to normal, and this eliminates many of the toxic materials, the carcinogens, and the mutagens that are formed otherwise, which are well-documented causes not only of osteoarthritis but also of cancer of the colon and atherosclerosis. The fiber also strengthens the bowel wall, making it thicker and healthier, and this creates more of a mucosal barrier between the colon's interior and the blood. Thus the diet should be more of a natural- and raw-foods diet if you want to get a good result."

Dr. Steenblock does warn, however, that people who have spent an entire lifetime eating refined, fiberless foods must approach a change to a raw, high-fiber diet with caution (excess dietary fiber can, for instance, cause calcium and zinc to be washed through the system so that calcium and zinc deficiencies result) in order to give their intestinal tract time to strengthen. A good physician with a solid background in nutritional therapy should be consulted before any drastic dietary changes are made.

CHELATION THERAPY

While atherosclerosis and arthritis often exacerbate each other, treatments other than diet that are directed at one condition often are beneficial in treating the other. For example, Dr. Steenblock discusses how chelation therapy, an intravenous chemical treatment commonly used for atherosclerosis and heart disease, can also benefit arthritic patients:

"One of the problems with osteoarthritis is that the capillaries of the synovium have become rigidified, or more rigid than they should be, as a consequence of the aging process and of atherosclerosis. This limits the blood flow through these joints; therefore, the heat that is produced when the joint is put in motion cannot be taken away because the circulation is poor. As a result, pain occurs when you exercise, and conversely, when you are resting, the blood flow through that tissue is poor and toxic materials accumulate and can cause pain. Anything that increases the diameter and the blood flow through these capillaries will aid in the restoration process. This is where chelation therapy is very valuable because it actually gets into these small blood vessels and capillaries and removes the cross-linkage of the collagen and elastin. This makes these small blood vessels more pliable and elastic, gives them more diameter so that more blood can pass through them, and thus helps in the healing process."

CHONDROITIN SULFATE

Dr. Steenblock also uses chondroitin sulfate as part of his treatment. Over the past decade, chondroitin sulfate has been used in both Europe and Japan for the treatment of osteoarthritis, rheumatoid arthritis, and atherosclerosis. "Again," he says, "there is a great similarity between osteoarthritis and atherosclerosis in the sense that both result from the wear and tear caused by irritative substances in the body. We need to protect these collagen surfaces from the irritative substances that circulate in the blood and ultimately get into the joint.

"Chondroitin sulfate appears to be one of the best treatments for both arthritis and vascular disease. When you take it orally, it actually enters into the body through the intestinal tract and will selectively go to the joints and all the areas of damage in the blood vessels. It not only acts preventively but also will help reverse the diseases that are present."

Dr. Steenblock says that while chondroitin is a promising treatment, it is not a miracle cure. "The treatment is not the sort of miracle-drug type of treatment where you give the person one pill and get immediate results. What we are dealing with is a natural substance, and it takes time for these natural substances to create the result we are looking for, namely, healing of the injured areas." He says that it may take from two to four months to see results.

Dr. Steenblock adds, "There is another substance, which is derived from the New Zealand green lip mussel. There are a number of trade names for it. This substance is also a mucopolysaccharide, and it is effective in treating osteoarthritis as well as rheumatoid arthritis. It is available in most health food stores.

"These mucopolysaccharides can also be used preventively to heal the small nicks and irritations that occur routinely in the blood vessels and joints. They immediately seal these little cracks and crevices so that they do not get larger. Our bodies are not really capable of doing that on their own, and we need to help them along."

CHAPTER 5

BIRTH
CONTROL

I n the United States today, few subjects are more volatile or politicized than birth control. My goal in this chapter is not to join the debate but to make sure that the information already available to some in the alternative health community is available to everyone.

No currently available form of birth control is 100 percent effective and risk-free, and no single method is right for everyone. A woman's fertility is a highly personal matter, so the more you are able to feel in sync with your menstrual cycle and fertility, the better able you will be to make the right decisions about birth control for you and your partner.

FERTILITY AWARENESS

Fertility awareness, which is also called natural family planning, the Billings method (named after John and Evelyn Billings, two Australian researchers who helped popularize it), and mucus observation, among other names, is an underrated but extremely effective method of pregnancy prevention. This is not the old rhythm method promoted by the Catholic Church in the past, which was notoriously ineffective; each woman has her own "rhythm" that may change from time to time and may not fit into an established pattern.

Actually, fertility awareness can be characterized not as a method of birth control but as a way of life. That is, if you have a more accurate understanding of the dynamic physiological changes that occur during your menstrual cycles, you will be more aware of exactly when you are likely to get pregnant and will be better able to take preventive measures or, if you are trying to become pregnant, enhance your chances.

Some years ago researchers at Princeton University reanalyzed a mountain of data that had been collected by the World Health Organization (WHO) on couples who used fertility awareness. They found that this method was 97 percent effective in preventing pregnancy for those who understood its principles and used it as their sole method of contraception. This research puts to rest the widely held myth that fertility awareness isn't very effective.

Two myths that prevent many people from using fertility awareness as their main method of birth control are that it is difficult to learn and that women have to take their temperature every day and laboriously chart their menstrual cycles for the rest of their lives. This is definitely not the case. You can learn the basic principles of fertility awareness over a few months, and by knowing what to look for, you can learn to identify your fertile period intuitively with a high degree of accuracy without having to deal with charts and thermometers on a daily basis.

Essentially, a number of specific bodily changes signal the onset of a woman's fertile time. These include changes in cervical mucus, body temperature, sexual desire, and an ovulatory pain called mittelschmerz (middle pain).

Getting pregnant requires three factors: sperm, alkaline fertile mucus to nurture and transport the sperm, and a ripe egg in one of the fallopian tubes. The menstrual cycle begins on the first day of menstrual bleeding, and the average cycle lasts twenty-seven to thirty days, although cycles as short as twenty-one days or as long as three to nine months are common. A viscous, "stretchy" mucous secretion manufactured in the glands of the cervical canal begins to ooze from the cervical opening at about Day 10 of the average cycle and increases daily, peaking at Days 14 to 16. Using a plastic speculum, you can actually see the clear mucus, which looks a lot like egg white, oozing from the cervical opening.

As production increases, the stretchy mucus seeps from the vagina and makes a sort of crusty secretion on your underpants or can be picked up by toilet paper.

At the same time that fertile mucus is beginning to develop, a ripe egg pops through the side of one of your ovaries and begins its trip of three to five days down the egg tube. As you approach ovulation, your temperature rises gradually and then, in most women, drops sharply on the day of actual ovulation. If fertile mucus is present and you have unprotected intercourse, the sperm slip easily along the liquid highway of mucus into the cervical canal, where they are kept alive for several days to regroup, as it were, and swim up through the uterus in search of an unfertilized egg.

The idea in using fertility awareness for contraception is to avoid having any sperm in the vagina at times when fertile mucus might be present. By carefully looking for the signs of ovulation (fertile mucus, a drop in temperature, mittelschmerz), you can identify pretty specifically when that time is. The first part of the cycle (including menstruation) is considered the "unsafe" time because fertile mucus can appear early or at low levels, but any fertile mucus presents the possibility of pregnancy. Couples who use fertility awareness as a form of birth control avoid penis-in-vagina sex at this time but may enjoy other forms of sexual activity. Others use a barrier method of contraception until they are sure that ovulation has occurred. After ovulation, however, another egg will not appear, so this is considered the "safe" time. After that time, according to researchers, it is perfectly safe to have vaginal intercourse without getting pregnant.

You can learn the tenets of fertility awareness from a number of excellent books, but many women and their partners find that taking a workshop with several sessions is the easiest and best way to learn. There are now a wide array of fertility detection devices that can be fun to use and are quite accurate.

METHODS OF BIRTH CONTROL

The Male Condom

Condoms, which are latex rubber sheaths that unroll to cover the penis, are 90 to 98 percent effective in preventing pregnancy and provide the best protection from sexually transmitted diseases (STDs). The effectiveness of condoms can be raised to nearly 100 percent by combining them with the cervical cap, diaphragm, vaginal contraceptive film (VCF), or fertility awareness. Many people—both men and women—are reluctant to use condoms because direct skin-to-skin contact feels better. However, that thin rubber membrane may be all that stands between you and pregnancy or a variety of annoying or serious diseases. If you think of the entire body as being available for sexual stimulation, maybe covering up 1 percent of it isn't all that bad. Some people also worry that condoms cut down on sexual sensations and make it more difficult for a man to achieve orgasm. From a woman's perspective, many men ejaculate too readily anyway, so delaying the man's orgasm may be an advantage.

Condoms are often thought of as a "male-controlled" method, but actually, the effective use of condoms requires the interest and willingness of both partners. Today both men and women buy condoms and keep them in their backpacks or at the bedside for ready use. Because of low cost and wide availability, condoms are the most commonly used barrier method in the world. Condoms come in a variety of styles, in different sizes, and with various aesthetic embellishments, with or without lubricants and/or spermicide.

To be effective, condoms must be used correctly. They should be unrolled along the shaft of the penis with a little space left at the tip to collect the ejaculate. Condoms may be lubricated or can be used with a variety of water-based lubricants (read the label), but they should not be used with petroleum-based lubricants such as Vaseline. When the penis is withdrawn after ejaculation, you or your partner should carefully hold the condom in place to ensure that no sperm are spilled into the vagina. For pregnancy protection, condoms should be used for all vaginal insertions. (For STD protection, you may want to use them in other types of sex play as well, such as anal insertions.)

Because of rumors about a high breakage rate, many people believe that condoms are not all that effective. To counter those fears, the U.S. Food and Drug Administration (FDA) has instituted more rigorous standards of testing, so breakage rarely occurs. Condoms that are old or have been exposed to heat are more likely to break. If you are worried about breakage, use two condoms at a time. Also, try to buy them in small quantities and at places where turnover is high, such as large discount drug stores. If a break occurs and you are aware of it, insert spermicidal cream or jelly into the vagina as soon as possible.

If you have a variety of sexual partners and vaginal or anal intercourse is a part of your sexual activities, you should consider using condoms at each and every sexual session.

The Female Condom

The female condom somewhat resembles the standard male condom and can be bought over the counter. It is more expensive than a male condom. It is a soft tube that is made of polyurethane, which is stronger and thinner than latex. It is inserted into the vagina like a lining. It has two rings. One is fitted around the cervix like a diaphragm, and the other remains outside the body and covers the labia. According to an article on the HealthWorld online website (www.healthy.net), the female condom has a failure rate of 5 percent when used under ideal conditions, but the average failure rate (since it is not always used in the most careful way) is 25 percent.

The female condom is said to provide effective protection against STDs, including AIDS, especially when it is used together with a male condom. It takes some learning to use properly, since it can get twisted if it is not inserted correctly. It may also reduce sexual sensation and the feeling of spontaneity.

The Cervical Cap

According to women's health and sexuality advocate Rebecca Chalker, the existence of the cervical cap is one of the best-kept secrets of modern times. This is an approach to birth control that is as safe and effective as the diaphragm but offers a good measure of spontaneity and the convenience of the Pill.

In Europe there are a handful of cervical cap designs. In the United States, the Prentif cavity-rim cervical cap made by Lamberts Ltd. of London has been approved by the FDA for general use. The Prentif cervical cap looks like a large thimble made of soft latex rubber. As Chalker explains in *The Complete*

Cervical Cap Guide, "a dollop of spermicide is placed in the dome. Then the cap rim is folded in half, tipped into the opening of the vagina, and guided with a finger to the back of the vaginal canal, where it readily slips over the cervix (the neck of the uterus). The cap stays firmly in place by gripping the cervix and forming a strong suction and provides a physical barrier to the sperm, while the spermicide affords an additional chemical barrier.

"Because it is smaller and more compact than the diaphragm, the Prentif has several distinct advantages. There is no large spring rim to press on sensitive vaginal walls, making it far more comfortable than the diaphragm. Thus, it can be left in place for longer than the diaphragm. The FDA recommends keeping the cap on for no more than forty-eight hours, but many women have reported keeping it in for three or four days with no problems. The cap stays snugly on the cervix, requiring no extra applications of spermicidal cream or jelly until it is removed. Consequently, it is not messy. Some women still prefer to use the cap more or less like a diaphragm, inserting it anywhere from a few minutes to a few hours before they anticipate having intercourse and removing it sometime the next day. Others keep it in for longer periods and especially like the convenience of being able to keep it in over the weekend."

Because of the cap's obvious advantages, many practitioners who fit the cervical cap now see it as the first choice among barrier methods and recommend the diaphragm only for those who cannot be fitted with a cap.

"Unlike the diaphragm," Chalker notes, "the cervical cap, with its greater freedom from spermicide applications and other inconveniences, can be associated with a greater enjoyment of sexuality. Of course, there is no perfect available birth control solution, and the cervical cap is no exception to that rule. The most vexing drawback associated with cervical cap use in the United States is that not everyone can be fitted with the four available sizes." According to Chalker, about 80 percent of women can be fitted: "If one of the four sizes fits you just right, then the cervical cap may be an excellent solution. In rare cases the cervical cap may develop an odor when left in place too long. Soaking for twenty minutes in water with 10 percent household bleach usually kills odor-causing bacteria. A well-fitting cap may occasionally dislodge. If you have repeated dislodgments, see your practitioner to reevaluate your fit."

About 200,000 women in the United States and Canada have been fitted with the cervical cap, and more than 2,000 medical practitioners who prescribe them are scattered across North America. Chalker notes that several new cap models are being studied and should be on the market soon.

The Diaphragm

The diaphragm is considered a barrier method of birth control, but the spermicidal cream or jelly used with it is actually what kills the sperm and prevents them from entering the cervix. A diaphragm is a shallow cup made of soft latex rubber with a flexible rim that fits neatly into the palm of your hand. Once very popular, the diaphragm was overtaken in the early 1960 by the heavy promotion and the flood of research dollars behind the Pill. The diaphragm is made in a variety of sizes, ranging from about 2 to 4 inches (50 to 100 millimeters) so that it may be fitted in accordance with the length of the vagina. When it is in place, one part of the rim is lodged behind the pubic bone, while the opposite part cups underneath the cervix in the back of the vagina.

A diaphragm with spermicide can be inserted up to six hours before vagina-penis contact. Between a teaspoonful and a tablespoonful of the spermicide is put into the shallow cup and then spread around, leaving a thin ribbon around the rim. Then, squatting, sitting on the toilet, standing with one foot raised, or lying down with your knees bent, you spread the lips of your vagina and insert the diaphragm into the upper vagina with the spermicide facing up. Then push the lower rim until the diaphragm locks into place. You should be able to feel the outline of your cervix with your finger through the rubber cup of the diaphragm.

The diaphragm should stay in place for at least six hours after intercourse to ensure that most of the sperm are killed. The maximum amount of time the diaphragm should be left in is twenty-four hours. If you have repeated intercourse while the diaphragm is in place, it is necessary to insert more spermicidal jelly or cream into your vagina with an applicator each time, leaving the diaphragm in place.

The standard for fitting the diaphragm is to use the largest size that is comfortable, but what is comfortable in the doctor's office or clinic may not be so comfortable after a few hours. If you are experiencing discomfort from a diaphragm, don't just put it in your drawer. Go back to your practitioner and ask for a smaller size. Then try using the smaller one, checking its placement both before and after intercourse for a month or so. If the diaphragm will not remain in place, you should consider another method.

The New Our Bodies, Ourselves recommends that when your doctor, nurse practitioner, or other women's health care provider fits you for a diaphragm, you want to make sure that you are correctly putting it in and taking it out by practicing before leaving the practitioner's office so that she or he can tell if you are doing it right. Alternatively, you can practice at home and then return to the practitioner's office with the diaphragm in place.

The diaphragm has few health risks. There is effectively no risk of it going farther inside than its correct position; if it pushes back against the rectum, it may be the wrong size. However, in addition to killing sperm, spermicide may kill off the lactobacilli in the vagina that keep yeast under control. To help counteract this, between diaphragm uses you can bathe the vagina with a solution of water and *Lactobacillus acidophilus* (available at most health food stores) by using a douche nozzle, a squirt bottle, or a plastic speculum. If a particular spermicide causes irritation either to your vagina or to your lover's penis, switching to a different brand may help.

About 20 percent of diaphragm users have occasional or recurrent bladder infections. This may occur because the rim bruises the urethra and makes it more susceptible to infection or because the spermicide alters the normal environment of the vagina and allows harmful bacteria to grow. If you are using the diaphragm and begin having recurrent bladder infections, you should look for a different method. If you have a prolapsed or otherwise displaced uterus, vaginal fistulas, or a protrusion of the bladder through the vaginal wall, the diaphragm is not an option for you.

As with other barrier methods, the diaphragm is effective only if you use it consistently and correctly. Studies have shown that the diaphragm is between 89 and 98 percent effective for women who use it during every session of intercourse (except during the menstrual period). However, the effectiveness of the diaphragm can be increased to nearly 100 percent by combining it with condoms or fertility awareness.

Your partner should not be able to feel the diaphragm, but if he does, it is usually only an awareness that something is there. Of course, using the diaphragm in no way compromises your fertility, and all you have to do if you choose to become pregnant is stop using it.

Vaginal Contraceptive Film

Another well-kept contraceptive secret is vaginal contraceptive film (VCF). This square inch of material that looks like plastic but turns into a viscous liquid after five to fifteen minutes in the vagina is 28 percent nonoxynol-9, the sperm-killing ingredient in commercial spermicides. The film was designed to be used alone and seems to be about 85 to 90 percent effective when used that way, but most practitioners recommend that it be used with a cervical cap, diaphragm, or condom. Combining VCF with these barriers should increase their effectiveness to nearly 100 percent.

Some people find the higher dose of nonoxynol-9—about three times as strong as regular spermicide—irritating. If this happens to you, you will probably have to stop using it. The other disadvantage of VCF is that it is somewhat expensive and not widely available in the United States. However, it is less messy than normal spermicidal cream or jelly and provides a stronger dose of spermicide.

The Pill

Birth control pills contain either a combination of synthetic estrogen and progesterone or progesterone only. In the first part of the menstrual cycle, higher-than-normal estrogen levels prevent the release of follicle-stimulating hormone (FSH). The absence of this hormone, which is manufactured in the pituitary gland, prevents an egg from developing inside the ovary. In the second part of the cycle, higher levels of progesterone thicken cervical mucus and inhibit the cyclic buildup of the uterine lining. If an egg were to be released or sperm were to get through the cervical mucus, the uterine lining would be too thin to support an implanted fertilized egg. The combination pills interfere with ovulation, thicken cervical mucus, and interfere with the buildup of the uterine lining. Progesterone-only pills, which are called minipills, only thicken cervical mucus and interfere with the buildup of the uterine lining.

In theory the Pill is an elegant solution to the age-old problem of preventing unwanted pregnancies, and it has some positive aspects. Many women like the Pill because its use can be completely separated from sex and there is no mechanical barrier to be aware of during sexual activity. Because the Pill suppresses the menstrual cycle, its users often experience less painful menstrual cramps, fewer premenstrual syndrome (PMS) symptoms, and a lowered risk of anemia. Women with endometriosis may experience a decrease in pain and other symptoms, and those who have a tendency to develop ovarian cysts are less likely to do so. Studies also show a lower incidence of pelvic inflammatory disease caused by gonorrhea as well as cancer of the uterine lining (endometrial cancer) and ovarian cancer.

However, the Pill, even in its current low-dose formulation, has some significant drawbacks. Higher-than-normal levels of hormones not only have the desired effect of preventing pregnancy but also travel through the bloodstream and affect other organs that have nothing to do with contraception, often precipitating or exacerbating serious underlying conditions. In addition, synthetic hormones can affect mood or exacerbate a tendency toward depression. They may decrease the desire for sex or cause hair loss or fatigue, a bloated feeling, and weight gain over time. Some women don't experience any of these symptoms and enjoy the freedom from contraceptive jellies and devices, but others say that they simply don't feel like themselves.

The Pill also interferes with the way vitamins are absorbed and utilized by the body. Sherrill Sellman, a leading women's health educator and writer, and author of *Hormone Heresy*, explains that the Pill causes major nutritional deficiencies of the B vitamins, vitamins C and E, as well as mineral imbalances. "The B vitamins are necessary to protect a woman's immune system, her fertility, her emotional well-being," she says. "The side effects from deficiency of these vitamins are fatigue, weakness, insomnia, aches and pains, weight loss, depression, irritability, lack of initiative, constipation, oversensitivity to noise, loss of appetite, circulatory problems, skin problems, gum disease, dizziness, depression, eye problems. Folic acid is an essential vitamin to help with the development of a healthy fetus. Women taking the Pill become deficient in folic acid. This compromises not just their own health and immunity, but also the health of their fetuses."

Vitamins C and E are key nutrients for the immune system and the heart. They help detoxify heavy metals out of the body. "These are also seriously depleted in women who take the Pill," Sellman says.

Mineral imbalances are not uncommon. "Copper goes way up and that causes migraine and hair loss and high blood pressure," Sellman explains. "Zinc goes way down, which causes poor resistance to infection, diabetes and infertility problems. The low-destiny lipids, the LDLs, go way up and the triglyceride levels also go up. So we are looking at serious, serious compromising of a woman's health and her ability to function."

One of the biggest problems that women have today with the Pill is fear that it may promote the growth of cancer. Medical studies on this issue are conflicting, but too many studies show an increased cancer risk to dismiss this issue. Some doctors grudgingly acknowledge an increased risk among Pill users in certain subgroups of women, especially women who have a mother or sister who developed cancer.

About ten million women in the United States use the Pill at any one time, but from 30 to 50 percent stop using it within a year because of undesirable side effects.

In the 1960s and 1970s high-dose pills caused serious problems for many women and are known to have caused a small number of deaths as well, but high doses equaled high effectiveness. The Pill got a reputation for being 98 percent effective. Today most women take the progesterone-only minipill, which is only about 96 percent effective in normal use. This is still quite acceptable in terms of effectiveness, but it's not really much better than condoms, the cervical cap, or the diaphragm when those barrier methods are used consistently. Failures with minipills occur when women forget to take them or decide not to take them because they cease to be sexually active for a time. You can't just take one pill and be protected; it takes several weeks for the hormones to build up in your system.

Other failures occur because of normal fluctuations in women's hormone levels. You must take the minipill at the same time each day to get maximum protection. If you miss a day or two, double up on pills for at least two days. If you miss more than two days, you need to use another method, such as condoms or VCF.

There are numerous caveats you need to be aware of if you take birth control pills. You absolutely should not take the Pill if you have heart disease, severe varicose veins, serious circulatory problems, liver disease, or breast cancer. You should seriously consider using another method if you have diabetes, hypertension, gallbladder disease, depression, epilepsy, migraines, irregular periods, or sickle cell anemia—the trait or the disease. A woman with these conditions may take the minipill safely but should do so only after a consultation with her doctor. You should stop taking the Pill if you are planning surgery or must have your leg in a cast. The Pill may interfere with the absorption of certain vitamins—including vitamins B1, B2, B6, B12, C, and E and folic acid—and may alter carbohydrate metabolism. If you smoke, the Pill becomes far more risky for you.

Contraceptive Technology, a leading family-planning handbook, has devised an easily remembered acronym, ACHES, to help make you aware of the danger signs of the Pill:

A—abdominal pain (severe)
C—chest pain (severe), cough, shortness of breath
H—headache (severe), dizziness, weakness, numbness
E—eye problems (vision loss or blurring), speech problems
S—severe leg pain (calf or thigh)

If you experience any of these signs, call your doctor immediately.

In an article in the magazine *Alternative Medicine,* Dr. Jesse Hanley reminds women that being in touch with the natural monthly cycle of hormones supports their intuition and creativity, yet women's lives today make it difficult for them to fully live out their female biological cycle. Taking birth control pills regulates their cycle to the point where they hardly notice that they're having a period. As Dr. Hanley puts it, "Many women become almost addicted to not being a woman, to not understanding the natural cycling of hormones and the feelings, increased sensitivity, intuition, and creativity this evokes." She sees this as a self-destructive tendency that will create health problems in the future. "Chinese medicine describes the uterus as the place where a woman's energy and essence reside, so we need to rethink our approach to uterine health," Dr. Hanley concludes.

Norplant

Norplant is a contraceptive that comes in the form of six silicone capsules about the size of matches that are implanted under the skin of the upper arm. The capsule releases a form of the hormone progestin (synthetic progesterone) that blocks ovulation and remains effective for as long as five years.

Dr. Hanley has noticed that the synthetic progesterone in Norplant interferes with women's hormonal balance and makes them upset and miserable: "Some patients tell me that using this form of contraception makes them feel as if a black cloud has settled over them." She adds that Norplant, like other synthetic progesterones, can cause irregular bleeding, weight gain, water retention, and depression. It disrupts thyroid function and has been linked to a greater risk of blood clots and cardiovascular disease.

In fact, about two hundred lawsuits involving more than fifty thousand women have been filed against the manufacturer of Norplant, Wyeth-Ayerst Laboratories.

Sterilization

Many people are surprised to learn that surgical sterilization—tying, clipping, or cutting the fallopian tubes in women or cutting the vas deferens in men—is the most widely used form of contraception both in the United States and in the rest of the world. About fifteen million women and men use this method.

Although it involves surgically altering parts of the body through snips and sutures, sterilization is the ultimate in "hands-off" birth control. Once the snips have healed, you never have to think about birth control again—unless, that is, you want to have a baby. Reversal rates for surgical sterilization are around 25 percent, depending on the type of procedure. This is a relatively low rate of success, and studies have found that regret is not uncommon among women and men who have had this procedure. Moreover, the surgery, which is not normally covered by insurance, may cost fifteen thousand dollars or more. Once again, no available form of birth control is without its drawbacks.

In women the surgery is most often done through a small incision below the navel. The abdominal cavity is inflated with carbon or nitrous oxide, and a laparoscope is inserted through the incision to allow the surgeon to see and manipulate the egg tubes with various instruments. This surgery is usually done on an outpatient basis, and a light general anesthesia or spinal block is commonly used. Most women have some abdominal discomfort for one to three days and feel fully recovered within a week.

CHAPTER 6

BREAST CANCER AND OTHER BREAST DISEASES

I n the summer of 2001 there was some good news on the cancer front: Death rates for eight of the top ten cancers in the United States were steady or down. The overall incidence of cancer also dropped, but unfortunately only for men. Among women, breast cancer rates have increased 40 percent since the 1970s, from 83 per 100,000 then to 118 per 100,000 today. Breast cancer remains the most frequently occurring cancer in women. Yet even the current "gold standard" conventional treatment for preventing breast cancer —the drug tamoxifen—is basically flawed.

CAUSES

Dr. Michael Schachter, a complementary physician from New York, describes some of the key factors in the development of the disease.

Estrogen

"Women whose menstrual periods start when they are relatively young have an increased risk for developing breast cancer, as do women who have a late menopause," explains Dr. Schachter. "This suggests that a woman who has a longer exposure to female sex hormones during her lifetime is at greater risk for developing breast cancer and that estrogen, the female sex hormone that stimulates cell growth, may play a role in its formation. Women who have no children and women who have children but do not breast-feed also have an increased risk. This suggests that the other female sex hormone, progesterone, may have a protective effect.

"Other known and accepted risk factors include an increased alcohol intake, a diet high in fat, being overweight, and a family history of breast cancer. This is because fat tissue can make estrogen and alcohol tends to stimulate its production. In summary, most risk factors seem to be associated with increased lifetime exposure to estrogen, decreased lifetime exposure to progesterone, or a combination of the two.

"Estrogen and progesterone tend to balance each other in the body. Excessive estrogen or reduced progesterone may lead to a condition known as estrogen dominance. The symptoms of estrogen dominance include water retention, breast swelling, fibrocystic breasts, premenstrual mood swings and depression, loss of sex drive, heavy or irregular periods, uterine fibroids, craving for sweets, and fat deposition in the hips and thighs.

"Estrogen tends to be transformed into two major metabolites in the body. They can be called the good and the bad estrogen, just as there are the so-called good and bad cholesterol. The bad estrogen, known as 16-alphahydroxyestrone, favors the development of breast cancer, whereas 2-hydroxyestrone seems to protect against it. Certain chemicals stimulate the formation of one or the other."

Xenoestrogens

"Now that we've seen that the role of estrogen is very important," Dr. Schachter continues, "this leads to a discussion of something called xenoestrogens. *Xeno* means 'foreign,' and xenoestrogens are chemical substances that are foreign to the body but behave like estrogens. These substances mimic estrogen's actions. Some xenoestrogens can reduce estrogen's effects. These varieties, which are rapidly degraded in the body, usually occur in plant foods such as soy, cauliflower, and broccoli. They protect against the development of breast cancer. Other xenoestrogens, typically synthetic ones, appear to stimulate cancer growth.

"We are living in the petrochemical era," Dr. Schachter says. Over the past sixty years, the amount of synthetic chemicals produced annually has jumped from 1 billion pounds to well over 500 billion. "Many of these compounds are toxic, mutagenic, and carcinogenic," he warns, adding, " the majority have not been adequately tested for toxicity, let alone for their environmental and ecological effects.

"Approximately six hundred chemicals have been shown to be carcinogenic in well-designed, controlled, and validated animal experiments. And within the scientific community the overwhelming consensus is that chemicals carcinogenic to animals are also carcinogenic to humans. In large-scale epidemiological human studies, approximately twenty-five chemicals have been proved to be carcinogenic. For each of these twenty-five chemicals, animal research established carcinogenicity one to three decades earlier, making the animal studies all the more significant.

"Many synthetic chemicals behave as bad xenoestrogens, particularly pesticides, fuels, and plastics. They do so in various ways. Some enhance the production of the so-called bad estrogens that I mentioned earlier, and others bind to estrogen receptors, inducing them to issue unneeded signals to increase cellular growth. Xenoestrogens may enter the body through animal fat, since they tend to accumulate in fatty tissue and tend to concentrate as you go up in the food chain.

"Xenoestrogens tend to be synergistic so that a mixture of tiny amounts of many chemicals may have dire effects."

Poor Lymphatic Drainage

Another possible cause of breast cancer is poor lymphatic drainage, which may be caused by constrictions such as those caused by wearing a bra. Dr. Sidney Ross Singer, a medical anthropologist who did graduate work at Duke University, specializing in biochemistry, has championed this point in his book *Dressed to Kill: The Link between Bras and Breast Cancer.* Dr. Singer explains: "The lymphatic system is so underemphasized by modern medicine. When I was in medical school, there was not even ten minutes' discussion of it. Yet it is a critical part of the body."

It's the circulatory part of the immune system. It consists of tiny vessels, like capillaries, microscopic in size and originating in all the tissues of the body. They drain the tissue of fluid, toxins, debris, cancer cells, bacteria, and so forth. The blood flowing through the blood vessels delivers oxygen and nutrition through capillaries under pressure. The fluid in the blood oozes out to bathe the tissues. This fluid is called lymph fluid. It is the medium of exchange through which nutrients are delivered to the cells.

As the cells take in oxygen and food and give off their waste, some of the cell debris is flushed out through this other channel, the lymphatic system. For the breast, most of the lymph nodes are located in the armpits. These nodes are tiny factories for white blood cell production in response to infection. They filter out the lymph fluid, which then goes back to the bloodstream and through the heart.

This pattern of flow is how the body works normally, Dr. Singer says. However, "when you wear a constrictive garment, the pressure of the garment, such as the elastic of a bra, presses on these tiny vessels, shutting them off and preventing them from draining. They have no internal pressure; they are passive drains. They are not like the blood capillaries, which are under pressure from the heart. As soon as they are constricted because the bra lifts the breasts and gives them a different shape—which requires pressure—there is a backup of fluid in the breast, which is a condition called lymphedema, or edema for short." This pressure and backup can cause pain and tenderness in the breasts.

Before a woman has her period, her estrogen level is very high, and this causes generalized body fluid retention. This is what premenstrual syndrome is all about, a generalized, all-over-the-body edema. That goes away after the hormones drop and the woman starts having her period. But during that time of elevated fluids she has typically been wearing the same size bra she wore all month, yet her breasts have been a little bigger. As a result of the constriction from the bra, which has become like a tourniquet, the breast cannot drain the fluid, and it backs up, causing congestion in the breast tissue.

The end result, Dr. Singer explains, is that "the cells are sitting in their own waste and debris. The pressure builds, there's tenderness, and cysts form. That's why women get cysts in their breasts. These cysts, which are filled with lymph fluid, eventually become hard. This condition is called fibrocystic breast disease. Eighty percent of American women have it, and it's because of the bra."

X Rays

Dr. John Gofman, professor emeritus of molecular and cell biology at the University of California, Berkeley, sounds the alarm on the harmful effects of X rays in his book *Preventing Breast Cancer.*

The effects of X rays take years, even decades, to manifest, which is why orthodox medicine does not pay attention to this danger. Indeed, X rays are standard practice for medical diagnosis and treatment. "The incubation time is what has led organized medicine exactly in the wrong direction," says Dr. Gofman.

"In the first half of the twentieth century medicine looked at treatments in this way: If you gave someone poison, the effects would be seen in weeks or months. They did not think in terms of years or decades. What we have learned about X ray–induced cancer is that a very small proportion occurs in the first few years after the X rays are administered. But most of them take ten, twenty, even fifty years. Women with breast cancer who are forty-five, fifty, or sixty are thinking, 'Why me? I haven't done anything wrong.' What these women are not thinking about is what they were exposed to early in life."

It is not the radiation itself that persists but chromosomal damage, Dr. Gofman says. "Inside the nucleus of every one of our cells is a string of DNA organized into forty-six chromosomes. That's a treasure. Damage to your chromosomes is going to be there for the rest of your life.

"A couple of years ago, I tried to answer this question—not whether X rays cause breast cancer but what part of all breast cancers are being caused by X rays? My estimate was about 75 percent. Everybody said, 'Oh, that's too high. It must be much lower.' Since that time I've done much more extensive work, and I have changed my numbers from 75 percent to more than 90 percent. Moreover, I now have enough data on a variety of other cancers to say that most cancers, not just breast cancer, are caused by medical X rays."

Whether Dr. Gofman is 100 percent right or just partly right, whether medical X rays are a primary cause of breast cancer and other types of cancer or merely an important secondary factor that until now has been ignored by our government and the medical establishment—in either case women need to recognize the seriousness of the problem and insist that radiation exposures be as minimal as possible.

Diet

Earlier, Dr. Schachter gave one explanation of how fat can cause breast cancer. Here Dr. Charles Simone, director of the Protective Cancer Institute in Lawrenceville, New Jersey, gives another reason why fats generate disease: "We know that fatty foods actually convert normal cells into problematic cells. Consuming high-fat foods, particularly unsaturated fats, increases free radical production, damaging the cell membrane. At this point the damaged cell has two choices. It can die. That's fine, because if it dies, you make another one. Or it can repair itself. In the repair process, a cell can go awry and metamorphose into a cancer cell. So fats cause free radicals, which damage cells, which in turn try to repair themselves and transform themselves into cancer cells."

Robin Keuneke, a natural food counselor and the author of *Total Breast Health,* points to another factor: essential fatty acid deficiencies. These fatty acids are found, for example, in extra-virgin olive oil. Many studies have linked Italian diets, which contain lots of extra-virgin olive oil, to lower rates of breast cancer. Italian women do not have a low-fat diet, but neither do they have trans-fats in their diets. (Trans-fats are unstable, highly reactive molecules that promote free radical oxidation and therefore can have mutagenic effects. They are found in margarine and other processed oils, shortenings, and confections such as cookies and candy.) A study of the relation of trans-fats and breast cancer in 1997 found that women with breast cancer have higher amounts of trans-fats in their body fats compared with women without the disease.

Other diet choices that seem connected to higher rates of cancer are cooked meat and fried foods. Keuneke notes, "One of the theses of my book is that burned meat and fried foods are linked to breast cancer. I found four studies linking burned meat, such as bacon, to cancer. Yet the so-called experts said there was not enough information to recommend changes in cooking."

This is not true. The first study was published in 1972. It was a population study looking at Seventh-Day Adventist women, who have a relatively clean diet. It found that women who ate the greatest amount of fried potatoes had the highest rate of breast cancer.

Hot, spicy foods, oily foods, and stimulants such as coffee, black tea, drugs, and alcohol should also be avoided. Water should be pure, free from fluoride, chlorine, pesticides, and other synthetic chemicals.

Tobacco and Alcohol

Dr. Simone cites two other factors as leading contributors: "We know that tobacco is the number-two cause of cancer in our country and the number-two cause of breast cancer as well. Regarding alcohol, we know that two to three drinks per week is enough to confer a twofold to threefold risk of getting cancer of the breast independently of everything else. So the number-one, -two, and -three causes of breast cancer—a high-fat diet, smoking, and alcohol consumption—are totally within our control."

SYMPTOMS

The initial symptoms of breast cancer include thickening, a lump in the breast, and dimpled skin. Later on there may be nipple discharge, pain, ulcers, and swollen lymph glands under the arms.

Once breast cancer is diagnosed, the prognosis depends on the course of the disease. Dr. Schachter explains: "The staging of breast cancer involves the size of the cancer in the breast, whether it has spread or metastasized to regional lymph nodes, and whether it has metastasized to distant organs. The more lymph nodes involved and the greater the size of the tumor, the worse the prognosis. Stage zero is limited to the topmost layer, and the five-year survival rate is about 90 percent. In stage four, in which cancer has metastasized to lymph nodes above the collarbone or has distant metastases to organs such as the liver, lungs, and brain, the five-year survival rate drops to 10 percent."

CLINICAL EXPERIENCE

Prevention

While the possibility of a positive diagnosis for breast cancer is terrifying, it is empowering to know that there are steps that can be taken to prevent the condition, that minimally invasive treatments are often beneficial, and that it is possible to avoid a recurrence.

Before we outline the steps you can take to prevent breast cancer, let's look at one step that is highly touted by conventional medicine, but which I would not recommend. This is the use of tamoxifen. We saw earlier that excessive estrogen production is held responsible by some for breast cancer. This is the rationale for prescribing tamoxifen. However, asserts Sherrill Sellman, psychotherapist and author of the best-selling book *Hormone Heresy*, this treatment is far from the panacea it is claimed to be.

THE TAMOXIFEN DEBATE

Tamoxifen has been used for more than twenty years as a treatment to prevent a recurrence of breast cancer. It has been only moderately successful in preventing new tumors, but even this moderate success has come at a cost. While tamoxifen may benefit some women with breast cancer, it is also a highly toxic drug with serious side effects.

Tamoxifen, Sellman explains, "is the leading drug being given to women with breast cancer. Millions of women are on it." Tamoxifen is in a class of drugs collectively known as SERMs, serum estrogen receptor modulators. Although the way these drugs work is not totally understood, it is believed that SERMs block the action of estrogen on the breast tissue, which in turn inhibits the growth of tumors.

So how does tamoxifen prevent breast cancer? Sellman says, "The theory is that it works like a weaker estrogen." Estrogen is a major factor in the growth of breast tumors. Many but not all breast cancers require estrogen to grow. These types of tumors have a site on the cell called an estrogen receptor. Tamoxifen competes with estrogen to reach these receptors, where it creates a barrier that prevents estrogen from binding to the cell.

In theory, then, tamoxifen acts like a phytoestrogen, although it has contradictory effects. In the breast it seems to reduce the effects of estrogen on tumor growth, yet in other parts of the body it acts like one of these estrogens, stimulating growth, for example in the uterus, where it can cause endometrial cancer. "It's unpredictable," Sellman stresses, "in the sense that we don't really know what are going to be the consequences in a woman's body."

HISTORY OF TAMOXIFEN

In the early 1980s American researchers began to speculate about whether tamoxifen might actually prevent breast cancer in women who had never had the disease. So in 1992 the National Cancer Institute initiated a $60 million clinical trial to test tamoxifen as a cancer preventative. Thirteen thousand healthy women who were at higher than average risk for breast cancer were enrolled in the trial. Half the women took tamoxifen (20 milligrams a day); the other half received a placebo.

From the beginning, the Breast Cancer Prevention Trial was controversial. Critics of the trial were outraged that healthy women would be exposed to the health risks associated with tamoxifen.

Results of the trial were made public in April 1998. At first glance, the trial results seem impressive. Women in the trial who took tamoxifen had a 44 percent reduction in breast cancers compared with the placebo group. But these results are misleading; tamoxifen also caused uterine cancer, blood clots, and cataracts. In fact, women who got tamoxifen had almost three times the rate of endometrial cancers and blood clots. Two prominent health groups, the National Women's Health Network and Public Citizen, have calculated that for every thousand women who take tamoxifen, there will be 2.9 fewer cases of breast cancer, but 2.8 more cases of extremely serious health problems. Even more important, results of the trial show there is no difference in overall survival rates or in the number of women who died of breast cancer.

In addition to cancers, blood clots, and cataracts, tamoxifen also caused strokes, hot flashes, vaginal discharge, mood changes, menstrual irregularities, and skin rashes.

In October 1998, the Food and Drug Administration (FDA) approved the use of tamoxifen to reduce the risk of breast cancer in healthy women. But even members of the FDA's own advisory committee voiced concerns about giving tamoxifen to healthy women. One committee member noted that every woman who took tamoxifen was exposed to the health risks, but only a few women would benefit from the drug.

Critics of the FDA say that approval of tamoxifen as an anticancer drug is premature. Two European studies found tamoxifen provided no benefit as a preventive measure. Still other criticism focuses on the statistical model (known as the Gail model) used to assess breast cancer risk for women considering taking tamoxifen as a cancer preventative. Opponents say this model greatly overstates risk, putting large numbers of women into a high-risk category and therefore eligible to take the drug.

HEALTH RISKS

The health risks associated with tamoxifen, some of which are mentioned above, are the same for women who have breast cancer as for those who take it as a treatment to prevent a recurrence. Tamoxifen may also cause liver damage and liver cancer. Animal studies found a link between tamoxifen and liver cancer in rats, but the results of human studies have been less conclusive.

A Swedish study looked at 1,327 breast cancer patients who took 40 milligrams of tamoxifen a day for two to five years. Comparing this group to one of the same size that didn't take the drug, it was found the tamoxifen users upped their chances for getting uterine cancer sixfold.

Strangely enough, many women's groups are supporting and advocating this treatment. Most of the time, however, these are groups that take money from the pharmaceutical industry. But other women's groups have been the primary activists opposing tamoxifen, the lead group being the National

Women's Health Network. And there have been so many false reports and so much misinformation that unless you really investigate the issue thoroughly, you will very seldom get access to truthful data. As Sellman says, "It's very easy to play with results, stats, and studies to make it look like something wonderful is occurring when in fact it is a scam. This drug has the potential to be such a big money spinner. It is already the number-one drug given to women with breast cancer. The industry will stop at nothing to get its drug out there. Health is not their primary concern."

DIET AND LIFESTYLE

Dr. Tori Hudson, a naturopathic physician in Portland, Oregon, says, "I believe that breast cancer is a preventable disease. Just look around the world. Women in our culture have one of the highest—if not the highest—incidences of breast cancer, while women in Asia have the lowest.

"The reason is diet. To make a big story simple to understand, cultures that have a vegetarian diet or are closest to a vegetarian diet have the least breast cancer. That's how it all pans out no matter how you look at it. This implies that cultures that eat less fat, especially less animal fat, have the least breast cancer. So the big picture is really clear. Eat a lot of vegetables, fruits, and whole grains and beans. Those foods provide protection."

Letha Hadady, an herbalist and educator in New York City, visited China to learn why Chinese women have such a low incidence of breast cancer compared with American women and those in other Western nations. While diet was a big part of the picture, she learned that other factors came into play as well. To prevent breast cancer, Asians build immunity through diet, cleansing herbs, and the avoidance of pollution, stress, negative emotions, smoking, alcohol, and radiation: "They have much cleaner habits than we do." In addition, Hadady made this important discovery: "I found it quite interesting that breast cancer is considered a disease of melancholy in China. That feeling of heaviness in the chest leads to poor circulation and excess phlegm. This leads to two conclusions: Increase circulation and you have a better chance of prevention, and reduce phlegm. The easiest way to reduce phlegm is to stay away from foods such as cheese, chocolate, fried foods, and milk. You will not find dairy in the diet in China. Their diet tends to consist of grains and greens."

Certain foods are medicinal in their ability to protect against breast cancer. They include soybeans, soy products, and lima beans. Isoflavones and phytoestrogens found in soybeans, soy products, and lima beans protect against cancer. The low incidence of breast cancer among Japanese women is largely attributed to the widespread eating of soybeans. Other cancer-fighting foods include flax, fish that is high in omega-3 fatty acids (salmon, tuna, sardines, mackerel, and herring), cruciferous vegetables (broccoli, cauliflower, and brussels sprouts), mushrooms (reishi, shiitake, and maitake), and onions.

Many herbs have been shown to help in both preventing and treating the disease. Some of these are listed in the next section.

In his book *Breast Health: A Ten Point Prevention Program,* Dr. Simone outlines the following plan for optimal breast health:

Optimize nutrition
Take antioxidant supplements
Avoid tobacco
Avoid alcohol
Avoid estrogens
Exercise
Minimize stress
Become spiritually involved
Increase your awareness of sexuality
Get a good regular physical examination starting at age thirty-five

Dr. Schachter states that trace minerals play a vital role in the prevention of free radical damage: "The body contains certain antioxidant proteins, such as SOD (superoxide dismutase), which help neutralize oxidatively induced free radicals. SOD requires three minerals—zinc, copper, and manganese—to function properly. Deficiencies of any one of these minerals may predispose to oxidation damage, with a resulting increase of susceptibility to breast cancer.

"Adequate amounts of calcium and magnesium are also important. Considerable evidence exists supporting the role of selenium in preventing and treating cancer. A dose of 200 micrograms daily is safe, and large amounts may be given with monitoring. Chromium and molybdenum may be supplemented as well, and these are also important.

"Recently I have begun to use the whole range of trace minerals in colloidal form as a supplement. That's a liquid form where the minerals are bound to organic chemicals. We use about seventy different minerals. Many of these minerals are in trace amounts, have already been shown to be essential, and are probably lacking in our synthetically fertilized soil. I believe these colloidal trace minerals will play an important role in bolstering the immune system."

Alternative Treatment Approaches

REEXAMINING CONVENTIONAL ASSUMPTIONS

When a diagnosis of breast cancer is made, minimally invasive therapy may be just as effective as more intrusive standard medical approaches, according to Dr. Robert Atkins, a well-known advocate of holistic medicine: "Women develop a lump in their breast and appropriately have a mammogram or biopsy, which leads to the diagnosis. At this point the trouble begins. The doctor gives the patient two choices: a mastectomy or a lumpectomy with radiation. A paper just published on this reported a third option that was every bit as good regarding survival rate and life expectancy. That was simply to do a lumpectomy without the radiation."

DIET AND NUTRITION

Dr. Atkins goes on to say that women don't realize that after the diagnosis and treatment there is much they can do to regain total health: "The biggest fallacy of all is when doctors tell patients after therapy that they've done all they can do and there is nothing left to do. This ignores the whole concept that people can get healthier by enhancing all their internal systems to make sure that the neoplasia, the process of forming cancer, no longer takes place. In other words, cancer is not the tumor itself; cancer is a process.

"Once you know that, you can ask, 'What can nutrition do?' You will learn that it can help in multiple ways. First and foremost, free radicals trigger the formation of cancer and the recurrence of cancer. Nutritional antioxidants can help slow down the formation of free radicals. Additionally, plant foods have antioxidant and immune-enhancing properties."

To prevent and reverse free radical damage to breast tissue, Dr. Steven Rachlin, an internist in Syosset, Long Island, New York, has his cancer patients follow this daily protocol:

> Emulsified vitamin A (up to 50,000 IU)
> Beta carotene (up to 100 mg)
> Vitamin B1 (400 mg)
> Vitamin B6 (500 mg)
> Folic acid (3,200 mcg)
> Vitamin C (up to 5 g)
> Coenzyme Q10 (270 mg)
> Flaxseed oil (1 tbsp)
> Cat's claw (1,800 mg)
> Melatonin (up to 10 mg)
> Shark cartilage (1 mg/kg of patient's weight)
> Pycnogenol (150 mg)
> Essiac tea (several ounces)
> Pancreatic digestive enzymes (up to 40 g)
> Aloe vera juice (9–12 oz)
> Minerals

HERBS

Natural herbal substances are a veritable gold mine for treating as well as preventing breast cancer. Some herbs to know about are listed below:

CARNIVORA (VENUS FLYTRAP)—This powerful herb is popular in Europe but less known in the United States. In Germany it is even used to wipe out cancer that already exists.

ESSIAC—Essiac is a Native American herbal combination that has a synergistic effect in putting an end to cancer and aiding in its prevention.

CAT'S CLAW—A cat's claw formula is used by the Peruvian Indians for the prevention and treatment of cancer.

EVENING PRIMROSE, BORAGE, AND BLACK CURRANT SEED OILS—All these herbs supply gamma-linolenic acid, which is known for its strong anticancer activity.

XIAO YAO WAN—This combination of digestive herbs increases circulation, builds blood, and breaks apart fibroids. The Chinese say it prevents breast cancer caused by phlegm and feelings of melancholy, which impede circulation to the chest. Xiao yao wan is available in Chinatowns throughout America.

DANDELION—Dandelion helps prevent cancer by breaking up phlegm and eliminating it from the system. Excess phlegm can turn into tumors.

ASTRAGALUS—Astragalus is a wonderful immune-system-strengthening herb that can be used in cancer prevention or as an adjunct to cancer treatments. Add a teaspoon of astragalus powder to some pure water and drink once or twice a day. Or try Astra-8, a combination of astragalus and other immune-system-strengthening remedies in capsule form that is found in health food stores.

ROSEMARY—Rosemary has been highly researched and is recommended even more than soy for its breast-protecting qualities. According to Keuneke, "Use rosemary in a vinaigrette or to marinate fish. Try to buy rosemary on a regular basis. Perhaps make a salad dressing with rosemary and garlic, fresh lemon, and extra virgin olive oil. All those ingredients are wonderful foods that are eaten throughout the Mediterranean."

MINT—Include mint in your diet on a regular basis. Mint has a phytochemical in it called limonene, which is effective in fighting breast cancer. In one study, it was found to reduce mammary tumors in animals up to 80 percent. The foods containing limonene are mint, dill, sage, celery seed, caraway, and organic citrus peel. The last item is also found in the Thai diet, which frequently uses lime peel.

TURMERIC—Turmeric also contains a vital phytochemical that has been found to prevent mammary tumors in animals.

ENZYMES

Enzymes are organic substances that help create reactions in the body, such as breaking down fats. They are linked to breathing and all the bodily functions we need to live and stay well. There are three thousand enzymes in the body. A healthy person can produce enough enzymes to fight off cancer cells, but substances such as free radicals from smoke, pollutants, junk foods, and medications interfere with enzyme production.

"So, as you can imagine," Robin Keuneke says, "there are many people who are low on enzymes. To combat this, people can increase the amount of raw foods in their diet and increase fresh juice—juice all kinds of fruits and vegetables."

Numerous studies, she recounts, link enzymes and breast health. More than ninety were conducted by universities throughout the world regarding the beneficial effects of enzymes. Much of this work has been done in Germany.

EXERCISE

Dr. Schachter notes, "Any activity that removes accumulated toxins in the breast reduces the chance of women developing breast cancer. Studies show that aerobic exercise is associated with decreased cancer risk, as exercise promotes lymphatic drainage and sweating helps remove toxins from the tissues.

"Although I am not aware of any direct studies showing reduction of breast cancer with a detoxification program using saunas and certain nutrients as is done with the Hubbard method of detoxification," says Dr. Schachter, "I do know that this procedure has been clearly shown to reduce pesticides and other toxic chemicals in the bloodstream and in fat tissues. Since high levels of these substances increase the risk of breast cancer in women, reducing them with this detoxification method should help reduce the risk of breast cancer to women."

MASSAGE

Lymphatic detoxification is aided by manual lymphatic drainage (MLD), a simple method of massage that uses light, slow rhythmic movements to stimulate the flow of lymph in the body. Massage therapist James Kresse notes that this is especially important for women suffering from lymphedema, a condition that often occurs after a mastectomy: "When our lymph nodes are not functioning properly or have been irradiated or removed, an excessive accumulation of stagnant waste occurs. The lymph system becomes overloaded, thus forming lymphedema.

"MLD should be applied directly after surgery rather than when a massive edema has formed. This will guard against any possibility of a blockage in the system or alleviate any that exists. Studies in Europe show that severed lymph vessels regenerate with constant MLD therapy. The therapy makes the scars from the mastectomy more subtle, which increases the mobility of the arm. It also lessens pain from surgery and the uncomfortable sensitivity that occurs."

IMMUNO-AUGMENTATIVE THERAPY

In the 1950s Dr. Lawrence Burton and a team of researchers discovered Immuno-Augmentative Therapy (IAT), a nontoxic, noninvasive method of controlling cancer by restoring the patient's own immune system. Although the therapy was successful, Dr. Burton left the United States after medical politics prohibited him from practicing here. In 1977 he opened the Immunology Research Center in Freeport in the Grand Bahama Islands, where thousands receive treatment for the disease.

Since Dr. Burton's death, Dr. John Clement, an internationally respected cancer specialist who studied with Dr. Burton, heads the center. Dr. Clement gives an overview of the treatment: "The intellectual basis of the treatment is that many cancers can be controlled by restoring the competence of the patient's immune system, as the body's complex immune-fighting system may well be the first, best, and last line of defense against many cancers.

"The method we use is similar in any type of cancer we treat, although each patient has her treatment tailored to the results of her own blood test. We do not deal with toxic chemicals in any way. We assay the blood for the factors we believe are aiding the patient's cancer. By identifying these factors, we are able to control them, put them back into balance, and hopefully destroy the patient's cancer."

Regarding breast cancer, Dr. Clement says, "We have had patients with breast cancer who have had no other treatment but IAT for upward of twenty years who have no recurrence of disease. While we are still claiming only to control their cancer, you will see that to all intents and purposes, by any kind of medical description, they have been cured."

Dr. Clement reports less success with patients who come to him after extremely arduous chemotherapy and those with advanced cancer where there is a loss of bone marrow and fluid collection in the abdomen or pleural effusions in the lungs.

THE MIND-BODY CONNECTION

Dr. Carl Simonton, medical director of the Simonton Cancer Center in California and coauthor of *Getting Well Again* and *The Healing Journey*, firmly believes that emotions drive healing systems and that the imagination and standard counseling can be used to increase a patient's will to live. "I would like to give an example of a patient I have worked with for more than twenty years," he says. "This thirty-six-year-old woman came to me in 1976 with metastatic breast cancer that had spread to her ribs and spine. Her father was a physician, and her husband's family had run a retail store for three generations. She was involved in helping her husband run the family business.

"Her religious and spiritual life was important to her. It was a great source of strength. She wanted more time to be involved in religious administration and spiritual counseling. As she began to pursue these areas, her beliefs about how she should be the good daughter, the good wife, and the good mother came into play. These beliefs were all quite rigid, allowing virtually no freedom for her own creativity. Over time we helped her make a shift in these beliefs and behaviors that was central to her recovery.

"She has been free of disease for fifteen years. Currently, she is weller than well and runs marathons. The family store burned down about ten years ago. Now she works primarily in church administration, doing religious and spiritual counseling, which is what she always wanted to do."

PATIENT STORIES

I have always been interested in holistic medicine, and I was a great fan of Carlton Fredericks. In 1989, when I discovered a lump in my breast, I sought help directly from a holistic doctor, Dr. Robert Atkins. I went to him before any diagnosis because I knew that if I had to have surgery, I wanted to see someone who was open-minded about alternative therapies.

The lump was malignant, and I had a modified radical mastectomy. Fortunately, my lymph nodes were clean, but the tumor was not a hormonal tumor and it was a very aggressive one.

I started therapy with Dr. Atkins that consisted of a low-carbohydrate diet. That meant absolutely no caffeine and no sugar of any kind. I was also on a program of vitamins and nutrients targeted to my specific problem. Once a week I was given an intravenous drip of an anticancer formula developed by Dr. Atkins that was largely vitamin C.

Soon after surgery I had a problem. The tumor grew back into the incision. Both the surgeon and Dr. Atkins advised radiation, which I was given for five weeks. While I was undergoing radiation, I did the IV weekly, and it alleviated any side effects of the radiation. I wasn't tired, and I was able to work half days.

A month or so after the radiation, the tumor came back again in the area of the incision, and again it was removed. I continued Dr. Atkins's therapy. That was almost seven years ago, and I haven't had a problem since. I am still on the diet and the vitamin program. The intervals between the IVs have been extended to two months.

There is no question in my mind that Dr. Atkins saved my life.

—Marylou

I got breast cancer ten years ago, when I was thirty-nine. I had conventional surgery but would not undergo chemotherapy or radiation. Since I had no positive node involvement and no metastases after surgery, I was told that I was fine and that there was nothing else to do. But because it was a very large tumor and an aggressive one, I was concerned about it. Since I had been involved with natural medicine for a long time and was pretty well educated in it, I started to search for ways to prevent the return of the cancer.

I discovered a lot of things. I went on a one-year program of injections of a formula that was mostly mistletoe. I had to get the prescription for the vials and send away to Switzerland for the formula. I injected myself with the herbal formula.

I did a lot of reading, and I took courses in Chinese herbology. I learned about several herbalists and studied with Letha Hadady over the years. I took several workshops with her where I learned about Chinese herbs and the whole philosophy of Asian medicine as well as the Ayurvedic and Tibetan systems. Over the years, I have taken formulas of Chinese and Western herbs.

The results are difficult to show concretely. All I can tell you is that I don't have cancer and that ten years later, after having had a very aggressive kind of tumor, I am still fine.

I believe in natural medicine. I also believe very firmly that it is important to have a practitioner, to not use the local health food store as your medical adviser. Everybody has to be examined individually.

—Rita

FIBROCYSTIC BREAST DISEASE

Causes

Fibrocystic breast disease is caused by overcongestion from foods that clog the system, such as wheat, dairy products, refined foods, and fats. Caffeinated products such as coffee, tea, chocolate, and soft drinks are hard on the body and add to the problem, as does a sluggish thyroid gland, which makes metabolism more difficult and leads to constipation, causing a buildup of toxins. Toxic accumulations worsen congestion and can manifest as breast lumps (cysts). Stress worsens the condition.

Symptoms

Fibrocystic breast disease shows up as single or multiple breast lumps. Cysts are usually harmless but are related to a higher than normal chance of contracting breast cancer later. Mammograms determine whether breast lumps are benign.

Drs. Ruth Bar-Shalom and John Soileau, naturopaths from Fairbanks, Alaska, add that the symptoms may also include tenderness and pain in the breast. In an article on the American Association of Naturopathic Physicians website (www.naturopathic.org) they stress the importance of learning breast self-examination and performing it every month, a week to ten days after the menstrual period starts. This enables you to recognize the cystic areas. If you are not sure whether a lump is a cyst or something else or if there is a discharge from the nipples, consult a physician.

Clinical Experience

DIET AND NUTRITION

A diet high in complex carbohydrates can make a difference; fruits, vegetables, grains, beans, and some fish are recommended. Red-hot peppers, cayenne pepper, and regular or daikon radishes cut through mucus and help eliminate breast lumps.

According to Drs. Bar-Shalom and Soileau, the most important dietary measure for reducing cysts is to eliminate from the diet all forms of caffeine, including coffee, tea, chocolate, and soda. Meat, especially the hormone-containing commercial type, should be avoided as much as possible. Finally, since constipation can aggravate fibrocystic breast disease, it is important to eat more vegetables, fruits, and whole grains and drink eight to ten glasses of water a day.

SUPPLEMENTS

The following nutrients offer extra help when combined with a cleansing diet: selenium, vitamins A, C, and E, magnesium, and iodine drops. Iodine speeds the metabolism of the thyroid gland. As the metabolism perks up, breast lumps tend to disappear. Iodine drops from seaweed can be obtained in the drugstore in a saturated solution of potassium iodide or Lugol's solution. There is also an Edgar Cayce remedy called Atomodine. In addition, health food stores sell iodine drops in the form of liquid kelp. Before you use iodine, a thyroid blood test should be done to check for thyroid antibodies. This ensures that there is no thyroiditis, an inflammation of the thyroid gland. Drs. Bar-Shalom and Soileau suggest the following supplements:

Multivitamin
Vitamin B complex—50 mg twice a day
Vitamin B6—100 mg twice a day
Vitamin E—600 IU a day
Flaxseed oil—2 capsules or 1 tbsp a day
Beta carotene—150,000 IU a day (if you are pregnant or of childbearing age, take no more than 15,000 IU a day)
Amino acids—1,000 mg each of choline and methionine a day to remedy the hormonal imbalance that is said to result in formation of cysts

HERBS

Herbalist Letha Hadady recommends the following plant remedies to break up congestion in the chest and release phlegm and mucus from the system before they lead to more serious problems:

XIAO YAO WAN—This formula is a combination of digestive herbs that increase circulation, build blood, and break apart fibroids. Xiao yao wan is available in Chinatowns throughout America.

DANDELION—Dandelion tea or capsules can be taken every day to break apart fibroids.

Drs. Bar-Shalom and Soileau recommend in addition poke root and iris versicolor taken as tinctures. Take 5 drops of each three times daily for up to three months. Do not take these herbs if you are pregnant.

EXTERNAL TREATMENTS

CASTOR OIL PACKS—According to the medical psychic Edgar Cayce, stimulating liver circulation ends constipation. Substances that clog the body and form breast lumps are then eliminated. To do this, rub castor oil on the skin over the liver. Cover this area with a towel and place a heating pad over it. Do this for twenty minutes each day.

PEPPERMINT OIL—Rubbing peppermint oil on breast lumps diminishes them by stimulating the circulation.

PHYTOLACCA OIL AND HYDROTHERAPY—Joseph Pizzorno has found success with this combination treatment: "We have a woman put a hot compress on her breast so that it gets real warm. She then covers the area with phytolacca oil. After the application, she covers it with a cold pack. We combine herbal medicine with hydrotherapy to help the cysts drain out of the breasts. I use that treatment with a lot of women and have had quite a good response."

HOMEOPATHY

Drs. Bar-Shalom and Soileau suggest the following homeopathic remedies. Choose one based on how well it matches your symptoms and then take it under the tongue three times a day, stopping when the symptoms are relieved.

PHYTOLACCA—Use 6c potency for hard, sensitive breasts or when you have multiple nodules.

CONIUM MACULATUM—Take 12c potency for sharp pain in the nipples and for breast swelling.

SEPIA—Take 6c potencey when irritability accompanies breast swelling.

YOGA

Dr. Gary Ross, a family physician and certified yoga instructor from San Francisco, recommends yoga poses, meditation, and breathing exercises to alleviate fibrocystic breast disease brought on by stress and a sluggish thyroid. These three postures increase blood flow to the thyroid and chest area:

SHOULDER STAND—On a mat or thick blanket, lie flat on your back. You may place a rolled towel under your neck. Raise your legs over your head so that your body is in a U formation. Rest the elbows firmly on the floor and support the back with both hands. Adjust your body so that it is completely vertical. Then press the chin against the chest. Hold still as you breathe slowly, concentrating on the thyroid gland. You may be able to do this for only several seconds at first, but then you will be able to work up to one minute. To come down, lower the legs slowly toward the head. Then lower the back to the floor one vertebra at a time. When the back is on the floor, continue to lower the legs gradually until you are once again flat on your back. Do this once in the morning and once in the evening. To get the full benefit, follow with the fish pose.

FISH POSE—Lie on your back with the legs straight or folded. If the legs are straight, place the hands under the buttocks with the palms down. Otherwise, hold on to the crossed feet. Resting on the elbow, arch the chest and neck back. The head should be on the floor, but do not apply pressure there. Support should come from the elbows. Do not bend the neck too far back as that can impede circulation. Focusing on the thyroid, breathe deeply in this position, holding for thirty seconds.

COBRA—Lie facedown with the elbows and palms down on the floor or mat and the palms beneath the shoulders. With a smooth, gradual motion, raise the eyes upward, then the head, neck, and spine, one vertebra at a time. Allow the area below the hips to remain on the blanket. Hold the pose and then come out of it using reverse motions that are equally slow and gradual. Breathe in as you come into the posture, hold the breath while in the cobra, and breathe out when coming down.

In addition, Dr. Ross advocates deep-breathing exercises to bring more energy into the chest area. Visualization creates a mind-set that helps make lumps disappear. Further, meditation creates spiritual and mental tranquillity that is conducive to healing.

LYMPHEDEMA

Lymphedema, a swelling of the limbs caused by an accumulation of lymph fluid, affects 1 percent of the U.S. population. Health practitioner James Kresse explains: "There are two types of lymphedema. The first is *primary lymphostatic lymphedema,* an inherent condition that predominantly affects women in their mid-thirties but can manifest at birth or during adolescence. The second is more common and frequently occurs in patients who have had mastectomies or the removal of malignant tumors. The large increase in the incidence of breast cancer and subsequent mastectomy operations is one of the major reasons for the rise in lymphedema today. Secondary lymphostatic lymphedema can occur from six months to three years after the initial surgery."

Symptoms

Lymphedema appears as a swelling or skin thickening in a limb. It is important to detect the condition early, and this can be done in several ways. Kresse advises, "Notice any jewelry becoming tighter on the affected limb over a short period of time. Or squeeze the affected limb for ten seconds. If an indentation is noticed, notify your surgeon immediately or measure your arm with a cloth tape measure around your wrist and forearm. If you notice an increase in the circumference of your arm, call your surgeon right away."

MANUAL LYMPHATIC DRAINAGE

Lymphatic detoxification is aided by manual lymphatic drainage (MLD), a simple method of massage that uses light, slow rhythmic movements to stimulate the flow of lymph in the body. "This type of therapy is very, very light," says Kresse. "It's almost featherlike. We're working on the parasympathetic nervous system. A regular massage stimulates the sympathetic nervous system. That is our fight-or-flight nerve. The parasympathetic nervous system is our night nerve, our rest and relax nerve. This is the nerve that lymph drainage affects in order to calm the patient down."

COMPRESSION BANDAGING

In addition to MLD, compression bandaging is used to apply pressure around the affected limb. Exercises performed with the bandage enhance muscular contractions that help with lymph flow.

LIFESTYLE CHANGES

Kresse states, "There are dos and don'ts that a person should be aware of. Just to mention a couple, as far as the dos are concerned, the person needs to practice meticulous skin care with the use of pH-balanced lotions and creams to protect the skin. Following a good nutritional program consisting of lots of fruits and vegetables is helpful. Salt and fatty foods should be eliminated, and protein intake should be limited. It is important to maintain an optimum weight, as obesity contributes to lymphedema. Exercise such as swimming, walking, and stretching is excellent. Incorporating deep diaphragmatic breathing techniques, along with specific exercises taught by an MLD therapist, is good. While sleeping, the patient can elevate the limb by tilting the mattress or by placing pillows under the arm. Antibiotic solutions should be carried at all times for incidental cuts, scratches, or bites. Infection should be treated at the first sign.

"Precautions to take include not subjecting oneself to extreme temperature changes such as hot tubs, saunas, steam baths, and other thermal treatments. Care must be taken when using instruments on the affected limb, such as the instruments used in manicures and pedicures. Pets must be watched to see that they don't scratch or bite. Blood pressure readings, injections, vaccinations, and acupuncture should be avoided on the infected arm. Constrictive clothing and jewelry should not be worn. Heavy prostheses can cause excess pressure on the affected limb. Care must be taken when cooking, gardening, and doing daily chores. Finally, heavy objects must not be lifted. This can cause a lymphedema right away or somewhere down the line."

Other therapies that help lymphatic conditions include rebound exercise, ozone therapy, enzyme therapy, colon hydrotherapy, deep breathing exercises, and a good vitamin and herbal program.

CHAPTER 7

CERVICAL DYSPLASIA, FIBROIDS, AND REPRODUCTIVE SYSTEM CANCERS

CERVICAL DYSPLASIA

Cervical dysplasia is an abnormal growth of cervical tissue caused by the sexually transmitted human papilloma virus (HPV), the same virus that is responsible for cervicitis, genital warts, and cervical cancer. These conditions can be detected with a Pap smear.

Causes

The likelihood of a woman contracting cervical dysplasia increases with intercourse at an early age, unprotected sex with several male partners, smoking, birth control pills, and weak immunity. Naturopathic physician Dr. Tori Hudson explains: "Women who have intercourse at an early age are more vulnerable to getting genital warts and cervical dysplasia because the cells of the cervix at that age are more susceptible to being infected by the virus."

"If you smoke, and you are exposed to the virus, you are much more likely to develop dysplasia, and you are much more likely to develop cervical cancer from your dysplasia," Dr. Hudson says. "We know that nicotine actually lodges in the glands of the cells of the cervix. When exposed to the virus, the DNA can change to take on more abnormal features. If you have genital warts and you smoke, it is much more likely that they will turn cancerous as well.

"Oral contraceptives are known for creating a folic acid deficiency, and folic acid deficiency is associated with acquiring cervical dysplasia and having the disease progress to cancer."

Symptoms

Dr. Hudson describes cervical dysplasia as a progressive syndrome that develops over time: "After initial exposure to the virus, there is no indication that anything has changed. Later, immune changes may occur. Warty tissue may develop, then mild dysplasia, moderate dysplasia, severe dysplasia, carcinoma in situ, and then invasive cancer." Since these symptoms are not evident upon physical examination, Pap smears are necessary.

Prevention

Since HPV is sexually transmitted, the conditions associated with it are preventable. Notes Dr. Hudson, "Cervical dysplasia, genital warts, and cervical cancer are all sexually transmitted diseases. That should make an impression on all of us, because it really dictates how we should protect ourselves.

"Obviously, we shouldn't smoke. We should protect ourselves by having safe sex and a healthy immune system. If you take birth control pills, it is advisable to take folic acid. A good maintenance dose would be 800 micrograms daily. Those are the main ways to protect against cervical dysplasia and genital warts." Additional preventive daily supplementation may include 5,000 milligrams of vitamin C and 25,000 units of beta carotene.

To catch the condition early, Dr. Hudson stresses yearly Pap smear exams. Statistics show that the longer women wait between Pap smears, the higher the incidence of cervical dysplasia and cervical cancer.

Diagnosis

Before treatment, it is essential to get fully diagnosed to determine the stage of the illness. If a woman has an abnormal Pap smear, her partner needs to be examined by a urologist for warty tissue. Otherwise, they will pass the virus back and forth, reinfecting each other. Diagnosis by a licensed, well-trained alternative practitioner will determine whether a woman is a candidate for natural treatments only or needs to integrate these approaches with conventional methods.

Conventional Treatments

Conventional medicine usually does nothing to treat mild dysplasias and genital warts. "Basically, they wait to see if it gets worse," says Dr. Hudson. "Often the body can reverse mildly abnormal states to normal on its own, as the body has an extraordinary ability to heal itself. But when it can't, then the disease progresses, and the downside of waiting becomes apparent."

In the later stages, aggressive measures may be taken. The preferred conventional treatment is known as LEEP (loop excisional electrosurgical procedure), which uses an electrical wire to cut out abnormal tissue. This is less expensive and less traumatic than the method of treatment previously used, called cone biopsy or conization. In advanced disease states, a hysterectomy may be needed to save a woman's life.

Alternative Treatments

NATUROPATHIC APPROACH

Women with cervical dysplasia often have excellent results using naturopathic approaches. Dr. Hudson notes, "In the results of a research study that I conducted at the College of Naturopathic Medicine in Portland, we treated forty-three women with varying degrees of cervical dysplasia. Through my treatment protocol, thirty-eight of the forty-three reverted to normal, three partially improved, and two had no change, meaning that they didn't get better and they didn't get worse."

Dr. Hudson's protocol consists of three parts: systemic, local, and constitutional treatment. She stresses that after a woman follows the protocol for three months, it is important for her to once again be examined by a health practitioner and to obtain another Pap smear. Sometimes a biopsy is also needed.

> **SYSTEMIC TREATMENT**
> Beta carotene—150,000 IU daily
> Vitamin C—10,000 mg in divided doses daily
> Folic acid—2.5–10 mg daily
>   (Note: High doses of folic acid must be prescribed
>   by a naturopathic physician. After three months,
>   the amount of folic acid is decreased.)
> Immune herbal formulation
>
> **LOCAL TREATMENT**
> Vitamin A suppositories
> Herbal suppositories
>
> **CONSTITUTIONAL TREATMENT**
> Diet: An optimal immunity diet is low in fat and
>   high in whole grains, vegetables, and fruits.
>   Immune system inhibitors such as coffee, sugar,
>   alcohol, and fat are omitted.
> Use of condoms
> Avoidance of smoking

HERBAL TREATMENT

Amanda McQuade Crawford, a medical herbalist, uses herbal infusions to treat cervical dysplasia. In her book *Herbal Remedies for Women,* Crawford also recommends herbal douches. Her favorite douche uses 1 ounce of wheatgrass juice for every 6 ounces of sterile water. If wheatgrass is not available, she recommends the following douche solution:

> 1 ounce marshmallow root
> 4 ounces periwinkle leaf
> 1 ounce goldenseal root
> 1 ounce gotu kola herb

Grind the herbs and mix with 4 ounces boiling water. Strain, and allow the mixture to cool to room temperature before using.

Here's another one:

> 1 cup warm, but not hot, sterilized water
> 15 drops thuja oil
> 1 ounce calendula oil
> 15 drops vitamin E oil
> You can also add:
> 4–6 drops blue chamomile oil
> 4–6 drops geranium oil

Dilute the oils in water and mix together well.

IMMUNO-AUGMENTATIVE THERAPY (IAT)

Treating cervical cancer by restoring the patient's own immune system has also proved successful at Dr. John Clement's Immunology Research Center in Freeport in the Bahamas. Dr. Clement specifies that success can occur if the treatment is begun early, even after surgery. (See chapter 6 for more information.)

FIBROIDS AND UTERINE BLEEDING

Fibroids are growths composed of muscle tissue that are usually benign. They attach themselves to the inner or outer wall of the uterus. One in five women over thirty-five has them; the majority of these women are African American. These tumors grow in response to estrogen levels. Medically, they are also referred to as fibromyoma uteri and leiomyoma uteri.

Complementary physician Dr. Robert Sorge says that fibroids are nature's way of encapsulating toxins that result from an unhealthy diet and lifestyle: "Most of our patients with this condition consume tremendous amounts of coffee. As far as I'm concerned, this is something that every person concerned about their health must stop drinking. Diet sodas, greasy fries, pizza, potato chips, doughnuts and Danishes, and other devitalized foods add to the problem."

Registered nurse and licensed acupuncturist Abigail Rist-Podrecca adds that Asian medicine sees fibroids as the result of blockage to the uterine area: "This can be caused by anger, emotional upset, or a history of problems with menstruation, where it is either late or prolonged. Sometimes, after an abortion, the endometrial wall will still have some cells from that particular pregnancy. Further down the line, that can develop into fibroids."

Symptoms

Small fibroids are symptomless, but when they grow, they may result in painful periods, bladder infections, and infertility. Uterine bleeding is another common symptom. Explains Rist-Podrecca: "If the fibroid is located on the inside of the uterus lining, then you will have this uterine bleeding, which usually sends women to the gynecologist, where she opts for hysterectomy. If the fibroid is located on the muscle wall, there is not so much bleeding, but the fibroid will continue to grow."

Dr. Sorge adds that bleeding is the body's attempt to restore balance, according to naturopathic medicine: "Circulation and oxygenation of the uterine muscles and blood vessels are diminished, and metabolic waste products begin to build up. Bleeding is the sign of a highly toxic condition attempting to correct itself."

Conventional Approach

Small fibroids that do not cause problems are sometimes removed by a procedure known as a myomectomy. This procedure removes the fibroid only and does not interfere with a woman's ability to have children.

For larger tumors or fibroids that cause heavy bleeding, hysterectomies are the standard treatment. Dr. Herbert Goldfarb, a gynecologist and assistant clinical professor at New York University's School of Medicine, reports that the majority of these operations are unnecessary, as well as dangerous. In addition, hysterectomies can be psychologically destructive.

"A new laser procedure, called myoma coagulation, has the potential to end the use of hysterectomies for fibroids once and for all, but most people don't know about it," Dr. Goldfarb says. "My book, *The No Hysterectomy Option*, was written in response to my frustration at having a technology to help women avoid hysterectomies but women not knowing about it. Sometimes women need hysterectomies but often they are told they need them for frivolous reasons. My book is designed to help women understand when a hysterectomy is needed and when other options are available. I always like to say that a hysterectomy may be indicated, but may not be *necessary*. Our best patient is an informed patient."

According to Dr. Tori Hudson, one alternative to hysterectomy is hysteroscopic surgery, which is used when a fibroid is protruding into the uterus. The surgeon inserts a hysteroscope (a tubular instrument that allows the surgeon to visualize the interior of the uterus) through the cervix and shaves away the fibroid with instruments passed through the hysteroscope. The hysteroscope is also used to shrink larger fibroids with lasers or electric currents.

An alternative for relatively small fibroids on the outside of the uterus is laparoscopic surgery. The laparoscope, an instrument used to visualize the interior of the abdomen, is inserted through an incision in the abdomen, and the fibroid is vaporized by an electric current or removed surgically, using instruments passed through the tube.

Dr. Vicki Hufnagel, using the new technique of female reconstructive surgery (FRS), has been successful in removing uterine fibroids regardless of the size or number of tumors, limiting both blood loss and surgical complications.

Alternative Therapies

MYOMA COAGULATION

Dr. Goldfarb lectures extensively to doctors on this new technology, which has enabled him to prevent hysterectomies in hundreds of women with fibroids and uterine bleeding. The typical candidate for this procedure is a woman uninterested in reproduction, since the uterine wall may become too weak to support a pregnancy. Also, the size of the tumor must be 10 centimeters or less (approximately 6 inches). If the fibroid exceeds this size, it can be reduced with the medication Lupron: "Lupron reduces estrogen levels in the body, and temporarily reduces the size of fibroids," Dr. Goldfarb says. "With Lupron, we get a 30 to 50 percent reduction in size."

Once the tumor has become smaller, coagulation can be performed, which shrinks it another 50 to 75 percent and puts an end to the problem: "When we do this procedure, we literally undermine the tumor by destroying its blood supply. As we put needles around the fibroid, it turns blue, showing that the blood supply has been interrupted. Fluid and blood go out, and the tumor shrinks. It becomes stringy tissue and just sits there, becoming very small, eliminating the need for removal. The patient has no symptoms and can go about her life without the need for further surgery."

DIET AND EXERCISE

Fibroids grow in response to estrogen, so nutritionist Gracia Perlstein advocates the natural lowering of estrogen through diet and exercise as a first-line defense against fibroid growth.

As Perlstein explains, "Research shows that an overfatty diet increases estrogen in the diet, and we know overweight women produce more estrogen. So the first approach would be dietary.

"The best diet for a woman attempting to decrease the size of her fibroids, or at the very least keep them from getting any larger, consists of whole foods and is semivegetarian or vegetarian. The best protein sources are from vegetables and include whole grains, especially millet, amaranth, quinoa, buckwheat, whole oats, and brown rice.

"Eat small quantities of legumes daily. Soybeans and foods made from soy, in particular, contain isoflavones that discourage tumor growth. Foods made from soy include tofu, fortified soy milk, miso, and tempeh. A variety of other beans can be used to make wonderful ethnic dishes: black beans, adzukis, pinto beans, chickpeas, mung beans, lentils, and lima beans. Grains and beans are your best source of proteins.

"The liver detoxifies excess estrogen, so you want to support liver function by avoiding all recreational drugs, alcohol, fried foods, coffee, and any processed or refined foods. Be sure to drink at least two quarts of pure water a day to help your bowels and kidneys. You are trying to remove excess estrogen from the system, and this is supported when your organs of elimination work properly."

Exercise is also very important, says Perlstein. "Regular exercise will reduce excessive estrogen levels. Most people are familiar with the fact that hard-training women athletes sometimes reduce their estrogen levels to the point where they stop menstruating. We are not after that kind of effect, but regular exercise is very beneficial."

For further uterine support, Perlstein recommends the following supplements and herbs:

> Balanced oil supplement (a mixture of flax, borage,
>   and other unrefined, natural, organic oils), 1 tbsp daily
> Multiple vitamin/mineral supplement
> Iron and herb supplement (This should be taken if there
>   is anemia from heavy bleeding. Avoid high doses of iron
>   as they are implicated in cancer and heart disease.)
> Vitamin E, 400 IU, twice daily
> Silica supplement
> Vitamin C with bioflavonoids, 1,000 mg five times daily,
>   divided over the course of the day
> Evening primrose oil, 100 mg three times daily
> False unicorn root tincture, 15 drops in a small amount of water,
>   taken every hour, for acute uterine problems
> Shepherd's purse tincture, 15 drops in a small amount of water
>   three times a day (may stop excessive bleeding)
> White ash (may reduce size of fibroids)

Perlstein asserts that such a comprehensive program of diet and lifestyle changes, geared toward reducing excess estrogen, gives the body the tools it needs to shrink fibroids or keep them from growing any larger.

NATUROPATHIC TREATMENTS

Complementary physician Dr. Anthony Penepent recommends fasting for excessive uterine bleeding, excluding life-threatening situations where a woman needs hospitalization: "This condition signals liver poisoning. During the course of the month, a little fasting might be in order, in addition to a very strict hygienic regimen, to straighten out the condition. I have had patients with all forms of dysfunctional uterine bleeding, and I cannot remember any woman who followed my instructions who did not have a good result."

Dr. Joseph Pizzorno, past president of John Bastyr College of Naturopathic Medicine, recommends oil-soluble liquid chlorophyll. He says this old natural therapy can quite effectively put an end to abnormal uterine bleeding. Oil-soluble liquid chlorophyll is available in capsules. Two to three are usually taken two to three times a day. Dr. Pizzorno says that for some reason, the chlorophyll seems to relieve this condition: "Many people think this works because it improves clotting, but it turns out that women with abnormal uterine bleeding do not have clotting abnormalities. So why it works is not clear, but the bottom line is, it works quite well."

HERBS

According to Judy Griffin, an herbalist from Texas and author of *The Woman's Herbal,* as quoted in *Positive Health* magazine, treating fibroids involves decongesting the liver by using safe herbs that can be taken over an extended period of time, including dandelion and vitex berries. Vitex is particularly beneficial for fibrocystic disease because it lowers estrogen levels.

Abigail Rist-Podrecca says the following herbs are good for stopping dysfunctional uterine bleeding when taken under the supervision of a Chinese herbal practitioner:

POO WHA—Made from bee pollen.

ER JOW—Made from the hide of an animal.

CHUAN XIONG (LIGUSTICUM WALLICHI)—Regulates bleeding by the amount taken. Too much causes uterine bleeding, and too little stops it.

HAN LIAN CAO (WARRIOR'S GRASS)—Helps tone the spleen and uterus and stops intense uterine bleeding.

ACUPUNCTURE

Acupuncture points that relate to the uterus are found on the ankle. Rist-Po-drecca explains how electrical acupuncture to this area helps reduce fibroids: "We use a small electrical current. This makes the uterus contract and expand. It palpates the area slightly to get the body to recognize that the fibroids are there, increase circulation, and start vibrating the fibroids so that they are released."

HOMEOPATHY

Beth MacEoin, a homeopath and the author of *Homeopathy for Women*, as quoted in *Positive Health* magazine, says that since fibroids are a chronic condition, they are best treated by a practitioner. For acute symptoms, however, a number of remedies may be effective; these must be chosen based on the specific symptoms a woman is experiencing at a given moment. "The idea is that for a remedy to be active, the remedy chosen must match the symptoms as closely as possible. So it would be very important to select that remedy with the help of either a practitioner's support or a very good, solid self-help manual."

With that in mind, consider the following remedies for uterine bleeding and fibroids:

IPECAC—Dr. Marjorie Ordene, recommends this remedy to stop acute hemorrhaging with bright red blood. "When given in the 200 potency, every fifteen minutes, Ipecac slows down the bleeding. That's two pellets under the tongue until the bleeding actually stops. I have had success with a number of patients, and other physicians have reported this as well."

SHINA AND SABINA—Dr. Ken Korins says the two remedies to think of first for heavy bleeding are Shina and Sabina. Shina is for heavy, dark blood that forms clots and leads to debility and exhaustion. Sabina is also for clots, but here the blood is bright red. When large clots are being expelled, there is a laborlike pain that radiates from the sacrum to the pubis.

SECALE—Women who need Secale have dark blood that is almost black. Periods are profuse and prolonged.

PHOSPHORUS—Phosphorus is indicated when there is bright red blood with no clots.

TRILLIUM—Trillium is indicated when bleeding is very heavy and bright red. The person characteristically feels faint and dizzy after bleeding. Periods occur biweekly, and the woman feels worse with even slight movement.

AURUM MURIATICUM—This remedy may reduce the size of fibroids. It should be used when there are no other symptoms, such as heavy bleeding, and there is no particular discomfort.

HYDRASTINUM MURIATICUM—This remedy has been known to cure large fibroids, especially when they seem to be on the anterior wall of the uterus, pushing on the bladder and causing symptoms of urinary frequency and pain.

REPRODUCTIVE SYSTEM CANCERS

Women are susceptible to ovarian cancer, uterine or endometrial cancer, and carcinomas of the uterine cervix. Of the three, ovarian cancer occurs most often and is increasing in frequency. Uterine cancers are easier to detect in the beginning stages and tend to be more treatable, whereas ovarian cancers are rarely discovered early on, and are terribly damaging to the woman's quality of life.

Ovarian Cancer

Women who are sedentary and don't exercise have an increased risk of ovarian cancer, explains Dr. Susanna Reid, a naturopathic physician in Connecticut. Dr. Reid also believes that being overweight, smoking—especially if you are postmenopausal—consuming alcohol and milk, eating meat (especially fried meat), and eating a diet lacking in fruits, vegetables, and fiber also increase the risk of ovarian cancer. The drug tamoxifen is associated with ovarian cancer, and hormone replacement therapy may also increase the risk of this cancer.

Ovarian cancer usually manifests after menopause, especially in women who have few or no children, were unable to conceive, or gave birth later than the average age. Other factors that place women at risk include a past history of spontaneous abortions, endometriosis, type A blood, radiation to the pelvic region, and exposure to cancer-causing chemicals, such as asbestos.

Women should look for the following early indications of ovarian carcinomas: abnormal vaginal bleeding, weight loss, and changes in patterns of urination and bowel movements. While a Pap smear will not detect ovarian cancer in the beginning stages, ovarian cancer can be diagnosed through annual pelvic exams.

Dr. Reid emphasizes therapies to help prevent reproductive cancers. Once reproductive cancer has appeared, she believes the role of natural medicine is to help heal the body after any surgery, for, she says, most reproductive cancers are not curable with natural remedies.

"I focus a lot on lifestyle. Fruits and vegetables have been shown in epidemiologic studies to protect against ovarian cancer, so I suggest that people put a lot of fruit and vegetables in their diet. Carotenoid-containing foods appear to specifically protect against ovarian cancer, carrot consumption in particular. Vegetable fiber is also important. Green vegetables and carrots seem to have a particular affinity for the ovaries and help protect them from reproductive cancers. Cruciferous vegetables in particular are very important in increasing natural killer-cell toxicity. Whole grains also provide protection."

One of Dr. Reid's guiding principles is to have people return to natural or raw foods as much as possible. She says that animal products have a strong association with ovarian cancer and recommends eliminating animal products from the diet. "That even includes yogurt, which many people think is one of the best dairy products to eat. I don't think a person can be too careful. Ovarian cancer doesn't have a very positive prognosis, so if anything, a person should do too many things rather than not enough.

"Legumes seem to help as well, and the woman should also help eliminate alcohol; wine consumption is associated with an increased risk of ovarian cancer. Although green tea isn't specific for ovarian cancer, it does act specifically on breast cancer, so that might be something a woman would want to add to her diet. Also, moderate exercise increases immune function and is an important aspect of treatment."

Dr. Reid says that women with ovarian cancer seem to have a problem with the antioxidative mechanism in their bodies, and suggests using antioxidants like vitamin E and selenium to help deal with oxidative conditions in the body. Indole-3-carbonyl may also be useful. "There is a new herb called *Camptotheca acuminata* that the National Cancer Institute is studying that seems to show some promise in the treatment of ovarian cancer."

Cervical Cancer

Cervical cancer is associated with cervical dysplasia, as discussed earlier in this chapter. Although not all cases of cervical dysplasia result in cancer, it can be the first stage of a malignancy.

Oral contraceptives and DES (diethylstilbestrol), reduced physical activity, multiple sexual partners or having the first intercourse at a young age, smoking, frequent douching, genital herpes, and multiple pregnancies are all associated with cervical cancer.

In the early stages of cervical cancer, symptoms are usually absent, although there may be a watery vaginal discharge or spotty bleeding. Signs of advanced cervical cancer include dark, odorous vaginal discharges, fistulas, weight loss, and back and leg pain. One's chance of survival increases with early discovery through yearly Pap tests.

Dr. Reid warns that cervical cancer can begin as a chronic inflammation that, if not treated, becomes cervical dysplasia and eventually becomes cervical cancer. She says that cervical conditions may be related to a virus. "Natural medicine has a really good track record in treating cervical dysplasia before it gets to cancer. I would not treat cervical cancer with natural remedies. A woman would normally have the cervix removed surgically.

"To treat cervical dysplasia, we use a diet high in fiber as well as flax seeds, olives, and avocados. There is some recent research that shows that olives contain immune-enhancing substances. And of course, I recommend a lot of fruits and vegetables."

Dr. Reid also recommends using supplements and botanicals. These include folic acid, beta carotene, and vitamins E and C with bioflavonoids. She also has a six-week set protocol that utilizes suppositories. It begins with mild herbal suppositories, which she alternates with more intense herbal suppositories followed by a healing herbal suppository. In one study, thirty-eight of forty-three patients with cervical dysplasia using this treatment had their Pap smears revert to normal.

Endometrial Cancer

Endometrial cancer is associated with hormones, including hormone replacement therapy with or without progesterone, a history of infertility, failure to ovulate, the use of drugs containing estrogen, and uterine growths. Tamoxifen is one drug that significantly increases the risk for endometrial cancer.

According to Dr. Reid, other risks include not having given birth to any children, beginning menopause after age fifty-five, being overweight, consuming alcohol, and eating a diet high in calories, especially when you are postmenopausal. Eating meat and saturated fats—even fat from fish, especially processed fish—and low consumption of vegetables, fruit, fiber, and legumes, are also risk factors. Other poor dietary habits that increase risk are drinking soft drinks and consuming sugar. Oral contraceptives seem to decrease the risk of endometrial cancer.

The symptoms of endometrial cancer are abnormal bleeding in the vaginal area, especially after menopause, and pain in the lower abdomen or back. A Pap smear does not always catch endometrial cancer early, but the cancer can be detected with a surgical examination of the uterus.

As with other reproductive cancers, Dr. Reid believes that endometrial cancer has to be surgically treated. "It's not something that we would ever treat in natural medicine."

Dr. Reid says that natural treatment is focused on helping the patient heal from surgery. She uses therapies that facilitate healing, such as zinc and antioxidants and anti-inflammatories such as bioflavonoids and quercetin and bromelain. The specific therapy depends on how the surgery was done. "If it was done vaginally, you can use hydrotherapy treatments on the abdomen. There is a time during which you have to be quiescent because clots are setting, so you don't want to encourage bleeding. Patients should drink lots of fluids and eat very light foods so that their bowels are minimally taxed and their digestive systems can rest as the abdomen is healing."

Combination Treatments

Gar Hildebrand, of the Gerson Research Organization in San Diego, California, says that more patients would triumph over reproductive system cancers if a combination of approaches were employed. This is the case because contemporary treatments for ovarian cancer are disappointing. While they can make cancers disappear for weeks or months at a time, they fail in the end, as the cancer returns with a vengeance to finish the job. In fact, orthodox survival rates for ovarian cancer patients are only between 5 and 10 percent.

Cancers of the uterine cervix initially exhibit higher success rates with surgery, which may involve the removal of the uterus (hysterectomy), as well as both ovaries and the fallopian tubes (salpingo-oophorectomy), in addition to X ray and hormone therapies. But there is no guarantee that the cancer will not return. He states, "No one should be treated by a single specialty, and then watched in hopes that the cancer will not come back. It's not scientifically justifiable, nor is it acceptable to the patient. Sitting and waiting just causes horrible, immune-suppressing anxiety."

Among the multiple modalities that work best for patients with ovarian and uterine cancer are nutrition, coffee enemas, hyperbaric oxygen, and Coley's toxins.

NUTRITION

"Let's say a woman with an ovarian cancer has just been admitted to Memorial Sloan Kettering Cancer Center," Hildebrand says. "The first thing the doctors will do is a laparotomy. She will be opened up, and a surgeon will get the bulk of the tumor out. I have no problem with that.

"But the second step would be to use drugs that kill tumors. Tissue damage always accompanies cancer; unless it is addressed, the cancer is sure to reappear. In other words, throughout the body tumor toxins cause cells to lose potassium and swell with extra salt and water. This state is worse around the tumor itself. Often a treatment that goes into the bloodstream fails to penetrate to a tumor effectively because the tissue next to the tumor has no immunity. What's really needed, then, is for the patient to be stabilized physiologically. The ideal treatment would be for the person to receive nutritional salt and water management, a diet that nourishes and corrects the water retention in the cells. We're going to feed the whole body to try to get the tissues back to normal functioning."

Hildebrand recommends a diet that detoxifies and stimulates cells back to health. "Doctors have long been aware that most cancer patients have an aversion to meat. They'll smell it and gag; that's a self-defense mechanism.

It's absolutely essential for these people to stop taking in heavy proteins—animal proteins and sometimes even heavy vegetable proteins like legumes—for a while, just to clear up. The tumor is converting that stuff into caustic chemicals, related to the ammonia we use in our laundry machines. It's those chemicals that create damage systemwide.

"We can also detoxify the body by supplying oodles of plant chemicals, called phytochemicals. These foods can be eaten cooked or raw, and should include vegetables of all sorts, fruits, and a few whole grains. Fruit and vegetable juices are especially important. You have to flood the system with nutritious fluids such as carrot and green leaf juices. Apple juice should always be added because apples contain a material that is very good for cellular energy. If you put those juiced phytochemicals into the body every hour, these cancer patients will have their cellular enzyme systems speeded up so that the individual cells can spit up toxins.

"Eating an excess of empty calories and proteins creates toxicity that causes the immune system to overproduce white blood cells that aren't very adept at what they do. Once you restrict protein and calories and get the nutrient level up, these patients' immune systems become intelligent again. They stop making excess stupid white cells and create more lymphocytes that are interested in more types of challenges. In other words, you get a very lean, mean immune system."

COFFEE ENEMAS

Coffee enemas have been used by thousands of cancer patients outside the realm of traditional medical care. Hildebrand explains: "Boiled coffee in retention enemas stimulates the liver's enzyme system, which in turn causes great relief from pain in cancer patients. The liver has more than a thousand documented medical functions. When we help it work better and faster, a cancer patient's overall physiological condition changes, sometimes within hours and certainly within the first several weeks of treatment. You have a whole different person. People come off gurneys and out of beds, excruciating chronic pain is eased, and addiction to morphine is broken.

"Every three minutes, all the blood in our bodies goes through the liver. Our livers and small intestine walls have an enzyme system with a fancy name that we will call GST for short [GST refers to the glutathione S-transferases]. This enzyme system naturally responds to cancer in the body by going up, and coffee enemas have been shown in laboratory experiments with rats, and in later experiments with humans, to produce increased liver bile flow and to stimulate the GST enzyme system. In fact, it's raised to 700 percent of normal levels of activity. When the GST system is running that fast, it can effectively remove tumor toxins from the bloodstream. And it doesn't take very long. The effects of these coffee enemas will last for sometimes four, six, or eight hours before a feeling of discomfort and pain around the tumor returns. They're that effective."

HYPERBARIC OXYGEN

Hildebrand states, "We're also going to try to increase circulation with full-body-immersion oxygen therapy. Hyperbaric oxygen treatment is given in a diving chamber that used to be used to treat the bends. There's been a lot of fascination with ozone in cancer treatment in the alternative field. But what we found is that ozone applications raise tissue oxygen only by 25 to 50 percent, whereas hyperbaric oxygen can predictably raise oxygenation by 800 to 1000 percent. This means that tissue around the tumor, which doesn't have enough oxygen to function, can get sufficient oxygen for energy production. This will also allow the tissue to repair itself by producing a high-potassium, low-sodium environment, so that this edema can come out of the tissue."

COLEY'S TOXINS

Hildebrand states that this treatment has the best record of any treatment in the cancer literature, especially when combined with the Gerson diet program. "I am hopeful that much interest will be sparked in this therapy because right now the only reports I've seen of long-term survival for ovarian cancer patients have been from a combination of these approaches.

"The word *toxin* is a little confusing, because Coley's toxin is not really a poison. It refers to a bacterial endotoxin that is an immune stimulant. I would put that directly into the abdominal cavity once the tissue around the tumor has been stabilized.

"Coley was a physician who searched the literature for cancer treatments after a heartbreaking experience of losing a child patient to the disease. Much to his surprise, he found a skin infection called erysipelas. Erysipelas is caused by a streptococcus that causes a skin fever of 105 to 106 degrees Fahrenheit. This fever causes an inflammatory infection which interferes with tumor action.

"Coley constructed a live erysipelas vaccine, which was too toxic at first. Some patients died, but others experienced a tumor regression. He went through a lot of trial and error and eventually settled on something that we now call *Serratia marsecens*. He mixed the *Serratia* and the strep in a ratio of 1,500 cells to one, and then crushed the mixture through a microfilter to liberate the internal toxins of the bacteria. This liberated antigens, which in turn caused the immune system of the patient to respond as if there were a chronic infection that had to be fought.

"The effectiveness of Coley's toxins seems to be due to the fact that the immune system, when turned on, can cause a lot of dust to rise. These patients need to be put into an intensive care unit and hooked up to monitors in case there is a problem, although there have never been any heart attacks or kidney failures reported in the nine hundred cases that have been thoroughly studied. Then a tiny amount of toxins is administered intravenously for four hours through a drip. About two hours into the process, the immune response begins. The patient will develop chills and shaking that last for about thirty to ninety minutes, followed by a rise in temperature of about a degree every ten minutes. Once that temperature hits 105 or 106, the ICU staff lays the patient down or puts in a suppository of Tylenol to stop it.

"The reaction is the immune system's response. This is not a poison. This is not a toxin. It's not like chemotherapy, which makes your hair fall out or causes bone marrow suppression. The Coley's toxins are much more like what happens when your immune system decides to cure you of an infection. So the symptoms are more flulike, without the nausea and vomiting. After the second or third IV application, patients usually get sleepy and actually nod off. The fever lessens progressively. In other words, there's a honeymoon period.

"Coley himself said that if you don't keep these up for at least three or four months, in booster dosages, you won't get a permanent response. The literature reveals that gains are lost when Coley's toxins are given in lower concentrations or for shorter durations. But when they are properly used, there is an extraordinary 50 percent cure rate in advanced, inoperable uterine and ovarian cancers."

THE BENEFITS OF A COMBINATION APPROACH

Hildebrand reemphasizes the importance of utilizing any and every cancer protocol that works: "We believe that it's time we stopped living in an either/or world where orthodoxy is over on one side and the marginalized alternative professions are in the trenches and foxholes, and nobody talks. We believe it's time to get the doors and windows of communication open so that we can find the context for each of these treatments and the way they fit together.

"Our own experience reveals that using the nutritional approach takes a toxic load off the immune system and speeds up intracellular enzymes so that they can repel toxins and pull them from the blood rapidly. Calorie and protein restrictions and a diet high in nutrients can lead to the sensitization of a tumor. Years of experience show that diet therapy alone can produce monthly fevers, and tumors may or may not regress through those fevers. But if you stimulate the immune system when those fevers are hitting, you have a much greater chance of tumor reduction. That's why we suggest the marriage of these disciplines and the respectful recognition of the role of every aspect of anticancer medicine that's ever been developed."

PATIENT STORIES

I still have cervical cancer, but I am working on overcoming it through a number of approaches. I watch my diet very carefully. I feel that my condition is in an early enough stage where I can handle it nutritionally. But it's not just nutrition that I have to deal with. I have to deal with all the emotions that help to create disease in the body. It's also a matter of detoxing. I do colonics and a lot of juicing. I take supplements. And I do meditation and exercise.

The major reason I started to see a nutritionist was, of course, the wake-up call, the cervical cancer, which was just diagnosed three months ago. But I had also had ulcerative colitis for almost twenty years.

I feel like I now have energy again. I exercise at least several times a week, which was literally impossible before. I even had trouble getting up a flight of subway steps without feeling exhausted at the top. So I have several different things that I am working with: nutrition, meditation, and detoxification. I'm working on it.

Now I have to find a gynecologist who is holistically oriented because my primary care physician dropped me after I refused to have a hysterectomy. I feel very lucky. I feel that someone else trying to deal with this would have followed the recommended course of action and would have given up her reproductive rights, allowing herself to be mutilated while always being fearful of having the cancer reappear.

Also, I feel that the cancer is nothing more than a wake-up call. Your body is saying, "Hey, something is wrong here. You're out of balance. You need to address this and this and this." If you don't, disease is the end result. Now I am vegetarian and doing a lot of things differently. If I didn't, I might not be alive now.

I might be at a higher risk for the cancer to spread throughout more of the body. This doesn't mean that I am 100 percent there. I still have a lot of work to do. But I feel very hopeful.

—Morgan

CHAPTER 8

CHRONIC
FATIGUE
SYNDROME

Chronic fatigue syndrome poses a major problem for traditional medicine. The medical establishment has fumbled in its treatment to the point of sometimes claiming that the illness does not exist, but chronic fatigue is a major problem in the United States, particularly among women. Millions of women lack the energy they once had, ranging from those who have just a little bit of energy to those who are maximally depleted, in bed and unable to function.

Chronic fatigue syndrome is the term used to describe a state of constant exhaustion. A syndrome is a disorder that includes a collection of symptoms but is not necessarily a disease entity. Although not labeled as such until the late 1980s, chronic fatigue syndrome is quite similar to other disorders that have been known for centuries. In the nineteenth century, for example, a common complaint of middle-class women was neurasthenia, which was characterized by chronic exhaustion and a variety of other physical symptoms.

Why is it that for years Americans with a debilitating illness were not recognized as having a disease? They were simply told that chronic fatigue syndrome does not exist. Dr. Dean Black says, "If you go back to the last century, you can read about women suffering from nervous disorders—so many of them that clinics had to be set up to care for them. There was always the search for a cause, but one couldn't be found, so doctors wouldn't say it was a disease. It had to be in the patient's mind. This is not a new way of sweeping things under the carpet.

"Medicine's power base is the idea of its basis in certainty, which hinges on the concept of a single linear cause-and-effect relationship. That's why medicine is always looking for a single causal factor. This is called the theory of specific etiology."

Dr. Black compares the situation of chronic fatigue syndrome to that of the Epstein-Barr (EB) virus, which was initially thought to cause chronic fatigue syndrome, although later this theory was challenged. "That is why they were so happy to discover this EB virus," he explains. "It seemed marvelous to them because it served to justify the single-cause idea. Yet, as has been frequently pointed out, everyone may have Epstein-Barr [it is so widely distributed]. Chronic fatigue syndrome is caused by many factors operating together. But this idea has been excluded by traditional medicine, which refuses to come to grips with multifactorially generated disease. Medicine is reluctant to accept this multifactorial explanation because it holds to this idea of absolute truth, which requires simplicity and must have one cause and one effect."

Dr. Andrew Gentile stresses that we need to differentiate chronic fatigue syndrome from other health problems: "Since chronic fatigue syndrome has no known cause, we need to rule out other disorders whose cause we do know. The working definition provided by the government for this disease says there is no other illness at the root of it. Differentiating it calls for great care, since fatigue is ubiquitous as a symptom of many diseases, such as anemia, low thyroid, hypoglycemia, and a variety of other illnesses. These other illnesses must be clearly ruled out."

POTENTIAL CAUSES

Viral Infection

A number of studies have looked at viruses in connection with this syndrome. One theory posits a single viral agent. Dr. Gentile states, "I have heard chronic fatigue syndrome being called a number of things from Epstein-Barr to mononucleosis.

"Epstein-Barr was brought into the discussion by way of a lab in Philadelphia that exclusively studies this virus. One of the lab assistants was negative for current and acute Epstein-Barr virus, but during the course of the study developed the symptoms of chronic fatigue syndrome. He was treated and found to be positive for Epstein-Barr virus. So we had the first studied case in which a person went from Epstein-Barr-negative to Epstein-Barr-positive at the same time that he had all the symptomatology for chronic fatigue syndrome. That began a flurry of studies investigating the Epstein-Barr connection. We now know there is not a high degree of correlation between the symptoms of chronic fatigue syndrome and Epstein-Barr serological titers. So Epstein-Barr is probably not the cause of chronic fatigue syndrome."

Dr. Gentile goes on to note that the Epstein-Barr virus is widely distributed in the populace. Most people have it by age eight. Thus, there is no clear distinction between those who have it and those who do not. We would expect many more people to be ill with chronic fatigue if it were indeed Epstein-Barr that was causing it.

Several other candidates have presented themselves, including human herpes virus 6 (HHV-6), a B-lymphocyte virus that was studied by the National Institutes of Health. "But again," Dr. Gentile says, "studies showed that this virus is very widely distributed and thus could not be the distinguishing agent responsible for the syndrome. Other studies are proceeding. Wistar, a renowned laboratory in Philadelphia, is looking at a retrovirus, HTLV-2 [human T-cell lymphotropic virus] as a possible cause."

Dr. Neenyah Ostrom, author of *America's Biggest Cover-Up*, believes that HHV-6 may be involved. "What is interesting is that there are two types of this virus. One form is found very widely in the general population, and the other is found in people with cancer, AIDS, chronic fatigue syndrome, and other immunological problems. This virus can attack the immune system very effectively, and I believe it will eventually be found to be instrumental in causing chronic fatigue syndrome, AIDS, and some forms of cancer."

Other viruses that have been thought to contribute to chronic fatigue syndrome are Coxsackie virus, adenovirus, enterovirus and the hepatitis virus, among others. Dr. Gentile states, "The consensus among practitioners is that a single virus probably does not cause this illness. We have to carefully distinguish between cause and trigger. Clearly, a virus may trigger a cascading set of events in various body systems: neural, endocrine, cognitive, hormonal. A variety of abnormalities may be found in these systems, but if viruses do trigger these imbalances, then they quickly hide within the normal cells—which is usually how viruses behave—while their effects wreak havoc in the body system."

It is as if the virus triggered something in the immune system that makes the system unable to self-regulate and find its way back to homeostasis. Thus, each time the immune system is stressed by a toxic load from the environment or from food allergies, or when infections are reactivated, there is a breakdown. The flare-ups and relapses occur and recur frequently, reproducing all the symptoms. These relapses then compound themselves. If a patient is not sleeping every night, symptoms such as exhaustion and lowered immunity crop up.

"We know, by the way," Dr. Gentile adds, "that the rhythms of this illness dovetail nicely with ninety-minute circadian rhythms. In sleep, we have a REM [rapid eye movement] cycle that occurs every ninety minutes, and this is the cycle by which our immune system is synthesizing proteins. The immune system works lock and key with this cycle. But if one has a sleep disturbance caused by a virus or a set of viruses from this disorder, one's sleep will be off and therefore the immune system will be off."

Environmental Factors, Nutrition, and Allergies

Dr. Majid Ali sees the surrounding environment and lifestyle as playing causal roles. He says that the immune system becomes injured by environmental pollutants such as mold, formaldehyde, and pesticides as well as by allergenic foods, poor nutrition, stress, and lack of physical fitness.

Dr. Shari Lieberman, a professor of nutrition, expands on this point. She has published articles and several books, including *The Real Vitamin and Mineral Book*. "We as a country are not healthy. We have all these discussions, lectures, books, and so on, concerning a healthy lifestyle. We have the information, but we are not actualizing it. I don't think people understand how all of the body's circumstances are impacted by the immune system."

Dr. Michele Galante also believes that allergies are important: "The patients I have seen have been very allergic not only to pollens and airborne agents but especially to foods and chemicals. These people are so sensitive and so debilitated that a short exposure to perfume, nail polish, gas fumes, carbon monoxide, or even just paint, such as from a freshly painted room, will give them headaches, make them weak, even make them emotionally upset. Chronic fatigue syndrome is closely connected to allergy."

Unfortunately, Dr. Ostrom adds, "some of these allergy-causing substances are unavoidable. Chemicals in our environment, aside from those in our foods (coloring, preservatives, and so on), are everywhere. There is chlorine in our water; the air is filled with pollutants—things that were not in our ecological system fifty or sixty years ago. Recent phenomena that accompany technological advances, such as the mercury in silver amalgam dental work, are weakening our systems. Each of these chemicals in itself does not necessarily have so strong an impact, but exposure to all of them together, day after day, for many years, overloads the liver and immune system. Electromagnetic influences, previously ignored, are now also under discussion. Many believe the cathode rays from computers affect the electromagnetic fields of the body, for instance, as does the electromagnetism of cellular phones, radio waves, and television waves—things relatively new to our environment."

Metabolic Regulation

Chronic fatigue syndrome can also be explained in terms of immune system depression related to a failure in metabolic regulation. When glucose production is up, it brings on hypoglycemia, with a high degree of glucose in the blood causing an increased level of insulin, which lowers the glucose level excessively.

Because of poor utilization of glucose, fatty acids increase in the blood to provide a sufficient level of energy. A high level of triglycerides will occur, and the immune system will be depressed because it needs a new army of T lymphocytes, which are not being produced because of derangement in lipid metabolism.

Vitamin, Mineral, and Hormonal Deficiency

Dr. Neil Block explains that lack of necessary vitamins, including C, E, and beta carotene, can also affect the immune system, as can a lack of minerals, particularly calcium, vanadium, copper, magnesium, potassium, molybdenum, boron, iodine, selenium, and chromium. The trace minerals are especially important for organ function.

Dr. Block also points to hormonal imbalances, particularly thyroid imbalance (especially hypothyroidism), which affects women six times as often as men. It tends to develop spontaneously between the ages of twenty and fifty, although it can come at any time, often from unknown causes. The rare causes, which are the ones known for this disease, involve either a superabundance or a deficiency of iodine in the body, although the latter is unlikely in our society, where we have iodized salt and other sources. Another rare cause is consuming too many of certain vegetables, such as cauliflower, broccoli, and brussels sprouts, which tend to bind the active ingredient and inhibit thyroxin production.

Other hormones frequently out of the normal range include the adrenal hormones and the gender hormones. It is not unusual to have imbalances in the estrogen that governs the ovarian function or in other governors, such as LH [luteinizing hormone] from the pituitary gland or progesterone." In fact, women frequently come to Dr. Block with lack of menstruation, milky discharge from the breast, breast tenderness, or more menstrual cramps than usual.

Drug Use

Dr. Galante remarks, "The allopathic drugs, conventional drugs, antibiotics, and steroids are major influences. The use and abuse of these drugs in childhood, for example, sets up chronically weakened conditions that will extend into adulthood and contribute to a predisposition for chronic fatigue. These drugs are suppressive in nature, not curative. They themselves impose an illness on the system. This may be one of the largest of the causal factors."

Dr. Ali talks about a young person suffering from chronic fatigue syndrome who went to a medical clinic and was given a prescription for steroids. We know steroids suppress the immune system, so why would anyone give these drugs to someone with this disorder? Steroids can create a sense of well-being and euphoria for a couple of days, but it is false.

Psychological Factors

Dr. Gentile tells us that chronic fatigue seems to reduce a person's tolerance to stress. He has had patients who were marathoners before contracting the illness. They report that they had been working hard and then got sick with fever and chills. The illness waxed and waned. They would feel better at times and go back to running but then quickly relapse. These patients cannot tolerate stress in either the physical or the psychological form. Stress will exacerbate the illness again and again.

According to Dr. Paul Epstein, a key tenet of naturopathic medicine is to treat the underlying cause. "A person diagnosed with chronic fatigue syndrome has a suppressed immune system, which can be documented by blood tests and other measures. But what caused this? It may be improper diet; then the patient will need to eat properly. But we also need to ask why she adopted that diet in the first place. If the answer is stress, we can then ask what caused the person to follow certain patterns of reaction to stress. As we treat the patient, going through all the different problems layered one on top of the other, we eventually get in contact with the person's core self.

"One way to make this contact is through the inner child. Many people have been influenced by John Bradshaw's work on recovering and healing the inner child and on seeing how the wounds and scars of childhood may have led us to create lifestyles that are addictive. Thus, even as I help the person medically by giving advise on diet, stress reduction, and so on, I remember this. If we do not touch deeper problems, healing may not occur."

SYMPTOMS

Chronic fatigue syndrome causes fatigue and usually begins after the onset of flulike symptoms. The fatigue is not a simple tiredness; it is an exhaustion accompanied by feelings of being unwell. Many people have difficulty getting out of bed and may become weakened to the point of needing to lie down all the time. Often patients are bedridden for months; extreme tiredness can last for years.

Chronic fatigue syndrome may be accompanied by depression, irritability, headaches, low-grade fever, infection, confusion, focusing difficulties, diarrhea, sharp muscle pain and weakness, swollen glands, and sleep disorders. The woman is not able to fall asleep or stay asleep and does not feel refreshed or restored even after much sleep.

Dr. Martin Feldman adds, "Immune system difficulty somehow pulls down hormonal function. Almost all patients with this syndrome have low adrenal function, and many have low thyroid function. So we have a hormonal mixup causing fatigue, but behind this is the viral disease pulling down the immune system."

Dr. Michael Vesselago uses laboratory tests to diagnose his patients and then treats them accordingly. He looks for viruses as well as allergies and stress: "I test the person for allergies with an IgE RAST [radioallergosorbent test] and get back a report showing how the body responds to more than one hundred tested foods. We adjust the diet so that the person is no longer eating allergy-causing foods, and that alone brings about a significant improvement in over 70 percent of individuals.

"If someone collapses unduly fast or wakes up tired and requires several cups of coffee to get going, then I will focus on the adrenals first. I do a test for adrenal function that involves checking cortisol, which is one of the main adrenal hormones. From that I get a picture of how well the adrenal glands are coping with stress during the day."

Dr. Martin Feldman says that the first step in the analysis of any woman who comes to him with fatigue, whether mild, moderate, or severe, is to profile the patient to see how she fits with the five major problems associated with the syndrome. Almost all people with chronic fatigue syndrome have at least one of these problems:

> Immune viral breakdown, leading to low adrenal function
> Thyroid imbalance
> Vitamin B deficiency
> Hypoglycemia
> Cerebral allergies

Dr. Feldman also tests the thymus, spleen, and lymphatic system. "You could test the T- and B-cell counts. That's easy to do, but it's very expensive, so in daily practice it's easier to test thymus electrical energy. You can also do this for the spleen. When we find a weak thymus circuit, we can try any aspect of therapy within the weakened circuit to obtain a resonance that will help strengthen that circuit."

Dr. Gentile is more concerned with self-diagnosis: "If you feel you have chronic fatigue syndrome, ask yourself these questions: Have I had debilitating fatigue for six months? Do I have flulike symptoms? Have I not found any physiological cause? Do I have pronounced sleeplessness? Do I have low stress tolerance so that if I take a short walk or try any sport, I feel vaguely ill and tired?"

Dr. Majid Ali states that most physicians have a tendency to focus narrowly on a problem. But, he says, "I don't think trying to find a diagnosis for one or two symptoms is terribly important. What is important is how the patient describes his or her suffering. We need to think of what we can do at a molecular and energetic level to relieve his or her suffering and restore his or her health.

"I've seen patients whose lives have been devastated by chronic fatigue syndrome. They've gone through all these drugs, antivirals, steroids. With each drug, they get better initially and then nose-dive. What do we do?

Alternative Therapies

The key to finding treatment for chronic fatigue syndrome, according to Dr. Gentile, is choosing the right expert. "It has reached the level of scientific respectability, and most practitioners and medical examiners believe it exists. It is important to have someone who is up to date on the literature and who has seen a minimum fifty to one hundred patients, someone who understands the ups and downs of the disease and is aware of the number of different treatments that have developed."

He points out several ways to locate a credible expert. For one thing, there are chronic fatigue syndrome support groups in every major town in our country, and now worldwide, that have lists of physicians who have specialized in the disorder. There are national groups, such as the Chronic Fatigue Syndrome Association. They maintain a list of doctors who understand the disease, have treated it, and are sympathetic.

"This last trait is so important," Dr. Galante explains, "because many sufferers have gone through scores of doctors. We're treating a woman now who has already seen seventy-five physicians all over the world. She was ready to give up because she feels people do not believe her. So a critical part of treating this illness is belief. A second thing to bear in mind is that because this is a chronic illness with a wide range of symptoms, it will tend to fall between the cracks of all the medical subspecializations. With this disease, it will not be adequate to go to a single physician. It would be worth considering putting together a team, which would include a GP/internist, one who works both with traditional and alternative therapies; an allergist/infectious-disease specialist; and a psychologist/psychiatrist. This team could coordinate to work out a treatment plan so that the client understands what is coming next. And if these treatments don't work, the team could determine why that might be and what would be worth trying next."

THE SPIRITUAL ELEMENT

Dr. Ali tells us that in dealing with a chronic, devastating illness like this, hope and the spiritual element are essential for long-term success. He has had case histories that truly stretch the bounds of credulity: "Creating hope is very easy to do; sustaining hope is difficult, but it is central to healing. By the time I see patients, they have each seen at least seven specialists. They've had biopsies, CAT scans. When they come to me, it's not that easy to simply reassure them, after they've seen the previous failures, that they'll get better. But fortunately, by the time they get to me, they've listened to some of our tapes, read our books, and, most important, talked to some of the other patients who have gotten better. So when they come in and they meet our nursing staff, our ancillary staff, they realize we are all serious. If they ask how my program differs, we say this: They do not have the option to remain sick."

VITAMIN SUPPLEMENTS

Another component of treatment is supplements. The hope, according to Dr. Shari Lieberman, is not only to repair damage and stabilize the weakened immune system, but also to overboost the system.

At Dr. Ali's clinic I watched a nurse making up an intravenous chronic fatigue syndrome protocol with vitamins and minerals. She said that patients who come in are very tired and have joint pains, headaches, and memory loss, and that these IVs help repair cell membranes and boost the immune system, which will then hopefully function better. About 90 percent of the patients have responded well. Dr. Ali will usually order a set of five to begin with, she says, and after that he can measure the patient's response, see how deep the problem is, and whether she requires further treatment.

"I see these drips as jump-starting the cellular enzymes," Dr. Ali says. "The enzymes, which are detoxification enzymes, are dependent on minerals and vitamins. If I feel there is enough time, when the patient is not acutely ill or has been chronically ill for a number of years, I will try to use a more conservative approach. But when I see people with severe, incapacitating fatigue, I use the IV. In fact, in one of our studies where we compared one group that had the IV and one group that didn't, we saw that the IV speeds up the recovery process."

Dr. Ali continues: "We have fourteen different formulations or protocols to manage different clinical problems in our IV drips. For chronic fatigue syndrome, we use vitamin C, magnesium, calcium, pyridoxine, pantethine, zinc, B vitamins, molybdenum, potassium, copper, and selenium. Most of our protocols have fifteen to eighteen items, and we change their quantities depending on the individual's state."

Dr. Feldman has found that "people suffering from chronic fatigue syndrome are deficient in such nutrients as vitamins A, B5, B12, and E; bioflavonoids; the essential fatty acids; zinc; selenium; and GLA (gamma-linoleic acid). All those must be put in order before we can proceed further."

Dr. Neil Block discusses his treatment: "If proteins or amino acids are low, we can try to individually supplement the amino acids. If minerals are lacking, they can be given individually or in tandem, trying to operate by an economy of scale so that a patient doesn't have to take from more than ten to fifteen bottles at a time.

"As for hormonal imbalance, I have 20 to 25 percent of my chronic fatigue syndrome patients on thyroid hormone. I prefer to use the more natural brands of thyroid hormone. Again, I believe in giving both the male and female hormones. We also have to try to adjust the pancreas and adrenals. For the pancreas I use chromium or chromium picolinate. For adrenals, the glandulars or homeopathics, and sometimes things such as licorice tend to help multiple hormones. If we are working on the pituitary, we use glandulars, the homeopathics, and on rare occasions I use a lot of the amino acids to try to build neurotransmitter activity. The amino acids to be used are arginine, tyrosine, and phenylalanine. Tryptophan was also once useful to me until they took it off the market. I'm also not afraid to use, correctly and in small doses, items obtained from the pharmacy. What I tend to shy away from are the tranquilizers, such as Valium and Librium. I do make use of antidepressants on occasion."

Often his patients have seen other physicians and holistic healers and may need only one or two things to turn the body around on multiple levels: "With neurotransmitters being easily adjusted nowadays, with items like the antidepressants such as Paxil and Zoloft, which lack drastic side effects and have a response beginning in two to four weeks, they're worthwhile. It's nice for a patient who has suffered two, four, or six years to take these new agents and within two to four weeks get at least some indication of the direction in which he or she is going."

ENZYMES

Dr. Steven Whiting, author of *The Complete Guide to Optimal Wellness,* tells us about enzyme supplementation. There are two forms of supplementation, he says, and it is important to understand the difference between them. One type of product you can get at health food stores consists of whole enzymes and actually contains such things as pepsin, rennin, and trypsin, the real enzymes. They have their place, and they have their drawbacks. Their primary use is for chronic disease and for people who are very debilitated. The big problem with using them is that the body can grow dependent on them quite rapidly. When they are taken orally in the form of supplements, the body is not always encouraged to make them on its own.

"The second group of supplements," Dr. Whiting says, "is called enzyme precursors. These are substances that not only contain the raw materials for the body to build its own enzymes but frequently contain the vital stomach acid hydrochloric acid, which helps the body build many of the protein digestants. Remember, proteins are digested in the stomach, and carbohydrates and starches are digested in the intestinal tract. This is why a very unique enzyme system has been created and needs to be maintained."

He continues: "For the average person looking for a good enzyme product, I recommend one that would contain at least the following things. First, hydrochloric acid. After years of eating junk foods and dead, lifeless foods, we need it to help with stomach digestion. According to a recent survey by the University of California at Berkeley, only 9 percent of the population eats the recommended number of fresh fruits and vegetables per day. This product should also contain protein digestants, which should include papain and pepsin. There should be fat digestants, ox bile and pancreatin. Also a starch digestant, which would be bromelain."

"The bulk of the five years of research I have done for my book is about what I call whole-spectrum nutrition. We have been able to isolate about 102 nutrients that the body needs every day. These include the 16 vitamins, the 3 fatty acids, 8 to 12 amino acids, and about 72 minerals.

"What we found out in working with patients such as those with chronic fatigue syndrome in a clinical environment is that the concept that has developed in the last twenty years of using potency to address chronic diseases may have been only part of the picture. In reality, we are finding that the ratio of nutrients to each other is as important as, if not more important than, potency alone."

HERBAL THERAPIES

Many herbs can help to heal the immune system and thus play a role in chronic fatigue syndrome. Herbalist Letha Hadady offers some recommendations. Strengthening agents include Chinese ginseng, dandelion, false ginseng, *Andrographis, Eclipta alba,* and honeysuckle. Honeysuckle flower, *Andrographis,* and dandelion may also help destroy germs. Chinese blood tonics, include han lien tsao, which is called *Eclipta alba* in Latin and grows wild in the American Southwest. It builds blood without any side effects, such as inflammation. You can take it every day in powdered form. Hadady also mentions fo ti, which builds blood while it keeps us cool.

There are three types of ginseng: American, Chinese, and false. The American type provides more moisture and more saliva and is good after a fever. Chinese ginseng, called ren shen, gives us energy. Dang shen, or false ginseng, makes us feel stronger without feeling hotter. All can be used in soups. When dang shen and astragalus are used together, the first lifts our energy and the second sends our defenses to the surface. Cayenne pepper increases circulation and makes us feel stronger.

There are also herbs for relaxing the nervous system. Siberian ginseng can be taken as an extract or in capsule form. Valerian, taken in capsules, can quiet the nervous system: "For people who are depressed," Hadady says, "we need to bring them to their center as a way to be grounded and to feel more whole. Use ginger and mint. Mint helps bring the worries out of the head, and ginger helps burn them away because it is digestive and heating, so it brings us warmly to our centers. They make a good combination."

High Energy preparation is an herb mixture that uses Western and Eastern ingredients: gotu kola, American ginseng, damiana, red clover, peppermint, and cloves. It strengthens the adrenals and lungs.

Hadady adds that cloves and hot water will increase your energy and make you breathe more deeply.

Dr. Lieberman has looked at American plants to find ones that can strengthen the debilitated immune system that accompanies chronic fatigue syndrome. "I'd say hands down that about the most important herb in this area is licorice root," she says. "A specific valuable compound found in this root is glycyrrhizin, available in health food stores as a supplement. It's not the easiest thing to find, but a few companies make it. Glycyrrhizin is just remarkable at boosting the lymphatic and immune systems, the white blood cells, and the thymus gland."

Glycyrrhizin can actually be therapeutic in relation to some of the viruses implicated in chronic fatigue syndrome. Glycyrrhizin stimulates the production of interferon naturally. It supports the thyroid gland and boosts natural killer cells and other aspects of immune functioning. A therapeutic dose ranges from 75 to 300 milligrams per day. It's important to monitor your blood pressure while taking this supplement. "I haven't seen many patients' blood pressure go up when taking this, but it will occasionally happen," Dr. Lieberman notes.

Another antiviral is echinacea. Dr. Lieberman believes that it is not used nearly enough for chronic disease and immune dysfunction. Many people use it for influenza, but it can be useful for other viruses as well. Echinacea has a remarkable ability to naturally stimulate interferon, natural killer cells, and phagocytes.

The liquid extracts of echinacea work best, Dr. Lieberman says. Use fifty drops once or twice a day, depending on the severity of your symptoms. "It's been recommended that you use echinacea four days on, four days off. There is some concern that if you use it all the time, you may adapt to it and it may stop boosting certain aspects of immune function. We don't know that for sure, but to be on the safe side, that's my recommendation. But I keep my patients on glycyrrhizin long term, though I gradually cut the dose down and maybe eventually have them on 75 milligrams per day as a prophylactic."

DIETARY CHANGES

Gracia Perlstein, an alternative health care practitioner with a private practice in New York, says that for chronic fatigue, food is the best medicine: "We really don't have any existing drugs on the market to help this condition. In fact, most drugs will weaken immunity and delay recovery further. It is best to approach this with natural supports to inherent healing processes." While there are no quick cure-alls, she makes the following recommendations to speed up recovery.

A diet of pure, nutrient-rich whole foods is imperative: "You want to include plenty of fresh organic vegetables. Cruciferous vegetables such as broccoli, cauliflower, and brussels sprouts are very important for their immune-enhancing properties. You want onions and garlic, the poor man's cure-all.

"Choose from a wide assortment of whole foods. Don't eat the same few over and over again. In this weakened state you can develop allergic responses to foods consumed repeatedly in large amounts. Eating different foods will ensure that you get a variety of nutrients and will keep you from developing allergic responses. Amaranth, quinoa, and other grains not commonly eaten by Americans are good to include.

"Really emphasize the green foods. Have a dark green salad daily. Super green powders are very helpful as well. Add them to juices, but do not emphasize sweet fruit and carrot juice.

"Eat an adequate amount of high-quality proteins. The best sources are vegetarian because of the low toxicity and ease of digestion. Good vegetarian proteins are tofu, tempeh, fortified soy milk, and legumes. You can benefit from small amounts of fresh fish because fish is high in omega-3 fatty acids. But there are some precautions you must take. Be sure to find a market that gets fish from clean, unpolluted waters and make sure they do not dip it in chlorine, which is a common practice. If you eat farm-raised fish, it should be organically raised. If you eat poultry, it should be naturally raised as well, free of hormones and pesticide residues. Consume only small amounts of animal protein, no more than three to four ounces a day.

"The best way to have protein is in a soup. An excellent old Chinese recipe for an immune-enhancing soup combines a whole astragalus root with onions, garlic, ginger, and free-range chicken, fish, tofu, or tempeh. Some fresh green vegetables and a handful of brown rice are added to that. The soup is brought to a boil and then simmered. Some miso is added for flavor. This is highly nourishing, easy to digest, and excellent for helping a weakened individual regain strength.

"Drink plenty of pure water daily. In colder seasons unsweetened herb tea, such as immune-supportive echinacea tea, is a very good source of liquid. Cold water is a little shocking to the digestive system for people with chronic fatigue syndrome, so you want warm liquids and plenty of them."

HOMEOPATHY

Homeopathy is Dr. Galante's specialty; it has been very effective against chronic fatigue syndrome. Homeopathic remedies, all made from natural substances, are given in microdoses. The essence of homeopathy is to select for each individual a remedy based on her or his unique physical constitution and manifestation of symptoms.

ACUPUNCTURE

Registered nurse and acupuncturist Abigail Rist-Podrecca points out that the *chi,* or bioelectrical energy, flows through pathways called meridians in the body. Disease, she says, is associated with an energy blockage. Acupuncture needles inserted in some of the 365 points that can be used open the blockages so that the energy can flow smoothly through the meridians. In addition, the needles dilate the blood vessels so that more blood flows through the area, bringing more oxygen and nutrients, which aid all aspects of health.

TAI CHI

A benefit of tai chi is that it increases one's awareness both internally and environmentally. "Then you can choose which to work on, whether there is something physically wrong or something in the environment that needs to be corrected," says Eric Schneider of the Northeastern Tai Chi Chuan Association.

According to Schneider, you have to cultivate a part of your body that can observe phenomena dispassionately without having to grab on to every experience and run with it, so that when you find yourself in stressful situations, you can say quietly, "Oh, so this is what is happening now. What can I do about it? What are my options, and how am I feeling?"

However, it takes ten years to achieve what is called the *gung chi*, which means that the body is able to contain energy. This is not a quick fix.

IMAGERY AND HEALING

Dr. Paul Epstein says imagery is a therapeutic technique that helps people explore themselves through words and symbols so that they can understand the language of the subconscious.

According to Dr. Epstein, "Usually what comes up is the issue that is at the core of what will be the healing. People may get in touch with childhood wounds or abuse from the past that needs healing. Perhaps they'll get in touch with the fact that the work they are doing is not real work.

"In one such case, with a person suffering from chronic fatigue syndrome, we found that the illness was a case of a person trying to get love. She had not let go of trying to get love from her mom and dad. She was still stuck at that place. And the pain and grief of not having that love were not only weakening her immune system but keeping her stuck in the unhealthy way she was living her life."

Dr. Majid Ali reiterates some of Dr. Epstein's message: "What I demonstrate to my patients is that the way you look at the world around you determines the biology under your skin. If you can be in a self-regulatory, healing mode, your brain activity, heart activity, muscle energy, skin energy will all be functioning positively. Or you can be trying to figure things out, think everything through in an overly intellectual way, and your biology will be as up and down as the New York skyline. This is the stress mode, and it causes disease. Another mode is an even, steady-state mode, a resting mode.

"Our goal is to perceive the energy in these modes and understand how the energy profoundly affects the electrophysiological profile. Can we allow this energy to guide us into the healing mode? We want a transition from an ordinary, thinking, nervous, stressful mode that causes disease to a nonthinking, meditative, deep-breathing mode that makes us well. That is our goal."

AYURVEDA

Dr. Nancy Lonsdorf of the Maharishi Ayurveda Health Center in Washington, D.C., and coauthor of *A Woman's Best Medicine,* defines fatigue as an imbalance in the body's rest-activity cycle. According to Ayurvedic principles, the natural structures of rest cycles allow the body to recover from activity cycles: "A state of chronic fatigue means that the body has not fully rejuvenated itself."

Dr. Lonsdorf reports that many of her clients overcome fatigue by adhering to the basic rules of Maharishi Ayurveda, which address rest, activity, digestion, cleansing, and meditation.

THE NOTION OF SELF-HEALING

Dr. Epstein wants to help patients listen, explore, and understand the message of their disease, which is the key that unlocks the door to recovery: "After the diagnosis and medications, natural or other, there still has to be an exploration of healing for this person. We might have conditioned immune-suppressant responses built into our attitudes, beliefs, the way we live our life, the way we think, and the way we eat. An illness cannot be fixed from the outside; there is no magic bullet for chronic fatigue syndrome.

"People heal themselves by engaging in a self-healing process, by looking at their life and its meaning. It may seem rather complicated, but it is not. It is based on the knowledge that we do not get sick overnight. The condition may manifest suddenly in certain symptoms, but it took years and years to arrive. And it was not from one virus, not just from Epstein-Barr or herpes or parasites, low blood sugar, or electromagnetic pulsations. It was a combination of all of them.

"What is needed in treating chronic fatigue syndrome or AIDS and similar problems is a new approach. We should be looking not for the quick fix or what will work for everybody but for an approach that is individualized and holistic and empowers the patient to get involved in the cure and gives that patient belief and hope that healing is possible.

"There are two points in my treatment that I've been told by patients have helped them most: that I have given them hope and belief that healing is possible and that I have shown them that there are things they could do to help themselves. I don't heal anybody. Doctors don't heal anybody. They support people as they heal themselves."

CHAPTER 9

DIABETES

D iabetes is a serious condition that affects nearly 16 million Americans a year. It is the third leading cause of death in the United States and a primary cause of new cases of blindness, renal disease, and nontraumatic amputations. It also contributes to heart disease. The prevalence of type II diabetes (see below) has jumped more than 40 percent over the last ten years. Overweight, sedentary people older than forty are among those at greatest risk. In the United States, African Americans and Latinos are disproportionately affected.

In 2001, a major study of more than 3,200 people at twenty-seven centers across the country confirmed what many of us in the alternative medicine community have known for years: moderate exercise and changes in diet can significantly reduce the risk of diabetes.

CAUSES

Diabetes is closely associated with heart disease, and the incidence of both conditions increased when Americans began to change their dietary patterns. "There is a wonderful book written about twenty-five years ago," says Dr. Robert Atkins, "called *The Saccharine Disease,* by Dr. Cleave. He made observations, one of which was 'the law of twenty years,' which says that after you introduce refined carbohydrates into a culture, two illnesses emerge two decades later, diabetes and heart disease. We know that a Third World diet without refined carbohydrates leads to no heart disease and no diabetes. When one illness emerges, so does the other. Studies of this sort have linked diabetes with heart disease. We know that a woman who is diabetic is three times more likely than women in the general population to get heart disease."

Under normal circumstances, insulin is released by the pancreas in response to elevated levels of sugar in the blood. It promotes the transport and entry of glucose to muscle cells and various tissues, thus lowering blood sugar levels. In a diabetic, part of the process is interrupted as a result of a deficiency in, resistance to, or insensitivity to insulin.

Insulin Deficiency

For many years, it was thought that diabetes is purely and simply a deficiency syndrome in which the body does not produce sufficient quantities of insulin for proper glucose metabolism and assimilation. More recently, it has been learned that many diabetics do produce enough insulin, but their cells do not take it in. The problem is, then, due to insulin insensitivity or resistance.

Insulin Insensitivity

Insulin enters cells at points known as receptor sites. When the receptor sites are plugged because of fat, cholesterol, inactivity, and obesity, insulin cannot enter. As a result, glucose stays in the blood and creates hyperglycemia, or high blood sugar. This excess sugar is diagnosed as diabetes. In such cases, there is no need to increase insulin production but rather a need to enhance insulin sensitivity. A person with diabetes needs to work at making his or her own insulin more efficient, and simply increasing the amount of insulin will not do that.

Insulin Resistance

Insulin resistance is a phenomenon that is closely related to insulin insensitivity. With insulin resistance, there is also a sufficient or even overabundant supply of insulin, but allergic responses prevent insulin from doing its job. Usually allergies to specific foods suppress the activity and efficiency of insulin. Different factors may be responsible for a disordered carbohydrate metabolism in different people. Wheat, for instance, may create symptoms of high blood sugar in one woman, whereas corn may affect another. Offending substances can be determined on an individual basis with food allergy tests.

TYPES OF DIABETES

Type I diabetes is the most serious form of the disease. Type I diabetes used to be called juvenile diabetes, because for many years it was believed that this type of diabetes only occurred in the childhood or teenage years. This form of diabetes is characterized by a true insulin deficiency. It results when the pancreas is damaged from some exotic viral infection or even a highly toxic state. The disease may also be a genetic condition. In type I diabetes the beta cells in the pancreas that produce insulin are destroyed. Since type I diabetics have an insulin deficiency, they have to take insulin by injection daily, and generally for life.

Maturity-onset, adult-onset, or type II diabetes is more of an acquired disease. It is often precipitated by chronic excess weight from poor diet and/or lack of exercise. It may also be brought on by overconsumption of stressor foods or other allergens that are insulin resistors.

Type II diabetes accounts for some 90 percent of all diabetes in the U.S. It occurs most frequently in adults over age forty. In type II diabetes, the beta cells in the pancreas still produce insulin, but for a variety of reasons there may be insufficient insulin production or the body may not be adequately using the insulin that is produced. Thus this form of the disease is characterized by complications of insulin resistance and insulin sensitivity rather than, in most cases, a true deficiency of insulin. For this reason, maturity-onset diabetes can frequently be non-insulin-dependent.

Some nondiabetic women develop a type of diabetes called gestational diabetes during pregnancy, usually in the last trimester.

SYMPTOMS

Often there are no symptoms present, especially in the beginning stages of type II diabetes. Obesity is sometimes a sign of a prediabetic state, especially when the excess weight is concentrated at the waistline and just above the waistline. Classic diabetic symptoms are more often experienced by type I diabetics and include frequent urination, especially at night, great thirst and hunger, fatigue, weight loss, irritability, and restlessness. Progressively, the eyes, kidneys, nervous system, and skin become affected. Infections and hardening of the arteries commonly develop. In type I diabetes, coma from a lack of insulin is a constant danger.

CLINICAL EXPERIENCE

Traditional Approaches to Treatment

MEDICATIONS

Before the development of insulin in the 1920s, diabetic patients had a bleak prognosis. Sufferers saw the condition rapidly go from bad to worse as complications such as blindness, gout, and gangrene developed. Overall life span was drastically shortened.

In the beginning, insulin appeared to be a miraculous drug, and it probably was. The life span of diabetic children was extended from months to decades. Today, many of these children live normal, productive lives.

Insulin is still the primary therapy for type I diabetes. Type I diabetics generally take insulin at least once a day, frequently several times a day.

While some type II diabetics require injections of insulin, many are given oral hypoglycemic medications. Many type II diabetics incorrectly believe that these pills are simply a form of insulin, but that is not the case. None of the oral medications used to treat type II diabetes contain insulin. They are designed to help your body use the insulin that is in your pancreas more effectively, or to stimulate better insulin production. Consequently, oral medications can only be used by diabetics whose pancreas still makes some insulin. In addition, some type II diabetics can control their diabetes entirely through diet and exercise.

In recent years, a number of new drugs have been introduced to treat type II diabetes. Some of these drugs are being rushed through the approval process without adequate review of their safety. One drug, Rezulin, was pulled from the market in early 2000. Some 500,000 Americans had been using the medication, which was approved for use by the Food and Drug Administration (FDA) in 1997. The FDA asked the manufacturer to withdraw Rezulin after it was linked to eighty-nine confirmed reports of liver failure, including sixty-one deaths.

COMPLICATIONS AND BLOOD SUGAR CONTROL

Although diabetes can cause a wide variety of complications, from kidney and eye problems to nerve damage, some of these complications can be reduced considerably by carefully controlling blood sugar. For many years doctors assumed that diabetics whose blood glucose levels were as close to normal ranges as possible reduced their risk of serious complications. In 1993, the Diabetes Control and Complications Trial (DCCT), one of the largest studies ever conducted, confirmed that diabetics in the intensive control group, with glycohumaglobin rates that averaged 7.1, reduced their risk of eye disease by 76 percent compared with the less aggressively managed group, with glycohumaglobin rates of 8.9 percent. Across the board, diabetics in the intensive control group had a 50 percent reduction in all serious diabetic complications. Although the trial was conducted only on type I diabetics, experts believe that the findings of the study apply to all diabetics.

CURRENT DIETARY RECOMMENDATIONS

The findings of the DCCT study make diet and eating habits even more important for diabetics than previously. Eating the right foods can help maintain proper blood sugar levels, as well as helping to boost your immune system. In 1994 the American Diabetes Association changed the dietary guidelines for diabetics.

In the past there was one standard diabetic diet, prescribed for all diabetics. Now the ADA recommends that diabetics work with experts in diet and nutrition to individualize their diets. In the past, complex carbohydrates, such as potatoes and bread, were restricted because it was believed they caused moderate increases in blood sugar. The new dietary recommendations recognize that complex carbohydrates are not the problem they were once thought to be. Emphasis is now put on the total amount of carbohydrates in a meal, rather than the source. Diabetics are frequently taught to count carbohydrates and to match medication requirements to carbohydrate intake. This is especially true for insulin-dependent diabetics.

Unlike simple sugars, complex carbohydrates are beneficial. Although both are broken down into glucose, the latter do not go directly into the bloodstream. While simple sugars immediately enter the blood, complex carbohydrates go through a long process of digestion and only very gradually release sugar into the blood. Therefore, they do not contribute to the high blood sugar levels, as do simple carbohydrates. Instead, they stabilize and improve health.

In addition, fat and protein are more carefully monitored than in the past. Diabetics who are overweight are told to keep fat intake to no more than 20 to 25 percent of total calories. Large amounts of protein may be related to accelerated kidney damage. This is because protein must be immediately processed by the body; it cannot be stored. This puts a great stress on the nephron cells, which filter the body's toxins. Many diabetics suffer from kidney deterioration as a result and must receive dialysis or a kidney transplant. Studies show that the elimination of meat from the diet is often enough to reverse kidney damage.

The Natural Approach

Despite its severity, diabetes need not be as debilitating as it usually is. While there is currently no cure, there are ways of enhancing the body's natural defenses through nutrition, avoidance of allergy-producing substances, and exercise. A healthy lifestyle and alternative approaches to treatment can decrease the amount of insulin or oral medications needed by some persons, although type I diabetics will need to continue taking insulin for life.

The goal of treatment can and should be to build up the body's ability to function as independently as possible. When changing to a more holistic approach to treatment, it is important not to immediately discontinue any of your diabetic medication. Instead, a preventive-medicine physician should assist in the gradual transition. With a doctor's guidance, medication may be reduced or completely eliminated with time. Complete elimination, however, is not always possible.

Physicians who practice alternative approaches to treating diabetes for the most part employ a program combining exercise and dietary modification aimed both at better nutrition and at weight loss, where indicated. Medications are used only as second- and third-line approaches. This sort of program usually controls the disease and its ancillary complications in a less invasive, more efficacious manner, in a short period of time.

While type II diabetics respond most dramatically, even type I diabetics may be able to reduce their insulin dependency. More important, they are able to alleviate many of the insidious complications that have come to be thought of as intrinsic to diabetes.

DIET

Since diabetes and heart disease are so closely related, Dr. Atkins recommends that some people with diabetes follow a Dean Ornish program, in which they drastically cut down on dietary fats. The best diet consists of organic vegetarian foods, eaten raw, sprouted, steamed, baked, or stir-fried with little or no oil. Those who have a true insulin disorder will not fare well on a high-carbohydrate diet, since diabetes is a carbohydrate metabolism disorder.

"It is important to know who needs carbohydrate restriction versus who needs fat restriction," Dr. Atkins says. "To determine that, there are a variety of tests, including a cholesterol profile in which we look at the ratio between the triglycerides and the HDL [high-density lipoprotein]. When a person has a blood sugar disorder leading to a lipid disorder, the ratio is extremely high. To be really safe, the number should be approximately the same, or the HDL should be higher than the triglycerides. It is perfectly appropriate to spend five or six weeks on one diet and then get all of your parameters checked again, and then spend five or six weeks on the other diet and get them checked again. In that way, you can make an intelligent decision."

EXERCISE

An exercise regimen is crucial for burning calories and normalizing metabolism, and is especially important for overweight adults, who are often inactive.

Exercise also heightens the body's sensitivity to insulin. By lowering cholesterol, it lowers triglyceride levels in the blood, making cells more available for glucose assimilation. This is why the insulin requirements of diabetic athletes always drop while they're engaged in swimming, soccer, and other sports. Athletes also notice an increase in their insulin requirements when they cease doing their physical activities for an extended period of time.

Athletes are not the only ones who benefit from exercise. Ten to twenty minutes of light exercise after each meal helps reduce the amount of insulin necessary to keep blood sugar levels under control. A brisk walk gets the body's metabolism working a little faster so that food is more easily absorbed. That prevents blood sugar from rising too high.

An exception to the rule involves diabetics with heart disease. In these patients, exercising after eating may precipitate an angina attack because of the transfer of blood from the intestines to the legs and other parts of the body.

ALLERGY TESTING

Testing for food allergies can determine which foods are responsible for insulin resistance. Clinical experience has shown that this approach to treatment is the most useful way to get to the root of adult-onset diabetes and reverse the condition. Patients can usually be weaned from insulin, since an insulin deficiency is not the cause of the problem. Eliminating allergy-producing foods may also foster weight loss. This occurs because people crave foods when they are allergic to them. When these foods are taken out of the diet, the desire for them eventually stops.

To determine whether a specific food is causing hyperglycemia, a doctor can monitor a patient's blood sugar before and after that food is eaten. Foods that raise the blood sugar cause allergic reactions and should be eliminated.

SUPPLEMENTS

In addition to diet and exercise, the following supplements are important to know about:

CHROMIUM PICOLINATE—Chromium helps normalize glucose levels in insulin-dependent diabetics.

MAGNESIUM AND POTASSIUM—These minerals also help to maintain a glucose tolerance level.

ZINC—Zinc is essential for normal insulin production.

ENZYMES—Enzymes useful in controlling insulin-dependent diabetes are digestive protylase, amylase, and lipase.

VANADYL SULFATE—Vanadyl sulfate may be the most important mineral for diabetes. It was discovered in France in the late 1800s and used to help diabetics before insulin appeared on the market. It works at the cellular level and is most effective when taken three times a day.

HERBS

Plants containing phytochemicals with antidiabetic properties include chicory, Indian snakeroot, thyme, safflower, Indian fig, dandelion, rice paper plant, jack bean, flax, kuzu, barley, evening primrose, oats, wheat, and alfalfa. Plants containing phytochemicals with insulin-sparing properties include coconut and the common plantain.

TOPICAL TREATMENT FOR DIABETIC ULCERS

Ulceration at various locations plagues many patients with diabetes and causes a condition that is often serious enough to warrant amputation. This tragedy may be averted with a simple solution. According to clinical studies, raw, unprocessed honey is an ideal dressing agent for almost every type of wound or ulcer. It sterilizes the ulcerated area, and often works even after antibiotics fail.

OTHER APPROACHES

Mucokehl (made from the fungus *Mucor recemosus*), which was originally developed in Germany, may actually reverse diabetic neuropathy. People using this remedy get feeling back in their extremities, and their eyesight improves. Many practitioners also recommend chelation therapy for reducing diabetic retinopathy and healing foot ulcers.

Monitoring and Preventing Diabetes

Diabetics and those who wish to prevent diabetes can do a great deal to monitor themselves. It's important to look for the presence of antibodies that attack some of the body to defend against an ingested allergen. This is easy to see if the symptoms are blatant, but not if they are subtle. The thing to look for is a general lowering of the body's immune response.

The best way to see this is to go five days without eating the food (or any of its relatives) you wish to test. If you want to test milk, abstain from cheese, ice cream, and all other dairy items or processed foods that contain milk as an ingredient. After five days, eat a meal consisting of just milk and eat generous amounts of it. Then tune in to your body's response. If you experience headaches, stomachaches, pulse rate changes, increased heartbeat or blood sugar, depression, lethargy, dizziness, or even delusions, you can see that your body has reacted negatively to this substance. In other words, you have an allergic response to it. You will have to back off from it. Leave it alone for twelve weeks initially. When it is reintroduced into the diet, it must be rotated with other foods. Eat it in modest amounts no more often than once every four days.

"Of course, there are a lot of good things about that four-day basis," says Dr. William Philpott, a prominent diabetes researcher and clinician. "You will eat thirty or forty kinds of foods instead of the half dozen you've been eating. This is a very wholesome thing. To have the necessary nutrition you will have a wide range of foods." It is a good idea to try introducing new foods into your diet, ones that you have never thought to eat. Try not to eat any foods more frequently than twice a week.

Dr. Philpott recommends that you invest in some diabetic equipment so that you can monitor your blood sugar an hour after each meal. "At least 110 is optimum," he says, "and 160 or beyond is high blood sugar. Before the next meal, test your blood sugar again to make sure it is at least 120 before starting your next meal. If it is not, wait and exercise. Get it down before your next meal. Monitor your pH from saliva; it should be 6.4. If it is below 6.4, you are having a reaction to the food. Measure your pulse; if it varies drastically, you are reacting to the food. Blood pressure is more significant. Physical symptoms, mental symptoms, and blood sugar are the most important. They are absolutely essential. It will take about thirty days to do this."

GESTATIONAL DIABETES

About 3 percent of nondiabetic women develop a type of diabetes called gestational diabetes during pregnancy, usually in the last trimester. Gestational diabetes is diagnosed with an oral glucose tolerance test. In many cases this type of diabetes can be controlled with diet and exercise. Although gestational diabetes disappears after delivery, as many as 50 percent of women with gestational diabetes will develop diabetes later.

Dr. Susanna Reid, a naturopathic physician at the Center for Natural Medicine in Connecticut, says that diet and exercise are the key to controlling gestational diabetes.

Diet

Dr. Reid advises women with gestational diabetes to learn how to eat on the low end of the glycemic index. The glycemic index was developed around 1982 by Dr. Sullivan, who gave people glucose and then measured how high the sugar level in their blood rose. He then established that level as 100 percent of the glycemic index. He repeated the experiment by giving people various foods and measuring how high their blood sugar would go just as he had with glucose, and then assigned each food a percentage.

Dr. Reid says that foods we don't normally associate with sugar may still be high on the glycemic index. "A baked potato and puffed rice are both 100 percent on the glycemic index, which means that they raise your blood sugar significantly. This is bad for your body; it goes into a state of alarm when your blood sugar rises so quickly and significantly, and it produces more insulin. Since the rate of rise is so rapid, the body tends to overproduce insulin, and people get what is called reactive hypoglycemia (low blood sugar). Then they have to eat sugar to get their blood sugars back up again. Therefore you need to eat foods low on the glycemic index to avoid either hypoglycemia or reactive hypoglycemia."

She explains that the position of some foods on the glycemic index may seem counterintuitive. These include fruits, nuts, and legumes. For example, peaches, plums, grapefruit, and cherries are between 20 and 29 percent on the glycemic index. But potatoes and even carrots and parsnips and rice are at the top level. She says, "When you eat foods that are high on the glycemic index, you need to have a healthy fat with them. Doing this seems to prevent the rapid rise in blood sugar. If you had a baked potato, for example, you'd want to have olive oil in it."

Foods you may think would be low on the glycemic index, such as vegetables, are often among the highest. "Peas are between 50 and 59 percent on the index and corn is between 60 and 69 percent. Yams are very high, but sweet potatoes are much lower on the index than yams. Brown rice and all the grains tend to be very high."

Exercise

Dr. Reid also tells her patients about the importance of exercise for gestational diabetics. She says that by exercising regularly, we can often keep our blood sugar levels within the normal range. "When a person exercises, it improves insulin's ability to remove glucose from the blood and also decreases insulin resistance. If you exercise sixty minutes a day at 60 to 70 percent of the maximum heart rate, then usually after just one week of exercise you'll see an improvement in the glucose tolerance test. But be careful not to overdo it and cause your blood sugars to drop too low."

Dr. Reid warns that a woman should not attempt to become a world-class athlete while pregnant. "But she should continue and enhance her current exercise program. There are some things she needs to be careful about. She should not lie supine and attempt to lift weights, she shouldn't get too warm, she should maintain adequate hydration, and she probably shouldn't take up a new sport in which balance is a main requirement because she is having to adjust daily to changes in the shape of her body and her orientation in space. She wouldn't want to do anything where she might fall, such as inline skating at top speed."

Dr. Reid's favored exercises are running and walking. "Women need to feel free to move when they are pregnant. It is not a pathological state. They are not ill."

Nutritional Supplements

Dr. Reid cautions against using some herbal supplements during pregnancy. "Most of the herbs are contraindicated in pregnancy, so one has to be cautious in treating gestational diabetes. For example, traditional herbs we would use to treat non-insulin-dependent diabetes, which gestational diabetes usually is, are bitter melon (*Mamordica charantia*), fenugreek, elecampane (*Inula helenium*), and garlic and onion supplements. All those are contraindicated in a pregnant woman. Ginkgo and Jerusalem artichoke are not contraindicated, and in all of the research that I've done I can't find a contraindication for *Gymnema sylvestre*, which is an herb that seems to increase the pancreas's ability to produce insulin, which would be advantageous in patients with gestational diabetes."

CHAPTER 10

DIGESTIVE DISORDERS

I n examining digestive disorders, one must realize that there are no special clinics where research and treatment focus exclusively on these disorders and that there are no particular pioneers in the field of digestion. One reason for this is that digestive disorders are not often clearly diagnosed as such. A determination may be made that a person has cancer, arthritis, or renal failure, for example, but not that the condition is related to a chronic digestive disorder that has gone undetected for a long time. While you may be undergoing extensive, costly, and perhaps toxic treatment for a diagnosed disease, it is possible that only the symptoms of your disease are being treated, not the underlying cause.

Furthermore, many people go through life with a chronic digestive problem and assume that it is a normal state of affairs. Any complications that result again are rarely understood as being connected to an underlying problem with the digestive mechanism. Some disturbances that obviously are related to digestion—diarrhea, constipation, and the like— are handled by taking over-the-counter drugs such as laxatives and antacids. Some people think they have a "weak" stomach or that these problems are just part of getting older, and so end up taking drugs habitually, unaware that they are likely exacerbating the real problem.

CAUSES

If any of the systems involved in digestion are faulty in any way, the efficiency of the absorptive process will diminish and the body will not be receiving the nutrients it needs.

Insufficient or suboptimal production of stomach acid, which is not an illness but a sluggish stomach, is the most common digestive problem, especially in people over forty. In the presence of low stomach acid, food digestion in the stomach is impaired and thus protein and minerals are not digested efficiently. Many people with this problem burp and belch after meals.

The pancreas is a gland that produces enzymes for digesting protein, carbohydrates, and fats. The enzymes neutralize the acidity of partially digested food (chyme). If the enzymes are inefficient, difficulties will result. Very often, when a patient complains of digestive problems two to three hours after eating, the pancreas is the culprit.

The liver produces bile, which is stored in the gallbladder and sent into the small intestine through the bile duct. This alkaline fluid is partly responsible for fat absorption, as it emulsifies or breaks down fats into smaller particles. The liver is a major workhorse of both digestion and the detoxification of the body, and it can be overtaxed by a poor diet or by any inefficiencies in the digestive process. If production of stomach acid or pancreatic enzymes is sluggish, this sub-par functioning can be a major stressor on the liver.

The pancreatic enzymes described above come into play when partially digested food moves from the stomach to the duodenum, which is the first part of the small intestine. The digested food then moves farther down the small intestine into the jejunum, where food absorption takes place. The nutrients are then carried through the bloodstream to various parts of the body. A malfunction in this part of the process, or anything leading up to it, can impair nutrient absorption.

The ileocecal valve is located between the small and large intestines. Diarrhea and constipation are often associated with malfunctions of this valve. The valve's job is to open when the contents of the small intestines are ready to pass through, to let a certain amount through, and then to close. However, if the valve stays open too long, or is too tight or closed, problems can occur.

If the ileocecal valve remains in the open position, it can enhance diarrhea, because everything is flushing through too quickly. Food passes through the digestive apparatus so rapidly that the absorptive process is impaired. In addition to the rapid transit due to the open valve, the movement of food may reverse, as the contents of the colon backflush. The colon is the "garbage disposal" area, whereas the small intestine is the "kitchen" area. Therefore, a backflush of waste material puts biochemical stress on the small intestine and irritates the liver as well. In short, the waste material makes a mess in the kitchen. The material may be absorbed into the bloodstream, causing various toxic reactions.

If the ileocecal valve is too tight or too closed, this can cause constipation. The tight valve, by not facilitating the passage of the small intestine contents into the colon, retards the entire digestive flow, which leads to infrequent bowel movements, or constipation.

When the stomach acid and pancreatic enzyme systems do not work properly, undigested particles of food or actual pieces of food may reach the colon, also called the large intestine. This not only irritates the colon but also leads to flatulence because the undigested food will be fermented by the friendly and not-so-friendly bacteria residing in the colon.

Finally, the colon may be irritated throughout its entire length or in any of its anatomical parts: the ascending colon, the transverse colon, or the descending colon. Often, the most common pattern is that all three parts are out of balance. In this case, the patient should consider how she handles stress because the colon may be the organ in which various stress elements are manifesting themselves.

There has been found to be a high correlation between food intolerances or allergies and irritation in the descending colon (see below). It's always a good idea to keep a careful food diary to identify frequently eaten foods and those you may suspect are culprits in allergic reactions. Foods that commonly prompt allergic reactions include gluten foods (wheat, barley, oats, and rye), sugar, peanuts, citrus fruits, dairy products, soybeans, corn, and caffeine.

Irritation of the ascending colon alone means that its ecology is off balance. For example, there may be an overgrowth of yeast because the ascending colon becomes a fermentation factory of sorts when undigested food particles reach it. The unfriendly bacteria that live in the small and large intestines may be especially likely to overgrow if the production of stomach acid is so low that the digestive system becomes underacidified or excessively alkaline. A highly alkaline environment favors the growth of yeast, which may then exceed the usual niche it maintains within the ecological population of the colon.

SYMPTOMS

Digestive system disorders can be placed into two main categories: those that are clearly and directly related to digestion, and those that are a step or two removed from the digestive process and therefore more difficult to connect with digestion.

Symptoms of disorders in the first category are more easily recognized. The most common include burping, belching, flatulence, a feeling of indigestion, undigested food in the stool, or a feeling of food "just sitting there." When such symptoms are present, it is relatively easy to connect the problem to some malfunction in the digestive process.

Problems that occur over time and are related to the long-term inefficient absorption of nutrients and/or an insufficiency of nutrients in the food to begin with are often not directly connected to digestive difficulties. Insufficient stomach acid production can result in malabsorption of calcium, leading to osteoporosis and osteoarthritis, for example. Periodontal problems may be caused by a deficiency of calcium and other nutrients. Anemia may be linked to low stomach acid levels, because iron is not absorbed efficiently. Poorly nourished skin is another common result of malabsorption due to digestive problems. The skin may show minor symptoms, such as blemishes, dryness, scaling, or a tendency toward irritation. These are often due to dietary deficiencies and/or poor absorption of calcium, zinc, vitamins A and E, and essential fatty acids.

CLINICAL EXPERIENCE

Traditional vs. Alternative Approaches

The differences between traditional and alternative medicine are particularly evident in the treatment of digestive disorders. In the traditional paradigm, a person is generally deemed healthy unless she has a major breakdown in the digestive apparatus or a major disease. In essence, the paradigm says that health is the absence of disease.

Traditional physicians are more used to treating symptoms than correcting causes. For this reason, one of the most common problems in digestion—a "cause" rather than a "symptom"—is one that is rarely considered in traditional medical practice. This is the *malabsorption syndrome*, or the failure of the body to absorb the nutrients that have been ingested. The problem here is that even though a food is eaten and goes through the digestive system, the nutrients, minerals, and vitamins do not get into the blood and hence do not penetrate the body at the cellular level.

Traditionally trained physicians are skilled at identifying and treating conditions when they have reached a disease state. Their approach to diagnosis and treatment is anatomical in nature. They use sophisticated technologies to evaluate the anatomy of the digestive tract—the stomach, pancreas, small intestine, colon, and liver—and look for evidence of tumors, polyps, ulcers, and other problems. They are less likely to search out or treat conditions such as underactivity, sluggishness, or suboptimal function. Even when such conditions are detected, they are often not considered significant.

The digestive process, like all body systems, produces a wide spectrum of symptoms when it is not functioning properly. Complementary physicians, who combine traditional medicine with alternative practices, consider mild or moderate symptoms to be signs of suboptimal functioning that should be addressed as such. These symptoms include burping, indigestion, and constipation. Complementary physicians often analyze the body biochemistry using sophisticated blood laboratory testing that goes beyond traditional medicine's use of the standard SMA-24 profile to identify major digestive disorders. They are very interested in the foods a person eats, and whether any specific foods cause irritation or other reactions. Thus they tend to test for food sensitivity as part of a complete analysis of body function.

In terms of treatment, complementary physicians tend to use natural substances such as foods, herbs, and homeopathic preparations. Supplements that contain concentrated forms of vitamins and minerals are fundamental elements of body rebalancing. Complementary physicians tend to be attuned to the concept of even the mildest malabsorption since they frequently see the end product of this condition, namely deficiencies of nutrients.

Dr. Martin Feldman's Approach to Digestive Wellness

Dr. Martin Feldman, whose ulcer protocol is described below, is a traditionally trained physician who practices complementary medicine. Over many years of practice, he has found that a surprisingly large number of health disorders are related to suboptimal digestion, which, as mentioned earlier, reduces the body's ability to absorb the vital nutrients needed for proper functioning. Rather than taking the traditional approach of waiting for symptoms to develop into full-blown disease states, Dr. Feldman strongly believes in treating sluggish conditions before they progress. By identifying and treating digestive system disorders when they first begin, he believes that many degenerative diseases can be avoided.

DIAGNOSIS

This approach makes use of standard medical procedures and tests. A complete medical history is taken, and comprehensive blood and laboratory analyses are conducted. Dr. Feldman looks for indicators of suboptimal functioning in the digestive system, such as a slight elevation of SGOT enzymes on an SMA-24 blood test. The SGOT, an enzyme found in liver cells, can double or triple in the presence of hepatitis. Traditional physicians will generally look for such extremely elevated levels and tend to disregard slightly elevated levels. Dr. Feldman, however, considers that even a small increase in the level of this enzyme can indicate that the liver, while not diseased, is off balance and in need of attention. As he explains, "I'm looking for the early evaluation of an imbalanced or a suboptimal liver, not a very diseased liver."

Lab tests can also disclose other indicators of malabsorption. These include low levels of minerals such as calcium, magnesium, zinc, manganese, chromium, and selenium, and deficiencies of fat-soluble vitamins such as vitamins A, D, and E. The water-soluble vitamins, including B complex and C, are generally less affected because they are more easily absorbed. Dr. Feldman also may test for bacteria and parasites.

In addition, Dr. Feldman uses a noninvasive technique, based on acupuncture pressure points, to test the strength of various internal organs and mechanisms. This technique can determine which components of a patient's digestion are sluggish by testing the level of electrical activity in their specific meridians. If the flow of energy in a given meridian field is deficient, that aspect of digestion is often suboptimal.

Dr. Feldman explains: "Acupuncture theory has taught us that there are many energy flows throughout the body. The energy flow is quite specific along anatomical pathways. A deficient electrical flow often reflects an organ weakness. Traditional acupuncture intervenes by inserting needles into specific acupuncture points to either improve the flow of electrical energy through that flow channel or meridian or to reduce the flow." Because he uses acupuncture theory only for diagnosis and not for treatment, Dr. Feldman has no need for needles. Instead, he uses meridians to profile the component parts of the digestive apparatus and pinpoint areas that are underactive or suboptimal in strength. In this way he can determine the energy flow or lack of flow and thus assess the body's function.

Once the areas of weakness are identified, Dr. Feldman may consult with a gastroenterologist to see if additional testing is needed, such as X rays or colonoscopy.

TREATMENT

Dr. Feldman then begins to formulate a plan to soothe, replace, repair, and rebuild faulty mechanisms. Treatment decisions are based on area of dysfunction, whether and where irritation is present, and whether any pathogens are present, such as parasites or unfriendly, harmful bacteria. To correct any of these problems, Dr. Feldman's treatment relies heavily on natural substances, including vitamins, minerals, herbs, and occasional homeopathic preparations.

The first step in this process is to soothe any parts of the digestive system that are irritated, whether the stomach, the small intestine, or the colon. Various herbal preparations, such as marshmallow, slippery elm, and aloe vera, may be used for this purpose. Aloe vera, in particular, can help soothe the ileocecal valve, the ascending or descending colon, or the entire digestive tract when it is irritated.

Next, it is important to replace whatever is insufficient or suboptimal. When deficiencies of stomach acid are determined, oral acid tablets (such as betaine hydrochloride or glutamic acid) may be prescribed in order to optimize the stomach-acid phase of digestion. Dr. Feldman warns that this therapy must be supervised by a knowledgeable practitioner. Other natural substances, including zinc, folic acid, intrinsic factor, and duodenal substance, can help get the stomach back on track to produce its own acid.

The most crucial step in Dr. Feldman's treatment is repair. The focus is on (1) eliminating negative influences on the organ in question, including foods that provoke allergic reactions, irritants such as caffeine, and poor food choices (such as fatty and denatured foods) that stress the digestive system; and (2) using natural therapies to rebuild the suboptimal or sluggish components of digestion. For example, the following substances may be used:

STOMACH—Cabbage juice, licorice, zinc, vitamin A, n-acetyl-glucosamine, marshmallow, ginger, and cayenne. Natural therapies such as goldenseal and a citrate bismuth can help to combat an infection of *Helicobacter pylori*, although an antibiotic may be needed as well to eliminate the bacteria.

ILEOCECAL VALVE—Lipid-soluble chlorophyll, aloe vera, slippery elm bark, and echinacea. Increased consumption of water can also help in the case of a closed valve.

COLON—For an imbalance of the ascending colon: bifido bacteria (which can help rebalance the ecology of the colon), fructooligosaccharides (FOS), insoluble fiber, and calendula. For a parasitic infection of the descending colon: grapefruit seed extract, black walnut herb, artemesia, and homeopathic antiparasite remedies. For a general irritation of the colon: aloe vera, lipid-soluble chlorophyll, butyric acid, Jerusalem artichoke flour, 1-glutamine, a mix of soluble and insoluble fiber, calcium, and magnesium.

LIVER—Choline, methionine, inositol, milk thistle, combination herbal formulas, and homeopathic solutions.

FOOD ALLERGY AND DIGESTION

Foods to which a person is allergic or sensitive are considered invaders by the body's immune system. Thus, they irritate and weaken the digestive apparatus. It is quite common to find that people consume large amounts of foods to which they are allergic. Reading food labels and choosing food correctly is a critical part of treatment.

Digestive malfunctioning can cause complications when allergens are present. If there is a deficiency of the gastric juices or pancreatic enzymes, for instance, a food will be in the system for a much longer time than it would if there were adequate amounts of acids and enzymes to break it down. If the food is one to which the body is sensitive, that sensitivity will be heightened by the delayed action of the digestive mechanism. Furthermore, if protein molecules are not broken down into small enough particles because of faulty digestive processes, the larger units entering the bloodstream will be treated like foreign invaders by the body's immune system, and an allergic reaction will ensue.

Children have less developed gastrointestinal systems than adults do, so they often suffer from obvious food allergies. Later in life, though, as the digestive system becomes more sophisticated, these allergies are manifested in less obvious ways. Even if the symptoms are not the same, the underlying allergy may be. A child who has suffered milk-associated asthma, for instance, may have severe acne as a teenager. The milk allergy is still there, but its symptoms have moved to a different organ system, often misleading the patient and physician into thinking that the original allergy has been outgrown.

High-Protein Diets

High-protein diets pose a special problem with respect to food allergies. People who consume a lot of protein usually tend to have it in their systems around the clock. This is because it takes at least four to seven hours for proteins to be digested, and if the protein is fried, deep-fried, or charcoal-broiled, it can take even longer. Consider the person who starts the day with bacon and eggs, has a sandwich of cold cuts and cheese at lunch, eats more meat and drinks milk at dinner, and tops it off with a late-night snack of ice cream. This person will have protein in his or her system all the time.

If any substance—in this case, protein—sits in the digestive system virtually all the time, two things will occur. First, the person will almost certainly develop an allergy to it because of overexposure. Second, the person will probably not be aware of the allergy because her system will never be without the substance long enough for her to notice changes due to its presence or absence. The negative symptoms then become cumulative and chronic, and are manifested as disease states. Digestion is usually strained, and the disorders that appear are generally regarded as signs of poor health, which becomes tolerated as unavoidable or is attributed to genetics or age.

Food Rotation

Food rotation is one way to help alleviate this problem. It can be combined with medical care. Don't eat the same foods day after day, because no matter how healthy and nutritious they are, you will not benefit from them if your body rejects or reacts negatively to them. Wheat, for example, is nutritious, but because it is found in practically every processed food, it is also a very common allergen. Therefore, it must be rotated in the diet with other grains. Eat it no more frequently than every fourth day and in no more than a 4-ounce portion at each meal. Then there is a good chance it can be eaten without causing an allergic reaction.

All foods should be rotated in this manner. Even if your body is not responding negatively in an overt way, you may be having hidden reactions to many different foods. Even if you are not, by overusing a food—eating it too frequently and in oversized portions—you may eventually develop an allergy to it. Try to make a routine of rotating all foods and avoid eating processed foods as much as possible because certain foods, such as corn and wheat, are ingredients in many of them.

LACTOSE INTOLERANCE

Lactose intolerance is a common digestive disorder. Probably two-thirds of the world's adults cannot tolerate lactose, which is found in milk and all milk products. When lactose-sensitive people continue to eat dairy products, they begin to suffer from a wide range of symptoms, which include abdominal cramping and bloating, chronic nasal discharge or postnasal drip, puffiness under the eyes, gas, and diarrhea.

Lactose intolerance is a malabsorption of lactose caused by a deficiency of lactase, the enzyme responsible for milk digestion. Lactase breaks lactose down into the readily digestible forms glucose and galactose. If it is absent or deficient, lactose remains undigested in the system. Some passes through the blood and is excreted in the urine, but most ends up in the large intestine. The lactose molecules draw water out of the tissues and into the intestinal cavity, while the undigested glucose is fermented by intestinal bacteria. Carbon dioxide is given off during this process, and diarrhea, bloating, flatulence, and belching may result.

The lactase deficiency can be caused by damage to the intestinal mucosa; this damage may be brought on by acute infectious diarrhea in infants. Malnutrition, cystic fibrosis, and colitis also have been known to cause lactase deficiency. Even in the absence of these traumas, lactose deficiency is very common.

The most obvious remedy for lactose intolerance is to stay away from milk and all milk products. Also, keep in mind that lactose is found in many vitamins and most processed foods, so it is best to avoid processed foods and request from vitamin manufacturers a full disclosure of their exact ingredients. It is important to eliminate lactose from the system completely in order to recover from its ravages. Another option may be to purchase a commercially prepared lactase supplement that boosts your supply of lactase and enables you to better digest the lactose. Some lactase-deficient people, however, can still eat a few fermented milk and dairy products without negative consequences. These items—primarily yogurt, buttermilk, and cottage cheese—must be tested on an individual basis to determine one's reaction to them.

GASTRITIS

Gastritis, another common digestive disorder, involves an inflammation of the mucosa lining the inner wall of the stomach. The inflammation is accompanied by symptoms such as nausea, vomiting, and loss of appetite. In the acute form, gastritis can be caused by infections and/or the ingestion of corrosive agents such as alcohol and aspirin. In the chronic form, gastritis is a serious condition that may be the cornerstone of degenerative diseases such as ulcers.

The treatment of gastritis should include the elimination of any substance (an allergen or anything else that is difficult to digest) known to be causing or aggravating the condition. The diet should include lots of liquids. Vegetables should be steamed to maximize their digestibility and reduce their acidity. A blood chemistry test should be performed to determine what, if any, vitamin deficiencies exist, since they often play an important role in this disorder. Vitamin deficiency related to gastritis is responsible for many complications, among which are a prickly sensation in the skin, loss of memory, depression, and general weakness.

PRESSURE DISEASES

Another group of disorders associated with the digestive system have been termed *pressure diseases* because they are caused by a pressure buildup that results from failure to eliminate waste efficiently. They include diverticulitis, hemorrhoids, hiatus hernia, and appendicitis, among others.

Diverticulitis

Diverticular disease is the most troublesome and widespread of the pressure conditions. It occurs when the muscle rings encircling the colon, which move along bulk matter, become clogged. Try clenching your fist and then imagine that mud is stuck in the creases of your hand. The creases can be thought of as diverticula, and the mud in them is food being trapped in the digestive organs. When bulk and fiber are lacking in the diet, the colon must deal with a mass of food too dry to be pushed along with ease, and so it becomes overworked, overstressed, and overstrained. Its membranes eventually herniate, or rupture, and it is these ruptures that are called diverticula. When there are many diverticula—and there can be hundreds—they tend to become inflamed and cause more acute symptoms. This condition is known as diverticulitis. Approximately one in four people with diverticular disease develop these acute symptoms.

Diverticulitis barely existed before the twentieth century, but now is said to affect one-third of all adults middle-aged or older, half the population over fifty, and two-thirds of the population over eighty. It is the most common digestive disorder of senior citizens.

Research on the genesis and development of diverticular disease has shown that it results from a gross lack of fiber in the diet. The refining of carbohydrates seems to be the main culprit here, since this condition is almost wholly absent in cultures where whole grains, legumes, vegetables, and such are the mainstays of the diet and where processed foods are not used.

The traditional treatment for diverticular disease has been to give the patient stool softeners to help the stool pass through the system and expanders to force it out. Antibiotics are also used. The patient is placed on a fibrous diet that helps the colon begin processing waste more efficiently and with less strain. Bran is usually prescribed, and patients are often told to avoid milk products and spicy foods, since these tend to produce abdominal pain, pressure, and gas.

Alternative treatments for diverticular disease may include the above suggestions but will add to the patient's diet other abdominal and intestinal cleansers taken orally. These include cellulose, hemicellulose, pectin, and noncarbohydrate lignin. Celery, brussels sprouts, broccoli, and especially beet juice will also help the condition. Bran should be unprocessed because this type has a shorter intestinal transit time and helps increase stool weight. The diverticula pockets may be cleansed with dietary supplements of chlorophyll, chamomile, garlic, vitamin C, zinc, nondairy acidophilus, pectin, and psyllium. Instead of medicinal antibiotics, natural antibiotics such as garlic may be used.

Hemorrhoids

Constantly straining to push dry, compacted stools out of the system causes the veins in the rectal and anal passages to become distended and engorged with blood. The veins become weakened, lose their elasticity, and can no longer carry blood properly. This causes the blood to pool instead, creating a ballooning effect known as a hemorrhoid.

When the hemorrhoids are internal, they can become obstructive to stool passage. With constant pressure being exerted against them, they may rupture and bleed and, in severe cases, hemorrhage. External hemorrhoids, also called piles, are very sensitive and may grow to the size of golf balls.

It is estimated that half of all Americans over fifty years of age have hemorrhoids and that hemorrhoidal treatment is a fifty-million-dollar-a-year industry. Most of the profit comes from sales of suppositories. Suppositories are given to shrink and lubricate hemorrhoids to prevent them from rupturing. Alternative treatments for hemorrhoids center on hygiene, diet, and exercise. Warm tub or sitz baths and ice packs may help. If you increase your intake of water, vitamin C, and fiber, and exercise regularly, the blood trapped in the hemorrhoidal veins will be reabsorbed into the body and the problem will be cleared up. However, it will recur unless you integrate these changes into a new, more healthful lifestyle.

Prevention of the recurrence of hemorrhoids is aimed at changing conditions associated with the pressure and straining of constipation. Doctors will often recommend increasing fiber and fluids in the diet. Eating the right amount of fiber and drinking six to eight glasses of fluid (not alcohol) result in softer, bulkier stools. A softer stool makes emptying the bowels easier and lessens the pressure on hemorrhoids caused by straining.

Eliminating straining also helps prevent the hemorrhoids from protruding. Good sources of fiber are fruits, vegetables, and whole grains. In addition, doctors may suggest a bulk stool softener or a fiber supplement such as psyllium (Metamucil) or methylcellulose (Citrucel).

In some cases, hemorrhoids must be treated surgically. These methods are used to shrink and destroy the hemorrhoidal tissue and are performed under anesthesia. The doctor will perform the surgery during an office or hospital visit.

Hiatus Hernia

Hiatus hernia is another condition related to constipation and low-fiber dietary regimens. Like the other pressure diseases, it is essentially a modern-day Western disorder affecting primarily middle-aged and older people. There are no warning symptoms until it causes a sharp pain just below the breastbone. It is a condition in which part of the stomach wall becomes distended and pushes up against the diaphragm and the skeletal system. Obesity may contribute to the condition, which also sometimes develops during pregnancy.

The traditional treatment for hiatus hernia usually includes antacids, a bland diet, and sometimes surgery. These steps are adequate to relieve the pain, and you certainly should follow the suggestions of your physician. The alternative (or even complementary) approach is aimed at going beyond alleviation of the painful symptoms by establishing a dietary regimen that can reverse the condition while ameliorating the source of discomfort. Since constipation due to a low-fiber diet is frequently the cause of this condition, make sure to get plenty of high-fiber bulk foods. Losing weight may also help.

Appendicitis

Appendicitis is an inflammation of the appendix, a small pouch that extends from the first part of the large intestine. The appendix has no known function. It can become diseased as a result of infection or obstructed from contents moving through the intestinal tract.

Appendicitis is caused mainly by troublesome elimination. The most common abdominal emergency in the Western world, it is often brought on by continuous constipation, straining during stool elimination, and anal retention—failing to evacuate solid waste when the body tells you to. By delaying your bowel movements, perhaps because you are too busy to be inconvenienced, you confuse your body. The water from fecal matter begins to be reabsorbed, and the dry, hard stool that is left will pass only with great pain and difficulty. In the meantime, you strain the muscles that must retain this mass and eventually train them to delay normal elimination.

Some people learn to have a bowel movement only once a day or even once every two or three days. You should have two or three bowel movements a day, depending, of course, on what and how often you eat. When there is not enough dietary fiber to move food and waste readily through the digestive system, pressure builds up and blocks the passage of stool. Bacteria accumulates and backs up into the 3- to 6-inch-long appendix, which is attached to the large intestine. The appendix becomes inflamed and infected, and an appendectomy must be performed.

To see how critical the issue of fiber is here, consider the six thousand appendectomies performed in the United States each week compared with only a handful per year in rural Africa, where processed fiber-depleted food is virtually nonexistent. This again is a pressure disease that can be avoided or even treated with a high-fiber diet consisting of complex carbohydrates.

ULCERS

Ulcers of the digestive tract afflict as many as fourteen million Americans. About one in twenty women suffer from ulcers. Digestive-system ulcers occur most often in the duodenum, which is the upper portion of the small intestine. The duodenal ulcer is usually found in the first few inches of the duodenum. The second most common type is the peptic or gastric ulcer, which affects the stomach.

Some ulcers are slight abrasions of the internal mucosal lining; others advance to the stage where they totally perforate the stomach or intestinal wall. Their three stages of development are known as perforation, penetration, and obstruction. In acute perforation, the ulcer eats through the wall of the abdomen. This is the most serious state and causes the greatest number of deaths. Surgery to close the perforation is virtually unavoidable.

Penetration is the stage where the patient usually awakens at night with severe pain in adjacent areas of the body—the back, liver, and so forth—not just the stomach. This transfer of effect to other organs makes the ulcer hard to diagnose. Obstruction is the stage in which swelling caused by inflammation affects the stomach and the opening to the small intestine.

The vast majority of ulcers are caused by the *Helicobacter pylori* bacteria. These bacteria take up residence in the lining of the digestive tract and then contribute to the breakdown of that lining, resulting in a lesion or crater. Doctors used to think that ulcers were caused by stress or the production of too much hydrochloric acid.

Traditional Treatment

Traditional physicians generally limit their treatment to the use of antibiotics to combat the bacteria, and acid-production blockers such as Tagamet and Zantac to prevent the stomach acid from irritating the broken-down tissues in the mucosal lining. The heavy reliance on acid-production blockers is troublesome for two reasons: The drugs do not address the real issue, which is why the bacteria have proliferated in the digestive wall; and since the natural stomach acid opposes the bacteria, the blockers may reduce the body's ammunition against the infection. In the process, these drugs may also lessen the effectiveness of the overall digestive process. The stomach's role in digestion is to produce acids that help to digest foods. When that mechanism is suppressed by acid-production blockers, the body may not digest foods efficiently and absorb nutrients. Thus, a patient may suffer from malabsorption.

Alternative Approach

As a complementary physician, Dr. Martin Feldman advocates a much more comprehensive approach to the treatment of ulcers. In addition to eliminating the bacteria, he says, the treatment should accomplish three goals: helping the stomach to heal the erosion; rebalancing the stomach acid production so that it works properly; and optimizing the immune system so that the body can protect against reinfection.

DIAGNOSIS

The mainstream medical community uses endoscopes and upper–GI X rays to determine if an ulcer actually exists. Dr. Feldman may call on these diagnostic techniques as well to obtain as much scientific data as possible on the status of an ulcer. He also uses tests performed by specialty laboratories to identify the presence of *Helicobacter pylori*. Dr. Feldman also draws on his clinical judgment in the diagnostic process. If the laboratory blood test is negative but his clinical experience suggests the presence of *Helicobacter pylori*, he may conduct a therapeutic trial by having the patient take some natural substances that combat the bacteria. He can use this technique because the substances are safe and well tolerated, producing very few side effects. Dr. Feldman then monitors the patient to determine if the therapy reduces the symptoms.

OPPOSING THE BACTERIA

Both antibiotics and natural substances can be used to fight the *Helicobacter pylori* infection. For antibiotic treatments, Dr. Feldman favors the use of amoxicillin because it is usually effective and well tolerated by most patients. In addition, he may combat the bacteria at a second level with natural therapies. These include goldenseal, an herb that has antibacterial properties, the mineral bismuth in a citrate form, and various combinations of homeopathic solutions. Because homeopathic solutions function primarily as transmitters of energy, Dr. Feldman can test the effect of specific homeopathic products on the body's acupuncture-meridian energy fields.

HEALING THE ULCER

In addition to removing the bacteria, it's important to help the body heal the ulcer irritation or erosion. Dr. Feldman uses a variety of natural treatments to heal the digestive lining. These include cabbage juice, aloe vera, licorice herb, and n-acetyl-glucosamine, a nutrient complex. Other substances that soothe the irritation and thus promote the healing process are marshmallow, ginger, cayenne, and an herbal combination called Robert's Formula.

TESTING FOR FOOD ALLERGIES

Food allergens tend to irritate the stomach, making it harder to heal an ulcer or any other irritation of the stomach or intestines. Therefore, any foods to which a patient is allergic should be eliminated from the diet. To identify such offenders, Dr. Feldman will test a patient's reaction to various food substances by placing them upon the taste portion of the tongue. The brain-taste mechanism, which is very highly developed, has the ability to ascertain if a given food substance is a danger to the body.

REBALANCING THE ACID-PRODUCTION MECHANISM

Paradoxically, many patients with ulcers have a low production of stomach acid. As Dr. Feldman notes, the low-acid environment allows the *Helicobacter pylori* bacteria to get a foothold in the mucosal lining, while a normal acid level would tend to provide some antibacterial protection.

In addition to allowing the bacteria to grow, a low acid production can cause other problems. One is that food will sit in the stomach for a long period of time and ferment abnormally due to the lack of sufficient stomach acid. This fermentation then produces abnormal acids that irritate the stomach and the ulcer. The result: People with low stomach acid experience the symptoms of a high acid production. They may take antacids to suppress the symptoms, but that remedy doesn't correct the true problem. The stomach must work efficiently so that food does not ferment abnormally.

Dr. Feldman has found that many patients suffer from this problem, so he puts a strong emphasis on reoptimizing the stomach's acid mechanism. Again, he uses a variety of natural therapies to get the acid-production system back on track. These remedies include zinc, folic acid, intrinsic factor, and duodenal substance. In some cases, he also prescribes oral acid supplements, which may assist the acid mechanism in strengthening itself. This latter treatment requires careful supervision to ensure that a patient takes the proper form of acid in the proper doses.

REPAIRING THE IMMUNE SYSTEM

As a final phase in his treatment of ulcers, Dr. Feldman focuses on rebuilding the immune system. The logic here, of course, is that the immune system must be working at its maximum level to fight the bacteria that cause most ulcers in the first place. This part of the treatment consists of nutrients that serve as the building blocks of the immune system. They include vitamins A, E and C, bioflavonoids, gamma linolenic acid (GLA), essential fatty acids, zinc, and selenium.

FOODS TO AVOID

As a final note, people who suffer from ulcers should avoid ingesting substances that exacerbate the condition. These include alcohol, nicotine, aspirin, coffee, soft drinks, salt, high-oil nuts, and even raw fruit (except bananas). Foods that are excessively spicy and difficult to digest should be avoided as well.

You don't want to eat a lot of high-protein foods, especially those that are high in fat. Animal foods require more gastric involvement and should be avoided if possible. If you do eat meat, at least trim off the fat; also avoid overcooking, deep frying, and charcoal broiling since these processes make the molecules bond more tightly so that more digestive effort is required to break them down.

Carbohydrate foods have their own protective buffer in the natural state (brown rice and whole grain and vegetables), but once they are refined (white flour and white rice, cakes and pastries) the buffer is stripped away. Therefore, avoid denatured, processed carbohydrates. Vegetables are usually quite acidic, so avoid those causing gas (turnips, cucumbers, brussels sprouts, broccoli, radishes, and cauliflower), especially in the raw state. Vegetables will be less acidic if you cook them, preferably by steaming since it does not destroy their fibrous structure.

CHAPTER 11

EATING DISORDERS

E ating disorders have plagued women in Western societies. Among the most common are anorexia, bulimia, and obesity. Anorexia involves compulsive dieting to the point where the woman eats so little that she becomes malnourished and may actually starve to death. It is marked by muscle wasting, loss of menstrual periods, body image problems, and an exaggerated fear of becoming fat. Bulimia is compulsive eating and forced vomiting or the use of laxatives or diuretics to eliminate the calories that are consumed during binge episodes. Obesity is an enormous increase in the ratio of fat to muscle, the result of eating to excess, far beyond what the body needs.

CAUSES

Carolyn Costin, author of *The Dieting Daughter* and other books, came to the study of eating disorders through her own experience: "I had anorexia myself when I was about sixteen years old. I had a pretty severe case, was seventy-nine pounds for a few years." In Costin's opinion, a number of seemingly benign factors, such as the emphasis on exercising and dieting in our culture, as well as interpersonal family pressures may cause a person to fall into any of these negative eating practices.

Eating Behaviors

The problem with diets is that they often disappoint their users. Costin explains, "The main thing I say to people about any kind of diet program is, 'Don't do anything to lose weight that you're not prepared to do for the rest of your life, because going on a diet certainly implies that you'll ultimately go off it.'"

So what happens when you go off it? This will lead to disillusionment and weight disorders, such as constantly going on and off trendy diets, unless a person realizes that a healthy lifestyle, not a temporary eating change, is the only answer to maintaining proper weight.

Another problem is that a healthy desire to exercise can be developed in the wrong way. This, Costin says, is "a little bit like an activity disorder. They can't not do it. There's an addictive component that makes them have to do more and more. Things in their life get put on hold in order to do the activity. They will continue to do it even if they've been injured or are in pain or it's snowing outside. And the way the eating disorders correlate with activity disorders, there are certainly a lot of anorexics and bulimics who also have activity disorder."

In Costin's view, eating disorders are also caused by the way people obsessively codify rules of eating, what she calls "the Thin Commandments." She notes, "Over the years I started to come up with these rules that people with eating disorders have, such as 'If I eat anything, then I have to exercise and burn it off' or 'I have to wear clothes to make myself look thinner. I have to punish myself if I've eaten anything fattening.'"

Interpersonal Relationships

Delving deeper, one finds that eating disorders in women are often rooted in relationships they had with their parents, particularly their mothers, though not the type of relationship that's commonly assumed to be at fault. "In the beginning," Costin explains, "anorexia nervosa was often blamed on over-controlling mothers. But that's way too simplistic." Rather, the problem is the type of role models that mothers sometimes provide for their daughters. Costin asks, "What are little girls learning from these role models about their bodies and about weight and about food?"

Not only those who actually end up with eating disorders but almost all young women and girls are influenced by these role models. Costin says, "When you have statistics that 80 percent of fourth-grade girls report that they're dieting and 10 or 11 percent of those girls report that they're vomiting on these diets, you've got to look at what's happening with their role models."

Costin describes a six-year-old girl in her waiting room who said she was really excited at having chicken pox. Asked why, she said it meant going to bed without any dinner. "I said, 'Well, what's so good about that?' And she said, 'Because it means I didn't have any calories.' The thing is, she's six. Her mother was a binge eater seeing me for treatment. But kids are little sponges. And she hears her mother saying that calories are bad, so she just learns that part of being female is trying not to have too many calories."

Fathers can also have a negative influence. "I talk to fathers a lot," Costin comments, "about being conscious about what they say about female bodies when they're reading magazines or watching television or things like that. I talk to them about not just praising their daughters for the way they look, which is a very common thing that fathers do with their little girls. A lot of praise and attention focus on appearance as opposed to internal validation. I also encourage them to pay attention to who their daughter is, and to do things with their daughter."

Genetics

There is mounting evidence that eating disorders have some basis in genetics. Costin states, "It's pretty clear from twin studies that we're going to learn more and more in the next few years about genes that predispose people to inherit this. It's probably going to turn out that there's a biological predisposition. And then maybe a cultural trigger sets it off. Thus, there's a swing back to a more biological basis of these illnesses and not as much of a focus on the big, bad culture. But I think there's no doubt that the culture plays a big role in it, which is why we see over the years an increasing incidence of anorexia and bulimia. But I think it's a combination of someone who has a predisposition and dieting, which is certainly a risk factor. So if more of the population is dieting, more people who have the biological predisposition are exposed to this trigger."

Zinc Deficiency

Some research has shown that anorexia nervosa, bulimia, and obesity may be the result of a zinc deficiency. Dr. Alexander Schauss, a clinical psychologist and eating-disorders specialist from Tacoma, Washington, reports that science has long been aware of this connection: "We've known since at least the 1930s that when animals were experimentally placed on diets deficient in zinc, those animals would develop anorexia. Our interest in eating disorders in relationship to zinc has to do with the observation that when humans are placed on zinc-deficient diets, they, too, develop eating disorders."

"By characterizing three of the most common eating disorders," Dr. Schauss continues, "you can see how vital zinc is. In morbid obesity, when people are significantly overweight in such a way that it could shorten their life span or increase their risk of disease, we know that there is an inverse relationship between the level of obesity and the level of zinc, meaning that the more obese they are, the less zinc they have in the body. We don't know yet whether this is cause or effect, but it is a very important observation because at the other end of the continuum, with anorexia nervosa, self-induced starvation, we also have individuals who are generally always zinc-deficient. We believe there is strong evidence today…that the lower the zinc status is, the more likely it is that the patient will not recover from any treatment plan to resolve the anorexia."

Stress is commonly associated with the onset and continuation of eating disorders and can also be understood in terms of zinc loss, since constant mental stress results in the depletion of this mineral. Women are more prone to stress-related zinc loss than men and therefore more likely to have eating disorders. Dr. Schauss explains: "The answer may lie in the fact that males have prostate glands and women do not. Zinc is highly concentrated in the prostate in males; it provides a mineral that is essential for the development, motility, viability, and quantity of sperm. If a male is under psychological stress, he can catabolize or seek out stores of zinc in the prostate. Since women don't have a prostate, they will catabolize the zinc from other tissue.

"In women, the richest source of zinc is found in muscle tissue and bone. A common feature of anorexia is muscle wasting and an increased risk of osteoporosis. Anorexics actually catabolize or eat their own tissue as a way of releasing nutrients they are not getting in the diet. The last muscle, and one that contains only about 1 percent zinc, is the heart muscle. When the body starts to scavenge zinc out of heart muscle tissue, it can interfere with the heart's function, which contributes to bradycardia, tachycardia, arrhythmia, and eventual heart failure. It is particularly dangerous when patients with damaged hearts are in recovery. As they put on weight, they add extra pressure to the heart. That is what killed the singer Karen Carpenter, for example."

CLINICAL EXPERIENCE

Nutritional Treatment

Carolyn Costin outlines some of the basic approaches to nutritional therapy. "There are many ways to do nutritional therapy with eating-disorder patients," she notes. "One is educational. A dietitian will do some educational sessions. The patients have a lot of myths about food, such as 'If I eat anything with sugar, it's going to turn into fat' or 'If I eat anything at night, it's going to turn into fat.' So you send them just to be educated."

Costin may also combine education with therapy. This is needed because "patients' food fears are related to some very deeply rooted psychological stuff. So you combine nutrition therapy and nutrition education."

There are various ways to do this. "For example," Costin explains, "I can send someone to a dietitian, and they get a food plan set up. They get some help, and they go for a few weeks, and then they continue with their therapy, but they don't go back for more nutritional sessions until they're ready to take the next step."

Psychological Counseling

The first step in counseling is to help the person analyze why she has this problem. Costin starts off by asking, "Why do you have this disorder? What's good about it? How has it helped you? Let's talk about the advantages of it.'

The person needs to understand how the eating disorder has "come to serve a purpose. And that's the whole psychological aspect of it.

"Getting to the emotional aspect is really, really important, and if you don't deal with that, I think you don't really deal with the illness."

Supplements

Costin finds supplements helpful in treating eating disorders: "We're using amino acids in some cases with patients instead of medication, and it's working. It's pretty interesting. We use tyrosine and tryptophan and glutamine."

More specifically she recommends "the use of tryptophan, particularly with bulimia nervosa. We use it for people who have trouble sleeping as well. Phenylalanine also, for depression. Tyrosine for depression. For people who are often given medications such as Ritalin, we use a combination of tyrosine, glutamine, and phenylalanine together."

Dr. Schauss adds that liquid zinc may have a positive effect in the treatment of eating disorders, as it is directly absorbed into the blood. Powders, tablets, and capsules, which must first be broken down by the stomach and absorbed by the small intestine, do not work as well because many eating-disorder patients are unable to digest nutrients properly. Dr. Schauss has found only one brand available in the United States, Zinc Status (supplied by Ethical Nutrients of San Clemente, California), to be effective in clinical trials. Other liquid zincs are not autoclaved (sterile); although they are cheaper, they have not proved effective. Once the patient shows marked improvement, a good zinc supplement will do unless deterioration occurs, in which case the more expensive Zinc Status is needed again.

While results are not usually immediate, taking from several days to weeks, once liquid zinc takes effect, its benefits are long-lasting. According to Dr. Schauss, "In fifteen years I worked with hundreds of eating-disorder patients. Until I saw this treatment, my colleagues and I felt that the best we could expect in long-term outcome in treating patients with either bulimia or anorexia was maybe a 20 to 30 percent recovery. In our five-year study, we found that bulimics had a 64.1 percent success rate after recovery on the liquid zinc treatment. In anorexic patients, our five-year follow-up study found an 85 percent recovery rate. These are extraordinarily high recovery rates for a condition that is considered difficult to treat and insidious."

Another favorable finding is that liquid zinc can lift the depression that is usually associated with eating disorders. Dr. Schauss reports, "In our eating-disorder studies, we used a multidimensional design and evaluated the mood state of our patients. One of the first things to improve was the degree of depression they were experiencing based on psychometric instruments such as the Beck Depression Scale and the Profile of Mood Scales, among other depressive indexes. The fact that we have discovered this antidepressive effect and could document it in patients under blind conditions is of great value."

Refeeding

People recovering from bulimia and anorexia need to return to normal eating patterns gradually. Carolyn Costin explains: "In fact, a lot of the deaths that happened early on with anorexia occurred during the refeeding process, because the heart just can't take the volume that you start giving it if you do the refeeding too fast."

In her practice, "We slowly raise the patients' calories. We get lab tests two to three times a week. We take their pulse in the morning and sometimes even during the day and after meals just to make sure their bodies are handling the stress that comes from refeeding. You can't just take someone who's emaciated and say okay, start eating."

Cognitive Therapy

Dr. José Yaryura-Tobias, an orthomolecular psychiatrist, also finds that because of the life-threatening severity of a condition such as anorexia nervosa, any nutritional approach must be preceded by a program of cognitive therapy: "Anorexia nervosa, from our perspective, is an obsessive-compulsive disorder that is related to self-image, the way that we perceive ourselves. Basically, anorexia nervosa is the process by which a human being self-starves. Thirty percent of the population who self-starve eventually die.

"In the vast majority of cases, when patients come for a consultation, they are already very emaciated. The chemistry we can measure is very altered. From the biochemical viewpoint, we know that there is a groove related to an area of the brain called the limbic system. This is the hypothalamic area, which regulates sugar, thirst, appetite, and so forth. This information can help us classify some of these patients but does not tell us how to manage and eventually cure the problem. The rest of the problem, we feel, has to do with body-image perception, the way these patients see their own bodies. They feel too fat. They have different perspectives than the rest of us do.

"How do we treat this condition? Basically, we use a nutritional approach after the patient has undertaken a behavioral program with cognitive therapy. Cognitive therapy is important because the idea is to educate the person about her problems and to discuss with her the many false beliefs she has about who she is, why she thinks this way, why her body looks the way it does for her, and so forth. So false-belief modification is an important part of treatment."

Breaking the Cycle of Food Addiction

Dr. Hyla Cass, a holistic psychiatrist who integrates psychotherapy and nutritional medicine, describes her experience as follows: "Some time ago, a psychologist who specializes in eating disorders began to send her clients to me because she had heard that antidepressant medications work for these patients. I had shifted to a more holistic way of looking at things, so I told the psychologist that before I did anything with antidepressants I would try some other things. With certain eating disorders, such as food cravings, the underlying problem is a food allergy. We often crave the very foods to which we are allergic. Typically, it's the very things we want to eat that are the most damaging, that create the symptoms. In fact, it's like an addiction to alcohol: As you abstain from the foods you're addicted to, you begin to have withdrawal symptoms and crave those foods even more.

"In order to break the cycle in cases of food addiction, just as in breaking the cycle with drinking (alcoholics are actually allergic to alcohol), you need to supply the body with the appropriate nutrients. When we correct the deficiencies and restore body balance, the food cravings and allergy symptoms will often be relieved. Rather than having to rely strictly on 'willpower,' it is possible for individuals to break addictive cycles by achieving metabolic balance through avoiding the offending foods and supporting the body with a balanced nutritional program of vitamins, minerals, and amino acids. Often the cravings will then simply go away. It's quite remarkable: With a good vitamin and mineral product, you can often put a stop to the food allergy and its accompanying symptoms.

"I may order a plasma amino acid analysis, a blood test to determine which amino acids—especially among the essential ones the body cannot synthesize by itself—are low. The amino acid glutamine, in a dose of 500 to 1,000 milligrams, is particularly useful for reducing cravings, including alcohol cravings.

"There are other things to do for food allergies as well," Dr. Cass adds. "Addictions and allergies are often related to magnesium deficiency and can be corrected by supplementation. There are also techniques that can actually eliminate food allergies through the use of acupuncture and acupressure."

"As we can see," Dr. Cass concludes, "there are many ways, other than psychotherapy and medication, to approach what at first seems like a psychological problem."

Carolyn Costin, however, disagrees with those who say that eating disorders such as bulimia are an addiction like alcoholism: "It's really, really important that you can be recovered from conditions such as anorexia and bulimia. With alcoholism, you have it and your body responds to alcohol differently. For your whole life you can't have a drink because you are then going to be off the wagon and compulsively drink." This is distinct from eating disorders: "For example, the approach to bulimia shouldn't be, well, okay, if you eat chocolate you binge on it, and therefore you can't eat chocolate. I think that instead we have to learn how to teach you that you can absolutely be in control of this. You have to learn how to have it without bingeing and purging it.

"The bottom line is that the new studies show that people become fully recovered from these illnesses. It takes a long time. The new research shows approximately five to eight years, but the recovery rates are high, much higher than originally thought. It's like 76 percent full recovery with anorexia nervosa. There's fewer studies on bulimia, but it's pretty good."

Food Cravings and Emotional States

Dr. Doreen Virtue, former director of a clinic and inpatient psychiatric unit specializing in eating disorders, has a Ph.D. in counseling psychiatry and is the author of several books on dieting and health, including *Constant Craving from A to Z.*

"Most nutritionists would have you believe that nutritional deficiencies are at the heart of all food cravings," Dr. Virtue says. "The problem with that approach is that it still leaves many food cravings unexplained. Food cravings tend to be so specific. For example, a person may crave a hard-boiled egg but not a soft-boiled egg. Or a person may want a chocolate candy bar but not chocolate pudding. It sounds bizarre and a little childish, but anyone who has experienced food cravings will understand how intense and specific they can be.

"Another reason why nutrient deficiencies may not be the only possible cause of these cravings is that not everyone satisfies his or her craving for food before the craving passes. Just as mysteriously as the food craving appears, it may vanish. A food craving can change as easily as a person's state of mind." Dr. Virtue has been researching food cravings for twelve years and has found patterns that correlate with people's personalities and emotional issues. Again and again, for instance, she found that someone who craved, say, bread was very different from someone who craved ice cream. It's similar to drug-taking behavior. Someone addicted to marijuana, say, has a very different personality and style from someone addicted to another drug.

Noting this, she says, "I investigated further to look at the correlation between personality, emotional and spiritual issues, and how they are connected to food cravings. I did a great deal of research in university libraries, looking at the psychoactive, that is, mood-altering, chemicals found in different foods. I'm not talking about chemicals such as pesticides. I mean the inherent properties, such as vitamins, minerals, amino acids, and so on, that can actually increase or decrease our blood pressure and trigger the pleasure centers of the brain and other areas, chemicals that really affect our moods and energy.

"What I found is that we all tend to act as intuitive pharmacists. We tend to crave foods that will bring us to a state of homeostasis, which means balance or peace of mind. Whenever we are upset, it is normal for us to do something to fix that. If we don't want to take direct action, for instance, by making changes overtly in our lives, a more covert way of dealing with the upset is food cravings, which are cravings for a chemical that will make the body feel at peace."

From this point of view, Dr. Virtue believes that food cravings should be dealt with by trying to understand their underlying emotional sources. Instead of getting angry at yourself for having food cravings, thinking, "Oh, I'm so weak. I should have more willpower," it's better and healthier to listen to those cravings, which are a form of intuition. As Dr. Virtue puts it, "Deciphering them is almost like dream interpretation. They can give us guidance in our lives and help us in many ways."

Just as a food craving is not due to a nutritional deficiency, neither is it due to physical hunger. Dr. Virtue explains, "Let's think about the difference between emotional hunger and physical hunger. They can feel identical, and actually, this is one of the most important points in managing the appetite: to know the difference between emotional cravings and physical cravings."

She notes several underlying differences. For one thing, emotional hunger comes all of a sudden, out of the blue. As she puts it, "You feel like you are starving. Whereas physical hunger is gradual, at one moment you might just feel a little pang in your stomach, then over the course of the next hour or so it grows into a voracious hunger."

The second difference is that emotional hunger is usually for a very specific food. It has to be Rocky Road ice cream or it must be a pepperoni pizza. Physical hunger, while it may have preferences, is open to different types of food. It doesn't require an exact type of food to be satisfied.

Third, Dr. Virtue says, "Emotional hunger is always above the neck, whereas physical hunger is based in the stomach. Emotional hunger is a kind of 'mouth hunger' where you get a taste for a certain thing. It's a very cerebral type of hunger. It is also very urgent. It has to be satisfied now, whereas physical hunger says, 'I am hungry but I could wait fifteen minutes or a half hour if I needed to.'"

The demanding nature of emotional food cravings is due to the urge's misguided attempt to fill an emotional hole: "One of the reasons emotional hunger is urgent is that it really is uncomfortable with the feeling and wants to make that feeling go away. Emotional hunger is also usually paired with some upsetting emotion. And if we stop for a moment when we are experiencing this emotion and ask, 'Could there possibly be something that upset me that I wasn't acknowledging?' as we go into introspection, we usually see that a clerk was rude or a driver cut us off on the road. We are upset, not really hungry."

Specific Trigger Foods

Usually, if you really look at it, Dr. Virtue notes, there are a few trigger foods that cause a voracious appetite. If you want to find out what your triggers are, you can ask a friend or someone who eats with you, "What kind of food do I seem to binge on?" If you are aware of your own food cravings, you can ask yourself, What's going on and how do I feel?, the same way you would about stress.

Dr. Virtue says, "What I've found is that several factors are involved that correlate the particular trigger food to the emotions. One is the texture. Is the food crunchy or soft or chewy? The next is the actual physical components and the underlying chemical properties that either increase or decrease blood pressure, elevate or lower mood, and create neurochemicals that alter mood. The last thing is the flavor or the taste, whether it's spicy, salty, sugary. All these things have to do with who we are as a personality."

Again, identifying your trigger foods is a way to understand what your underlying fears and other emotions are expressing. "Instead of getting mad at ourselves for craving these things," she counsels, "we need to see our cravings as a blessing in disguise. It's the body's way of talking to us. It's just like when a person puts his or her hand on a hot plate. Then the body talks back and says, 'Get that hand off that heat.' Our appetite is trying to do the same sort of thing and give us a message."

Insulin Reaction and Overeating

Colette Heimowitz has a master's degree in nutrition from Hunter College, is certified in health and nutrition by Pratt University, and has twenty years of clinical experience in weight management. The number-one biological cause of obesity in our sedentary population, she maintains, must be understood in terms of insulin resistance: "In a normal homeostasis, an individual ingests a carbohydrate and it raises the glucose levels in the blood. When someone eats protein or fat, by contrast, this doesn't happen. Once the glucose level rises in the blood, it sparks an insulin response from the pancreas. What the insulin does is take the glucose to the peripheral tissues, either to the fat cells, the liver, or to muscle as storage. As a result of years of eating refined carbohydrates, maintaining high-sugar diets, and living a sedentary life, when we age, the insulin is no longer efficient at taking the glucose to the peripheral tissue.

"One of two things happens. Either the glucose levels remain high or the insulin is constantly being produced—overproduced in a prediabetic state—and fat is constantly being stored. When we are sedentary, the process of burning glucose for energy is not happening. It will even provoke the reaction more."

Among the factors that contribute to insulin resistance, "one, of the utmost importance, is lifestyle, a sedentary lifestyle. Some research was done with retired master athletes. Glucose tolerance tests with insulin levels were studied before putting them on bed rest for only one day. The glucose tolerance factors were normal, and the glucose in the blood was normal, because they were still leading an active life, not an elite athlete life, but still one that was active. After one day of bed rest, the glucose tolerance test was repeated and the glucose levels were much higher."

Equally important, Heimowitz says, was a history of eating refined foods, which "the American public is known for—taking the bran out of food, taking the fiber out of food, and replacing the essential fatty acids with hydrogenated fats. This causes a complete stress on the insulin level. The glycemic index of foods [a measurement of the amount of glucose found in the blood as a result of eating a specific food] is much higher, provoking more of an insulin response. The pancreas eventually gets trigger-happy."

There is also a genetic component. It has been shown that people whose parents have a history of diabetes or cardiovascular disease have a weak gene that makes them susceptible to this particular condition. She says, "They have to be especially careful and have an active lifestyle and a low-saturated-fat, higher-protein, lower-carbohydrate diet."

TREATMENT

To alter this continuous fat-and-flabby syndrome, a lower-carbohydrate diet is needed to give the pancreas a rest. Heimowitz recommends eating "low-glycemic-index-type foods, that is, complex whole foods such as fruits and vegetables." She also recommends specific supplements for the insulin-resistant individual.

Alpha lipoic acid is the biological spark plug in converting glucose to energy. She states, "It can lower and stabilize glucose levels and stimulate insulin activity. Some research was done with diabetics being given 600 milligrams daily, and it stabilized their glucose levels without any medication. A nondiabetic or hypoglycemic person could probably use 200 to 300 milligrams a day."

The mineral vanadium, found in vanadyl sulfate, also reduces insulin resistance; 15 to 30 milligrams a day is appropriate.

Chromium is a component of the glucose tolerance factor, a molecule essential for normal insulin function in glucose metabolism. Usually 200 to 1,000 micrograms daily is the range for a beneficial effect.

Heimowitz also emphasizes "essential fatty acids, which are grossly lacking in the American diet and also improve insulin sensitivity and reduce insulin resistance. So supplementing the diet with 3,000 to 6,000 milligrams of the omega-3 fatty acids is appropriate."

Vitamin E is also important. It relieves some of the oxidative stress caused by excessive glucose, which results in free radicals. It will also reduce the risk of cardiovascular disease. Heimowitz adds, "Excessive insulin also causes a lipidation of the triglycerides, and that causes free radical pathology. The excessive insulin also thickens the aortic valve. You are at a higher risk of cardiovascular disease. The vitamin E should be anywhere between 400 and 800 international units [IU] daily."

Zinc also influences carbohydrate metabolism, increases the insulin response, improves glucose tolerance, influences the basal metabolism rate, and supports thyroid function; 50 to 100 milligrams of zinc a day is important.

Magnesium helps maintain tissue sensitivity so that insulin is more effective at taking that glucose to the peripheral tissues. Magnesium helps control glucose metabolism and also decreases sugar cravings; 500 to 1,000 milligrams a day is recommended. "Sometimes," she cautions, "when you go as high as

1,000 milligrams, it may cause diarrhea, so the dose should be determined individually. People should start at 500 and work up slowly."

Heimowitz notes that manganese has been shown in studies to be important for insulin activity: "Manganese-deficient rats showed reduced insulin activity and impaired glucose tolerance. This lack also lowered glucose oxidation and the conversion of triglycerides in the rats' adipose tissues. However, the manganese should be dosed in relation to zinc and copper because they will compete at the cell site. So as little as 35 milligrams of manganese is all you need. The proportionate amount of zinc would be 100 milligrams."

She notes further, "If someone has hypotension because of the insulin resistance, the amino acid tyrosine could also help control the hypotension; 1,500 to 3,000 milligrams daily is appropriate. Hawthorn berry, an herb, can also help control hypotension; 240 to 480 milligrams is a good range.

"When there is cardiovascular involvement, with a high risk, especially with low HDL [high-density lipoprotein] and elevated triglycerides in individuals with insulin resistance, coenzyme Q10 is also appropriate. I suggest 100 to 200 milligrams a day."

Lack of exercise also causes blood sugar problems. Thus, exercise is key. Heimowitz recommends that "for exercise, we look at the fitness level of the individual. I wouldn't tell someone who has been a couch potato to go out and exercise an hour a day. The fitness level needs to be increased slowly so that the body can adjust to the different mechanisms that are going on.

WHY POPULAR DIETS DON'T WORK

The High-Protein, Low-Carbohydrate Scam

The multifaceted approach to combating eating disorders presented so far combines assessing your emotional state, exercising, eating right, and taking supplements. This is in contrast to the faddish, highly touted wonder diets that appear in the media every season. These diets are more often feel-good panders to eaters' worst cravings than scientifically sound practices.

Dr. Joel Furman is a board-certified physician in private practice in New Jersey who specializes in preventing and reversing diseases through nutritional methods. He is the author of *Fasting and Eating for Health.*

"High-protein, low-carbohydrate diets have become increasingly popular over the past few years," he notes, "and doctors who promote these diets list a number of reasons why people with weight problems need to get onto this type of diet. One reason they give is that these people's bodies do not metabolize carbohydrates properly, a condition popularly referred to as insulin resistance."

"In fact," Dr. Furman cautions, "such diets, promoted in some of the most heavily promoted, best-selling diet books, are among the most dangerous.

Among these books are *Enter the Zone* by Barry Sears, the [Dr. Robert] Atkins books, and *Protein Power* by Michael Eades."

The problem is how these books recommend breaking the habits: "All these people who read these books, wanting to lose weight by eating a high-protein, low-carbohydrate diet, remind me of people who want to lose weight by snorting cocaine and smoking cigarettes. In other words, there are lots of ways that may work to help you lose weight, but we are interested in more than just having a person temporarily lose weight. We want a diet that is going to enable us to lose weight and protect our health simultaneously, not something that will end up making us look thin in a coffin or increase our cancer risk."

These diets, he goes on, counsel replacing one bad food, refined carbohydrates, with another, animal fats: "You know, some of these high-protein-diet gurus claim that they have the truth [about the value of eating meat and animal products] and that there's a conspiracy among the 1,500 scientific studies that continue to point to the association between the consumption of meat, eggs, and dairy products and cancer, heart disease, kidney failure, constipation, gallstones, and hemorrhoids, just to name a few. They are overlooking the fact that you must pay a price with your health for eating increased animal proteins as a way to lose weight."

"Of course, there is one good point in what these people say," he adds. "It's true that refined carbohydrates such as pasta, bread, sugar, sweets, candies, bagels, croissants, potato chips, and all the junk food that Americans eat are not doing us any good. This junk now constitutes about 50 percent of the American diet. We know that this food is linked to heart attacks, cancer, obesity, and diabetes. That is absolutely true."

However, the gurus "are taking the fact that these highly refined, low-fiber carbohydrates can cause increased insulin levels, obesity, and insulin resistance, showing that those are dangerous foods and then saying that therefore the diet should be low in carbohydrates and high in animal protein.

"But that's a jump that the nutritional and scientific literature doesn't make. As a matter of fact, there are no data showing that a person on a high-carbohydrate diet rich in unrefined carbohydrates, such as mangoes, cabbage, beans, legumes, and squash, is in any danger. In fact, many studies show that a diet centered on unrefined carbohydrates—vegetables, whole grains, legumes—will not raise blood sugar or insulin levels."

What people don't realize, Dr. Furman continues, is the value of plant protein. "Compare a steak to broccoli, for example. Let's look at the protein comparison for 100 calories of steak and 100 calories of broccoli. Sirloin steak has 5.4 grams of protein for 100 calories, and broccoli has 11.2 grams. In other words, green vegetables are very rich in protein. Beans are very rich in protein. We can devise a diet that is very low in animal fat or totally vegetarian, but with a good, satisfactory amount of healthy protein.

"People have to realize that there is a big biochemical difference between animal and plant protein. Plant protein lowers cholesterol; animal protein raises cholesterol. Plant protein is a protector against cancer; animal protein is a cancer promoter. Plant protein promotes bone strength; animal protein promotes bone loss. Plant protein has no effect on aging or kidney disease, and animal protein accelerates both of them. In other words, plant protein is packaged along with fiber, phytochemicals, vitamin E, and omega-3 fatty acids. Animal protein is packaged with saturated fat, cholesterol, and arachidonic acid."

Therefore, "if you are on a diet such as the Atkins diet or another high-protein diet in order to lose weight, you are paying a price with, for example, the risk of increased cancer."

In Dr. Furman's opinion, after studying the food recommendations of these diets, "I suspect that a person really following one of these high-protein diets that restrict fruit and carotenoid-rich starches—found in foods such as sweet potatoes, corn, and squash—could be more than doubling her risk of colon cancer.

"There are studies that show a clear and dose-responsive relationship between increased cancers of the digestive tract and low fruit consumption. High fruit consumption has a powerful dose-response relationship to reduction of mortality from all causes of death. The only other food that even approaches this powerful effect of reducing cancer is raw vegetable consumption. So I suggest that if you are going to average 60 to 70 percent of your calories from fat and animal products with no fruit, you have to consider that diet exceedingly dangerous."

The Blood-Type Diet

Other popular diets advocate eating according to a person's blood type. These diets have sold many books, and the authors have appeared on all the shows. The authors say, "It's your blood type. You have to eat this for your blood type." I've seen a ton of scientific evidence that could disprove that and show its lack of validity. So why is that approach not being challenged by the American public or the media?

According to Dr. Furman, these diets are popular because they give free rein to people's ingrained bad habits: "I think it reinforces what people want to believe. People are addicted to their rich diets. They are looking to hang on to any reason, however irrational it may be, not to have to change.

"If you talk to smokers, you'll see the same thing. You'll hear how irrational are the reasons they give for why they must still smoke and how they have diminished in their own minds the strong reasons against smoking. The same is true with eating. People want to rationalize why it is okay to do whatever they are addicted to.

"The American addiction to such things as junk foods is such that when you stop doing it, you get uncomfortable. The problem is that the American diet is so toxic and so unhealthy that when people try to go off it, when they skip a meal and start eating fruits and vegetables, they feel sick. They get headaches and abdominal cramps. They get shakes and confusion. Then they think that it must be this new diet. It must be that eating healthily is making them sick. They must need this rich animal-fat protein and the junk food. In other words, they don't see that this is a temporary phase that lasts a week or two, when they are withdrawing from caffeine and the rich nitrogenous waste. You might feel a little ill when you change your diet. That slight resistance to change is one basis of people's addiction to harmful foods, and it makes them turn to these quack diets."

CHAPTER 12

ENDOMETRIOSIS

Endometriosis is a condition in which the glands and tissues that line the inside of the uterus (the endometrium) grow outside the uterine wall. Normally, cells build up in the uterus each month in preparation for pregnancy, serving as a nest for an incoming embryo. When pregnancy does not occur, the lining is shed and appears as menstrual flow. In endometriosis, endometrial-type cells may attach themselves to the fallopian tubes, ovaries, urinary bladder, intestinal surfaces, rectum, part of the colon, and other structures in the area.

About 7 to 15 percent of American women have endometriosis. One of the goals of medical treatment is to reduce the stimulating effect of estrogen on these cell "implants." Since there is no cure for this illness, the most that natural care can do at present is to work on relieving the pain.

CAUSES

The exact cause of the condition remains a mystery, though several theories exist as to why it happens. These are some possible explanations:

RETROGRADE MENSTRUATION—Blood flows backward instead of downward through the cervix and out of the body. It is thought to go out the fallopian tubes and into the pelvic and abdominal cavity. Once it is there, cells from the exiting blood implant themselves outside the uterus onto other tissues.

LYMPHATIC CHANNELS—Cells of the endometrium lining pass through lymphatic channels or migrate via blood and then implant themselves outside the uterine cavity.

GENETIC PREDISPOSITION—Certain families are predisposed to the condition.

IMMUNOLOGIC DISORDER—The immune system is deficient in some way, causing tissue to proliferate in abnormal areas. The idea is that through some type of immune deficiency, hormonal and chemical influences cause endometrial tissue to become activated at different times in the cycle.

CHILDBEARING—Childbearing in combination with methods of contraception may be responsible.

SYMPTOMS

Dian Shepperson Mills, a nutritionist and tutor at the Institute for Optimal Nutrition in London, is the author of *Endometriosis: A Key to Healing through Nutrition*. She explains that endometrial implants cause a problem "because the endometrium is designed to shed blood at the end of every month if a pregnancy has not been achieved. So these endometric implants, which are scattered around on the bowel and the bladder and so on, do likewise; they shed blood. When you are having a normal period, the blood comes out of the body down the vagina. However, with endometriosis, the implants bleed into the abdominal cavity, and the blood is trapped there because it has no exit. Thus, people with endometriosis have considerable pain.

"We also think that the reaction going on in the body, which is trying to remove the implants that the body's immune system knows should not be there, may affect people's fertility in some way, although we don't know how. It's believed that it is mainly the chemical secretions by the immune cells that are trying to remove the endometrium that are affecting the sperm or the ova."

Endometriosis can produce slight to severe pain, ranging from mild cramps to agony and dysfunction. About 70 percent of women with endometriosis have severe, chronic symptoms. Endometrial implants produce chemicals, including prostaglandins, which cause the uterus to contract, resulting in cramping. Pain also results from swelling, inflammation, and scarring of affected tissues. It is usually cyclical and most commonly occurs just before menstruation. Some women have pain during sexual intercourse any time in the month.

Where and to what degree pain is felt depend on the location of the endometrial tissue and the degree to which it has spread outside the uterus. Some women have pain during urination as a result of implants on the bladder. Some have pain during bowel movements because of colon and rectal implants. There can be ovarian pain or pain radiating to the back or buttocks or down the legs. Upon manual gynecological examination, there may be pelvic pain.

Internal bleeding may occur as well as nose bleeding or bleeding from another orifice at certain times of the month. Any cyclic bleeding is suspect for endometriosis. Other symptoms that sometimes appear include aggravated premenstrual syndrome (PMS), bladder infections, fatigue, and lower back pain.

Diagnosis

Endometriosis may be suspected in the presence of one or more of the symptoms listed above, but the only real way to confirm a diagnosis is with a surgical procedure known as laparoscopy, which allows the doctor to actually see and biopsy tissue. Sonograms and magnetic resonance imaging (MRI) scans may be helpful, but they are not definitive in making the diagnosis.

The proper diagnosis is important, notes Dr. Anthony Aurigemma, because while endometriosis is considered benign, it can become malignant.

Conventional Therapy

Treatment usually consists of medical prescriptions for pain control and reduction of endometrial growth. Antiprostaglandin medicines such as indomethacin, ibuprofen, and naproxen are often given to reduce pain.

Another popular pharmaceutical, danazol, is also used for this purpose, but in some women it does not provide total or lasting relief. Studies show that danazol has a good effect after surgery to remove adhesions. After some of the adhesions have been removed, it may help an infertile woman become pregnant. A side effect of the drug is that it may increase cholesterol, especially the low-density lipoprotein (LDL) variety, which is implicated in accelerated arteriosclerosis. The adverse effects of all these drugs can include weight gain, edema, decreased or increased breast size, acne, excess hair growth on the face, and perhaps even in a developing fetus, and deepening of the voice.

Hormones are sometimes given to fool the body into believing it is pregnant, since pregnancy seems to retard or prevent the development of endometriosis. This method appears to have some benefit, but the side effects include depression, painful breasts, nausea, weight gain, bloating, swelling, and migraine headaches. Since the side effects can be fairly severe, this is not a popular method.

Newer drugs, called gonadotropin-releasing hormone compounds, are sometimes given by injection. These agents suppress pituitary gland release of the female hormones follicle-stimulating hormone (FSH) and luteinizing hormone (LH), causing what is called a clinical pseudomenopause. They help reduce pain in many women and decrease the size and volume of endometrial tissue after surgery.

Through the advanced surgical technique of female reconstructive surgery (FRS) developed by Dr. Vicki Hufnagel, the uterus and ovaries can be repositioned, thus reducing the deep pelvic pain that is associated with endometriosis.

Alternative Therapies

PAIN RELIEF

"When I started looking at nutrition for the endocrine system," Mills says, "I came across a lot of research that suggests that if you are deficient in various nutrients, it may affect the way your body deals with pain. These nutrients would be the essential fatty acids, such as evening primrose oil, fish oil, linseed oil, safflower oil, and vitamins C, E, and K. All these are important in the body's control of pain. The B vitamins, particularly B1, seem to be important in building up the endorphins, which are the body's natural painkillers. There is also an amino acid called DLPA, which is DL-phenylalanine, which seems to help in dulling pain, and there are zinc, selenium, and magnesium."

If you are deficient in many of these nutrients, your body may not be able to cope well with pain. Mills says, "If we look at, say, magnesium, we see that it is very important in allowing muscles to relax. Calcium and magnesium balance one another. Calcium causes muscles to contract, and magnesium allows them to relax. Seeing that the uterus is one of the largest muscles in the body, it would be quite important to make sure you are getting enough magnesium-rich foods, such as green leafy vegetables, nuts, and seeds. The same is true of B vitamins. There are lots of those in vegetables and fruits. That's also where you'll get vitamin C. Zinc is found in nuts and seeds. Selenium is in seafood."

DIGESTION AND THE REPRODUCTIVE SYSTEM

"Once I have a patient who has a major endometriosis problem," Mills says, "the first thing I look at is her digestion. If she doesn't get the nutrients from food or any supplements she takes, nothing will work. So you have to heal the digestion first. If she has constipation or diarrhea or heartburn indigestion, I will give her digestive enzymes, acidophilus, and possibly slippery elm. Then, once we've got that healed, you can try a digestive supplement, such as a multivitamin, and some magnesium, zinc, and vitamin C.

"You have to analyze what is wrong with each individual person and tailor the treatment specifically to her needs. Generally, for endometriosis, I try to ensure that the woman is taking evening primrose and fish oil. The supplements must also be wheat-, yeast-, sugar-, and dairy-free. By taking magnesium, zinc, the probiotics, and the digestive enzymes, you are working through the body system from different angles to try to relieve the pain while supporting the endocrine and immune systems."

NATUROPATHY

Dr. Tori Hudson, a naturopath from Portland, Oregon, believes there is most support for the immunological weakness theory of endometriosis because women with this condition have altered immune cells and fewer T lymphocytes. By improving immune function with supplements, diet, and botanicals, she claims to help many patients: "I've seen women with severe pelvic pain who were scheduled for surgery one month from the date I saw them. My treatment helped them recover completely without the surgery." She adds that most, but not all, women respond to her protocol, which is designed to stimulate a maximal immune response. The basic program consists of the following:

> Antioxidants
> Vitamin C—to bowel tolerance, up to 10,000 mg
> Beta carotene—150,000–200,000 IU
> Selenium—400 mcg
> Vitamin E—800–1200 IU

Changes in the diet are made to further stimulate the immune system. This is accomplished by lowering fat; adding whole grains, vegetables, and fruits; and eliminating immune system inhibitors such as coffee, sugar, alcohol, and high-fat foods. Foods such as cheese and meat have high amounts of estrogen and are omitted, because estrogen aggravates the disease. A mostly vegetarian diet is best for lowering estrogen and stimulating the immune system.

Two botanical formulas are included. One contains chaste tree berry, dandelion root, motherwort, and prickly ash in equal amounts. One half-teaspoon is taken three times daily. The other formula contains small doses of toxic herbs that must be carefully prescribed by a naturopathic physician.

In addition, Dr. Hudson sometimes prescribes natural progesterone made from wild yam. The wild yam extract is converted in the laboratory to natural progesterone.

OTHER NUTRITIONAL RECOMMENDATIONS

Dr. Susan M. Lark, a physician who is the author of *The Women's Health Companion: Self-Help Nutrition Guide & Cookbook*, recommends vitamins, herbs, and minerals that will decrease estrogen stimulation of the endometrial cells.

VITAMIN A—In the form of beta carotene, a maximum daily dose of 5,000 IU to help decrease the excess menstrual bleeding that may occur with endometriosis.

VITAMIN B COMPLEX—50 to100 mg with an additional dose of up to 300 mg daily of vitamin B6. These vitamins help the liver convert excess estrogen into less stimulating forms.

VITAMIN C—1000–4000 mg of bioflavonoids daily. Vitamin C not only regulates estrogen levels but reduces cramps and bleeding by strengthening capillaries. You can get bioflavonoids by eating citrus fruits (including the inner peel), berries, the skins of grapes, alfalfa, buckwheat, and soybeans and taking 800 mg a day of vitamin C as a supplement.

VITAMIN E—400–2,000 IU daily. If you have high blood pressure, begin with 100 IU and work up to the higher levels gradually. Vitamin E helps even out the effects of high levels of estrogen.

ESSENTIAL FATTY ACIDS—Essential fatty acids (EFAs), including linoleic and linolenic acids, are the source for the manufacture of prostaglandins, which prevent cramping of muscles and blood vessels. Good sources of EFAs are raw seeds, especially flax seed, nuts, salmon, mackerel, and trout. They can also be taken as dietary supplements.

HERBS—100 mg daily maximum dose of fennel, anise, blessed thistle, black cohosh, and false unicorn root works to restore hormonal balance. You can also use white willow bark and meadowsweet to reduce pain, fever, cramps, and inflammation of the endometrial implants. Be sure to follow the directions on the label, since these herbs can cause an upset stomach and diarrhea.

ASIAN MEDICINE

Dr. Roger Hirsch, a naturopathic doctor in California who specializes in Asian medicine, says that the Chinese diagnose endometriosis by looking at the way the blood flows in the body, specifically in the pelvic cavity. This is determined by the appearance of the root of the tongue, which represents the pelvic cavity. "If a woman has endometriosis, there will be raised bumps and papillae in the back of the tongue and perhaps a greasy yellow coating," Dr. Hirsch says. "If you look at the back of your tongue in the mirror and see raised bumps that are red and fiery, especially during the time of menstruation, you may well have endometriosis."

HELLERWORK

Hellerwork is a bodywork technique derived from Rolfing. Both modalities use deep tissue work to improve body structure, but Hellerwork is different in that it is not painful. Certified Hellerwork practitioner Sarah Suatoni gives an overview of the process: "There are three components to Hellerwork. There is a hands-on part, which feels much like a massage; a movement educational aspect; and a mind-body dialogue aspect.

"In the hands-on process, we analyze the body much as a chiropractor would, looking at the posture, or the structure, as we call it, to determine which parts of the body are out of balance. We look to see which myofascial tissue connections are creating this misalignment. Then we work with our hands to release it.

"The second part of the work is movement education, in which we do very simple everyday movements. We look at how a person sits or stands. In the case of computer programmers, we look at how they sit at the computer and use their arms. We look at whatever it is that may be contributing to the dysfunction in the body, and then we begin to look at how we can have the person move in a way that will not create the same problem.

"Last but certainly not least is mind-body dialogue. We work under the belief that our emotional patterns, memories, and attitudes are reflected in our bodies. In the same way one needs to look at a movement pattern in order to shift some sort of physical dysfunction, one needs to look at emotional patterns or beliefs in order to shift those as well.

"This work is a process where people come in for eleven sessions. Once a week for an hour and a half is ideal, although other time frames are possible. Each session touches upon a different part of the body and different aspects of the being."

Suatoni tells how she began using Hellerwork to treat endometriosis and similar chronic conditions: "I met Dr. David Kaufman, a urologist, who determined that women with interstitial cystitis had severe spasm of the pelvic muscles. He has since started working with patients with endometriosis, vulvodynia, vestibulitis, and a number of other conditions that show the same symptoms of severe spasm or contraction. Dr. Kaufman was using biofeedback and felt that he needed someone who did hands-on work to accompany the biofeedback treatments. That's how I began.

"Although this process deals with mind-body relationships, this does not imply that these diseases are imaginary. Some women have been told for years that their disease is all in their head, when there are all kinds of physical evidence for the disease. Rather, the disease is the result of a set of relationships between the mind and body. Hellerwork and other forms of bodywork help because they are process-oriented and look at relationships. Once women start understanding these relationships, they find that they have a whole lot of power to overcome disease and regain health."

HOMEOPATHY

Homeopathy is another holistic therapy that addresses underlying emotional causes. Dr. Aurigemma has been treating his patients homeopathically for ten years and claims that the therapy is completely safe and highly effective. "There is no doubt in my mind that something actually happens and that it helps people," he says. "I utilize the remedies because I see them work. What spurs me on is the continuous improvement of most of the patients I see."

PATIENT STORY

One woman came to see me who was on prescription narcotic medication for the pain. The medicine gave her no relief, and she was at the point of wanting a hysterectomy to get relief from the pain. I put this woman on a natural hygienic regimen for a couple of weeks. First she fasted for five days. Then she followed up with a nutritional plan.

Let me briefly describe a typical hygienic regimen. The patient has a breakfast consisting of a vegetable juice or a vegetable and fruit juice combination, a blended salad, a piece of fruit, perhaps some hot cereal, and a couple of soft-boiled egg yolks. Lunch is a vegetable juice or vegetable and fruit juice combination, a blended salad, a cup or a little more than that, a piece of fruit, and then some raw nuts or unsalted raw-milk cheese. For the evening meal the patient starts with juice again, blended salad, tossed salad, and steamed vegetables such as string beans, broccoli, or escarole. Then she goes on with the main course, which includes a steamed potato or yam, natural brown rice or another whole grain, and a legume. I also might supplement the meal with egg or cheese, depending on the protein needs of the woman. Of course, there are variations for individual patients.

After following this general plan, this patient was pain-free at the end of a month. That was ten years ago. Right now she is pregnant with her second child, whereas before she was infertile. Natural hygiene has tremendous implications for endometriosis. There is absolutely no reason why a woman should have pain or be infertile because of such a simple condition.

From my perusal of the literature I can see that endometriosis is plainly a condition of liver toxicity, where the liver is failing to completely break down the estrogen hormones the body is manufacturing. These breakdown products wreak havoc in the form of endometrial tissue in the pelvic cavity.

—Dr. Anthony Penepent

CHAPTER 13

ENVIRONMENTAL
ILLNESS

Environmental illness was first recognized three decades ago, but mainstream medicine still generally disregards this syndrome. When patients come in with the symptoms of sensitivity to a toxic environment, doctors often do not know the correct protocol. Standardized blood tests appear normal, leading doctors to assume that no problem exists.

Another problem is that most doctors today are not trained to work with a disease that affects the whole body. Heather Millar, author of *The Toxic Labyrinth* and former sufferer of environmental illness, notes, "In the medical community we have created a world of specialists. Physicians are now neurologists, cardiologists, rheumatologists, and so on. We have gotten away from the old-fashioned approach. We no longer have general practitioners. Before, you would go to a doctor's office and tell him your history from start to finish. He would look at you as a whole individual, checking the psychological as well as the physical aspect of the body. Only then would he make an assessment.

"Now technology has compartmentalized the body. The neurologist looks only at the symptoms of numbness, tingling, and headaches. The rheumatologist looks only at arthritis, joint pain, and aches. The infectious disease doctor looks only for infection. What happened to me was, I would go in and give a detailed history of what was happening. The doctor, according to his specialty, would look only at one specific area. He or she did not want to hear about the other symptoms I had.

"What we are failing to realize with all this supertechnology in medicine is that the body works in harmony. You do not have one body system that works separately from something else. They all work together. So if you are having symptoms in one system, you are probably having symptoms elsewhere."

CAUSES

Dr. Stephen M. Silverman of Port Washington, New York, says that thousands of poisons in our food, water, and surroundings are responsible for environmental illness: "The first thing you must realize is that what you eat can have a tremendous effect on your immune system. One of the most toxic foods that people expose themselves to unknowingly, for example, is hydrogenated oil. People don't realize how widespread that ingredient is. It's in crackers, all commercial breads, potato chips, pretzels, and cookies, and it has a very strong damaging effect on the immune system.

"Along with what you eat, you must consider what you drink. Most people are being exposed to tap water, whether directly from the sink or outside when they buy a cup of coffee or tea. Probably one of the highest exposures to carcinogens comes from this source. In 1989 Ralph Nader's group identified over 2,000 chemicals commonly found in people's drinking water. When water is tested over the course of the year, it is tested for approximately 120 chemicals. When you are told that the water is safe to drink, it means that it is safe with respect to what it was tested for. You have no idea about the other 1,900 chemicals. Insecticides and pesticides in the water have been associated with Long Island's high rate of breast cancer. Certainly, if they can create cancer, they can cause immune system damage.

"Among the other factors that can set you up for illness are the things you put on your body. I am talking about cosmetics, moisturizers, and hair sprays. We know through medical applications of the nicotine and estrogen patches that what you put on your skin will be absorbed into the bloodstream. If you were to take a look at the ingredients in your cosmetics, hair sprays, and underarm deodorants, you would see that they are loaded with chemicals. You have to realize that when you use these chemicals every day, they eventually get into the bloodstream. When you think about it, is it possible that these chemicals have no effect on your immune system? It's almost impossible.

"In addition, there are environmental factors. One of the most important rooms to be safe in is the bedroom. If you happen to have a carpet that is outgassing, by which I mean releasing chemicals at a very low level, and some of those chemicals are suspected carcinogens, despite how well you may be eating, you are going to get sick from that carpet. When we sleep at night, we are supposed to detoxify. Your body attempts to purify itself at night of any additives or toxins in foods you may have eaten. If you have a toxic bedroom where the carpet, the paint on the wall, or a mattress loaded with formaldehyde is releasing gas, and if you're reacting to these chemicals, then eight hours a night, instead of restoring your immune system, you may be causing it severe damage."

According to the environmental medicine specialist Dr. Marshall Mandell, "There is absolutely no question that environmental factors play a major role in many diseases; where they do not actually start the disease, they can complicate it. Anything that makes your illness worse is important for you to know about."

In the same way that cocaine goes right from the nose of the user to the nervous system in a matter of seconds, producing a wide variety of effects, toxins in food or air produce a range of effects in the systems of highly sensitive individuals. Conventional physicians and traditional allergists simply miss this phenomenon by recognizing only a very limited range of symptoms. If their patients aren't sneezing or itching, they will not recognize the possibility that an allergy may be present. But logically, once a doctor recognizes that minute flecks of animal dander or pollen in the air can produce marked symptoms, is it so difficult to see that chemical toxins in meat or milk or air pollution, among a host of other possible causes, might also have an adverse effect? Simply put, the human race has evolved over millions of years and has adapted to most of the conditions on this planet. But many of the pollutants and toxins we are dealing with have arisen over the last thirty to fifty years. Our bodies just haven't had time to evolve in response to these changes in our environment. Unless we act sensibly by at least recognizing this discrepancy, we may cause great damage to our environment and ourselves.

Whatever you breathe in enters your body along with the oxygen. If your home, work, or school environment is polluted, the pollutants will travel through the walls of the lungs, go into the blood vessels of the lungs, and ultimately reach the heart through the pulmonary circulation. Similarly, chemicals, additives, and contaminants in our food and beverages will pass through the digestive system and reach the heart. Once there, they will be pumped through the bloodstream. Every tissue in your body is exposed to what you eat, drink, and breathe. That is why so many people are sick today.

"Research shows that women are more prone to environmental illnesses," says Heather Millar. "The reason is that many chemicals, such as formaldehyde, benzene, phenols, and chlorine, have estrogen-mimicking properties. These chemicals take the place of estrogen in the body. The body thinks it has enough estrogen and doesn't make enough. Estrogen is responsible for reproduction as well as many other vital functions in the body. Problems occur when the body calls upon the estrogen it thinks it has but doesn't.

"Silicone breast implants are making women terribly ill. They have a tendency to grow fungus inside the implant, which adds a problem to an already existing one. Fungus is extremely hard to get rid of once it starts to grow.

After breast implants are removed, women do not feel better. This indicates that their immune systems have been damaged. It will probably take a very long time for them to recover, and we do not know the long-term effects."

SYMPTOMS

Symptoms vary with a woman's constitution and may include fatigue, aching muscles, a flulike feeling, ringing in the ears, burning eyes, headaches, migraines, disturbed sleep, shortness of breath, food allergies, a heightened sense of smell, loss of balance, inability to concentrate, memory loss, anxiety, panic attacks, depression, and irritable bowel syndrome. There is a marked progressive debilitating reaction to consumer products such as perfumes, soap, tobacco smoke, and plastics.

CLINICAL EXPERIENCE

Diagnosis

In her book, Heather Millar has a checklist to help people determine whether they may be suffering from environmental illness. These are some questions she asks people to consider:

Do I have a toxic lifestyle?
Does my environment contain chemicals that could be making me sick?
Do I feel ill at work?
Do I feel ill at home?
Do I live in a new home?
Have I recently painted or installed a new carpet?
How much plastic do I have in the home?
Does my neighborhood contain chemicals that could be making me sick?

"Discovering the cause of the problem is a detective process," Millar says. "It involves taking a close look at your home, workplace, and neighborhood.

"Start with your home. You may ask, 'Why didn't we have these problems before? We always painted our house and put new carpet in.' What I'd like to suggest is that technology has changed a lot of chemicals and manufacturing processes. Since the 1980s we have added more synthetics and are now seeing their effects. A lot of these products emit gas. The newness smell is a gas that is coming off. Basically, it's a chemical soup that is very hazardous to our health. Also, since we live in energy-efficient buildings, we do not have the ventilation needed to lessen the concentration of these gases.

"Plastics present further problems. They have a lot of these estrogen-mimicking properties. Softer plastics have more toxicity. We used to live with metal, wood, and glass. These are far safer alternatives. When replacing plastic with wood, consider the type of finish on it. Does it smell?

"Then look at the workplace. Ask yourself, what are you doing as an occupation? Are you working with chemicals on an ongoing basis? Or are you working in an energy-efficient office building that was recently renovated? Is it currently being renovated? Does it have no open windows? Do other people in the office frequently get colds and flu or feel unwell?

"Finally, examine your neighborhood. Where do you live? Do you have chemical manufacturing in your backyard? Is there some kind of toxic incinerator nearby? What is in your water supply? What kinds of pesticide regulations does your neighborhood have?

"You may react differently to toxins in your environment than your coworkers do. For example, in my workplace, which was extremely toxic, my symptoms were mainly neurological. Other colleagues were diagnosed with chronic fatigue. Still others experienced asthma or fibromyalgia, which is an aching of the muscles. We react differently depending on our genetic predispositions."

Fortunately, there are physicians who do recognize the illness, and there are tests available to pinpoint the condition. Occupational health doctors and environmental physicians prescribe tests that look at solvent levels in the blood. They look at pesticide levels in the blood and check mineral levels, which are usually low in people who suffer from chemical exposures.

Four Clues to Proper Treatment

Dr. Michael Schachter, a clinical ecologist, or environmental medicine specialist, identifies four contributing factors that he considers key in his examination and in determining a course of therapy: the quality of nutrition generally and the identification of any nutritional deficiencies, infections, psychological stresses, and toxicity. According to Dr. Schachter, the course of therapy should be determined by the condition of the patient in regard to these four criteria.

Dr. Schachter is also concerned with improving the oxygenation and energy utilization of the body at the cellular level. Anything we can do to improve that process is going to strengthen the immune system and thereby help reduce a person's tendency toward sensitivity and reactions. Thus, Dr. Schachter encourages the use of oxidant therapies, but only up to a point, since oxygen in too great quantities can have a damaging effect. The key here, as in virtually every area of health, is balance.

The first and foremost oxidant therapy must be aerobic exercise. Keeping in mind that oxygen is the main nutrient of the body, it is easy to understand that as we improve oxygenation, we improve the body's ability to detoxify and enhance the immune system. Beyond exercise, a number of new nutrients are available to enhance oxygenation, such as germanium and ubiquinone, as well as a variety of traditional oxygenation techniques.

Vitamins and minerals are another key component in Dr. Schachter's approach. He sees vitamin A as a major protective factor that guards against both chemical sensitivities and infections. Thus, cod liver oil, which parents once gave automatically to children, is indeed an excellent preventive medicine with its high concentrations of vitamins A and D. In treating children with recurrent ear infections, Dr. Schachter has found that by simply enhancing their diet, removing most of the sugar and refined foods, and adding a spoonful of cod liver oil, the ear infections can be controlled and prevented in many cases. Other useful vitamins include vitamin C, vitamin B12, and vitamin E, which is an antioxidant. Selenium and beta carotene are also important antioxidants. Vitamin B12 can help counteract the adverse effects in the body of pesticides in the environment. Moreover, while conventional physicians may test for vitamin B12 levels in the bloodstream, normal levels may be present in the blood while there are deficiencies at the cellular level.

According to Dr. Schachter, infections are a key factor in going from troubled to good health. Frequently, infections will yield to nontoxic treatments.

Take candida, for example. Women who have repeatedly used antibiotics, include a lot of refined carbohydrates in their diet, and may have been exposed to steroids or birth control pills tend to develop a chronic overgrowth of *Candida albicans,* a yeastlike, funguslike organism that we all have in our bodies. In certain cases the infection will give off toxins that may impair the immune system and produce a variety of symptoms. Some of these symptoms will be the result of food and chemical sensitivities that have been aggravated by the infection.

Dr. Schachter has found that starting the patient on a special diet that excludes refined carbohydrates, especially sugars and alcohol, and includes various nutrients, especially certain fatty acids that inhibit candida growth, will go a long way toward controlling the infection in many cases. He also notes that garlic has strong anticandidal properties.

Chronic viral syndromes are another key problem. A previously healthy individual suddenly gets a flu and instead of recovering completely experiences frequent fatigue, exhaustion, swollen glands, sore throat, night sweats, anxiety, and loss of appetite. However, conventional testing shows nothing definite. More sophisticated testing may show exposure to various viruses, but the main problem here may be that the person's immune system just isn't responding as it should. Dr. Schachter has obtained excellent results in patients with this profile by using nutrients to bolster the immune system. Intravenous vitamin C may be used, along with germanium and a variety of other vitamins and minerals given orally. In cases of herpes virus, for example, he may use high doses of the amino acid lysine, which has antiviral effects for the herpes virus and certain other viruses. For short treatment periods, he may administer as much as 10 to 15 grams of lysine per day.

Psychological stress is another key factor, according to Dr. Schachter. Environmental medicine specialists, he warns, must be careful that in emphasizing the importance of the physical environment they do not underestimate the importance of psychological factors in determining the strength of an individual's immune system.

As for toxicity, Dr. Schachter feels that hydrocarbons and other chemicals are already playing a major role by damaging our immune systems, as are heavy metals. He sees chelation therapy as a valid treatment to detoxify our systems of the effects of heavy metals. Chelation therapy has also shown impressive results in patients with cardiovascular disease.

Detoxifying the Body

Without detoxifying the system, all other steps to repair the body will be of no avail.   Dr. Zane Gard, an expert in toxicology, explains some methods of detoxification that have had impressive results in the reversal of environmental illness: "Heat stress detoxification includes wood saunas, hot sand packing, steam baths, and sweat lodges. The history of these approaches goes back several thousand years. Careful supervision is required. Heat stress detoxification can be effective but requires knowledge of toxins and their potential effects on the body. If it is not administered properly, there can be a lot of complications, and the patient can actually end up worse.

"The biotoxic reduction program was designed with the toxic-chemical-syndrome patient in mind. It is a comprehensive, medically managed program that addresses toxicology, psychology, neurology, pathology, and immunology. The program must be followed seven days a week, one to two hours a day, for a minimum of two weeks. It would be nice to have Saturday and Sunday off, but patients actually regress one or two days every time they take a day off during the first two weeks. So it has to be every day during that initial period.

"The program consists of increasing niacin, aerobic exercise, sauna therapy, and other therapies as necessary. With those who have neurological damage, other therapies will be needed, including one that stimulates the myelin sheaths of the nerves to regenerate. As a result, many peripheral neuropathies completely reverse. In more than eighty peripheral neuropathies, including multiple sclerosis (MS), we have only two patients who did not fully recover.

Detoxifying the Environment

It is no longer enough to watch what we eat or the medicines we take; environmental toxins have become an unavoidable reality, especially for those living in densely populated urban areas. The very air we breathe on the streets or in our homes and offices can attack our health; noise pollution and artificial lighting add to the physical and mental stress of urban life.

The myth is that you should look for the big toxin. But it's the chronic, day-in, day-out exposure to small toxins that are really the concern. It may take decades—none of these environmental toxins, even asbestos, will knock you out right away—but you may pay for your lack of awareness with lung cancer, leukemia, arthritis, or heart disease down the line. Perhaps worst are the subtle symptoms of fatigue, anxiety, and minor nagging physical problems that many of us come to accept as a normal part of life.

Elimination of the unseen substances that attack your system stealthily, over time, is half of achieving good health. If you never use any supplementary vitamin, mineral, or herb but simply eliminate those factors that depreciate your health, you should be able to live to one hundred years of age in a healthy way. One group of people, nearly seventy thousand in number, in the north of Pakistan at the base of the Himalayas, often live well past ninety or even a hundred, putting in full days of work daily until they die. It may not be possible for all of us to live in the pure atmosphere of the Himalayas—not to mention emulating the diet, activities, and social structure of these people—but we can alter our environment realistically and functionally. A good place to start is where we live.

Dr. Alfred Zamm, a fellow of the American College of Allergists and the American College of Physicians, has written a book, *Why Your House May Endanger Your Health,* which explores the relationship between our homes and our well-being more thoroughly than we can here; much of the following discussion is indebted to information he shared on my radio show as well as to Dr. Richard Podell.

The Sick Building Syndrome

The "sick house" is a relatively new development. Materials and methods used to construct houses have changed considerably since World War Two; an extreme example is the energy-efficient office buildings built during the energy crisis of the 1970s, about which we'll have more to say later in this chapter. But not only are houses built with more emphasis on energy efficiency—which means heavy insulation and minimum ventilation to the outside—the construction materials themselves, as well as the furnishings (carpeting, fabrics, furniture) are new, often more convenient, cheaper, lighter synthetic compounds unheard of in prewar houses. The particleboard that is so useful in modern house and furniture construction exacts a price for this convenience; it is a silent time bomb, giving off invisible, odorless—but no less dangerous—vapors years after it is installed.

Formaldehyde is a major culprit in the modern house or office building. Particleboard, new synthetic carpets, insulation, many interior paints, and even permanent-press fabrics can give off formaldehyde. It is invisible and odorless except in high concentrations, but even quite low chronic levels can cause symptoms ranging from burning eyes and headaches to asthma and depression. New houses may be built largely of materials that vaporize formaldehyde for years; the worst culprits are mobile homes, which also are often poorly ventilated.

Another important factor in a house's potential toxicity is its source of heat. Combustion-heating appliances using natural gas, oil, coal, kerosene, or wood can all create afterburn by-products even if you can't see or smell them. Good ventilation can help, but this makes it harder to keep a house warm. Electric heat, though expensive, is the safest source.

What can be done about a toxic house? Some changes can be made in the furnishings, floor coverings, and ventilation and heating systems, but often much of the problem lies in structural components that would be expensive and difficult, if not impossible, to alter. Building your own house or having it built with attention to all the materials used is one solution if you can afford it or have the time and skill. If you are looking for a place to live, consider an older home. Prewar houses were often constructed of bricks, plaster, and hardwood, not the chemically treated plywood, composite board, and other synthetic materials used almost universally now. If synthetic materials were used in an older house, they will have had years to emit their toxins. Often a house built before the energy crisis will allow more air circulation. Ceilings are often higher, allowing fumes to rise away from the inhabitants.

There may be disadvantages in an old house, however; molds and mildews may have accumulated over the years. Old carpet is a fertile ground for mold as well as accumulated dust, animal hair, and whatever toxins have been tracked in or sprayed over the years, but it can often be pulled up to reveal a hardwood floor. Outdated heating systems can usually be replaced without too much trouble.

If moving or rebuilding your house is not an option, you can still do a lot to detoxify your home. We'll identify the weak spots room by room.

THE GARAGE

An attached garage is like a toxic waste dump stuck to the side of your house. Many garages have heating and cooling systems that lead directly into the house; anything that can be absorbed through any crack or ventilation system will end up in the house. What's in the garage? The car, of course, and gasoline. Gasoline vaporizes. The afterburn fumes caused by inefficient burning of gasoline are mostly carbon dioxide, which has no odor and is invisible. Breathing these fumes results in headache, dizziness, and mood swings. (Think of people stuck in traffic jams, breathing the afterburn of all the cars around them for hours at a time.) When you park a hot car in the garage and close the door behind it, the hot oil in the engine is volatile and gets into the air. Park the car outside and wait for it to cool off before you bring it into the garage.

Other things you may keep in the garage—paint thinners and removers and turpentine—also vaporize easily and stay in the air for months at a time. If you smell a rag that was used for paint thinner three months ago, you will see that it is still giving off these fumes. Try to minimize the number of these substances in your garage. If you must keep them, use a small shed or garbage can outside the garage to store them. And the garage should be ventilated out, not into the house, with a suction fan. There should be no ducts from the garage into the house.

Your garage is probably where you keep chemicals you use on your lawn and garden: pesticides, fungicides, or herbicides, for instance. In the first place, do you really need them? Look at it this way. If it's going to kill an insect, a plant, or a mouse, it's a toxin and it can affect you, your pets, and your children. If you spray a weed killer on your lawn and then walk around on the lawn, you will repeatedly be bringing it inside on your feet. It doesn't just go away. Think of all the things you bring in on your feet and think, for instance, of your kids playing on the carpet, perhaps putting things into their mouths that have been on it.

Taken individually, none of these things is going to kill you, but be aware that everything you spray outside is likely to be in the air you breathe or will make its way back into your house and settle there. There's no real need to run this risk: We can use diatomaceous earth and natural biological controls or just weed without spraying.

THE BASEMENT

A typical basement in a private home is often damp. People like their lawns unencumbered by debris that might wash down from the gutters of the roof through the downspout, and so the downspout is kept close to the house. Thus the water runs off the roof, down the downspout, and into the ground directly by the foundation of the house. You might just as well run this water directly into the basement, since its walls are rarely waterproof. A little dampness in the basement is enough to support a healthy growth of mold, which can then permeate the house. A forced-air system of ventilation, which has ducts running to the basement, will create a vacuumlike effect that will suck particles of mold into the system, to be dispersed around the house.

Many people react to mold whether it is eaten or inhaled, a point that is obvious to anyone who begins to sneeze as soon as she walks into a damp basement. More insidiously, though, mold that is inhaled even in small quantities cross-reacts with mold that is ingested in food. This effect, known as concomitancy, means that a small quantity of inhaled mold that in itself would hardly cause a noticeable reaction will enhance sensitivity to foods that contain mold.

Any food made by fermentation can induce this reaction. Wine and vinegar are fermented fruit juice, cheese is fermented milk, yeast in bread ferments, and even mushrooms are in the mold family. Thus, it is easy to ingest mold three times a day, exacerbating our inability to tolerate the mold that has circulated upward from a damp basement. Obvious symptoms are sneezing and watering eyes, but allergic symptoms can also be systemic, making them harder to pin down to a specific source. Fatigue, headaches, depression, and even arthritis can have a basis in chronic allergic irritation.

In addition to water coming into the basement from the downspout, groundwater can flow down a hill toward the house, which then serves as a dam. You can place a drain field around the house using deco-drain piping in two tiers. Contact your local hardware store for more information. If a high water table is the problem, a sump pump is needed. Thoroseal, a dense cementlike material, can be applied to the outside block foundation as caulking to keep water out.

If the basement is still damp, a dehumidifier can help, but these work well only above a temperature of 50 to 60 degrees Fahrenheit. Chemicals such as baking soda are only temporary measures. The best way to remove the mold is to scrub the area with sulfur water. The basement can be hosed down and the water removed with an industrial vacuum.

THE KITCHEN

What's the most dangerous toxin in most kitchens? Gas. You should always have a vent in the kitchen; it has been shown that cerebral allergies are often directly attributable to the gas burnoff of pilot lights on stoves, which leak constantly. If you often have headaches and suspect that they are more common when you're spending time in the kitchen, try disconnecting your stove when you're not using it. If this makes a difference, you should consider replacing the gas stove with an electric one. Not only are gas ovens a health risk, microwave ovens can leak; a defective microwave creates a very unhealthy environment within about eight feet around it.

The freon in the condenser of the refrigerator is a highly volatile, dangerous chemical. It is a very good idea to replace refrigerators that are more than ten years old.

The refrigerator contributes to another seldom-considered form of pollution found especially in the kitchen: noise pollution. You should be able to tolerate background noise of about 30 to 35 decibels. Noise higher than 50 decibels becomes uncomfortable. Above 80 decibels, you become substantially irritated, and noise above 100 may cause ear damage or central nervous system overstimulation. The compressor in most refrigerators is up to 60 decibels. You don't appreciate this until you turn on a refrigerator when everything else is totally quiet. But think of a kitchen with a television or a radio on, things cooking, telephone conversations—you can't even hear the refrigerator, and the noise level may be up around 100 decibels. The kitchen is one of the most stressful places because of this level of background noise. Even if you are unable to replace appliances such as refrigerators and air conditioners with less noisy ones, you can cut down on the number of noise-makers you are using at the same time.

Street noise can be irritating in any room. Noise-buffering double-fold drapes can keep noise down as well as insulate.

Mold and mildew are common invisible toxins in a kitchen. When was the last time you changed the water tray in your refrigerator? Under the condenser coil is a tray to collect water, but it can also collect all kinds of mold. Mold spores are in the air all the time, and you're inhaling them. If you're sensitive and your immune system is low, you'll feel it: Your eyes will get puffy, your nose will clog, and your throat will get sore. Keeping this area clean and dry could make a big difference.

Look under your kitchen sink; you'll be amazed at the range of toxic chemicals you keep there, so close to your food. Cleansers, for instance, especially ammonia-based products, often vaporize easily. Ammonia is very toxic and will stay in your blood for hours after you've smelled it. When you wax the kitchen floor, the floor wax will evaporate and you will breathe it in. Try to install floors that will not need waxing, but if you don't want to tear up your current floors, you might want to settle for a matte finish rather than a high sheen if you have to constantly apply volatile chemicals to maintain that sheen. As with the weed killers and insecticides in your garage, there are alternatives to chemical cleaners in the kitchen. Apple cider vinegar and hydrogen peroxide mixed half and half in cold water do the same job as ammonia. This preparation will clean windows and glassware perfectly too.

Roach sprays are very stable. They can last for months and vaporize constantly. A dog or cat licking the floor can pick them up directly. A safer alternative is to use boric acid. You can mix it with sugar as a bait, but be sure pets and children can't reach it; line all the counters and fittings underneath with a strip of this no thicker than a pencil. This mixture is not volatile and is safe as long as it's put only in inaccessible places. Diatomaceous earth is safe and works well too. Or use the roach motels that use resin instead of poisons.

Aluminum-based cookware in which the aluminum can come into contact with food should not be used. Aluminum has been implicated in Alzheimer's disease. It is a heavy metal that lodges in the blood, brain tissue, and central nervous system, where it can cause motor problems. Aluminum foil is all right to store cooked food but should not be used in cooking, where it can oxidize in microscopic amounts. You can't see this, but it can get into your food and your body. Teflon and all other nonstick coatings should also be avoided. They easily scratch or flake off with age, getting into food as well as exposing it to the often inferior metal underneath.

Water from the kitchen tap may contain over a thousand chemicals, including those which the government puts in, such as fluoride; traces of herbicides and pesticides that have leached down into the water supply from fields; and traces of metal, rust, and molds from the inside of your pipes. Most water filtration systems can remove only a portion of these; the finer particles, including toxic chemicals such as pesticides, come through. If you live in a polluted area and your water supply is from underground streams, buy bottled water. I would buy plain distilled water. You get minerals from food; you don't need them from water. Since 72 to 74 percent of our bodies consists of water, we should be sure it is the purest water possible.

THE BATHROOM

One of the most common causes of allergy is what we put on our bodies: soaps, deodorants, and cosmetics. We use these things day in and day out, rarely thinking about their effect on us. For example, women who wear lipstick every day and lick their lips are absorbing chemicals never meant to be eaten. Perfumes vaporize and get breathed in. Read the ingredients of your antiperspirant; most likely it contains an aluminum-based compound that can be absorbed through the skin and carries the risks of aluminum outlined above. You can minimize these sources of toxins by using natural soaps and shampoos made out of vegetable ingredients, a nonfluoride toothpaste such as Dr. Bronner's or Tom's, and mouthwash you can make yourself with a little ascorbic acid in water.

It's important to air out the bathroom after a shower or bath and let it dry out. A window fan to evacuate the moist air is a good idea. Bathrooms are too often closed up most of the time and can be like little chambers that trap the perfume, deodorant, and cleaning-fluid fumes in a small space. Odor disguisers such as pine- or lemon-scented aerosol sprays are worse than useless; the odor is a molecule floating around in the air that can be removed only by letting the air escape. Products that claim to take away odors only cover them up with a chemical that probably smells worse and is certainly worse for you.

The "disinfectant" cleaners so popular for bathroom tiles and tubs are virtually useless. To disinfect something, you have to boil it for twenty minutes, but within one minute it will be covered with germs again. Those germs are not going to kill anyone despite the fear tactics used to market these cleaners. Their heavy aromatic odors are often more of a problem than the germs; pine, for example, is a resinous material that is quite troublesome to allergic or sensitive people.

Never store medications in the medicine chest; it's hot and humid in the bathroom, and this can cause them to go bad. Store medicine and vitamins in the refrigerator.

As in the kitchen, look around the bathroom and think about potential toxins: cleaners for the tiles and sink, toilet fresheners, and so on. Do you need all those things? Can you substitute natural, nontoxic products?

THE BEDROOM

We spend a third of our lives in the bedroom; if you live seventy-two years, that means twenty-four years in bed. An ecologically ideal, safe place to spend all this time should be as free of dust as possible. Many bedrooms have wall-to-wall carpeting, which is an ecological disaster. Carpeting is toxic in several ways. Whereas new synthetic-fiber carpeting contains chemicals, such as formaldehyde, which will vaporize for a year or more, old carpets collect dirt, yeast, fungus, and mold. Dust mites live in rugs. Through an electron microscope these mites look like tiny dinosaurs; their diet is chiefly composed of the shed human skin cells that are another large component of dust. House dust mites can be wafted into the air by currents and breathed into the lungs. People who are allergic to them react as they do to cat or dog dander. Like dander, they can get into your eyes and make them red and puffy.

Think about ripping up your old carpet and putting in nice hardwood floors. They're easy to maintain and nontoxic. The Japanese have never had polyvinyl fluoride or no-wax floors; they use natural resins on wood, and some of these floors are five hundred years old. If you feel you must have carpets, buy wool or natural fiber rugs with natural dyes. Stay away from synthetic carpets. And learn to vacuum efficiently. Most people just zip the vacuum over the carpet; by the time the dust has had a chance to get up through the nap into the air, the vacuum has moved on and has only raised the dust. You've actually increased the pollution in the air. Run the vacuum very slowly over the carpet, giving the dust you raise time to get into the vacuum.

You may be sleeping on foam-filled synthetic pillows and using synthetic-fiber pillowcases and sheets. Replace them with down-filled pillows and comforters and pure cotton sheets. Be aware of what you're putting in your sheets when you wash them; bleaches and fabric softeners are potential irritants. Many manufacturers of bedding use chemicals to which many people are allergic in order to fireproof the material. The way to test for this is to sleep on bedding that is not treated to be fireproof and see if your symptoms disappear. Again, if you feel better when you are sleeping away from your house on vacation, it should alert you to the fact that something in the bedroom is causing trouble.

Sleeping on clean sheets that are changed frequently reduces possible reactions to dust and dust mites. When you wash bedding, it's best to avoid perfumed detergents, antistatics, and softeners and to use biodegradable brands. Bleach should be oxygen bleach, not chlorine, which leaves an irritating residue. Miracle White, made by Beatrice Food Company, works well. If you suspect that a pillowcase, for example, is bothering you, wash it with a simple unscented detergent, rinse it three or four times, and try it again to see if the problem goes away.

Even your closets can affect your health. Mothballs emit a dangerous gas. Try a mixture of rosemary, mint, thyme, ginseng, and cloves, which has the additional advantage of smelling good.

AIR QUALITY

If you ever see the sun slant into a room at a certain angle, you know how much dust and smoke are in what you thought was clear air. It's there all the time. An air purifier with a negative ionizer is the best way to eliminate air-borne toxins: spores, dust, cigarette smoke, hydrocarbons and pollutants from the street, cat hairs, and positive ions. The ionizer bombards the room with negative ions that attach themselves to the positive ions of pollutants, which then drop to the ground and can be filtered out by the filtration system.

Humidifiers are fine for improving air quality as long as you use distilled water in them. Otherwise mineral deposits from the water will end up all over your carpet, floor, and furniture.

PLANTS

One efficient and natural air-quality *improver* is living greenery in your house. The more plants in your environment, the better. A large number and variety of houseplants will increase the oxygen level in the air. Green, nonflowering varieties are best, since they will not give off pollen. Plants are also a great natural air pollution filtration system. They help maintain humidity levels and a proper electricity balance in the air. They also create a living energy field that we can share and be invigorated and calmed by.

LIGHT

Your visual environment is more important than you might realize. If you feel tired, ill, or depressed inside in the winter, especially if you live at a high latitude where the days are very short, and if you spend most of your day indoors, you may be suffering from seasonal affective disorder. In this condition the hypothalamus of the brain is deprived of full-spectrum natural sunlight—most artificial lights use only a part of the spectrum. The best solution is to allow plenty of natural light into your house; use double-glazing rather than small windows or heavy drapes if insulation is a concern. Try to spend time outdoors or arrange your activities so that you're near a window.

If getting more daylight is beyond your control—the days are short, your house is dark, and you must stay indoors—the situation can be improved with full-spectrum light bulbs. Full-spectrum incandescent lighting works on a completely different principle from that of fluorescent lighting (discussed in the section on the workplace below) and is more natural for the eyes. These bulbs are available in health stores in all sizes; using them in your office as well as in your home can make a big difference in your energy level and mental state.

HEAT

In cold areas we shut down for the winter, closing and sealing the windows to avoid ventilation from the outside. These practices contribute to the toxic state of the air inside.

Oil heaters often burn inefficiently and release unburned oil fumes into the house. An afterburn catalyst that is available on the market can now recycle these fumes, creating a clean air burn. Electric stoves are not a problem. Gas or oil space heaters are one of the worst offenders. Dry radiated heat can dry up your nose and skin. Wood-burning stoves may seem rustic and natural but can be one of the worst sources of indoor pollution.

In forced-air combustion heating systems that use gas or oil, a little pinhole not infrequently develops between the heat exchanger, which is next to the combustion chamber, and the air going past it to be heated. As the air that you're going to breathe goes around that heated chamber, it sucks in the partially combusted gases. You may not even perceive this in the air, because it's at a very low level, but over a six-month period this air can produce severe illness. Therefore, you must have your forced-air system checked out electronically for these pinholes every year. The smell test is not satisfactory. If you don't do this, you're at risk.

THE WORKPLACE

The energy crisis of the 1970s led to a generation of very well insulated but poorly ventilated office buildings. People who work in these buildings often complain of fatigue, nasal congestion, dizziness, and a host of other mysterious symptoms, yet there has been clear-cut documentation of toxic levels of pollutants in very few cases. The levels of toxins in these buildings are rarely high enough to provoke official alarm, but they are high enough to cause fatigue and illness through long-term, chronic exposure. Even low levels of organic chemicals, pesticides, formaldehyde, carpet cleaners, and tobacco smoke can affect those exposed to them for a long enough period.

The individual pollutants can be located and reduced, but the single most important factor is ventilation. Monday is the worst day for headaches and stress, at least partly because the ventilation systems have often been shut down over the weekend; you're breathing old, stale air. The ducts of your office air-venting system probably haven't been cleaned in years. Dust and molds have built up inside them and are coming out into the air you breathe when the system is restarted. Ask the maintenance people to clean them; if they won't, get a heavy-duty charcoal filter and put it in the vent with a thick white insulation pad over it. These filters can be bought inexpensively at any hardware store. In one week the insulation pad will be covered with black particles large enough to see.

If it's noisy where you work, wear earplugs. You can also make your desk more pleasant with a small portable ionizer. The ionizer can actually fit in your pocket and is also useful in airplanes or on the dashboard of your car.

The fluorescent lighting often used in offices flashes on and off rapidly and constantly, placing great stress on your central nervous system. Although you are not consciously aware of this very rapid flickering, your eye and nervous system are overstimulated by it; two or three hours of work under fluorescent light can have the effect of three or four cups of coffee. At a certain level of overstimulation the central nervous system will shut down, and you will find yourself deeply fatigued. Replace the fluorescent lighting at your desk with a lamp that uses incandescent bulbs and use natural full-spectrum light bulbs. It's best to have an office with a window or skylight for true natural lighting; if you don't have one and can't arrange it, it's especially important to have natural—and sufficiently bright—lighting.

Stay away from the photocopier at the office as much as possible; it uses volatile chemicals. Don't leave typewriter ink or correction ribbons lying around open; put them in a sealed plastic bag when they are not in use. An exhaust fan on the ceiling will help draw away vaporizing fluids.

PATIENT STORY

I started becoming ill a year before I realized what was happening. At first I just thought I was tired. I was having trouble getting out of bed. I was dragging myself to work. I would come home feeling exhausted. Sometimes I had asthmalike symptoms and couldn't quite catch my breath. I wondered why this started all of a sudden when I was thirty years old, because my understanding was that most people develop asthma as children. I attributed these symptoms to working and living a fast-paced lifestyle, and I ignored them. One day my wrist started to ache for no apparent reason, which made me wonder if I was getting arthritis. But I ignored that as well and thought it would go away. I had these warning signs for a year before collapsing at work in September 1993.

I had woken up feeling as if I had the flu but thought I was well enough to go to work. I had gone shopping with my mom that morning and had had difficulty walking up stairs. When I arrived at work, I realized that I was feeling quite unwell and that I would be able to work only part of my nursing shift. At the end of the first hour, I needed to go home because I was too ill to walk down the corridor and deliver medications to my patients. It was then that I returned to the nursing station and collapsed. I could hear, but I couldn't move. I felt as if I were paralyzed. I couldn't communicate with the other nurses who came to attend to me.

They took me to the emergency room, but I started to feel better and went home. I decided that I had the flu and that I would be better in three days.

Three days of flu evolved into a year and a half. During this time, I experienced many difficulties. The problem with environmental illness or chemical sensitivity is that you have a wide array of symptoms that come and go. You don't really know where to start and what connections to make. These are some of the symptoms I experienced:

Flu symptoms plagued me every day and became worse with time. As time passed, I was having more difficulty getting out of bed and walking around the house. I was extremely tired. No matter how much I slept, I just could not seem to get enough sleep. Even small tasks that shouldn't take much energy overwhelmed me. Cooking a meal was too much to even think about.

I also started having disturbed sleep. Despite my fatigue, I would wake up between 2:00 and 4:00 each night with numb hands. Sometimes I would have an incredible thirst. And sometimes I would wake up shaking as if I had a very high fever.

At one point I lost sight in my right eye. This happened for a short time but was extremely frightening nonetheless. All of a sudden, the vision in my right eye became completely silver, as if I were trying to look through a piece of tinfoil.

I had headaches with stabbing pains in my temples and a burning sensation in the back of my neck that made it difficult to turn my head. If you try to drive a car or move to do something, you realize how important it is to have range of motion in your neck.

The next month, I started to experience food allergies. It started with a few things. First I wasn't tolerating wheat very well and stopped eating it. Then I noticed that I did not feel well after drinking coffee and milk, so I eliminated them also. As the months progressed, I was unable to tolerate more and more foods. By January, I was virtually down to two foods: lamb and yams. By February, I lost my tolerance for everything. I was caught in a vicious cycle. I knew I needed to get nutrition in order to turn my health around, but eating these foods would make me even sicker.

As I became increasingly ill, my sense of smell became more and more acute. All of a sudden perfumes were a problem. I absolutely hated going to the department store and passing the perfume counter. I couldn't stand the smell of car exhaust either. I even avoided the hardware store because of the strong smell in there. Going to public places became difficult, as many people wear scented products such as clothes washed in scented laundry detergents, perfumes, and aftershaves. I would walk into a room, and if someone had perfume on, I would suddenly feel like I had the worst flu. My shoulders and muscles would start to ache. I would feel short of breath. I would get a headache.

A heightened sense of smell is part of the illness. People who are not affected need to understand what is happening when individuals with environmental illness ask, "Please do not wear that fragrance because it makes me feel sick."

I also started to have ringing in my ears. That would come and go, so I never could associate it with any particular event. Sometimes it would affect one ear, sometimes both. It was bothersome trying to have a conversation with somebody and trying to hear that person over the ringing in my ears.

Additionally, I felt dizzy. I had days when it was even difficult for me to stand up and navigate my way to the bathroom. Several times I fell over.

One of the most disturbing symptoms I had was difficulty concentrating. I could no longer read something from start to finish. It would take me three to four tries to read material I should have comprehended in the first reading.

I also noticed that I was forgetful. Previously I had had an exceptional memory. All of a sudden I noticed that I couldn't remember things that were extremely important. At age thirty I was wondering if I was getting the beginning stages of Alzheimer's disease, the loss of memory was so apparent. Some days my memory was better than others, and some days my ability to concentrate was better than others.

Then there were the panic attacks. My heart would race while I was driving my car on the interstate. I did not understand why I felt better on residential streets. Later, I realized that I had difficulty on the interstate because the exhaust was so much more prevalent there. Every time I was exposed to exhaust, my heart raced; I felt anxious and had difficulty concentrating.

I also felt extremely anxious in shopping malls. I have since learned that there are extremely high levels of chemicals in shopping malls, such as formaldehyde, emitted by new building materials. These synthetics are highly toxic. What I couldn't understand was why I felt anxious at some times and not others. The reason was that some shopping malls are less toxic than others, and some stores, because of the types of merchandise they carry, are also better than others.

The day I collapsed at work was the last day I worked as a nurse. I kept assuming that within a month I would feel better and go back to my job. One month rolled into two, two months into three, and three months into a year and a half.

Being a nurse, I felt that I would receive the support I needed. After all, I was a medical person myself. What I experienced instead was how a patient feels when he or she is told that nothing is wrong. I had always been on the other side of things. I found this new perspective extremely alarming.

The medical community has become technologically based. Everything relies on a diagnostic test. I would go in, and they would run a gamut of tests. As with most people with environmental illness, the standard tests would come back negative. The doctors would then tell me that there was nothing wrong. This was disturbing because I was extremely ill. I was so sick that I could hardly get up off the couch. Nor could I make myself a meal. Going to the bathroom was an effort. How, on a diagnostic test, could I look perfectly normal?

When the doctors could not diagnose me, they said that I was suffering from stress. But this was not the case. Before I got sick, my life was wonderful. I had one of the least pressured jobs I had ever had, and I was enjoying what I was doing. At the end of a contract I would go on vacation to Europe for a month. I was about to get married. My life couldn't have been better.

Stress is becoming the catchall diagnosis in the medical community. We must ask why so many people in our society are being told that they have stress, panic disorder, anxiety, and depression. That category is growing larger and larger. People have to ask, Why is this happening in our society? Is something chemical bringing this on? Do we need to make changes in the environment?

If you are feeling some symptoms of toxicity, it is time to take action now. Don't wait until you end up, as I did, in a wheelchair, bedridden, and completely intolerant to food.

—Heather Millar

EVERYDAY HEALTH

DIET AND NUTRITION

It has finally become conventional to associate good nutrition with good health. Mainstream medicine and the public at large now acknowledge that a good diet can not only promote health, but also prevent disease. Today it is customary to talk about how food choices affect our overall well-being and help ward off heart disease, cancer, diabetes, stroke, osteoporosis, and other ailments. Most people are also aware that a healthy diet can decrease the risk of disease by reducing predisposing conditions such as obesity, high blood pressure, and high cholesterol.

Eating a balanced diet is the most effective way to ensure that our bodies receive the nutrients we need. Unfortunately, the typical American diet does not meet many of the requirements for good health. Part of the problem relates to the types and proportions of foods people eat. Just as important to our health is how the foods are grown and processed as they make their way to our grocery shelves and kitchen tables.

Eating properly means selecting unprocessed or minimally processed foods. You want to avoid pesticides, dyes, and wax coatings. Many of our diets need to be adjusted to include more complex carbohydrates, fewer proteins, and less fat. A wide assortment of whole grains, legumes, vegetables, fruits, nuts, and seeds supplies multiple nutrients. Sometimes supplements are necessary. Juices from watermelons, raspberries, pomegranates, and tomatoes are filled with phytochemicals that help repair DNA and prevent cancer. We should be thinking about our diets as part of our daily health routines. In this chapter, and throughout the pages of this book, there is information on how diet and nutrition help promote everyday health and prevent and/or manage health problems.

Toxic substances abound in our air, water, soil, and food. A healthy person can often eliminate harmful substances through the liver and other organs. But a person whose health is compromised, or on a diet that is too high in fats, processed proteins, sodium, refined sugars, and other refined foods has a reduced capacity to rid the body of toxins. When this happens, the toxins accumulate.

Frances Taylor, coauthor of *The Whole Way to Natural Detoxification,* tells us more: "As we journey through life the way most people do, we become over-loaded with the toxins that absorb in the body. Unless we do something to get rid of these things, our bodies become overloaded and our health suffers. We de-velop symptoms such as headaches, digestive problems, sluggishness, after-meals fatigue. Many health benefits can be obtained by simply detoxifying the body."

Taylor says there are many ways to detoxify at home. Her guidelines are presented below:

Water

One of the first things people need to do is make sure they consume enough water. Taylor says, "Some people do reasonably well with city water, tap water, which of course contains a number of additives. Most people will do consid-erably better if they use some type of filtered or ionized water or reverse os-mosis water."

Detox Bath

"We use a lot of detox baths with our patients," Taylor says. "We jokingly refer to detox baths as a poor man's sauna. Hot water increases the blood flow in the capillary action near the surface of the skin and causes a faster release of toxins."

Anybody who has a bathtub can do a detox bath. Taylor explains the pro-cedure: "First of all you need to start off with an absolutely clean bathtub. You wash your body thoroughly before you take your bath. Then you fill the bath-tub with water as hot as you can tolerate it without burning your skin. You need to cover the overflow valve so the water will be high enough for you to immerse your body up to your neck.

"This next step is very important. You begin with a five-minute soak in the hot water. Some people say, 'Oh, gee, it felt so good I stayed in for fifteen minutes.' These people frequently cannot get out of bed the next day be-cause their body releases toxins more rapidly than the liver can detoxify them, so they don't feel well. It's very important that you stay in the plain hot water bath for five minutes only the first time.

"After your bath you must take a shower and scrub every square inch of your skin to get off any toxins that may have been released. If you don't do this, these [toxins] will be reabsorbed into your body."

If you don't have any symptoms after the five-minute bath, increase bath time by five minutes more the next day. Gradually increase your time until you can sit in the plain hot water for thirty minutes. Most people need to do a detox bath only about three times a week. It's a good idea to drink an eight-ounce glass of water during your bath because you are going to be sweating. You can even take some vitamin C both before and after your bath because this will help your body remove the toxins that are released into your blood-stream.

Taylor recommends the use of Epsom salts in the bath. "The sulfur component in Epsom salts helps detoxify," she says. "It works as a counter irritant on the skin to increase the blood supply and it changes the pH of the skin surface. Begin with only a fourth of a cup of Epsom salts and gradually increase it over time until you are using about 4 cups per tub of clean hot water."

Again you want to do things very gradually so that your body won't detoxify too rapidly. You don't want to exceed the capacity of your liver and your detox system to get rid of the toxins.

Apple cider vinegar, baking soda, clay, and herbal teas may also be added to a detox bath, following the same principles as Epsom salts. With apple cider vinegar, Taylor says to start with the plain hot water bath first, then add 1/4 cup of apple cider vinegar, and over a period of time increase this to 1 cup. Baking soda baths are particularly beneficial for people with weeping open sores. Combining baking soda and salt is effective if you have had an X ray or been exposed to radiation. "We routinely have our patients take a salt and soda bath if they have to have any X rays done," Taylor says. "You will use equal amounts of the soda and noniodized sea salt and you build up until you use a pound of each."

For clay baths, Taylor recommends a cup of clay to a tub of water. Clays can be purchased at many health food stores.

Among the herbal teas that can be used in a detox bath are catnip, peppermint, blessed thistle, and horsetail. Use 1 cup of brewed tea per tub of hot clean water. Taylor says use only one of these teas per bath. In addition, "some sensitive people may not tolerate the tea."

Diet

Taylor says, "You want to eat clean food. Food that has not been pesticided, has not been dyed, doesn't have a wax coating on it. If you have food allergies, of course, you don't want to eat your food allergens. Rotation diets will help people with allergies. Some people even find that fasting is helpful. One word of caution about fasting: if you do have numerous food allergies and you start fasting, you could have withdrawal symptoms because people are allergic to the foods or they are addicted to the foods to which they are allergic. If a person has a very heavy load of food allergens, they may not feel very well if they try a fast."

Following are some foods that can help build good health:

SPROUTS—Sprouts are one of the most nutrient-rich, powerful, health-building foods in nature. They will help cleanse and rebuild your entire system.

What kind of sprouts should you try? Don't stop with just common sprouts like alfalfa or mung beans. Expand your cuisine. Try high-protein buckwheat sprouts; the sweet sunflower sprout; the aromatic fenugreek sprout; clover sprout; and for a little bite and pinch, try a radish sprout. A mustard sprout tastes as good as mustard, and yet it has that nice salad feel to it.

More than fifteen different seeds for sprouting are available commercially. They're inexpensive and versatile. You can make salads out of them, put them into pita bread, use them in casseroles, and put them in soups.

MISO—Miso should also be on the list of detoxifying and rebuilding foods. For more than three thousand years, this nutritionally superior food has been helping people build better health. Miso is a fermented product. Like yogurt, its bacteria work well in the intestines. Miso should be used sparingly, however, because it does have a high sodium content.

VEGETABLE JUICES—Vegetable juices are important detoxifiers. Generally speaking, Taylor says, drink no more than one glass of carrot juice per day. Beta carotene is a precursor of vitamin A in the body. If you drink too much carrot juice, you'll be overloading the liver with vitamin A and your skin may turn yellow or orange. One glass will give you all the benefits of the vitamin. Celery, cucumber, cabbage, parsley, and sprouts can be added. For people who've never really enjoyed vegetables, juices are another way to get good-tasting, high-quality nutrition into the diet.

GRAINS—Grains are another group of foods that help the body cleanse itself and rebuild its strength. It is unfortunate that most Americans never taste whole grain. They eat refined carbohydrates in white bread or white rice, but not brown rice or whole grain bread. Whole grains are loaded with far more nutrition than their refined counterparts. The grain family includes rice, corn, buckwheat, rye, oats, and millet, as well as less well-known, newly available grains like triticale, amaranth, and quinoa (pronounced *keen-wa*), a light, fast-cooking grain from South America.

SEA VEGETABLES—The next group of foods to include as part of your health-rebuilding program is the sea family of vegetables. These include hijiki, a form of seaweed that tastes salty like fish. You can buy seaweed dry and store it for months. There are many types, including kombu, wakami, and nori. You can cut it into pieces, flake it, or put it into casseroles or soups. Include seaweed in your miso soup to increase its nutritional value. You can wrap seaweed around rice like grape leaves. Seaweed is so versatile that entire books are devoted to its use in cookery.

Seaweed is loaded with minerals. By dry weight, hijiki has ten times more available calcium than cow's milk.

BEANS—Beans, or legumes, are a group of healthy, detoxifying foods that many Americans deliberately avoid. The main reason we have kept ourselves away from one of nature's most important sources of vitamins, minerals, and fiber is that we have never really understood how to cook it. Most people, and most restaurants, do not soak beans overnight. This diminishes their digestability. During digestion, gas forms in the colon, causing indigestion and flatulence. That uncomfortable feeling needn't be. All you have to do is soak beans overnight and then boil them for one or two hours. That usually takes care of most gas-producing properties. Then be sure to combine them with the right foods: Don't eat fruit or sugary foods with a bean meal.

Legumes have more protein than grains or seeds. They are also high in fiber. There are more than 60 different legumes.

Nutritional Supplements

Taylor also recommends supplements. "We encourage our patients to take bowel tolerance vitamin C," Taylor says. "I'm talking about a clean, pure vitamin C that is free of the common allergens such as wheat, yeast, corn, and sugar."

Taylor explains the procedure: "To do bowel-tolerance vitamin C, you start off with a gram, which is 1,000 milligrams, with each meal, and at bedtime. The next day you would add another one at breakfast. Then the next day you would add another one at lunch. The next day you would add another one at bedtime and so on. You know when you have reached bowel tolerance when you develop diarrhea. Most people can take much larger amounts of vitamin C than they would ever imagine. If a person is very, very toxic or has a lot of allergies they may be able to take 10 to 20 grams, that is 10,000 to 20,000 milligrams, of vitamin C a day. Between meals we encourage people to take buffered C, which is an ascorbic acid to which calcium, magnesium carbonate, and potassium bicarbonate have been added. This helps with detox but also helps with digestion. You would continue adding vitamin C, a gram a day, until you develop diarrhea and then you would back up 1 gram and that is the amount you would take in divided doses throughout the day."

Other nutrients are important for detoxification. These include the B vitamins. "You need to take a multimineral also because detoxification in the body is an enzymatic process and all of the enzymes require a metal to make them work," Taylor says. "Organic germanium is also good because it helps the body oxygenate at the cellular level. It is a little expensive but is very, very well worthwhile."

NATURAL MEDICINE CABINET

Many times we want to be able to go to our home medicine cabinet and find what we need for our day-to-day ills and problems. In this section you will find some of the components of a well-stocked natural medicine cabinet.

Herbal Antibiotics

The widespread use of antibiotics in this country has created a serious problem. The danger now is that bacteria have become immune to some of our most common antibiotics. The way this happened is that bacteria communicate with each other and actually teach each other how to become immune to medications. Now that they have become resistant to so many antibiotics, what does this tell us about further attempts to create stronger antibiotics? Steven Harrod Buhner, author of *Herbal Antibiotics*, explains: "Five million people a year are coming down with antibiotic resistant infections. The Centers for Disease Control and many epidemiologists are warning that in the next ten to fifteen years most of our antibiotic arsenal will fail. People will have to turn to more natural alternatives that are more ecologically sound, as herbs are. Things that naturally stimulate the immune system, that help keep us from getting ill in the first place.

"As our antibiotic arsenal fails, it becomes more and more important for everybody to stimulate their immune system and to keep it healthy and balanced. Whether it is bubonic plague or Ebola river virus, some people never become ill because their immune system is potentiated and healthy.

"We only get sick when our bodies are out of balance. Our natural immune system should deal with almost all diseases we encounter. Plant medicines are not something bacteria can become resistant to. Herbal medicines are so much more effective than antibiotics and are a lot gentler on the body."

To identify the most useful herbal antibiotics, Buhner studied each individually. "When I assessed the most powerful herbs, I had three criteria. One was the length of time it had been used in different cultures. Second was the degree to which it was used by indigenous and folk practitioners around the world. Third was the effectiveness in clinical trials and laboratory studies." Below, Buhner describes some of the herbs that met all three criteria:

ALOE—"Aloe comes from a Southwestern American plant. It is directly effective against staphylococcus bacteria, even resistant staph bacteria. Staph bacteria like to infect burns because the skin is not available to protect them. When aloe is used on burns, it also softens the skin, keeps it moist, and is soothing. Honey can be used almost identically. In China they have been using honey on second- and third-degree burns and seeing healing with no scarring or muscle loss."

ECHINACEA—"Echinacea is exceptionally effective against streptococcal bacteria, those that cause strep throat. It is well known and popular."

GOLDENSEAL—"Goldenseal is good in the mucous membrane system. It is an amazing plant for *E. coli* infections, which can cause severe, sometimes bloody diarrhea that can be fatal in children."

CRYPTOCOCCOIS—"This is a West African plant used traditionally for malaria for thousands of years. It is effective against all antibiotic-resistant bacteria as well as malaria. It is equally as good as the pharmaceuticals that are used for malaria, but it doesn't have any of their side effects."

GARLIC—"Garlic is effective against every antibiotic-resistant bacteria except for malaria. If you eat it regularly, it helps stimulate the immune system, so that helps prevent infection. Use it raw as a juice or eat the raw cloves when you have a bacterial infection. Many clinicians who are using herbs for difficult diseases such as AIDS use juiced garlic. They give people between two to nine bulbs of garlic a day, not just the cloves. It is usually taken in 1/4 to 1/2 teaspoon in about 12 ounces of a binder such as tomato or carrot juice. You drink it throughout the day."

LICORICE—"Licorice is one of the most potent herbs. It is an immune stimulant and immune modulator, which means it helps the immune system become more functional. By the way, the rubbery candies we call licorice candies often contain no licorice and are mostly flavored with anise or fennel."

ESTONIA—"Estonia is a lichen that grows on trees throughout the world and has been found to be more powerful than penicillin. In dilute concentrations of 1 to 20,000 it completely inhibits both tuberculosis and resistant staphylococcus bacteria. It is two plants in one, a symbiotic plant. The inner white thread is an immune enhancer and an immune stimulant, and the outside green part is strongly antibacterial. You not only fight bacterial disease directly but also enhance your immune functioning."

Homeopathic Remedies

A number of homeopathic remedies also belong in the natural medicine cabinet. Homeopathy is based on the idea that the cure for an illness is similar to its cause. Homeopathic remedies, all made from natural substances, are given in microdoses.

According to Food and Drug Administration regulations, a natural remedy cannot be labeled safe and effective for treating a specific ailment even if study after study has proven that it is more effective than over-the-counter or doctor-prescribed medications. Therefore the average American will only see television commercials for products such as Anacin or Tylenol to treat a headache, even though a simple homeopathic remedy may be safer and just as effective.

Millions of Americans suffer from a myriad of everyday health conditions and do not know about natural remedies. Dr. Lynn Page Walker is a doctor of homeopathy and has a master's degree in Chinese herbology and acupuncture. She has specific recommendations for what ought to be in everyone's medicine chest, especially if your access to a doctor or medical care is limited:

TEA TREE OIL—Dr. Walker's first recommendation—although this is not, strictly speaking, a homeopathic remedy—is tea tree oil. "Tea tree oil is an oil from Australia, also called melaluka oil. It is a strong antiviral, antifungal, and antibacterial. You could use it on any cut, for any kind of fungus in the mouth, and for fungus under the nail. It works as a gargle for sore throat and for gum problems. There is a tea tree oil toothpaste for those with ongoing gum problems. It works on canker sores, cuts and abrasions, insect bites, and even as an astringent for the face. Tea tree oil is a good basic remedy to have around the house."

RESCUE REMEDY—"The next thing I recommend is rescue remedy, a Bach flower essence that is a combination of five different flower essences. It is excellent for relieving stress, so it can be calming in emergency situations. It is safe for small children and animals. When there is a crisis, I recommend that every member of the family, not just the sick one, take Rescue to see things a little bit more clearly."

BITING INSECT—"The next useful remedy to have around the house actually prevents insect bites. It is Biting Insect by Molecular Biologicals. It is good for flea bites, mosquito bites, and any kind of bug bites. Although it helps with some spider bites, it is not as effective. If you know you will be exposed to bugs, take 10 drops three times a day."

PEPPERMINT OIL—"I recommend peppermint oil for a number of things. You can mix it in warm water and drink it for a stomachache or rub it directly on the forehead for a headache." Again, although not strictly speaking a homeopathic remedy, peppermint oil is an enteric coated herbal remedy Dr. Walter recommends.

BLACK OINTMENT—"Black ointment is made by Nature's Way and some other companies. Anytime you have a splinter or any little sliver that won't come out, black ointment can draw it out. It is also a very healing salve for any kind of cut."

ARNICA—Dr. Walker also recommends "arnica homeopathic in low potency, either a 6x or 30x, for any kind of trauma to the body. It stops the body from overreacting to the trauma. It's good for muscle aches and pains, such as on days when you have worked really hard physically. Some people take it before surgery, but just take one dose to help your body not overreact."

TRAUMA OINTMENT OR TRAUMED OINTMENT—These are "combinations of homeopathic remedies specifically for trauma. They are nice combinations to use on your muscles if you are sore."

CALENDULA TINCTURE—"Calendula tincture is a healing oil made from marigold flower. It is good for cleansing wounds and promotes healing. I've seen wounds heal in a day or two."

NUX VOMICA—"Nux vomica in a low potency, 6x or 30x, is for hangover and also for upset stomach from overeating or overdrinking. When you feel bloated and your digestion feels off, nux vomica is a good remedy. It also works well for hemorrhoids."

CALENDULA HYPERICUM—"Calendula hypericum ointment, especially the brand made by Boron, promotes healing. The cholangiole promotes the healing and the hypericum helps with any kind of pain. Together they work for cold sores, any kind of sore on the face or mouth, cuts or abrasions to heal them fast and take away the pain."

GUNPOWDER 6X—"One of my favorites is not well known. It is called gunpowder 6x. This is for any minor infection like tooth abscesses or any infection on the skin. I find it useful for those who are getting their ears or bellybuttons pierced and they get infected. You can't get any sustainable antibiotic levels at those sites if you get an infection there. Take three gunpowder pills three times a day and the infection will resolve in two or three days."

VACTICIME DROPS—"Vacticime drops are a combination made by Complemed that stimulates your body to fight bacterial infection. If you had an abscess or sore throat or any kind of bacterial infection take 10 drops three to five times a day. This will clear the infection in a short period by boosting your own immune system."

ABC DROPS—"ABC drops is a combination of aconite, belladonna, and chamomile homeopathic medications. Popular in Europe, it is good for colds and earaches."

COLDS

So far there has been no cure for the common cold even though lots of money has been spent on medical research. Keeping healthy in the first place is the best defense. A healthy immune system can tackle the bacteria and viruses better than any antibiotic or medication. Dr. Ray Sahelian is a board-certified family practice physician and graduate of Thomas Jefferson School of Medicine. In his book, *Finally the Common Cold Cure*, he recommends an approach for getting rid of the cold.

Immune System "Busters"

As Dr. Sahelian points out, the primary cause of the cold is a virus. There are at least a couple of hundred types of viruses that cause colds. But, as we know, not everybody comes down with the common cold when they are exposed to the virus. The most likely reason people don't get sick is that they are maintaining healthy living habits.

Dr. Sahelian has identified four immune system "busters" that cause some people to come down with a cold when they are exposed to the virus. The first is lack of sleep. "People come down with a cold when they are not getting six to eight hours of restful sleep. It is during the time of our deepest sleep that the immune cells are regenerated. One particular type of immune cell, called the natural killer cell, is very important. It is during deep sleep that the natural killer cell is activated. If it is not activated, then we are more vulnerable to getting a cold. Everyone is going to be exposed to the virus sooner or later, by shaking the hand of someone who has a cold or being exposed to children who are sneezing or coughing. If we have a good, activated immune system it is going to knock out that virus.

"Besides lack of sleep, stress is another immune system buster, whether it be from relationship difficulties, financial worries, stress at work, physical stress, intense athletic competition—sometimes running a marathon can do it—or from illness. Stress can temporarily lower the immune system, and that can allow the virus to get a foothold. Poor diet, particularly a lot of sugars, potato chips, cookies, pies, and junk foods, interferes with the immune system."

The third immune system buster is smoking. "Smoking damages the lining of the respiratory tract," Dr. Sahelian says. "There are hairlike structures called cilia that are constantly sweeping out the germs that we inhale. If the cilia are damaged from smoking they are not going to be able to sweep out the bacteria or viruses, which then settle in to start a cold or another type of infection."

The final immune system buster is taking antibiotics when you don't need them. Dr. Sahelian explains: "Whenever someone comes down with a cold, as a rule they wait it out a day or two, take some over-the-counter pills if they are not into natural medicine, and then go to their doctor. The doctor examines them, says, 'You have a cold, take some more over-the-counter medicines, and you are going to be okay in a week.' Well, the patient is not satisfied if they made the effort to go all the way to the doctor, wait in the office waiting room, pay sixty to two hundred dollars to see a doctor, and then be told to use an over-the-counter medicine. So they are going to request an antibiotic prescription.

"So, even though 90 percent of all upper respiratory infections are caused by a virus, over 50 percent of the time the patient will come out with a pre-scription for an antibiotic. *Antibiotics do not kill viruses.* And antibiotics are harmful because they can cause side effects, such as yeast infections, killing all the good bacteria in the gut. They can also cause fatigue, allergic reac-tions, diarrhea, and sometimes even more harmful things. So that is not the answer."

Immune System Boosters

What is the answer, then? "In addition to having a good healthy diet, taking some supplements on a regular basis, such as vitamin C, vitamin E, juices, and fish oils will help you stay healthy," says Dr. Sahelian.

Gail Ulrich, founder of Blazing Star Herbal School in Shelbourn Falls, Massachusetts, and the author of *Herbs to Boost Immunity*, tells us more: "Our culture's diet is high in fats, refined sugars, and sodium. We now know that these foods produce free radicals in the body that create toxicity and weaken immunity. It is important first of all to eliminate refined sugar and flours, as well as caffeine, cigarettes, alcohol, and processed or deep-fried foods. It goes without saying to avoid tobacco, commercially raised red meats, especially be-cause of the high pesticide and hormone content in these products, and to minimize alcohol consumption.

"An immune-enhancing diet would include a wide variety of organically grown fruits and vegetables or wild fruits and vegetables as well. You also need whole grains and legumes along with adequate amounts of protein from soy, grains, or fish. The more you get back to a simple diet based on whole foods as they occur in nature, the better off you will be. It is important to include superfoods or nutrient-dense foods such as miso soup, garlic, and sea vegetables such as kelp. Wild foods are important, as are greens such as dandelion greens, mustard greens, watercress, astragalus, and steamed nettle greens. There are some delicious medicinal immune-enhancing mushrooms such as shiitake and reishi. Yogurt that contains acidophilus is important for balancing the garden of the intestinal flora, if you don't have lactose intolerance. Other immune-enhancing foods include dates, almonds, buckwheat, chicken soup, chickpeas, burdock root, and parsley."

Other lifestyle changes may be in order. "They always say, eat like a king at breakfast, a prince at lunch, and a pauper at dinner. Drink at least eight glasses of pure water daily and exercise adequately.

"There are many herbs we can use to enhance immunity. Echinacea is well known. I also recommend garlic, osha root, and milk thistle. These protect the mucus membranes and stimulate production of white blood cells. There are also deep immune tonic herbs that would be helpful to build the bone marrow and increase deep immunity. These are astragalus, Siberian ginseng, and shiitake and reishi mushrooms. These are especially helpful when we have immune deficiency and long-term stress on the immune system.

"There are also herbs called adaptogens that help the body cope with stress on many levels, including not only physical stress but environmental and emotional stressors. In this category is Siberian ginseng, panax ginseng, which is American, and Korean ginseng, licorice, borage, and milk thistle, to name a few."

Natural Remedies

What should you do at the first signs of a cold? "Sometimes a cold can come on mildly—a scratchy throat, a runny nose, or even just a tingling sensation in the nose or throat," Ulrich explains. "But as soon as you notice the very first symptom, do not wait to act. Immediately take between 3 to 5 grams of vitamin C. You may wish to keep the 500 milligram capsules on your kitchen counter and take about six to ten of these, which would equal about 3 to 5 grams of vitamin C. Right after that immediately put a zinc lozenge in your mouth. The zinc lozenge should contain between 10 to 25 milligrams of zinc. Many people chew it and within a brief period swallow it, but this is a mistake. The zinc is fighting the cold by acting locally in the throat and palate and the nasopharyngeal area. It has to stay in the mouth for as long as you can tolerate it, generally five to ten minutes. You can bite it, but keep the pieces in your mouth before you swallow it. Keep these at home because you never know, a cold can start at two in the morning and by the time you have gone to the health food store in the morning to buy these supplements, the cold might have gotten a foothold.

"Another common mistake is stopping the medications too soon. The symptoms may have eased and then you forget to take the supplements. They have to be taken continuously. With the vitamin C you can lower the dose from 3–5 grams to 1–2 grams every few hours. I recommend the zinc at least every hour or two for the first half day and then every two to three hours after that. The problem with the zinc lozenge is that it can irritate the palate and cause soreness. But I would rather have that than allow the virus to settle in. These suggestions are crucial, and timing is very important here.

"You may travel somewhere where zinc and vitamin C are not available, so I recommend taking them with you. I also recommend using the zinc lozenge right before you go to bed. If you wake up, take it again. Don't let six or eight hours pass without doing it.

How can you tell the difference between a virus, bacteria, or allergy? "Even doctors have trouble differentiating them because the symptoms overlap," Ulrich says. "Viruses and bacteria will give fever but allergies do not. Runny nose is common with the common cold virus and allergies, but bacteria will rarely if ever give you a runny nose. Nasal congestion is common with the virus and allergies, but bacteria rarely. Another way to differentiate viruses from allergies is muscle aches and pains. If you have bad muscle aches and pains, it is more commonly a virus and hardly ever an allergy. Allergies will rarely give you yellow-green mucus, but bacteria commonly will as all the viruses.

"I want to mention children and zinc. One study done recently did not show zinc to be effective in children. The kids probably swallowed the zinc tablets and didn't let it stay in their mouth and throat long enough for it to kill the viruses. I still feel that in a clinical sense older children can use zinc effectively when used appropriately.

"It is not inevitable that we all come down with colds. By eating the right foods, getting a good night's rest, reducing stress, not smoking, taking some of the supplements on a regular basis, like vitamin C and fish oils, garlic, onions and then taking the immediate steps right away when coming down with a cold, you can, as a rule, either eliminate or greatly decrease the frequency of viruses."

HEADACHES

A pounding headache afflicts most people at some time in their lives. It interferes with daily activities and keeps us from functioning at our best. If you are a migraine headache sufferer, you know what I'm talking about. (See chapter 24 for a discussion of migraines.) Doctors offer powerful medications that may or may not help and have side effects of their own. What causes our headaches? And how can we get rid of them without making ourselves sicker?

In her book *No More Headaches, No More Migraines,* Dr. Zuzana Bic has some of the answers. Dr. Bic is an assistant adjunct professor of medicine at UCLA at Irvine and is in private practice. In her research and work using integrative lifestyle medicine in the prevention of chronic diseases, she has been able to identify headache "triggers." There are many things that trigger headaches. If we know what they are, we can avoid them and cut down on headaches without pain medications. She describes changes we can make in our day-to-day lives to make headaches a thing of the past.

"Where my research is unique," says Dr. Bic, "is in trying to identify the common denominator for all the lifestyle factors. I have a group I call diet-related triggers. In this group belong all food that is high in fat, high in refined sugar, most processed or refined food, and food that is low in complex carbohydrates. A related group is obesity, which is connected to not eating properly, and also hypoinsulinemia or insulin resistance, one of the first signs of diabetes. Hypoglycemia, which means low levels of sugar, is another trigger for headaches. Prolonged hunger and dehydration can cause headache, as can alcohol and caffeine intake.

"So what could be the common denominator of all these things that lead to headaches? This is the question I have addressed in my studies. What I have found I try to explain to the patients. As you know, the cells in the blood—platelets, red blood cells, and white blood cells—all coexist in the blood vessels. A high level of fat in the blood will crowd up the vessels, similar to a crowded freeway with one car bumping into another car. A process like platelet congregation occurs and there is a little bit of damage to the platelet, causing it to release serotonin. The body acts to excrete this excess serotonin and thus you have lower levels of serotonin. Serotonin is a very important neurotransmitter, and its lack is an important factor in triggering headache.

"There are other lifestyle triggers. These include smoking, a sedentary lifestyle, and exhausting physical exertion. Some patients who suffer from anorexia nervosa or bulimia exercise excessively, and this is the type that can result in headache. Stress and oral contraceptives or hormone replacement also trigger headaches."

But Dr. Bic points out that some types of headaches are caused by things other than triggers and these types of headaches are unaffected by lifestyle changes. Headaches caused by head trauma, infection or tumors in the brain, or problems with eyes or ears cannot be resolved with lifestyle modification.

She hits the nail on the head by identifying imbalanced diet as one of the main headache triggers. It makes sense that if you eat an unbalanced, unhealthy diet, your body will react by giving you a headache. In Dr. Bic's research she found it effective to put her patients on a low-fat diet and combat their hunger with fruit, vegetables, grains, beans, and a higher amount of fiber helps. She also recommends increasing the daily intake of water. "They think they drink enough water, but if they monitor it in their food diaries, they find that there is not enough water. They are always surprised.

"I also recommend starting an exercise program or increasing the level of physical activity. Start walking ten minutes in the morning and ten minutes in the evening. Or park the car as far away as possible and walk to the office. To cut down on stress, I recommend meditation or one-minute relaxation techniques such as breathing exercises or changing how they perceive situations to a more objective point of view."

In her research she also elucidates the timing of the trigger and the headache. "Some of my patients are more sensitive and can have a headache immediately, one hour after the trigger. For others it can be seventy-two hours after the trigger. I think it is the accumulation of unbalanced lifestyle factors. It is possible for a person to be sedentary, eat a high-fat diet, have a very stressful situation, and not be drinking enough water. All these things accumulate and they can have that headache from three hours to seventy-two hours."

So a good plan to avoid headache triggers is a low-fat diet, lots of water, exercise, and stress-reduction.

HANGOVERS

The alcohol hangover is an old problem. It's even referred to in the Bible: "Woe unto them that rise up early in the morning, that they may follow strong drink" (Isaiah 5:11). It may not happen too often, but there are always those big celebrations—weddings, graduations, office parties, New Year's Eve—when we may drink too much. The doctors call it by a fancy name: veisalgia, meaning "uneasiness following debauchery" and "pain." The symptoms are headache, nausea, diarrhea, and fatigue, combined with decreased cognitive and visual-spatial skills and work loss.

Alcohol in high doses can be toxic. It can dehydrate the body and have effects on the heart. Anyone who drives a car or has to operate machinery is going to have a problem when they have a hangover. Anyone who has to run a meeting or get the chores done is going to have a problem the next day. These people are going to feel lousy even after the alcohol is gone from their bodies. The alcohol leaves behind its toxic effects when you drink too much.

We know it has something to do with what's in the alcohol you overdose on. Dark-colored liquors, like brandy, wine, and whiskey give a much worse hangover. Drinking vodka, gin, or other clear liquors does not cause the worst symptoms. Sulfites found especially in dark wines can make you sicker. Alcohol causes a diuresis, meaning dehydration, meaning you go to the bathroom and the fluids in your body are depleted.

Are there any ways to prevent hangover? In a nonblinded study, an herbal preparation called Liv.52 from the Himalaya Drug Co. in Bombay decreased hangover symptoms. How did it work? The investigators thought it might be because the herb blocked the conversion of ethanol to acetaldehyde. Acetaldehyde is created from the by-products of ethanol (which is alcohol) in our stomachs. It can act like a poison in some people. Women are more susceptible to this because they have lower levels of the enzyme needed to convert alcohol to something less toxic.

In another study, vitamin B6 was given before, during, and after parties where the participants drank enough to get intoxicated. Those who took the vitamin reduced the number of hangover symptoms by 50 percent.

One thing everybody agrees on is to drink lots of fluids before, during, and after drinking alcohol. It helps to dilute the alcohol in the first place and replaces the fluids that are excreted by the kidneys. The diuresis, or excessive fluid excretion caused by the alcohol, causes the dehydration that leads to a lot of the symptoms of the hangover. And, of course, limit the number of times you get intoxicated with alcohol in the first place.

INSOMNIA

Insomnia is a common problem, affecting one-third of all adults and accompanying many of the disorders discussed elsewhere in this book. People with sleep-onset insomnia have difficulty falling asleep, while those with maintenance insomnia wake frequently throughout the night or very early in the morning.

Insomnia can be caused by a variety of physical, mental, and behavioral conditions. Among the common causes are pain, anxiety, tension, illness, indigestion, caffeine, and drugs. A major cause of insomnia, especially if it's chronic, is reactive hypoglycemia. This is frequently exacerbated by eating late at night, especially foods with a high glucose level, such as pastries, candy, or even fruit juice. Such foods cause blood-sugar levels to go up and then plummet, a fluctuation that can contribute to insomnia. Also, overindulging late at night in highly fatty foods can cause sleeplessness. That's because foods with a lot of fat take four to five times longer to empty from the stomach and be digested than simple or complex carbohydrates do.

Another important cause of insomnia is intake of stimulants. Most of us are aware of the caffeine in coffee, tea, chocolate, and colas. Alcohol, although generally considered a depressant, can have stimulant effects in some cases. In addition to food and drink, certain medications can be culprits in insomnia. Drugs that can interfere with the natural sleep cycle include Prozac, the newer drugs related to it, and Xanax.

Exercising in the late evening is another possible bane for the insomnia-prone in that it can overstimulate adrenal levels and excite the musculoskeletal system, resulting in difficulty getting to sleep. Likewise, stress and overstimulating the mind by thinking about unresolved conflicts can be a problem when the goal is sleep.

Conventional Treatment

Many people with insomnia often use over-the-counter or prescription drugs to help them sleep. Benzodiazepines and tricyclic antidepressants are among the medications that may be prescribed by a doctor. Potential side effects include daytime sleepiness, loss of muscle coordination, and addiction.

Herbal Remedies

A variety of herbs can be a real help to those challenged by insomnia. Unlike sleeping pills, herbs won't leave you in a fog in the morning, or feeling like you haven't really slept. Most of these herbs address the underlying cause of the insomnia, a depleted nervous system that cannot settle itself down.

Herbalist Terry Willard, in an article posted on the HealthWorld Online website (www.healthy.net) offers some recommendations:

REISHI MUSHROOM (*GANODERMA LUCIDIM*)—This herb provides daytime calm, decreases anxiety, and adjusts sugar metabolism. It helps to resolve what the Chinese call disturbed *shen qi* (a disturbed mental spirit). It has also been found to boost the immune system and reduce cholesterol and hypertension. Take three 1-gram tablets three times daily.

HOPS (*HUMULUS LUPULUS*)—This age-old sedative can be taken as a tea or combined with other dried herbs in a sleep pillow. To make the tea, mix 1 teaspoon whole hops into a cup of boiling water. Some people may have an allergic reaction to hops.

VALERIAN (*VALERIANA OFFICINALIS*)—Valerian has been used as a sedative for more than two thousand years. In Europe it is the most commonly used over-the-counter drug for sleep disorders. Willard recommends that valerian be taken only for short periods or intermittently, when insomnia is at its worst. This is because the herb can become habit-forming, and increased doses may be required if used for a long period. Too much valerian can also make you nauseous. About an hour before going to bed, take a dose of 300–400 mg of valerian product standardized to 0.5 percent oil.

SKULLCAP (*SCUTELLARIA LATERIFLORA*)—This is a powerful nerve tonic and sedative herb. It can be taken as a tincture of 15 to 40 drops two to three times a day; in combination with reishi, hops, and valerian; or as a tea, using 1 to 3 teaspoons of the root for every cup of water.

PASSIONFLOWER (*PASSIFLORA INCARNATA*)—This is an important relaxant herb. You can find tinctures and extracts in health-food stores. You can make a cup of tea by pouring 1 cup boiling water over 1/2 teaspoon dried passionflower. If you're being treated for depression, Willard issues a warning: this herb can reduce the effects of monoamine oxidase inhibitors.

LEMON BALM (*MELISSA OFFICINALIS*)—Lemon balm is used to relax the body and help with sleep. It can be taken as a tea, by steeping 1 to 2 tablespoons in a cup of hot water.

KAVA KAVA (*PIPER METHYSTICUM*)—This powerful anxiolytic (antianxiety agent) and sedative "will probably become one of the most important healing herbs in the next few years," Willard says. Its active compounds, called kavalactones, apparently work directly on the limbic system, which regulates emotional feelings and behavior. A clinical study in Germany found that patients receiving 100 mg of kava extract three times daily experienced a significant reduction in anxiety symptoms after only 1 week of treatment. Willard cautions that you should not take this herb if you are depressed, pregnant, nursing, or operating machinery.

CHAMOMILE (*MATRICARIA CHAMOMILLA*)—Chamomile not only relaxes and calms the body, but also strengthens the nervous system. Chamomile tea is a commonly used before-bedtime sedative. You can also take it as a tincture, 10–40 drops three times a day; or in capsule form, six 300–400 mg capsules daily.

HERBAL SLEEP PILLOW—Rosemary Gladstar, former director of the California School of Herbal Studies and author of *Herbs for Reducing Stress and Anxiety*, tells how to make an herbal pillow that can be placed next to your head while you sleep: Fill a 4-by-4 inch piece of fabric with dried hops, rose petals, lavender blooms, and chamomile flowers. You might want to put a few drops of lavender oil on top of the pillow as well.

Nutrition and Supplements

Foods with naturally occurring tryptophan in high amounts, such as turkey, eggs, fish, and dairy products, may help you sleep. Other options include calcium citrate and magnesium citrate—1,200 milligrams of each taken any time after dinner; 50 milligrams of the B complex; and 200 milligrams of inositol. Also, 200 micrograms of chromium in the evening will help stabilize your blood-sugar level. Melatonin, 1 to 3 milligrams before bed, and niacinamide, 70 to 280 milligrams daily, have been found to help some people.

Dr. Robert Atkins points out the efficacy of tryptophan, which has been banned from public sale in the U.S., in the treatment of insomnia: "Tryptophan is very valuable for sleep disorders because serotonin is the sleep chemical. If you take it right when you are ready to go to bed, when your serotonin level is on the upswing anyway, you are really fitting in physiologically with your body's chemical rhythms."

Homeopathy

Homeopathy is based on the principle that "like cures like." Homeopathic remedies are prescribed in minute doses. The homeopathic remedy chosen should correspond to the symptoms described; only one should be used for best results. Sometimes it's a matter of trial and error; if one does not work, try another. Judyth Reichenberg-Ullman and Robert Ullman, naturopathic and homeopathic physicians, describe some of the most commonly used remedies for insomnia in an article posted on HealthWorld Online (www.healthy.net):

ARSENICUM ALBUM—Recommended for insomnia caused by anxiety, with waking after midnight and restlessness.

NUX VOMICA—Used for insomnia from overuse of stimulants, stress, worries about work. The person usually wakes up in the middle of the night and stays awake.

COFFEA CRUDA—Recommended when you find yourself wide awake at three o'clock in the morning, feeling jubilant, excited, with a racing mind.

Other Natural Therapies

A gentle neck and head massage for fifteen minutes may do the trick in conquering insomnia, and fifteen minutes in a warm bath may be helpful as well. Along the lines of positive affirmation, writing in a diary shortly before bedtime can be extraordinarily beneficial. It can be a way of really seeing what you've done that's affirmed your mental, spiritual, and physical health, as well as any deeds you've done that have had positive effects on others. If a woman spends some time at the end of each day reflecting on what she's done in the past twenty-four hours that's been positive, and on plans for the next day, she gains a sense of completeness about the day. In a sense, then, diary-writing legitimizes going to bed; it's as if you can now see that you really deserve the good night's sleep you're about to get.

Judyth Reichenberg-Ullman and Robert Ullman also say it's important to prepare for sleep. Choose a time for bed and stick with it. Get ready for bed by unwinding slowly. Your bedroom should be "soothing and comfortable, dim and quiet." Make it a "peaceful sanctuary" used simply as a place for sleeping.

APHRODISIACS

Aphrodisiacs enhance sexual desire, arousal, and performance. There are foods, herbs, vitamins and minerals, amino acids, hormones, and aromatic oils that can directly affect our biochemistry and hence could affect our sexuality. There are over a dozen herbs that act as aphrodisiacs, but they work in various ways and produce different results. For example, there are fast-acting herbs, which affect one or more of the stages of sexual response. Then there are herbs that, if taken over a long period of time, boost a person's overall physical and emotional readiness. Although herbal preparations do not carry the same risk as pharmaceuticals taken to enhance sexual performance, it is important to understand how to take them for maximum effectiveness. Overall, herbs can vary tremendously in their strength and effectiveness depending on where they are grown, when they are harvested, how they are processed, and so on. It can be challenging to sort it all out.

Nancy Nickel, the author of *Nature's Aphrodisiacs*, has studied food, nutrition, and alternative therapies for over twenty-five years. Using her expertise as an educational writer, lecturer and researcher in nutrition and molecular therapy, she offers a review of nature's aphrodisiacs.

She says, "Natural aphrodisiacs have been a source of legend for centuries. Oysters and shrimp actually contain nutrients that benefit the reproductive system. There have been some scientific studies of natural aphrodisiacs but not too many. Most research is done by pharmaceutical manufacturers and it doesn't pay them to research a product they cannot patent. But we have some scientific evidence on why several natural products and natural aphrodisiacs work."

As we all know, sex is hardly ever just about sex. Emotions and psychological health have a direct impact on sexual health. Feelings such as anger, worry, tension, and depression all affect sexual encounters for both women and men. There are quite a few herbs that are useful for addressing this aspect of sex and pleasure.

Nickel helps us to identify what they are and how they work: "To reduce anxiety and elevate mood, there is kava kava, valerian, which is widely used in Europe, gotu kola, lemon balm, angelica, skullcap, and vervain. These work quickly. (St. John's wort is also very good but takes several weeks to have an effect.) Kava kava tea has a physical effect on sexual performance; however, it is also an unbeatable tension reducer. It makes you feel happy, relaxed, and sociable. You can buy tea bags or make it from an extract. Put 10 to 30 drops in juice or water. It is fairly safe although slightly narcotic. Because it affects the nervous system, it should not be used by people who have Parkinson's disease or those taking an antidepressant.

"Gotu kola is an excellent nerve tonic. It stimulates the central nervous system, decreases depression and fatigue, and stimulates the sex drive. If you take it regularly, which you can do, gotu kola tea has a cumulative effect as a sex drive booster. Unlike herbs that contain caffeine, it doesn't cause insomnia or nervousness. You can take one to three capsules a day. As an extract, you can mix 5 to 10 drops in a liquid and drink it. Take it about three times a day. Excessive doses can make you feel faint and sometimes it can cause a headache.

"Lemon balm can be grown in your own garden. It relaxes the nervous system and elevates your mood. It is one of the gentlest herbs and one of the most pleasant tasting. In Europe it is customary to drink lemon balm tea to calm stress and frayed nerves. It is available as a tea, a dried herb, and an extract. If you buy it as an extract, mix 1/2 to 1 teaspoon in liquid. Use the dried herb to make tea. Avoid lemon balm if you have a thyroid condition because it could interfere with a hormone that stimulates the thyroid. They are not sure about this, but I say be on the safe side.

"Angelica is a versatile herb that increases blood circulation. It acts as an aphrodisiac and is especially good for tension headaches. The dose is between 10 to 30 drops in a liquid. It should not be used by pregnant women because in strong doses it can bring on a period. And because it contains sugars, diabetics should not use it.

"Another excellent tranquilizing herb is skullcap. It is called skullcap because the flower looks like a little cap. It is excellent for relieving stress or nervousness associated with sex, or any kind of performance anxiety. It is very safe and mild, relaxes the muscles, and produces inner calm."

Other useful herbs are damiana, yohimbe, and muira puama (also called potency wood).

"Just one more reminder," Nickel says. "Because these herbs are potent and have chemical compounds that work, there are side effects, so you have to be careful."

SKIN CARE

The state of your body on the inside has a direct effect on the appearance and texture of your skin. Certain nutrients, foods, and herbs are important for healthy skin. Stephanie Tourles, a certified herbalist, aromatherapist, and reflexologist, and the author of *Naturally Healthy Skin*, tells us more:

"Nutrition is very important for skin care. I don't care what you put on the skin topically, if you are feeding yourself garbage, your skin is going to reflect that. What you eat is reflected on your face and body. In my daily quest for natural beauty, health, and vitality, I am in awe of what Mother Nature has to offer us. She provides everything you need to encourage and support the healthy functioning of your skin, but it is up to you to partake of these offerings.

"My personal recommendation is that you try to eat a very balanced diet, preferably vegetarian with minimally processed whole foods in their natural state. Include approximately 40 to 60 percent complex carbohydrates, 20 to 30 percent lean proteins, and 10 to 20 percent fat. This all depends on your activity level and your state of wellness."

Tourles also recommends a number of essential vitamins, minerals, and fats.

Vitamins

She starts by describing the vitamins: "Five essential vitamins provide a potent combination of antioxidants and healing agents that boost your skin's ability to make you look your best. The first one is vitamin A, or beta carotene. It is a fat-soluble antioxidant…. Vitamin A is essential for growth and maintenance of epithelial tissue, which is your skin tissue, and for the proper functioning of the mucous membranes. This vitamin helps prevent dry, rough skin, and premature aging. It speeds healing, especially of acne and impetigo, which is caused by staph or strep infection that results in pustules around the nose and mouth. Vitamin A also boosts your general immunity. Deficiency symptoms of this vitamin include premature wrinkles; acne; pimples; blackheads; cirrhosis; and dry, rough, itchy, scaly, or cracked skin, especially on the feet and the hands, and slowed healing. An early symptom of deficiency is what I call chicken skin, small raised bumps on the back of the neck, upper arms, back, and the shoulder."

The next vitamin group is the B complex vitamins. Tourles explains: "These are water-soluble nutrients and they are always grouped together in a complex when naturally occurring. You would never find just one of the B vitamins isolated like you see in the health food store. If you must supplement, be sure that you take a supplement that supplies the entire complex. Outstanding vegetarian sources of this vitamin are brewer's yeast, whole grains, alfalfa, almonds, sunflower seeds, all the soy products, green leafy vegetables, blue-green algae, fresh wheat germ (make sure you get it in the refrigerated section as it tends to go rancid rather quickly), molasses, peas, and beans. This is your antistress vitamin. It helps prevent premature aging and acne, and promotes healthy circulation and metabolism. It is very essential to wound healing such as sunburn, bruises, and infection. It aids in new cell growth and increases your vitality. Deficiency symptoms of this vitamin include a sore mouth and lips. Where your top and lower lip meet will get cracks and become red and very sore. Other deficiency symptoms are eczema, skin lesions, dandruff, a pale complexion, pigmentation problems, and premature wrinkling."

"The number three vitamin is vitamin C. This is a water-soluble antioxidant. Outstanding sources are rose hips, citrus fruits, fresh tomatoes, all kinds of berries, pineapples, apples and persimmons, bell and hot peppers, and papayas. Vitamin C helps to produce collagen in your connective tissue. Collagen is what keeps your skin plump and firm, and keeps you from getting wrinkles. Vitamin C also strengthens the capillary walls, speeds healing, and helps battle environmental stress and toxins. If you have a deficiency in vitamin C, you will probably bruise more easily, your gums can become spongy, wrinkles form more quickly, you will notice sagging skin, premature aging, pyorrhea (which is a gum disease), and slowed healing."

Vitamin D is the fourth essential vitamin. "Vitamin D is a fat-soluble nutrient," Tourles says. "Most people think it has to come from milk or fish liver oils. These are good sources but vegetarian sources include fortified soy milk, alfalfa, watercress, and sunshine. Skin care benefits when you combine vitamin A and vitamin D to treat acne. It also treats herpes simplex, the little sores that show up around and just inside your lips. It helps slow premature aging and enhances bone mineralization and calcium absorption. This is great for your fingernails. Deficiency symptoms of vitamin D are a lack of vitality, very slow growth and bone problems.

"Vitamin E, our last vitamin, is a fat-soluble antioxidant. Outstanding sources are the cold-pressed vegetable oils, not the vegetable oils you normally find in your grocery store. Those have been heated too high and heavily processed, so you need to get the cold-pressed oils. Whole grains, alfalfa, parsley, sprouted seeds, nuts, fresh wheat germ, and green leafy vegetables are good vegetarian sources. Skin care benefits for vitamin E are that it oxygenates the tissues and increases body stores of vitamin A, slows premature aging, helps to block the formation of tumors, and speeds healing of severe burns and chronic skin lesions. It may also decrease scarring.

"It also promotes red blood cell formation. If you are deficient in vitamin E, there will be a degeneration of epithelial cells, which are your skin cells in the organs, and skin germinating cells. This results in tissue-membrane instability and collagen shrinkage, which leads to premature aging and the sagging of your skin. Your skin can look very lackluster. You can be very tired because you are not getting oxygen in your body. Remember I said vitamin E helps to oxygenate the tissues. You will also have an increased tendency to bruise as a result of the fragility of the red blood cells."

Minerals

Tourles also recommends four minerals for healthy skin. "The first one is iodine," she says. "Outstanding vegetarian sources for iodine are blue-green algae, sunflower seeds, kelp, iodized salt, and sea salt. If I use salt at all, it is sea salt. Fish and shellfish are also great sources. Skin care benefits of iodine are that it aids in healing skin infections, increases oxygen consumption and the metabolic rate in the skin, and helps prevent roughness and premature wrinkling. Deficiency symptoms of iodine include slow growth and healing, slow metabolism, very poor skin tone, and dry skin. There is a contraindication for iodine: It may aggravate acne. If you have acne you may want to drastically decrease fish, cut down on your blue-green algae, and maybe switch over to barley grass instead. You may see good results by doing that.

"The next mineral is silicon. A good source for that is horsetail herb, which is very good to combine with nettle and blue-green algae in capsule form. Echinacea root is very good; dandelion root, alfalfa, kelp, flax seed, barley grass, wheat grass, all varieties of apples and berries, onions, almonds, sunflower seeds and grapes are all good sources. Silicon aids in collagen formation, helping to keep the skin taut, tight, and uplifted. It helps to strengthen your bone and skin tissues and aids in wrinkle prevention. Deficiency symptoms include premature wrinkling, lack of skin tone, and sagging skin."

The third mineral is sulfur. "Sulfur can be found in turnip greens, dandelions, greens, radishes, horseradish, string beans, onions, and garlic," Tourles says. "All of these foods have a strong flavor. Cabbage, celery, kale, soybeans, and asparagus are milder. Asparagus is particularly high in sulfur. Sometimes sulfur is called the beauty mineral. It really helps to keep the skin clear and smooth. Deficiency symptoms of sulfur include dry scalp, rashes, eczema, and acne."

The last mineral is zinc. Tourles says, "Good sources are blue-green algae and barley grass, alfalfa, yellow dock root, echinacea root, any of the seaweeds such as kelp, fresh wheat germ, all variety of seeds, brewer's yeast, and all kinds of nuts and green leafy vegetables. Zinc aids in wound healing, promotes cell growth, and boosts immunity. It helps treat acne when combined with vitamin A and B. Deficiency of zinc includes slow healing, dandruff, and lowered resistance to infections."

Essential Fats and Fatty Acids

Tourles goes on to describe the essential fats and fatty acids that are important for healthy skin. "Fat in the diet is very vital to your skin's health and beauty," she says. "Without fat your skin has no contour, no roundness. It cannot be beautiful without at least a thin layer of padding to support it and give it shape. Fat is a necessary requirement if you desire radiant and moisturized skin.

"As far as proper skin care goes, there are two types of essential fatty acids that are greatly beneficial. These are omega-3 and omega-6 fatty acids. The first one is omega-3, and people usually think of coldwater fish such as bluefish, salmon, mackerel, or tuna as good sources. If you want a vegetarian source, use ground flax seeds or flaxseed oil. Flaxseed oil is sometimes called the vegetable alternative to fish oil. Walnuts and walnut oil and Brazil nuts are other sources. Omega-3 helps with proper wound healing, is reported to relieve arthritis symptoms, aids in healing eczema and cirrhosis, and helps to balance the sebum or the oil production in the skin. A deficiency symptom of omega-3 is dry, scaly skin, eczema, inflammatory skin conditions, and slow healing.

"The main constituent in omega-6 is gamma linolenic acid or GLA for short. Good sources for this include evening primrose oil, borage oil, black currant seed oil, and blue-green algae. Skin care benefits are a smooth, healthy, moisturized skin and proper joint function and flexibility. Deficiency symptoms include dry, flaky skin; eczema; and painful stiff joints."

Herbal Formulas

HERBAL TEA

Stephanie Tourles has formulated an herbal tea that is "a delicious way to boost your energy levels as well as your natural immunity." This tea contains 2 tablespoons lemon balm, 1 tablespoon lavender flowers, 1 tablespoon peppermint leaves, 1 tablespoon chamomile flowers, 1 tablespoon rose petals, 1 tablespoon nettle, 1 tablespoon alfalfa, 1 tablespoon rose hips, 2 teaspoons dandelion leaves, 2 teaspoons raspberry leaves, 1/2 teaspoon gingerroot (or you can substitute cinnamon bark).

"Combine all of these herbs in a medium-size bowl," Tourles says. "Blend the ingredients and store this mixture in a tightly sealed tin, jar, or plastic tub and store it away from light in a very cool, dry location. It is best if used within six months.

"For each cup of tea you need 1 teaspoon of the dried herb. Bring a cup of water to a boil in a small saucepan. Remove this from the heat and add 1 teaspoon herbs. Cover this and allow it to steam for ten or fifteen minutes and strain before you drink it. You can add honey, lemon, cream, or maple syrup to enhance the flavor. This recipe yields approximately 30 cups of tea if you use 1 teaspoon of formula per cup."

SKIN OINTMENTS AND CLEANSERS

Tourles describes an herbal ointment you can make yourself for soothing skin irritations, cuts and abrasions, and even diaper rash. It has four simple ingredients: 1/2 cup vegetable shortening, preferably 100 percent hydrogenated soybean oil; 10 drops calendula essential oil; 10 drops everlasting or spike lavender essential oil; and 5 drops orange or lemon essential oil.

"Start with the vegetable oil at room temperature and add all the essential oils all at once," Tourles says. "Whip all the ingredients together until thoroughly combined. It can be stored in a glass or plastic container with a tight lid and will keep, if refrigerated, for up to 1 year. To use, clean the infected area and apply the ointment; use as necessary to help heal and prevent infections. It is great for a nightly treatment for dry hands and feet and also as a cuticle treatment. It will have a beautiful orange color and it smells really nice, too."

Regular use of sunscreen is the most effective way of protecting your skin from sunburn, aging effects, wrinkles, and cancer. Start with a sunscreen with an SPF of 15 or higher. SPF stands for sun protection factor. It means that you can stay out in the sun fifteen times longer before burning than you would be able to without sunscreen. Put it on your face and hands after you wash your hands. If you are older and beginning to see age spots, use an even higher SPF. Use it every day all year round.

Psoralens are chemicals found in certain foods that make your skin more sensitive to the sun so that it burns more easily. Psoralens are found in foods such as parsley, limes, and parsnips. Be sure to use a sunscreen with a high SPF if your diet includes a lot of psoralens.

Some perfumes cause age spots, especially those with musk or bergamot oil. Small age spots can be bleached away with hydrogen peroxide. With a cotton swab use 30 percent hydrogen peroxide daily for several weeks. Another choice is hydroquinone, which interferes with your skin's production of melanin. It works very slowly but can fade age spots.

Tourles has another herbal formula for cleansing the skin. "I call it my Pure Cream Cleanser," she says. "This is great for all skin types except oily. It is a wonderful emollient, leaving skin soft and hydrated, and removes eye and lip makeup if you happen to wear those. It has only two ingredients: 1 tablespoon heavy cream and 1 drop carrot seed essential oil or rose essential oil. Rose oil can be very expensive. Mix the ingredients in a tiny bowl and apply the cream with a flannel cloth or a very soft washcloth in gentle circular motions over the entire face, neck, and chest. Rinse well, pat dry, and follow with your favorite herbal toner and moisturizer if you desire. There is so much fat in heavy cream that frequently you won't need an additional moisturizer unless it is the dead of winter and the air is very dry. This amount yields one or two treatments."

Cosmetic Laser Surgery

Cosmetic surgery continues to increase in popularity, for women as well as for men. What are the pros and cons of the various procedures? Dr. Debra Sarnoff, a graduate of Cornell University and George Washington University's School of Medicine, is one of the premier laser surgery experts in North America, specializing in cosmetic dermatology and dermatological surgery. She sees lasers as a great new tool. "New methods and uses for laser surgery are emerging almost every month. Lasers can't do everything, but they have truly made a difference in cosmetic surgery, particularly in relation to what may seem minor problems, such as broken blood vessels on the face and around the nose, brown spots, age spots, liver spots, whatever you'd like to call them, on the tops of the hands or in the chest area." Lasers have proved helpful with problems such as removing tattoos. They are also useful for spider veins on the leg, acne scars, and wrinkles.

Lasers are essentially beams of light applied to the skin. Unlike a scalpel, which actually cuts the skin and causes some bleeding, a laser beam will pass through the skin without causing any bleeding. It has a particular target that it is trying to eradicate. There are certain problems that only lasers are capable of solving, just as there are certain problems only scalpel surgery can solve. For example, Dr. Sarnoff says, "There's no way that pulling and stretching and tightening the skin, through surgery, can change the quality of the skin. If your problem is that something is wrong with the quality of the skin, very often a laser can help that."

One cosmetic surgery procedure that can be done well with lasers is skin resurfacing. We all develop wrinkles as we get older. After smiling, laughing, and expressing ourselves with our faces for all these years, most of us develop lines around the eyes—crow's feet—as well as lines on the upper lip.

Dr. Sarnoff says that even the best face-lift in the world will not eradicate those lines. Something has to be done to resurface the skin. "In the old days, we used a machine called a dermabrader, which was like a little sanding machine that people used to try to peel off the top layers of the skin. In other cases, doctors used acid as a chemical peel. The theory was that when the skin healed, it would be much smoother and the wrinkles would not be as apparent.

Then, says Dr. Sarnoff, "Along came this generation of lasers. The laser can be used to peel off the top layers of skin as opposed to using a chemical or a dermabrading machine."

This procedure involves going to a reputable physician, preferably a dermatologist or plastic surgeon who is experienced in this technique, and having the top layers of skin removed in a controlled way with a laser. Healing will take at least ten days, during which the recovering patient has to lie low. She will look like she had the worst sunburn ever. The skin will be red, moist, and chapped. She won't be able to put on makeup for at least ten days.

The cost of resurfacing the entire face can be between four and five thousand dollars. There may be some added costs for the operating room, as well as charges for anesthesia.

AGE SPOTS

Many people have sun spots or age spots, what is called photodamage, from all those years of baking in the sun before we knew that ultraviolet rays are potentially harmful. Dr. Sarnoff explains: "A lot of that sun damage will be entirely reversible if the beam of light can be used to strip off those top layers of skin. That type of laser resurfacing is a fairly involved procedure that really takes a commitment and a healing time. It's not the kind of thing you just pop in to have done as if you were going to the deli and do a little laser over your lunch break. That laser resurfacing is a bigger deal."

BROKEN BLOOD VESSELS, HAIR REMOVAL, TATTOO REMOVAL

Dr. Sarnoff adds, "We are also using lasers now to help lighten stretch marks and to deal with birthmarks. The costs for these procedures are usually more in the hundreds of dollars. It depends on how large the discoloration or the tattoo is and how much time is required. For something like a tattoo, usually several visits are needed. They would be spaced about six to eight weeks apart, and it would not be unusual to need up to eight treatments to clear a tattoo completely."

Procedures such as zapping broken blood vessels and removing little brown spots are simpler; the side effects are usually no more than a little bruising, crusting, or scabbing, something you might want to wear a small bandage over or apply a little antibiotic ointment to, but nothing that would keep you out of work or prevent you from functioning. Many times people have these procedures and go right back to work.

Lasers can also be an alternative to electrolysis for hair removal. The procedure can be done very rapidly, and the patient can immediately return to her activities.

KNOW WHAT TO ASK

Dr. Sarnoff warns that a savvy consumer must ask the right questions. You must learn whether a procedure is a one-shot deal or will have to be repeated. And you should ask how long the improvement will last. Certainly you want something that is going to be cost-effective. Some laser treatments are really long-lasting. Laser removal for wrinkles has been around for about five years, and people who had the treatment when it was first introduced still look good. With hair removal, by contrast, very often the hair will grow back in a few months. Dr. Sarnoff stresses that you have to know that before you commit. "I think it is very important to ascertain ahead of time approximately how many treatments are needed and what you should expect."

KNOW THE RISKS

There are risks, Dr. Sarnoff cautions. One is that you will pay good money and be disappointed because your underlying problem will still be there. "Something else that consumers have to be aware of is scarring. It's usually not the case that scars occur, and with a doctor who is well trained and experienced, I think the technique is very safe. Nonetheless, it is a topic that definitely needs to be addressed before the procedure is done."

Sometimes there are some temporary changes in pigment. As the skin is healing, it can become a little darker or lighter than the surrounding skin. You must be aware how often this happens and know whether it is in fact only temporary or could be permanent.

There are very different types of lasers. Each beam of light accomplishes a different purpose, and the potential hazard from each is different. Still, there are some universal precautions that all competent laser providers follow. You need the correct eyewear, for example. Each laser is set at a very specific wavelength, and the protective eyewear needs to be specific to that wavelength.

Postoperative instructions make a difference, too. If you're removing tattoos or broken blood vessels, there is usually nothing else to do. However, with skin resurfacing, Dr. Sarnoff cautions that it is extremely important that patients follow the protocol afterward so that they do not get any kind of infection and heal properly.

LASERS AND RADIATION

The number-one fear people have about lasers is that they involve harmful radiation. But, as Dr. Sarnoff explains, the word *radiation* in the spelled-out version of laser actually refers to the verb *radiate*, meaning "to give off light." Most of the beams of light used in lasers are in the visible light range. That is, they are part of normal light. The only unique thing about lasers is that they are monochromatic. You might have a red beam or a yellow or green one, as opposed to natural light, which is a blend of all the colors of the rainbow. Laser light is nonionizing; it's basically safe, as opposed to X rays or ultraviolet light from the sun, which are ionizing. Ionizing radiation may change our cells and damage our chromosomes. We can get in real trouble with that type of radiation, but most lasers are not in that part of the electromagnetic spectrum.

FINDING THE RIGHT PERSON TO DO THE PROCEDURE

Another fear that people express to Dr. Sarnoff involves whether the specialist they are seeing is qualified. Physicians don't need any board certification to perform laser surgery, and, in fact, one doesn't even have to have a medical degree to use lasers. Lasers are relatively new; many have been around only about fifteen to twenty years. There are many wonderful doctors who trained at reputable universities and passed their boards in their respective fields, but the advent of lasers came after they graduated. Not every doctor has kept up with the technology and really understands it. A doctor might be board-certified in one particular field, know relatively little about laser techniques, yet could get a laser this afternoon and start to do any of the procedures. Consumers have the right to know about the doctor's actual experience in laser surgery.

In Dr. Sarnoff's opinion, if you are considering cosmetic laser surgery, "The best thing to do is to ask around in your community. Start by asking your regular doctor, your neighbors, your friends, and anyone you know who might have had a laser procedure done similar to the type you are interested in. You can also call groups for a recommendation, such as the American Academy of Dermatology, the American Society of Plastic and Reconstructive Surgeons, or the American Society of Laser Medicine and Surgery."

She suggests that you make more than one consulting appointment. You want to meet the doctor and ask how many procedures like yours he or she has performed. Ask if you can see photos of the doctor's work. This may not be necessary for some of the minor procedures, but if you are thinking about resurfacing your face, it is very important to know that the doctor is experienced and is going to do it correctly.

DENTAL CARE

Famed dental researcher Weston Price wrote a book, which he worked on in the 1920s and 1930s, based on studies of the teeth of people in native cultures. People who followed traditional ways, eating simply prepared food indigenous to the region where they lived, had healthy teeth. As soon as they adopted a Western diet of canned, processed food with white sugar and white flour, their dental health deteriorated. Children born to parents on a Western diet had occlusion and malformed teeth. Price even saw that children born before the introduction of Western foods had healthy teeth, while children in the same family born after the new diet was instituted had poor teeth.

The first thing to think about when it comes to healthy teeth is diet. A good diet will be reflected in the condition of the gums and teeth. Think of the general practitioner of yesteryear. One imagines this doctor making a house call on an ailing patient. His first request on seeing this patient was "Stick out your tongue." He wanted to see the tongue's color.

Dr. Victor Zeines, the author of *The Natural Dentist*, reminds us that this practice, far from being quaint and outdated, can still be used to make a good first diagnosis of medical problems. In fact, Chinese doctors, who also ask to see the patient's tongue, have a book that discusses 280 diseases that can be detected from the state of the tongue. For example, a white tongue indicates that toxins are coming out of the body (this will be observed in people with a cold or the flu), cracks in the tongue indicate vitamin deficiency, a yellowish gray or yellowish green tongue indicates gallbladder or liver trouble, and a brownish or grayish green tongue indicates intestinal or stomach problems.

The mouth is indicative of the body's general state of health. If you have a cavity, it is the end result of general physical problems of the whole body, not just the isolated tooth. When a person is not eating properly, the body becomes acidic. Minerals are pulled out of the mouth to travel into other parts of the body. The teeth weaken in an acid environment, while acid-based bacteria increase. A cavity may arise from a mineral deficiency followed by an invasion of bacteria.

Sugar is a main culprit in this process, though not in the way popularly understood. Many people believe sugar gets in the mouth and sits on the tooth, wearing it down. The real problem with sugar is that it reverses the fluid flow. This flow normally goes from the tooth's pulp chamber into the mouth. Sugar alters this process, sending materials in the mouth into the tooth's internal environment, irritating the inside of the tooth.

Many Americans contend daily with high levels of stress, pollution, and a deficient diet. Food often comes to us shipped over long distances, losing many of its nutrients along the way. We need to make up for those lost qualities with vitamins and minerals.

Calcium and magnesium are especially important for healthy teeth. Folic acid can help the body utilize nutrients. Coenzyme Q10 and vitamin C are also recommended.

Green leafy vegetables and carrot juice are high in calcium. Traditional culture held that chewing on kale was the fastest way to get white teeth. This idea is probably based on a recognition of kale's high calcium content. Kale can be juiced and mixed with carrot or apple juice, perhaps with a drop of lemon.

The Truth About Mercury Fillings

Mercury is widely used in common dental fillings. The "silver" filling is actually a mixture of silver, tin, copper, and mercury. Mercury makes up about 50 percent of the filling. Eighty-five percent of the American population has these fillings.

For over 150 years we have been told these fillings are safe, the most durable available. This is not true. Until 1985, the American Dental Association (ADA) repeatedly declared that mercury never escapes from fillings. Then they had to acknowledge that it did leak. Still, even with the leakage, the ADA still declares the fillings safe.

SYSTEMIC EFFECTS OF MERCURY

Dentist Flora Para Stay, in an article posted in the HealthWorld Online website (www.healthy.net), summarizes some of the research on the mercury in dental fillings going back at least thirty years. One of the first reports, published in 1970 in the *Journal of the American Dental Association*, concluded that mercury is not stable but rather "vaporizes at ordinary temperatures." In 1985, a report in the *Journal of Dental Research* stated that mercury vapor from fillings travels through the body and accumulates mostly in the brain, kidneys, and gastrointestinal tract.

According to Dr. Stay, researchers have also described a "battery effect" that occurs when mercury gets into the saliva. She explains that "currents are generated, causing mercury molecules from the surface of the fillings to be released into the tissues."

Mercury can also damage the immune system. Dr. Stay cites another report from the 1980s that concluded that amalgam- and nickel-based fillings are associated with a reduction in the number of T lymphocytes, a type of white blood cell.

The effects of mercury toxicity range from a metallic taste in the mouth, brittle nails, and dry skin, to fatigue, anxiety, depression, headaches, memory loss, gastrointestinal problems, kidney disease, heart problems, and more. Mercury can stop nutrients from entering the cells and prevent wastes from being eliminated. High mercury levels have been found in people with multiple sclerosis and other autoimmune diseases. Mercury can also produce spontaneous abortions. Because of these wide-ranging symptoms, mercury toxicity often goes undetected.

REMOVAL OF FILLINGS

Many people aware of the dangers of amalgam fillings have had them removed and replaced with safer alternatives. Gold, porcelain, or composite restorations may be used. Upon removal of the silver filling, they often see improvement, although it may be constrained by the mercury already in the body. Complementary physician Dr. Michael Schachter has seen patients whose blood tests have gone from abnormal to normal once silver fillings were removed. He has also seen people with multiple sclerosis and chronic fatigue syndrome markedly improved once fillings were taken out. Dr. Zeines has seen improved memory, better sleep, and less nervousness in patients following removal of mercury fillings.

Removing these fillings is not an easy task and the process is potentially dangerous since taking out the amalgam could accidentally release mercury.

Dr. Howard Hinton, a holistic dentist, stresses that the removal must be done under the care of both a physician and a dentist. The patient must be on a good diet and should undergo laboratory tests to determine how he or she is eliminating the mercury. Ideally, the removal should be carried out in a sterile, bubble chamber—a round room with a Laminar Air Flow or hepafilter circulating through the space; negative ion generators, to charge particulates in the air; and processed water and air. A rubber dam is used in the mouth to reduce exposure, and the filling is removed with extreme care. (The highest absorption in the body is in the mouth.) During the procedure, high suction and a lot of water are used to reduce the presence of mercury vapor.

Once the fillings are removed, the body should be detoxified. A lack of health improvement may be due to the fact that mercury is still in the body.

Dr. Elmira Gadol, another practitioner of holistic dentistry, says that garlic supplements will help the body eliminate the existing mercury toxins, and selenium can be taken to neutralize the metal. Once the fillings are removed, hair analysis should be done to see what other heavy metals are in the body. These metals interfere with cell processes, such as the oxygen going in and the carbon dioxide going out. These metals also have to be drawn out or problems will remain.

Some patients can be helped by taking intravenous vitamin C. Also, various chelating agents can be prescribed. These agents will attach to the mercury and take it out of the body in urine or feces.

Hot baths with Epsom salts and baking soda are also recommended as a way of bringing out the mercury. In working on detoxification, various methods should be tried alone and in combination.

The Fluoride Debate

We don't have to look too far to find fluoride these days—it's there in our toothpastes, our mouthwashes, and much of our drinking water. In fact, 50 percent of the people in the United States drink fluoridated water. Proponents of fluoride say we need it to prevent tooth decay. But many health experts say otherwise.

Dr. David Kennedy, from the International Academy of Oral Medicine and Toxicology, puts it quite well when he states that fluoride is a poison. It kills rats and insects so, certainly, it will kill bacteria if it is scrubbed on the teeth.

Dr. Taylor, in an article posted on the HealthWorld Online website (www.healthy.net), adds that fluoride is retained in the body, where it amasses over time. Small exposures now may not pose problems. But gradually, "you accumulate levels that may be dangerous to your health."

Many people are concerned about the lack of scientific research in this area. To date, there have been no long-term studies exploring how fluoride affects the body over time. Furthermore, Dr. Taylor says, the beneficial effects of fluoride have not been proven.

Dr. Mark Breiner, the author of *Whole Body Dentistry*, who has been practicing holistic dentistry for twenty years, says that putting fluoride into toothpaste or mouthwash will probably cut down on decay somewhat because it is such a potent toxin. However, he asks, while it may cause a decrease in tooth decay, what else is it causing? "I think there are better ways to prevent tooth decay, the main way being proper nutrition and if need be, some supplementation. But to go and use a potent toxin like that just doesn't make any sense."

TOXIC EFFECTS OF FLUORIDE

The health hazards of fluoride are known, and have been for some time. In 1977, an executive of the National Cancer Society documented that there was a 5 percent increase in cancer in communities that began fluoridating their water. An even more notorious study, and an attempt to suppress it, involved Dr. William Marcus, a senior science advisor at the Environmental Protection Agency's Office of Drinking Water. He read a study that was done to test the dangers of fluoridation. It concluded that there was an increase of bone cancers in animals that were given fluorides. In April 1990, Dr. Marcus went to a meeting where the National Toxicology Program was to review the study and found that the program's staff had downgraded every cancer reported. An investigation found that scientists at the program had been coerced into making these downgrades.

Dr. Taylor lists some of the ailments that may be caused or exacerbated by the accumulation of fluoride in the body: a depressed immune system, musculoskeletal problems, genetic damage, cancer, and kidney and thyroid problems. Other effects of fluoride include abdominal distress, tremors, convulsions, skin eruptions, headaches, increased thirst, and disturbances of calcium metabolism. Mottling of teeth, marked by white and brown patchy areas, may also occur.

HOW TO AVOID FLUORIDE

To limit your exposure to fluoride, drink bottled or filtered water and use nonfluoridated toothpaste. Dr. Breiner offers some additional recommendations. "As far as toothpaste, I like a toothpaste that has no fluoride in it and has natural ingredients. Same thing with the mouthwash. I like something called Tooth and Gum Tonic, which is made without alcohol or any chemicals. It is an herbal product and has a number of really good ingredients such as echinacea, peppermint, thyme, and eucalyptus. This will also kill bacteria."

For a mouthwash, you can also use plain salt water. Dr. Breiner says, "Use nonfluoridated water and take some salt and swish that around in your mouth. It is good for the gums. You can take some baking soda and mix that with a little peroxide and make your own toothpaste. You don't have to go to the store and buy something."

HAIR CARE

A beautician who has treated hundreds of people's hair is asked whether she sees any connection between a woman's diet and lifestyle on the one hand, and hair health on the other. She says, "Definitely, I see that when people eat well, the hair is healthy looking. It's a reflection of what they eat and the habits they have. Everything is shown in the hair."

Another hairstylist adds, "Your hair is fed by the bloodstream, so if there are any difficulties in that area, it will be carried through into the hair and skin. You could be losing your hair, it could be brittle or dull. Nutrition has an effect on everything in your body, and your hair is an appendage of what is going on. It is a reflection of who you are."

Nutritional Approaches to Better Hair Health

Dr. Danise Lehrer, a licensed acupuncturist and a doctor of homeopathy, confirms the statements quoted from the hairstylist, above. She notes that in traditional Chinese medicine, hair health is viewed as a sign of the health of the kidneys, liver, and blood.

One clinical nutritionist tells us that for hair and overall body health, we should consume six freshly prepared green juices a day with organically grown vegetables. Increased circulation to the scalp is important, so exercise should be part of any program.

I recommend the following four-stage program to provide increased vitality to your hair and scalp:

STAGE 1
DAILY PROTOCOL FOR THE FIRST THREE MONTHS
B complex (50 mg)
B12 (100 mcg)

Garlic (500 mg twice)
Aloe (1 oz three times)
Protein (0.9 g per kg of body weight)
6 glasses dark green vegetable juice or 6 scoops chlorophyll-rich powder

STAGE 2
DAILY PROTOCOL FOR THE SECOND THREE MONTHS
Sea vegetables (1 serving)
Flaxseed oil (1 tbsp)
Evening primrose oil (500 mg)
Choline and inositol (500 mg twice)
PABA (100 mg)
Folic acid (400 mcg)
Biotin (500 mcg)

STAGE 3
DAILY PROTOCOL FOR THE THIRD THREE MONTHS
Sea vegetables (1 serving)
Zinc (50 mg)
L-cysteine (500 mg twice)
Evening primrose oil (300 mg twice)
Pantothenic acid (100 mg twice)
Vitamin E (400 IU)
Coenzyme Q10 (100 mg twice)
Biotin (500 mcg)
Choline and inositol (500 mcg)
B complex (50 mg of each)
B12 (100 mcg)
Silica (150 mg)
PABA (250 mg)
Folic acid (800 mcg)
6 glasses dark green vegetable juice, or 3 glasses dark green vegetable juice plus 3 glasses green plant extract, or 6 scoops chlorophyll-rich powder

STAGE 4
DAILY PROTOCOL FOR THE FOURTH THREE MONTHS
PABA (500 mg)
Pantothenic acid (500 mg)
Garlic (1,000 mg)
Onion (1,000 mg)
Sea vegetables (6 oz)
Biotin (500 mcg)

Choline (1,000 mg)
Inositol (1,000 mg)
Niacin (250 mg)
Borage oil (500 mg)
Omega-3 oil (1,000 mg)
Cayenne (5 mg)
Protein (0.9 g per kg of body weight)
6 glasses dark green vegetable juice, or 3 glasses dark green vegetable juice plus 3 glasses green plant extract, or 6 scoops chlorophyll-rich powder

CHAPTER 15

FOOD
ALLERGIES

t is a classic case of overreaction. Your body incorrectly senses that the food that has just been eaten is a foreign substance to be repelled. Cells begin to exhibit diseaselike symptoms as they react and overreact to the food.

Allergists conservatively estimate that up to 15 percent of the population suffers from a minimum of one allergy, frequently one that is serious enough to warrant medical attention.

Symptoms can range from a mild tension headache or irritability to criminal actions and full-blown psychotic behavior. Most common are fatigue, headache, insomnia, rapid mood swings, confusion, depression, anxiety, hyperactivity, heart palpitations, muscle aches and joint pains, bedwetting, rhinitis (nasal inflammation), urticaria (hives), shortness of breath, diarrhea, and constipation. Reactions can be immediate following exposure to the allergen or delayed for many hours after contact.

Allergic symptoms are so diverse that the reactions can occur in virtually any organ of the body. Reactions in the brain or central nervous system may lead to behavioral changes and to paranoia or depression. A response in the gastrointestinal tract may translate into bloating, diarrhea, or constipation. Different food combinations can cause multiple reactions in the same person. If a person has an allergy to wheat that manifests itself in the brain, while their gastrointestinal tract is sensitive to milk, they may experience both fatigue and irritable bowel syndrome from a breakfast of whole wheat toast and milk.

All forms of a potentially offensive food can cause an allergic reaction, not just the whole form. Corn sugars and syrup, including dextrose and glucose, for example, will cause symptoms in many corn-sensitive patients. In many instances, researchers find, corn sugars will cause a more immediate reaction than will corn starch or corn as a vegetable.

Environmental medicine experts, also known as clinical ecologists, say that one reason people are developing sensitivities to certain foods is their widespread occurrence in our diets in both the natural and processed forms. Just because you only rarely treat yourself to corn on the cob, for example, doesn't mean you're not eating corn every day. On a typical day you might eat corn flakes, a corn muffin, and processed food products containing both cornstarch and corn syrup. Also, many of the daily vitamin C supplements are derived from corn.

TYPES OF FOOD ALLERGIES

The foods we eat most frequently are also the most common causes of allergies. These include milk, wheat, corn, eggs, beef, citrus fruits, potatoes, tomatoes, and coffee. Food allergies can be divided into several categories:

FIXED FOOD ALLERGY—Each time you consume a specific food, you react. For example, whenever you eat beef, a reaction occurs.

CYCLIC FOOD ALLERGY—This is the most prevalent type of allergy. It occurs when you've had an abundance of a particular food. If exposure to the food can be reduced to no more than once every four days, little or no reaction occurs. The food, in other words, can be infrequently tolerated in small amounts. So, in a cyclic allergy, a person can remain symptom-free as long as she eats the offending food infrequently.

Of course, other factors can influence the degree of this sensitivity. Infection, emotional stress, fatigue, and overeating can increase susceptibility. The condition of the food (raw or cooked, fresh or packaged) may also be an important factor. Pollution, the presence of other environmental allergens, or marked environmental temperature change can also help trigger or subdue a reaction. A food eaten by itself may be tolerated. But if it is combined with other foods at the same meal, an allergic response may develop. The length and severity of the symptoms will depend in part on how long the allergens remain in your body after ingestion.

ADDICTIVE ALLERGIC REACTION—Here the person craves the foods to which she is allergic. In essence, she becomes addicted to the foods. When made to go without the food, depression and other withdrawallike effects may appear. Moreover, eating the food may momentarily alleviate the symptoms, only to aggravate them later. Over time, the symptoms of the addictive allergy may grow increasingly complex.

This type of allergy often remains hidden or masked—even to the individual who is suffering from the problem. Because of its insidious nature, the person never suspects that the foods that seem to alleviate the symptoms might contain substances to which she is allergic.

But allergies do not always fit neatly into one of the three categories. A fixed allergy in infancy can develop into an addictive allergic reaction later in life. Milk is a good example of such a food. When first introduced to a baby, it may cause an acute reaction in the form of hives or spitting up. However, if the parents don't recognize this as an allergic reaction and continue to keep milk in the diet, the symptoms may take on a more generalized and less obvious form.

What is first experienced by the body as an acute reaction will—in the body's attempt to adapt by assimilating the new foreign substance—lead to more chronic symptoms such as arthritis, fatigue, depression, or headaches. For example, if you drink milk or eat milk products every day, symptoms of allergic reactions may blur with your natural personality traits and may become an accepted, even unnoticed part of your everyday life.

Eventually, you may develop a chronic condition, such as arthritis, migraines, or depression. Your daily dose of milk would never be suspect at this stage. Your body has upped its tolerance levels in trying to adapt. At the same time, milk's harmful effects have been subtly registered. You keep on with a daily dose of milk, your own substance for abuse, to keep withdrawal symptoms at bay. Acute reactions are gone—except when the milk is withdrawn completely. Chronic reactions have replaced them.

Hidden or masked food allergies, no different from allergies generally, tend to be to the very foods we eat most frequently. In the United States, dairy products, including milk and eggs, are high on the list. Corn, wheat, and potatoes are also common allergens, as is beef. Yeast, which occurs in many foods, is often a cause. Finally, many people have a hidden allergy to coffee.

CAUSES

Impaired Digestion

Most food allergies can be traced to an impaired digestive system. Proper digestion requires that the body secretes sufficient hydrochloric acid and pancreatic enzymes into the stomach to process foods. These substances break down large protein molecules into small molecules so that they can be absorbed and utilized. When too few digestive juices or enzymes are secreted, the large protein molecules go directly into the bloodstream. The immune system reacts to these large molecules as if they were foreign invaders—the allergic response.

Environmental and Emotional Stresses

In addition, other stresses can affect a person's "allergic threshold." These include environmental stresses such as air, water, and food pollution; inhalants such as perfume, aerosol hair spray, or room freshener; and emotional stress.

The less healthful the physical and mental environment, the less likely are our chances for achieving and maintaining a state of well-being.

Environmental pollution poses a particular problem. Over the past two centuries the barrage of chemicals introduced into our environment has disrupted the balance of our ecosystem. Residues of many toxic chemicals such as pesticides, herbicides, and insecticides are ingested into our bodies along with food additives and preservatives that are added during commercial food processing.

In many cases, the contamination of food is an irreversible result. Foods such as oranges, sweet potatoes, and butter can be dyed. Other processed and packaged goods, such as Jell-O, ice cream, sherbet, cookies, candy, and soda can contain large amounts of food additives.

Most of our commercially raised meats and poultry are riddled with residues of antibiotics, tranquilizers, and hormones. It is even common practice to dip certain fish in an antibiotic solution to retard their spoilage. A person allergic to these antibiotics and drugs may be unknowingly ingesting them continuously, provoking either long-term or short-term reactions or illnesses, the source of which might remain unidentified. It is estimated that more than 10 percent of all Americans are sensitive to food additives. But remember, even when a person eats only organically grown foods, they may still be food allergic.

In most cases, the more severe a person's food sensitivity becomes, the more numerous the allergens that induce it. One clinical study reported that the average person suffering from hay fever was allergic to five foods as well. A total picture of a person's allergen exposure, environment, habits, and history are vital for effective treatment.

The end result of repeated or prolonged sensitization of the body by recurrent allergic reactions is termed "breakdown"—the point at which diseaselike symptoms appear. They may be erroneously diagnosed as the onset of an illness. But the biochemical breakdown, although it manifests itself suddenly, was actually initiated years before by prolonged exposure to allergens.

Genetic Makeup

You can inherit allergic sensitivities. If both parents suffer from allergies, their children have at least a 75 percent chance of inheriting a predisposition to this hypersensitivity. When one parent is allergic, the chances of an inherited allergy remain as high as 50 percent. The child does not have to inherit the same allergic response. What is inherited is a genetic makeup that is more likely to have allergic reactions in general. For example, the mother may have chronic indigestion while the child's allergy manifests itself as acne. A mother may be sensitive to corn while her child is sensitive to yeast. Infants can develop allergies to the same foods as their mothers while still in the womb, through the placenta, or through breast milk after birth.

The Mechanisms of Food Allergy

Conventional allergists believe that the mechanism of food allergy is triggered by direct contact of the food antigens—the substances the body produces to fight the "foreign food invader"—with immune system antibodies in the gastrointestinal tract. The usually swift reaction that results is called an immune system–mediated response. This is the only kind of allergic reaction conventional allergists recognize.

But there is a second mechanism recognized by clinical ecologists, through the absorption of the allergen from the gastrointestinal tract into the bloodstream. Circulating in the blood, allergens can react with elements other than antibodies. The resulting reaction can occur in the blood, in the nervous system, or in the musculoskeletal system. Sometimes referred to as a sensitivity or intolerance, to distinguish it from a classic allergic reaction, this second mechanism can be extremely complex. However, tests to uncover these more subtle intolerances are available.

Hypersensitivity to foods can come at any time of life and continue to any age, although the onset occurs most commonly in infancy and early childhood. This is largely because the gastrointestinal systems of the very young are less efficient than in the adult. One researcher refers to the progression of allergies from childhood to adulthood as the "allergic march." Symptoms can move from one organ system to another. A child may suffer from asthma as a result of drinking milk. During teen years the allergy may take the form of pimples. Unfortunately, many people erroneously believe that they have outgrown their allergy because they no longer suffer from the original symptom. They don't consider that their current problems may have the same underlying cause. Their allergic symptoms may continue to vary throughout their lives because of an underlying imbalance that remains constant. Hyperactivity as a child may be the result of ingested food additives. In later years, these same ingredients may cause migraines and fatigue.

CLINICAL EXPERIENCE

Testing for Food Allergies

In some cases, a comprehensive medical history will provide significant clues about a person's allergic profile. A trained clinical ecologist may find the needed information from such a medical history alone.

The skin test performed by the traditional allergist has minimal use in identifying food allergies. In some cases, however, it may be helpful. A similar test takes another approach, putting extracts of food mixed with glycerin under the tongue, instead of into the skin by injection. A technique called applied kinesiology is based on the principle that there is a reflex response between a suspected allergen and the patient's body, in the patient's muscles. In this test, a doctor offers food to the patient and then measures or evaluates the energy or muscle function after the food is ingested. Here many foods can be tested in each session. However, the results may not be highly accurate depending on the nature and experience of both the person administering the test and the person being tested.

Newer tests are being developed. Some, such as the cytotoxic test, mix blood samples with food extracts and measure how many white blood cells burst. In allergy smears, samples of different body fluids or secretions are evaluated in the laboratory to look for a specific type of white blood cell. The various immune system cells may also be evaluated. In the Arest program, radioactive atoms are used to determine how antibodies respond to particular antigens.

There are also less technical tests, some of which can even be done at home. A fasting test, which should be done under medical supervision, begins by cleansing the system. Symptoms may subside, remain unchanged, or, if the allergy is an addiction of some sort, worsen by the second or third day of the fast. Then foods are reintroduced one at a time to check for symptoms.

Another test that can be performed at home is the Coca Pulse test. First find your normal pulse range by taking it every two hours. Then take it again at specific, regular intervals after eating the suspected allergen. If your pulse rises more than ten points, the food eaten last becomes suspect. The pulse is rising as a reaction to increased adrenaline in your system. The adrenaline may be released in reaction to an allergy.

Another home test involves keeping a food diary and recording everything you eat for a week. Record symptoms and when they occur as well. After the week, look for a relationship between symptoms and the food eaten.

Elimination testing is yet another approach. Eliminate the suspected allergen until symptoms clear up over a twelve-day period. Reintroduce the food on an empty stomach. Usually, if symptoms are to develop, they will do so within an hour of testing. A variation on that is the elimination of all common allergens—wheat, corn, dairy foods, citrus fruits, food colorings, sugar—and foods you may crave, over the course of a week. Then reintroduce the foods, one per day. If symptoms develop, the food may be an allergen. Don't eat it for five more days and then reintroduce it to double-check the result.

A final home test—perhaps among the most effective and sensible of all tests—also doubles as a treatment for food allergies. It is called the rotary diversified diet. Plan a diet in which you eat no individual food more often than once every four days. After five days, start a food and symptom diary. After reviewing correlations that may crop up through your recordkeeping, eat any suspected food the next time it comes up in the four-day rotation alone as one full meal. Note symptoms. Eliminate foods that stimulate adverse symptoms from your diet—permanently. The theory here is that food sensitivities become even more pronounced when a food is eliminated and then reintro-duced into the diet. With this diet, your symptoms—and with them the re-sponsible food—are clearly highlighted. This approach is also useful as a maintenance diet, enabling people who are prone to food allergies to pre-vent the emergence of new allergies, since they never eat any food too fre-quently. And even then, if a new food allergy does develop, it is spotted and quickly eliminated.

Alternative Treatments

ELIMINATION AND ROTATION DIETS

Elimination and rotation diets as described above can be used to treat food allergies.

NEUTRALIZING-DOSE THERAPY

Neutralizing-dose therapy is a treatment method that is especially useful in cases of multiple food allergies, and when avoidance of chemicals and medi-cinal inhalants is difficult, as during the pollen season. A neutralizing dose is determined for each allergen, and when it is injected or administered under the tongue, this dilution can bring about relief from the allergic symptoms.

These treatments are administered in a series during which the dose of the allergen is progressively increased, causing desensitization to this substance. (They work on the same theory as allergy shots or vaccines. The only differ-ences are in the dilution of the substance and the wide variety of the substances that can be tested in this way.) Eventually, the person can tolerate contact or in-gestion of the allergen with only a mild reaction or no reaction at all.

With the neutralizing-dose treatment, the allergist is first determining the amount of a particular allergen that causes an allergic reaction. The physician can work with many substances that the traditional allergist would be unable to treat, including foods, chemicals, perfumes, and cigarette smoke. The neu-tralizing-dose approach seems to be effective in eight out of ten patients.

Like the traditional allergy shot, the neutralizing dose can be adminis-tered by injection. However, it can also be given as drops under the tongue. Instead of taking approximately six months to find the optimal dose, the physician can usually determine the correct dosage in one or two sessions using this technique. Another advantage of the neutralizing dose is that the patient can be given the drops to take at home. It not only works as a pre-ventive measure but can also block a reaction that has already started.

BOOSTING THE IMMUNE RESPONSE

Strengthening the immune system should improve resistance to current al-lergies and reduce susceptibility to new ones. There are several ways the immune system may be strengthened. Getting sufficient rest is essential, as is regular exercise. Keeping stress levels to a minimum will also help. You must also be receiving the right nutrients in the right amounts.

Many nutrients have been found to enhance the effectiveness of the immune system. These include vitamin C, beta carotene, vitamin E, selenium, and glutathione. These are all antioxidants, which help to eliminate free radicals from the body.

Garlic has been found to be an immune stimulant, having both antifungal and antibacterial qualities. Garlic is most effective when eaten raw. It may be added to food or taken as a supplement in tablet or capsule form.

The essential fatty acids are also important to a proper immune response. Many researchers recognize the importance of omega-3 fatty acids, which are found in such oils as linseed and walnut, and in many fatty fishes, such as salmon.

It has been noted that 200 to 500 milligrams of pantothenic acid plus 50 milligrams of B complex vitamins can be useful in people with allergies. Vitamin C, in addition to its antioxidant properties, also has an antihistamine effect, which may benefit those with allergies by reducing the swelling of tissue and cell membranes. One study found that people with asthma who took 1,000 milligrams of vitamin C daily had 25 percent fewer asthmatic attacks than those receiving a placebo. Another study found that asthmatic children benefited from magnesium supplementation.

STRESS MANAGEMENT

A number of techniques are available to recondition the body to learn a new, more healthful way of responding to and dealing with stress, including that associated with food allergies. These include progressive relaxation, biofeedback, self-hypnosis, visualizations, meditation, yoga, and tai chi. Stress management techniques can improve the digestion of allergy sufferers.

The Link Between Food Allergies and Chronic Disease

If food and chemical sensitivities were routinely considered in each case of chronic disease, there would be a tremendous increase in well-being in this country.

An overly analytical medical system insists instead on classifying patients into narrowly defined disease states. Environmental aspects, including a patient's diet, are considered to be nonmedical. The person's whole experience—including diet, environment, lifestyle, emotional life, and work life—may also be considered to be outside the physician's domain, although few physicians would deny that the cause of almost any patient's illness will involve one or more of these factors to some degree.

FOOD ALLERGIES AND MENTAL HEALTH

It may be that up to 70 percent of symptoms diagnosed as psychosomatic are probably due to some undiagnosed reaction to foods, chemicals, or inhalants. Different allergic reactions occur. There are localized physical effects, such as gastrointestinal disorders, eczema, asthma, and rhinitis (nasal inflammation). There are acute systemic effects, such as fatigue, migraine headaches, neuralgia (nerve pain), muscle aches, joint pains, and other generalized symptoms. And there are acute mental effects, such as depression, rapid mood swings, hallucinations, delusions, and other behavioral abnormalities. It has been estimated that over 90 percent of schizophrenics have food and chemical intolerances.

Researchers now believe that food allergies may directly affect the body's nervous system by causing a noninflammatory swelling of the brain, which can trigger aggression. Despite studies at various correctional centers clearly showing the connection between diet and behavior, little is being done to change the dietary standards of correctional facilities throughout the nation. Routine screening programs for food allergies and nutritional deficiencies in chronic offenders do not exist.

While many other factors—not food alone—mitigate criminal, antisocial behavior, or mental illness, a case can be made for testing for and evaluating food sensitivities in any overall treatment, prevention, or rehabilitation program. (For more on mental health concerns, see chapter 23.)

FOOD ALLERGIES AND HEADACHES

Migraines are an example of a condition in which recognition and elimination of food allergens can make a tremendous difference. The trick is to recognize the possibilities.

Right now, about 25 million people who consult their physicians each year complain of bad headaches. Although there are various types of headaches, about 50 percent of these people suffer from migraines. While conventional medicine has very little to offer the migraine sufferer, clinical ecologists see migraine as a disorder frequently resulting from food allergies. The nontraditional medicine offered by the clinical ecologist may offer a unique opportunity to relieve the suffering.

Headaches due to food or chemical sensitivities can often be treated simply by eliminating the allergy, once it has been identified, with an elimination or rotation diet. Yet, as a rule, food sensitivities are not investigated in the diagnosis and treatment of headaches.

While the pain may sometimes appear immediately after eating a particular food, it may also be delayed until hours afterward. For this reason it is not unusual for a person to fail to identify the correlation between what they're eating and the onset of their headache. A food may even seem to relieve migraine symptoms temporarily—a classic example of an addictive allergic reaction.

Of course, allergic headaches typically occur as the result of combinations of factors, rather than from food allergies alone. Emotional stress, for example, may play a large role in triggering an episode. Thus, even when a food allergy is at cause, the specific food source may not produce the same symptoms on every occasion, depending on the array of associated circumstantial factors. In some individuals stress may be compounded when the allergic reaction triggers further emotional symptoms. A vicious cycle is created. Sudden changes in temperature or light may also affect one's susceptibility, as well as the presence of any other health problems.

Environmental-medicine specialists have found that some of the foods that occur most frequently in the typical American diet are also the foods most commonly implicated in food allergy–related headaches. The list includes wheat, eggs, milk, chocolate, corn, pork, cinnamon, legumes (beans, peas, peanuts, and soybeans), and fish. Moreover, individuals with food allergies should avoid or limit their intake of fermented products, such as red wine, champagne, and aged cheese, because of the presence in these foods of a substance called tyramine. Tyramine has been associated with migraine occurrence in some cases.

Too often, conventional medical practitioners tend not to look toward nutritional solutions in cases involving allergies, including allergy-related migraines. In part, this is because the medical training they have received does not extend deeply into nutrition. And yet, a preponderance of evidence continues to point to the importance of nutritional solutions for an increasingly wide range of health problems. (Migraines are discussed in greater detail in chapter 24.)

FOOD ALLERGIES AND FATIGUE

Probably no allergic disorder is more puzzling and pervasive than tension fatigue syndrome. Indeed, for many of us, varying daily levels of tension and fatigue are the norm, tranquillity and energy the rare exceptions. To compensate, we choose artificial solutions for moderating energy, from the first caffeinated gulps of coffee in the morning to the quick sugar, caffeine, or drug fix during the day, and the alcoholic "equalizer" in the evening. The result is that energy levels are either depressed or falsely elevated most of the time. In many cases, these quick pick-me-ups are responses to allergic disorders with their roots in food and nutrition.

Next to headaches, tension fatigue syndrome is the most common manifestation of cerebral and nervous system allergy. Yet, too often, this far-reaching malady is not even recognized by physicians or allergists. Its symptoms are usually assigned a psychiatric origin and treated with drug therapy or some other conventional modality when, in fact, a simple elimination and rotation diet is the best medicine.

There are several reasons for this all too common oversight. First, there are similarities between tension fatigue syndrome and psychiatric disorders. And second, there is the failure of standard scratch tests to identify many food and chemical reactions. The scratch tests simply have not been shown to be effective in the diagnosis of food and chemical sensitivities. And yet they continue to be used by allergists.

Of course, tension, extreme nervousness, irritability, depression, and emotional instability may be symptoms of psychological disorders in some cases. But too often this is the only possibility that is considered. The allergy may be due to any number of foods, and it is only through careful testing that a definitive diagnosis can be made. In all cases where such symptoms appear, food allergies should be ruled out first—before further traditional medical sleuthing occurs. This can save a lot of trouble and mistaken diagnoses.

Symptoms

The symptoms experienced in tension fatigue syndrome can include fatigue, weakness, lack of energy and ambition, drowsiness, mental sluggishness, inability to concentrate, bodily aches, poor memory, irritability, fever, chills and night sweats, nightmares, restlessness, insomnia, and emotional instability. Mental depression is another common symptom, ranging from mild to severe episodes of despondency and melancholia. Generalized muscle aches and pains, especially in the back of the neck or in the back and thigh muscles may also be present, as well as edema (fluid retention), particularly around the eye, and tachycardia (rapid heart beat). Gastrointestinal symptoms often associated with this syndrome are bloating, abdominal cramps or pain, constipation, diarrhea, and a coated tongue. Chills and perspiration are also frequently experienced in association with fatigue during food testing of symptomatic patients.

The disorder can begin at any age. It can last from several months to several decades. In some adults the extreme fatigue, bodily aches, depression, and mental aberrations that come from this continuing allergic state can be so severe that they interfere with work and domestic life.

As headaches or gastrointestinal upsets caused by allergy increase in frequency, the fatigue is more likely to remain even between episodes. Fatigue soon becomes the allergic individual's major complaint. The allergic origin of the fatigue and weakness commonly remains a mystery.

It's not unusual for allergic individuals to sleep up to fifteen or more hours for several successive nights to try to overcome their fatigue. Unfortunately, in most cases, these efforts prove futile. The fatigue experienced in allergic fatigue is quite different from the fatigue that naturally follows physical exertion. It cannot be relieved by normal or even excessive amounts of rest. It can be relieved only by eliminating its cause—the allergen.

Differential Diagnosis

Before the diagnosis of allergic fatigue can be defined, a complete medical workup should be done to exclude both organic and functional origins. This should include a comprehensive case history, complete physical examination, and diagnostic laboratory blood testing. Other causes for nervous fatigue include chronic infections and metabolic disorders, including diabetes, hypoglycemia, hypothyroidism, neurological disorders, heart disease, anemia, malignancy, and various nutrient deficiencies. Even if another disease is found, allergic fatigue may still be a causal factor. In some cases, fatigue is caused both by an allergic reaction and an underlying chronic disease state.

FOOD ALLERGIES AND OBESITY

Many obese women believe that they are overweight due to heredity, because they have a thyroid or metabolic problem, or because they simply eat too much. They may blame it on a lack of self-control, or become convinced that they have psychological problems. However, some experts believe that roughly two out of three obese individuals suffer from some form of allergy.

Of course, allergy may be only one of several factors affecting an obese person's weight. The presence of a thyroid condition or psychological problems can cause or aggravate a weight problem. Obesity is also related to many diseases including high blood pressure, heart disease, kidney problems, and diabetes. For obese individuals with allergies, the problems of each condition may adversely affect the other. Typically, someone who is obese will have allergic responses more often than a person who is not obese. The extra weight is a burden on the immune system, and the weaker the immune system, the greater the effects of allergies. People who are obese may also have difficulty breathing.

We store chemicals in the body in fat. Very often, allergies are triggered by a response to chemicals stored in this way. Because the obese person may naturally hold more chemicals in the body, she may tend to experience more frequent allergic responses. This may also explain why she feels worse, or has strong food cravings, at the beginning of a diet. Chemicals are stored in fat, and as the fat is burned, a large quantity of chemicals is passed into the bloodstream, often causing such cravings.

The mechanism by which an allergy can trigger obesity may be that of the hidden addictive allergy, whereby a person is addicted to the very foods to which she is allergic. Often, these are high-calorie foods, such as chocolate, cheese, or sugar. So the person may gain weight because she eats these high-calorie foods too frequently.

Hunger itself can be an allergic response, and compulsive eating and intense cravings for particular foods may also result from hidden allergies. In some cases, compulsive eating of the food one is allergic to may really be an attempt to stave off withdrawallike symptoms induced by going without the food for too long. Such withdrawal symptoms might include headaches, drowsiness, irritability, or depression.

Allergies can cause weight problems if they interfere with the body's natural ability to regulate itself. As noted by Dr. Arthur Kaslow, physician and author, both humans and animals naturally attempt to maintain their bodies in a state of biochemical equilibrium known as homeostasis. Unless there is a flaw in their regulatory system, human beings will maintain their proper weight by eating the amounts and types of foods their bodies need to function properly. When the body needs food, it will send out a hunger signal. When it needs water, it sends out a thirst signal. If this mechanism breaks down, an individual may feel hungry when she does not really need food. It is possible that allergies can temporarily impair the cells responsible for sending out these signals. (For more on obesity, see chapter 11.)

FOOD ALLERGIES AND ARTHRITIS

Some clinical ecologists estimate that 80 to 90 percent of all cases of arthritis are either allergy induced or are allergylike reactions to some food the patient has eaten. The arthritis may also be related to an environmental factor to which the patient is sensitive, such as gas inhaled from constant proximity to a gas stove. Examining arthritics for both food and environmental allergies may help reduce current symptoms, prevent recurrences of symptoms, and minimize the damage that eventually results from joint inflammations.

Dr. Marshall Mandell has successfully treated hundreds of arthritis patients by putting them on a five-day distilled-water fast and then allowing their usual foods, one at a time, back into their diet. If a food causes the arthritis symptoms, the symptoms will return when it is reintroduced into the diet and should be permanently eliminated. (For more information on arthritis, see chapter 4.)

CHAPTER 16

HEART
DISEASE

I n nearly every year for which we have records, heart disease has been the number one cause of death in the United States. Every thirty-three seconds an American dies of heart disease. Heart disease among women is a much greater threat than many people believe: According to the American Heart Association, women accounted for 53 percent of heart disease deaths in 1998. Twice as many women die from heart disease as from all forms of cancer combined.

CAUSES

"Overall, there are 247 risk factors that can damage the heart," states Dr. David Steenblock, a complementary physician from California. "A risk factor is anything that injures the inner lining of the blood vessels that supply the heart with oxygen and nutrition. Any agent that injures this inner lining, such as tobacco, air pollution, food additives, high blood pressure, and gasoline fumes, can initiate atherosclerosis, the so-called hardening of the arteries. Then the accumulation of such things as cholesterol, calcium, scar tissue, and fat causes atherosclerotic lesions, which gradually go on to occlude, or block, the arteries to the brain and the heart. When the arteries to the brain [the carotid arteries] are blocked, you have a stroke, and when the arteries to the heart [the coronary arteries] are blocked, you have a heart attack."

High blood pressure (hypertension), which affects some fifty million Americans, increases the risk of heart attack and stroke. Dr. Michael Janson, former president of the American Preventive Medical Association and author of *The Vitamin Revolution in Health Care* says, "High blood pressure can be the result of dietary habits; lack of exercise; high stress; being overweight; having too much caffeine, sugar, alcohol, or, in particular, salt in the diet. In the past few years, some reports have said that salt does not make much of a difference for most people. The fact is, that's not true. Even a slight elevation in blood pressure is enough to increase the risk of heart disease."

Among the more recently identified potential risk factors for heart disease are high levels of the amino acid homocysteine, high fibrinogen (a blood-clotting protein), and certain viral and bacterial infections. An elevation in the level of C-reactive protein, a substance in the blood that indicates the presence of inflammation, is also thought to be involved.

Dr. Janson describes other common heart ailments, some of which are precipitated by atherosclerosis. In angina pectoris, he explains, "clogged arteries leave the heart muscle with inadequate oxygen. As everyone knows, muscles hurt when exercised beyond their oxygen capacity. When not enough blood flows from the coronary arteries to the heart muscle, people experience pain in the chest. Sometimes they feel pain in the jaw, the shoulder, or even the wrist. Often they do not realize that this is referred pain coming from the heart itself."

Congestive heart failure is another common heart problem. "Hardening of the coronary arteries can lead to a number of other problems," Dr. Janson explains. "When heart muscle tissue functions inefficiently, more blood comes in than is pumped out. In other words, with each beat the amount of blood being returned to the heart is more than the heart muscle can handle. Fluid backs up, and other tissues, such as the lungs and legs, can get congested. Congestive heart failure leads to shortness of breath, water in the lungs, and swelling of the ankles."

SYMPTOMS

Heart disease is a gradual process that takes years to develop into a serious condition. At first there are no warning signs. If the coronary arteries become severely blocked, a woman may experience shortness of breath or chest pressure and pain (angina pectoris) that is relieved by rest. Other signs of an impending heart attack may include light-headedness, sweating, nausea, and pain spreading to the shoulders, neck, or arms. Unfortunately, many people are unaware of or overlook these signs: Fifty percent of all people who have heart attacks wait two hours or longer before seeking treatment, and many die before reaching the hospital.

Diagnosis is an important first step. Before anyone begins a cardiovascular health program, a doctor should take the following factors into account: family history, blood pressure, cholesterol level, weight, and stress electrocardiogram (ECG) tests. After assessment of a woman's risk factors, the program can begin.

Conventional Treatment

Conventional treatment of heart disease often involves the use of medication to address symptoms such as high blood pressure and high cholesterol. And every year, about 1 million Americans undergo surgery such as coronary bypass and angioplasty (in which a balloon catheter is used to open clogged arteries) to restore their hearts.

Dr. Janson believes the general public is being misled into believing that medications for high blood pressure are safe and always necessary: "We all hear advertisements on the radio telling us to stay on these medications for life. They say that no symptoms tell you whether or not your blood pressure is high. Therefore, if you are taking medication for high blood pressure, you must stay on your medication and never, ever stop. That so-called public-service announcement is really a sales pitch from the drug companies that make the medications. We know that these medications actually cause more heart disease and that they create side effects in addition to the high blood pressure."

Dr. David Steenblock warns, however, that patients who depend on medication to control high blood pressure should not self-discontinue: "Many people have this idea that since the doctor is not getting at the cause of their high blood pressure, it is somewhat illogical for them to take their blood pressure medicine. True, doctors often do not have the answer. Still, if you fail to take your medicine and your blood pressure gets out of control, you can develop heart disease and go on to have a stroke."

In the 1990s, many doctors began prescribing hormone replacement therapy (HRT) to help prevent heart disease in women. A Harvard study of about 46,000 female nurses had found that those who had taken HRT had a lower incidence of heart disease by up to 50 percent. However, when that study was more fully investigated, it turned out that the women with lower rates of heart disease were actually women who were healthier in general. Compared to the group who were supposed to have a greater incidence of heart disease, they were wealthier, more likely to exercise, and had better diets; fewer of them had diabetes; and they smoked less. The women who didn't take HRT were more likely to have diabetes, smoked, were poorer, and didn't visit their doctors. Also not reported in the study was the fact that the women who took HRT had a 50 percent increase in strokes. This, then, was a flawed, biased study.

"The rationale for giving HRT to postmenopausal women is that when you arrive at menopause, your risk of getting heart disease or stroke will skyrocket and, therefore, you need protection," says Sherrill Sellman, international seminar leader, psychotherapist, and author of numerous articles on women's health and of the best-selling book *Hormone Heresy*. "But studies from reputable researchers show that this is a myth. There is no rapid increase of heart disease in postmenopausal women. There is simply a rise in heart disease as women move on in life in general. The doctors who push HRT as a preventive for women's heart disease seem not to take into account the fact that men also have a higher incidence of heart disease as they age.

Recent studies have challenged the theory that hormone replacement therapy is beneficial to the heart. A study published in 2001 found that postmenopausal women with heart problems who took hormone supplements for less than one year actually had a greater risk of another heart attack or death from heart disease than women who were not on HRT. An earlier study, sponsored by Ayerst, the company that manufactures the number-one replacement estrogen, Premarin, yielded similar results. Sellman explains, "They gave half the women hormone replacement therapy and the other half a placebo. After five years, they discovered that in the first year of treatment, the women taking the HRT had a 50 percent increase in heart attacks. Over the five years, the risk decreased. The conclusion was that women who already had heart conditions got no overall benefit from HRT. But this glossed over the horrible fact that HRT increased heart problems the first year. What was more, women taking it had three times as many blood clots in the legs than women taking the placebo. There was also an increase in gallbladder disease.

"The manufacturers' own package inserts warn that these drugs should not be taken by women who have current problems with or a past history of clotting, thrombosis, stroke, cardiovascular disorders, high lipoproteins (a specific type of blood fats), severe hypertension, or lipid metabolism disorders. Estrogen and progestin will increase the possibility of strokes and clotting, since they thicken the blood and raise blood pressure. And these factors all contribute to the possibility of heart disease."

In 2001, the American Heart Association finally took heed of the growing scientific evidence and shifted its stance, advising against the use of hormone replacement therapy to prevent heart disease in women.

The Complementary Approach

The solution here is to work with a complementary medical physician until your heart health is restored. In some cases, medication may be needed long term, even for a lifetime, but no one can fail to benefit from improving lifestyle and diet. A number of full alternative therapy programs are available to combat heart disease, including those developed by Dean Ornish, Julian Whitaker, John McDougall, and Eric Braverman. To varying degrees, these and other programs incorporate the following approaches.

Diet

The power of a vegetarian diet in a cardiovascular health program was recognized in a now-famous study by Dr. Dean Ornish. The Ornish study placed heart patients on a protocol of healthy vegetarian foods, daily aerobic exercise, and relaxation. At the end of a year, a significant number of patients showed improvement in their heart condition, and in some the disease was even reversed.

Dr. Paul Cutler, a complementary physician from Niagara Falls, New York, says, "Medicine in general owes Ornish a great deal of gratitude. He showed that a drastic reduction of fats was most important. I believe that the total dietary fats should be well below the typical average of 40 percent. Modern nutritionists are saying 30 percent. I try to get fat content down to 10 percent of the total calories. I see improvement in angina just by reducing the fats to that degree."

There is not much controversy about what is wrong with the standard American diet with its high amounts of animal proteins, saturated animal fats, dairy products, deep-fried foods, and refined carbohydrates. The average American diet consists of 43 percent fats and 14 percent proteins and the rest is mainly carbohydrates. The average daily intake of cholesterol is 450 to 500 milligrams. But there is controversy over the proper foods for those with heart disease. There are more than sixty thousand dietitians in the United States, and they have been a primary source of information on what a sick person should eat. After all, physicians graduate from medical school with only an hour or two of learning about nutrition. However, even though dietitians are well trained, there is a split in the field. Only a very small percentage believe the standard American diet plays a large role in causing the diseases we are beset with, including heart disease.

The American Heart Association recommends that we cut fat intake to 30 percent, with only 10 percent of this in the form of saturated fats (fats found particularly in land animals, palm and coconut oils, and hydrogenated vegetable oils). We have been told that margarine, made from "polyunsaturated fats," is good for the heart and will lower cholesterol. That is simply not true; margarine is loaded with the fatty acids that contribute to heart disease. Instead of margarine, use olive oil, canola oil, or flaxseed, almond, safflower, sunflower, or soy oil. Of these, olive oil would be at the top of my list. But don't have margarine.

No more than 10 percent of the oils you eat should be polyunsaturated fats, such as those found in some vegetable oils, including corn and cottonseed oils. According to the American Heart Association, we should get the rest from monounsaturated fats such as olive oil and take in less than 300 milligrams of cholesterol each day.

While the dangers of saturated fats to heart health are well known, Dr. Ray Peat, a distinguished scientific researcher in Eugene, Oregon, says unsaturated fats can be just as damaging: "Many people have been soaking their bodies in unsaturated vegetable oil diets for years. As a result, every time they get hungry or face stress, their blood sugar falls, their adrenaline rises, and these unsaturated fats are drawn out of storage. Once released, they immediately start poisoning the lining of the blood vessels and all the cellular energy-producing systems. In 1960, this effect was demonstrated by a group in England, which saw that adrenaline, either natural or synthetic, caused damage to the circulatory system. It turns out that this occurs after unsaturated fats become mobilized. They hit the lining of the blood vessels, where they cause lipid peroxidative damage."

Dr. Janson adds that people should avoid foods such as sugar, salt, white flour, white rice, and particularly any shortening or hydrogenated vegetable oils found in products like margarine and vegetable shortening: "Whenever you see vegetable shortening, hydrogenated vegetable oil, or partially hydrogenated vegetable oil on a label, avoid that product. These are not foods. In fact, I consider margarine an industrial waste product that is fashioned to resemble food."

HEART-HEALTHY FOODS

Dr. Janson continues, "The diet should be high in complex carbohydrates, including whole grains, beans, vegetables, and fruits. Remember, flavonoids, which are plant pigments, are present in fruits and vegetables and in some beans and grains. These are very protective, and most of them are not available as supplements.

"I think the diet should be largely vegetarian, although a number of studies show that fish also reduces levels of heart disease and cancer. Fish may or may not be the reason for this. It may be that eating more fish means eating less chicken and meat. Cutting those foods out of the diet helps cut down on heart disease."

Broccoli and other vegetables are the first foods to turn to. Broccoli and all kinds of produce, seeds, legumes, and grains provide necessary vitamins, and they also contain important phytochemicals. These phytochemicals include beta carotene, alpha carotene, ascorbic acid, ash, boron, caffeic acid, calcium, chlorophyll, chromium, citric acid, copper, glycine, iron, linoleic acid, lysine, magnesium, niacin, oleic acid, phosphorus, potassium, riboflavin, selenium, thiamin, tryptophan, and zinc, among others. These chemicals have all kinds of healing properties. Chlorophyll, for instance, helps purify the blood and acts as a detoxifier.

You can lower your blood pressure by eating vegetables such as garlic, broccoli, and asparagus. You should have at least five servings of vegetables and three of fruits each day, raw, steamed, or juiced. Once you start, you will notice a world of difference in your overall vitality. Other valuable heart foods are rice and beans, which are complete proteins rich in fiber and B-complex vitamins.

Many people grow up with the pernicious myth that if it is not an animal protein, it is not a complete protein, so is not really nutritious. I did studies at the Institute of Applied Biology that proved conclusively that beans, legumes, and all grains contain complete proteins just like animal proteins, without the saturated fats. They are not high in calories and are rich in vitamins, minerals, and essential oils.

Nuts, despite their high fat content, are being found to have some important benefits as well. Not only do they provide protein, they also contain nutrients that can protect against heart disease, high blood pressure, and stroke. The protein in peanuts, hazelnuts, and walnuts, for example, is a good source of arginine. This amino acid is noted for its ability to produce nitric oxide, which helps blood vessels to widen and may stop or even reverse plaque buildup. These nuts also contain folate, which has been found to lower blood levels of homocysteine. High levels of homocysteine are associated with increased blockage in the arteries.

A recent Harvard study of 86,000 nurses found that those who ate more than 5 ounces of nuts a week were 35 percent less likely to develop heart disease than those who rarely ate nuts. Other studies have reported similar findings.

Exercise

"Aerobic exercise and an improved diet should go hand in hand," notes Dr. Paul Cutler. "Aerobics help the good cholesterol go up significantly, which in turn helps remove cholesterol from arterial walls after the cells are through with it, so it is less likely to form plaque." Exercising aerobically means getting the heart rate up three or four times a week. A doctor can help determine how much exercise is needed.

Dr. Michael Janson adds that people should stretch before and after an aerobic workout: "The stretching has another benefit in that it relaxes the body and keeps people limber and more flexible. That makes it easier to continue an aerobic exercise program."

Exercise is, however, not a panacea. Some people mistakenly assume that cholesterol can be burned off by exercise and activity and that as a result, people who engage in athletics and body building can eat more meat and eggs without suffering ill effects. There is no scientific basis for this notion. To the contrary, studies have shown that good conditioning and muscle tone do not necessarily put a person in good cardiovascular condition.

Dr. Julian Whitaker refers to "studies done on marathon runners in South Africa in which five of them died of heart attacks. These were conditioned long-distance runners. They all had cholesterol levels of 270, 290, et cetera. They were very fit but not very well."

Supplements

Supplements provide wonderful support for the heart and sometimes help eliminate or reduce dosages of medication. Antioxidants help protect the heart from free radical damage, also known as oxidation. Antioxidant nutrients include vitamin E and vitamin C (see below), beta carotene, and selenium. Free radicals damage the tissues lining the arteries, which leads to atherosclerosis and plaque deposits. Antioxidants, particularly vitamin C, can prevent this from happening by protecting the lining of the arteries. The following are nutrients you should know about:

L-ARGININE—L-arginine is an amino acid that has been receiving well-deserved attention in the medical literature for its ability to produce nitric oxide. Nitric oxide benefits the arterial walls in several ways. It helps the smooth muscles in the arterial walls relax, promoting an antianginal, antihypertensive, and antistress effect. Additionally, research shows that L-arginine reduces the activation of platelets, the small bodies that can initiate arterial spasm and plaque development. Other studies show that L-arginine slows plaque development and even reverses small amounts of plaque buildup. "I've seen it work," says Dr. Cutler. "Taking 2 to 3 grams of L-arginine per day has quite a marked antianginal effect. L-arginine is now a must in my protocol for nutrients. Usually I start with about 1,000 milligrams per day, and raise the levels if that amount isn't helping."

L-CARNITINE—The heart muscle needs to burn fat for energy, and L-carnitine allows this to happen. Dr. Janson explains: "L-carnitine gets fat into the little engines inside the cells called mitochondria. These little mitochondrial engines are where fat is burned for energy. Your heart muscle needs to burn fat for energy, and the only way it can get the fat into that little engine is with the amino acid L-carnitine. At the same time, that inner mitochondrial membrane requires another nutrient to burn the fat: coenzyme Q10." Dr. Janson recommends that people take 500 milligrams L-carnitine two to three times a day. You should take L-carnitine along with vitamin E, because they work together synergistically.

CHROMIUM PICOLINATE—Chromium picolinate has been shown to be beneficial both for the heart and for blood sugar levels.

COENZYME Q10—Coenzyme Q10 is a nutrient that should be taken by anyone who has heart problems or who wants to avoid getting them. Along with L-carnitine, it helps prevent angina and protects the heart muscle by letting it burn fat for energy more easily. It also improves heart health by reducing blood pressure and arrhythmias. As an antioxidant, it prevents the damage to blood vessels that leads to hardening of the arteries. Therapeutic levels are between 50 and 200 milligrams for mild heart disease. More severe heart disease may respond to 200 to 300 milligrams.

LECITHIN—Lecithin is made from soy. Not only does it keep the arteries strong and healthy, but it also helps emulsify fats, helps the brain, and is good for memory.

MAGNESIUM—Magnesium increases blood flow by allowing muscles in the arterial wall to relax. Usually 1,000 milligrams are needed.

MAXEPA—MaxEPA, a combination of EPA (eicosapentaenoic acid) and DHA (docosohexaenoic acid), also known as fish oil, is part of the omega-3 and omega-6 fatty acids found in salmon, sardines, and mackerel. Since many people do not eat these fish, they should be getting these fatty acids in fish oil. The recommended daily dose is 500 to 1,000 milligrams. Clinical and epidemiological experience as well as scientific studies have found that people who eat a lot of fish have less heart disease than people who do not.

NIACIN (VITAMIN B3)—A fifteen-year study on the effects of niacin published by the American Heart Association in the mid-1980s connected the use of niacin to a significant reduction in heart attacks and death from heart disease. Long-term niacin use has also been associated with decreased rates of cancer. Niacin should be taken under medical supervision, since it can affect liver function.

TAURINE—Taurine, an amino acid, is another important antioxidant that helps prevent atherosclerosis. Additionally, it can avert heart failure by improving the strength of the heart's contraction. That increases the outflow of blood from the heart and reduces congestive heart failure. Generally, 500 milligrams are taken twice a day.

THYROID SUPPLEMENTS—Thyroid supplementation may normalize high cholesterol. According to Dr. Ray Peat, "High cholesterol indicates a thyroid hormone deficiency. A clear demonstration of this was seen in the 1930s in patients whose thyroid glands were surgically removed. After the operation, cholesterol levels became abnormally high, but they returned to normal with thyroid supplementation." He adds that thyroid extract is linked to fewer heart attacks: "One of the foremost American researchers in the field, Broda Barnes, wrote *Solved: The Riddle of Heart Attacks* after finding that patients in one group had far fewer heart attacks than did patients in another group. All the low-heart-attack group did differently was take thyroid when they needed it."

VITAMIN B1 AND OTHER B VITAMINS—Vitamin B1 (thiamine) is the most important B vitamin for the heart: 25 to 50 milligrams daily are recommended. Dr. Janson adds, "Other B vitamins, such as folic acid and B12, can help lower blood levels of homocysteine, a risk factor for heart disease."

VITAMIN C—If there is one vitamin everyone needs to take every day, it is vitamin C. Get over that old-fashioned idea that all you need is one glass of orange juice to get the necessary vitamin C. Now we have thousands of studies of the valuable properties of vitamin C, which can help with everything from cancer to heart disease and diabetes. I would take 500 to 1,000 milligrams, five times a day. Vitamin C washes out of the system, so you need to take it throughout the day. Two well-known specialists in coronary heart disease recommend that their patients take vitamin C before going to bed at night because they find it helps prevent heart attacks during sleep and in the morning, which is when the majority of heart attacks occur.

VITAMIN E—Vitamin E has several functions. Aside from being a protective antioxidant, it reduces the stickiness of the platelets, little blood fragments that initiate blood clots. This effect is helped by the addition of essential fatty acids and garlic to the diet. Minimizing free radical damage and keeping platelets from clogging the arteries give arteries a chance to heal and recover. There is more room for oxygen to flow through the arteries to reach tissues. It is estimated that between 400 and 800 international units (IU) are useful in preventing stroke. You may go higher, up to 1,200 or 1,600 units, unless other medical conditions preclude a higher level. I believe we would cut the incidence of stroke by 20 percent, saving 50,000 to 100,000 people a year, just by having everyone take this little, inexpensive supplement.

In addition, two other beneficial supplements are chondroitin sulfate A and evening primrose oil (1,500 mg/day).

Herbs

In addition to the herbs listed below, consider taking barberry, black cohosh, and butcher's broom.

BUGLEWEED—Bugleweed is a remedy for heart palpitations and elevated blood pressure. It may also alleviate anxiety, since elevated blood pressure is frequently associated with a rapid pulse rate, anxiety, and agitation.

CAYENNE—Capsaicin, the active ingredient in cayenne, helps the heart in many ways. It stimulates circulatory function, lowers cholesterol, reduces blood pressure, and lessens the chance of heart attacks and strokes. By decreasing blood levels of fibrin, it also reduces the risk of forming blood clots that cause heart attacks and strokes.

GARLIC—Among its many benefits, garlic helps lower blood pressure and decrease cholesterol. When combined with vitamin E, it lessens the frequency of blood clots in arterial walls, which in turn helps prevent heart attacks and strokes. The recommended amount is 2,000 milligrams per day.

GINKGO BILOBA—Ginkgo biloba helps improve small blood vessel circulation.

HAWTHORN BERRY—Hawthorn is an overall heart tonic that works against arrhythmia (irregular heartbeat), angina, high blood pressure, and hardening of the arteries. It aids circulation and ameliorates valvular insufficiency and an irregular pulse. Hawthorn berry can also correct acid conditions of the blood. It can safely be taken every day.

MISTLETOE—Mistletoe is a cardiac tonic that stimulates circulation. Fifteen drops of tincture taken three times a day or three cups of tea daily can help lower blood pressure and alleviate heart strain. Mistletoe should not be overused, nor should the berries be eaten.

MOTHERWORT—Motherwort helps stabilize the electrical rhythm of the heart. The amount taken should be monitored by a doctor.

WILD YAM—Wild yam stimulates production of DHEA. Low levels of this hormone have been related to higher incidences of heart disease.

Chinese Herbal Therapy

Letha Hadady, one of the leading herbalists in the United States, says most Americans do not go to the doctor when they are a little sick; they wait until they are really suffering. They may have chest pains or difficulty breathing, but they generally don't go to the doctor nor, of course, to the herbalist. They say, "I'm tired; I'm under stress," and ignore it. That is a problematic approach because some of the associated conditions of heart disease are the ones they are complaining of: fatigue, stress, and poor digestion. Poor digestion and fatigue lead to cholesterol buildup, which leads to pain and heart congestion. People try to breathe more deeply and reduce stress when they experience these early symptoms, but that does not help. However, changing your diet, taking herbs and foods that reduce cholesterol will definitely help.

Hadady's clients often have conditions that they believe are unrelated to heart disease; but her special training as an herbalist enables her to see a connection to the heart. Mind, body, and spirit are interconnected, and the heart is affected by all of these. Depression, for example, is related to a weak heart. Insomnia, poor concentration, and palpitations are all signs that poor circulation could be affecting the heart.

Many Western doctors will say that herbs have not been tested. But when you go to a public library or consult an on-line medical search and reference service such as Medline, which is available free to any interested person, you find 3,500 studies on Chinese herbs alone. The majority of the research is done in Asia.

Quite a number of these remedies are available in health food stores, by mail order, or in your local Chinatown. The ingredients are always in English or Latin on the back.

Hadady points out that one of the major underlying problems associated with heart disease is fatigue. Chinese doctors link the heart's health to the strength of the adrenal glands—not an obvious connection. Hadady states, "If I had a patient complaining of fatigue and being overweight, I would suspect heart problems—if not then, somewhere down the line, so I would work on the adrenals. To strengthen the adrenals, you can get the herbal preparation from Chinatown called Goldenbook. It adds to immune energy and will help with kidney and heart problems. We strengthen what is weak so that the heart will not falter."

Hadady explains that clove is a strong stimulant. A pinch in the late afternoon will act like coffee. Coffee is a major problem because it increases painful, sluggish circulation in the gastrointestinal tract that affects the whole circulation, meaning that the heart will not run smoothly. A pinch of clove will replace coffee better than anything else can.

Siberian ginseng, a blend of various ginsengs, is beneficial. The ginsengs are adaptogens; that is, they help us maintain energy as well as aid us in living under a high level of stress. They support the nervous system. Raw Tienchi ginseng, one that Americans are less familiar with, comes in powdered form. A half teaspoon in cool water, taken every day, will reduce cholesterol and pain around the heart.

One Chinese remedy that is especially valuable in relation to heart pain and blood vessel congestion is dan shen wan, which combines salvia and camphor. The camphor dilates the blood vessels while the salvia increases the heart's action. Another valuable remedy is guan xin su he wan, which contains frankincense. Both frankincense and myrrh improve circulation. Frankincense increases blood flow around the heart. You can take it once a day to prevent heart attack. It can be chewed and swallowed. Hadady recommends it even if you have no heart symptoms. It has healthy ingredients such as liquid amber and sandalwood, which keep the esophagus and chest cool.

Yans shen jia jiao wan is a combination of ginseng and other herbs that free the circulation of the blood in the brain. This is not just for victims of heart attack but also for those with stroke and hemiplegia (paralysis of one side of the body). People with high cholesterol and those at high risk of heart trouble can take one dose a day as a preventive measure.

Baoxin wan is a remedy for heart attacks. If you feel faint and experience pain and weakness, you sniff it like a smelling salt. If the pain is great and you feel the onset of an attack, take it orally. It includes ginseng and liquid amber. It treats the congestion of the blood vessels around the heart and opens them up.

Some of the underlying problems leading to a heart attack, such as excess weight and cholesterol, are well countered by herbal remedies. One preparation whose name is self-explanatory is Keep Fit, Reduce Fat. The ingredients are ginseng, hawthorn, and other herbs that are good for the heart. Hawthorn, a slightly bitter, slightly sour berry, works as a digestive. You can take a capsule of Keep Fit after meals. Cholesterol is reduced, and the muscle of the heart is made stronger.

Evening primrose oil is another useful herb for reducing cholesterol. Chinatown is an excellent place to purchase this remedy since the prices are apt to be considerably lower than those for comparable items in health food stores.

Another popular remedy in Asia is green tea, which has been reported in the popular press as being very good for reducing cholesterol. "This is a good alternative to other caffeine teas," Hadady notes, "because the caffeine in it is very low. It gives the satisfaction of a bitter tea while reducing cholesterol."

Bojemni slimming tea protects the heart. It includes hawthorn. Xiao yao wan, a digestive remedy that boosts circulation and combats depression, contains ginger, mint, and other herbs; it eases the flow of bile, eases the digestive process, and reduces chest congestion.

Digestive Harmony is an American-made product that contains Chinese herbs, one of many such products that are now on the market and sold door to door or through mail order. "This is part of a trend now," Hadady explains, "a very important trend in herbalism, of using Asian herbs manufactured with American standards. Digestive Harmony can be ordered from Oakland, California. It will ease the underlying troubles related to heart disease.

"Remember that depression is in part a heart problem," Hadady goes on. "The heart is not just a circulatory center, but is related to our emotions. Depression is rightly associated with heart disease since it affects the heartbeat. When we are not happy and our emotions are not smooth, we feel it in the heart.

"Some remedies that combat depression come to us from China. Schizandra strengthens the energy level and keeps us from losing the energy we have. It is good for both the adrenals and the heart. It fights against poor memory, poor concentration, and depression. Also try anshen bu nao pien, available in all the Chinatowns in the United States. It is for depression, blood deficiencies, and heart-related problems such as panic and anxiety.

"Also useful is mao dong qing, which is the Chinese name for holly, and it comes in capsule form. It is for chest pain and prevention of heart trouble. You can take several of these capsules each day as a preventive. If you already have heart problems, it reduces cholesterol, congestion, and pains.

"In general," Hadady concludes, "Chinese remedies for the heart treat not just pain but also emotional problems: sadness, anxieties, and other mental suffering."

Chelation Therapy

Chelation therapy, which is being administered to hundreds of thousands of heart disease patients, is proving quite successful and is considerably safer and substantially less expensive than bypass surgery. It is not new, having been in use for more than forty years.

Chelation involves the infusion into the bloodstream of the amino acid EDTA. The EDTA bonds with toxic metals and calcium and carries them out of the bloodstream through the kidneys, slowing or reversing some plaque formation in the arteries and thus retarding the degenerative process. EDTA enhances blood flow, permitting more essential oxygen and nutrients to circulate and be absorbed by the body. As chelation therapy is more commonly used, chelation specialists feel that it will become the most important heart disease therapy offered in the future.

As Dr. Steenblock describes it, "EDTA binds with calcium that has deposited in artery walls and is excreted from the body through the kidneys. In addition, it breaks down scar tissue and allows the arteries to become softer. In other words, it takes the *hard* out of *hardening of the arteries.*"

When deciding whether or not to administer chelation therapy, Dr. Cutler tests patients for heavy metal buildup. "I look for elevated iron and copper levels in the blood. I also measure something called the serum ferritin, which reflects artery tissue levels of iron. If I start chelation, as the iron levels come down in the blood, there are also clinical improvements in angina and exercise tests. And there are angiogram and treadmill test improvements as well.

"If I do not find any abnormality in these metals, I do what is called a challenge, which means I give one chelation treatment, collect urine for twenty-four hours afterward, and observe the metals that come out. Based on these results, I make the decision as to whether I want to chelate the person."

Dr. Steenblock, who has administered chelation therapy for more than twenty years, uses the treatment more extensively. He explains why it is so valuable for most individuals: "In their forties most people develop some degree of atherosclerosis due to cholesterol, scar tissue, fat, and calcium, which accumulate in the artery walls.

"You have to try to prevent all these risk factors by keeping your diet low in fat and cholesterol and by exercising, thinking properly, avoiding chemicals, and taking antioxidants to protect the inner lining of the blood vessels. In addition, you can break down scar tissue and remove calcium with chelation.

"Studies show that if you start chelating in your forties, you can actually reverse all the atherosclerosis as soon as it starts to develop. If you have done things that have not been perfect in your life—you haven't eaten right, you have been under too much stress, you have smoked—by the time you are forty, you will have some degree of atherosclerosis. Chelation can reverse this process and keep those arteries more pristine.

"By the time you are sixty, the amount of calcium that has been deposited in your arteries is ten times what you had in your arteries at ten years of age. Al Fleckenstein, a leading cardiovascular drug researcher, says in one of his books that the amount of calcium present in the walls of the arteries is the single most important risk factor in the development of atherosclerosis. In other words, as calcium accumulates in the arterial walls, it promotes the development of atherosclerosis; atherosclerosis develops because you are gradually accumulating this calcium. If you can remove the calcium somewhere between the ages of forty and sixty, you can change that ratio, reverse the whole process, and put off the development of atherosclerosis for a number of years. That's for prevention.

"Of course, if you have outright disease, you can be helped as well. I have been doing chelation since 1977, so I have treated thousands of patients, and most do not come for prevention. They come for treatment of disease. They come in with angina or claudication [lameness due to leg pain]. With chelation, most of the time these symptoms disappear. If they do not, it is usually because the person has advanced disease and needs more than the standard thirty treatments. When people who are seventy-five or eighty years old come in with advanced disease, I tell them that they need to start out with thirty treatments—that's one treatment twice or three times a week. They wait a month or two, and then come back and do another thirty. This process continues until we clean out these arteries, because it takes time to reverse all of the terribly occluded blocked arteries that develop over many, many years of bad living."

Stress Management

Virtually all the authorities agree that if you want to get a handle on heart disease, you have to deal with stress. Stress or distress is a major problem for the American psyche.

For a long while we have known that stress is a contributor to heart disease, but only recently have we begun to understand the physiological basis of the connection.

Richard Friedman, Ph.D., of Harvard Medical School, remarks that when we are confronted with stressful situations, most of us try to oversolve the problem. We constantly try to fit square pegs into round holes, and when we find that is not going to work, we turn inward, brood, and look for ways to dissipate stress, frequently by acting inappropriately, such as overeating, drinking, or taking inappropriate drugs or medications. This contributes to the disease process.

Dr. Friedman says there is a link between stress and cardiovascular disease. When we are stressed by a fear of physical or psychological danger, the body exhibits a fight-or-flight response as it prepares to deal with an enemy. Very recent research indicates that the body readies itself not to bleed if it is cut or injured, which makes a lot of sense from a biological and evolutionary perspective. However, if the threats are psychological and you have a bad diet, you may be going through stressful incidents twenty or thirty times a day, triggering the fight-or-flight response. Each time this happens, the body prepares not to bleed by making the blood platelets stickier. This internal clotting takes place every time you get angry, whether on a supermarket line or in a traffic jam. Over time this continual clotting can contribute to plaque buildup in the arteries.

Stress also contributes to heart disease by increasing free radical damage to tissues and increasing spasms in the arterial walls.

When you are exposed to a biochemical or psychological stress, a host of changes take place in addition to platelet stickiness. The body's ability to fight off viral and bacterial infection is lessened by the weaknesses induced by stress. Stress compromises the immune system's ability to fight off opportunistic diseases.

There is some good news, though, about our ability to fight off the debilitating conditions that lead to a heart attack. Dr. Friedman notes that just as continued stress leads to a weakening of the system, there is an opposite effect, one that has been labeled by his colleague at Harvard, Dr. Herbert Benson, the "relaxation response." Eliciting this calming response on a daily basis makes it less likely that you will have high blood pressure, arteriosclerotic plaque buildup, or a heart attack down the road.

The relaxation response should be combined with other behavior modifications to create a healthier response to stress, and all these techniques should be combined with the best medical care. That is the way to optimize your health.

Dr. Friedman tells us how the relaxation response is induced: Use whatever strategy you have available to let go of any muscle tension you may be experiencing. Make sure your muscles are loose and your jaw lets go. After you feel a bit more comfortable, focus your attention on your breathing. If you find yourself having any distracting thoughts, do not let them bother you or take you away from the process. As soon as you have a distracting thought, simply say to yourself, "Oh well," and return to a concentration on your breathing and to a thought or image that allows you to stay calm, peaceful, and relaxed. Become aware of the cool air coming into your nostrils and the warm air going out. Keep this up till you are deeply relaxed.

Other ways to overcome stress are exercise, deep breathing, visualization, tai chi, yoga, meditation, qi gong, mantras, massage, Reiki, biofeedback, and aromatherapy. An essential oil blend of ylang ylang, lavender or peppermint, and marjoram added to oil and applied during massage helps calm the system and may even lower blood pressure.

Treatment of Helicobacter pylori

Dr. Paul Cutler says that recent research links the *Helicobacter pylori* bacterium to high incidences of heart attacks and strokes. "*Helicobacter pylori* causes ulcers and chronic gastritis. Most practitioners are well aware of the higher incidence of stomach complaints in patients with heart disease. Apparently, this little bacterium, which comes from contaminated foods, burrows its way into the stomach wall. In its attempt to fight off the body's defenses, it produces toxins that initiate plaque development and thickening of the blood. This points to a strong correlation between stomach ulcer disease and coronary artery disease."

Fortunately, this problem is simple to cure, says Dr. Cutler: "You can use one particular type of honey that is high in hydrogen peroxide or cider vinegar, bismuth, and extracts of licorice. Or you can take a one-week course of three antibiotics to kill this bacteria, probably 97 percent of the time. It is very gratifying as a physician to see not only stomach symptoms but angina improve, sometimes dramatically, with the treatment of this common bacterial parasite."

Homeopathy

Dr. Ken Korins explains how his specialty, homeopathy, seems to get results with heart disease: "Homeopathy works by giving very small doses that are extremely individualized to the person's symptoms and physical state. These doses work by means of a type of vibration or energy that stimulates the body much as acupuncture does."

Many traditional practitioners dismiss homeopathy. These physicians say this therapy has never been proved by randomized, double-blind studies in the way more scientific procedures have been. Dr. Korins argues that is absolutely incorrect. He tells us that a 1991 *British Medical Journal* article by Kleijnen reviewed 107 clinical studies of homeopathy. About 80 percent of them found that homeopathy had positive effects. Many of these were extremely rigorous studies. A double-blind study in the *Journal of Pediatrics*, for example, showed extraordinary results from homeopathy.

What kinds of heart problems improve with homeopathy? Hypertension is one. Homeopathy can also help people recovering from congestive heart failure, cerebrovascular accidents, arteriosclerotic heart disease, and a wide range of other conditions.

In classical homeopathy, the specialist selects a single remedy. Korins elaborates: "We don't rely on a lot of tests and the high technology that goes with them. We prefer to look at what symptoms a person has and how they present themselves. For example, if a person is having angina, tightness, a squeezing sensation, a remedy such as hawthorn cactus, which is extremely effective in treating angina, is called for."

Qi (Chi) Manipulation

An Asian treatment that has some success with heart patients is the manipulation of *qi (chi)* energy. This term refers to all the nonliquid, biological energy that circulates through the body. Dr. Jeie Atacama uses *qi* to accomplish healing. He estimates that in twenty years of practice he has helped between three thousand and five thousand people. Rebalancing *qi* energy can help greatly with heart disease by rebuilding the body's health and restoring its self-healing powers.

This practice works exactly like acupuncture. It does not use needles, but it shares with acupuncture a focus on the meridians of the body. In a technique he learned from his father, Dr. Atacama uses his fingers directly on the patient's skin. Points are found on either side near the base of the spine. The treatment session should be done three times a week for as many weeks as are called for by the condition. If the problem is cramps in the leg due to poor circulation, ten sessions will get rid of the problem.

Healing practices such as tai chi and qi gong depend on channeling internal *qi* energies to rebalance the body.

Psychological, Social, and Spiritual Factors

Most healing programs focus on physical modalities. We look at diet, exercise, supplements, and substances to avoid, but people are beginning to understand that more subtle factors have a powerful influence as well. Dr. Ron Scolastico, a spiritual counselor and author of *Healing the Heart, Healing the Body*, believes that the process of remaining healthy involves four important elements: "The first element is our physical life, which most people know a great deal about. The second element looks at our mental life. It is becoming clearer and clearer that our thoughts promote or hinder health and in some cases actually cause disease. The third element addresses our emotional lives. Feelings, particularly love, have a profound effect. The fourth element addresses spiritual factors. I believe those energies come from the soul, which is an incredible source of power, love, and wisdom inside each of us."

Dr. Scolastico says we must draw on each of these factors as needed. Sometimes we must take physical steps such as seeing a doctor and taking medications or herbs, but sometimes that is not enough. "For example, one of my clients developed congestive heart failure after a painful divorce, along with pericarditis, which is an inflammation of the membrane surrounding the heart. She failed to respond to medical treatment, and her condition began to worsen. As I worked with her, she realized that she had lost touch with her soul. The divorce had wreaked such havoc in her emotional life that she could no longer feel love.

"Every day for six months she took an hour to connect with her soul. By doing this, she was able to regain a feeling of deep love for her body and herself. Today she is symptom-free and believes that without inner work she might be dead. So, many times, we need not only physical treatment but mental, emotional, or spiritual work to augment that process."

To promote health at every level, Dr. Scolastico advises the following:

Connect with your spiritual nature. Religious or not, we need to accept the existence of some benevolent, healing force larger than our personality and physical being. Once we realize we are never alone or abandoned, amazing changes can happen.

Be mindful of your thoughts. We all have negative thoughts, but this alone does not cause illness. Swallowing them and actualizing them does. We must learn to release negative ideas. This work takes time, and we should not be hard on ourselves when our thoughts are less than perfect.

Follow the physical principles of health. Living in a healthy way includes eating the right foods, exercising, and getting enough rest, play, and social activity. Giving to others has a beneficial impact on health.

Create love in your life every day. This is perhaps the most important principle of all. Research shows that love affects every aspect of our beings, including the physical. When we feel love, all body systems work better. The endocrine system produces beneficial hormones. Muscles relax, so that the flow of oxygen to the cells increases. Immune system function is enhanced. When we are filled with self-love, our health is strongest and our lives improve all around. Recent studies show that self-esteem improves academic performance and promotes emotional stability and greater health.

"A powerful way to enhance self-love," advises Dr. Scolastico, "is to notice when you are creating negative thoughts and feelings about yourself. Then consciously create an experience of love for yourself right at that moment, using the power of the word to augment the process. You can say, 'I just noticed I'm creating these negative thoughts and feelings about myself. I now choose to use my imagination, my creativity, and my will to create an inner experience of love for myself right now, in this minute.'"

Another way to build love into our lives is to set aside time each day for cultivating loving energy. Dr. Scolastico says, "For at least five minutes, use your mind, open your heart, and create love in your feelings. You can do that by imagining a person you love. Let your feelings for that person fill you as you bring that loved one fully into your thoughts and feelings. Let the corners of your mouth lift up in a smile. Just let your heart swell with love. You won't need a scientific test to prove the benefits."

Equal in importance to self-love is the love we share with others. Connecting with family, friends, and community gives us a sense of belonging that is invaluable to our well-being. Recently, a link between social bonds and heart health was reported in *Natural Health*. The magazine summarized thirty years of research on the town of Rosetto, Pennsylvania, and concluded that the most important risk factor for heart disease is a lack of community and intimate relationships. In this town, people lived in three-generation households with grandparents, parents, and children. There was a lot of interaction among families and much participation in community organizations. The incidence of heart disease was virtually nil even though residents ate high-fat diets and did not go out of their way to exercise. In fact, there was less coronary heart disease in Rosetto than in any other population in the United States.

CHAPTER 17

HERPES

$\int$ ome viral infections, such as a cold or the flu, are like bad party guests you can't persuade to go home. They seem to hang around forever, although you know they will eventually leave. After a few weeks of misery, the cold and flu depart. But there are other viruses, notably herpes, which come to the party with a bedroll and tablecloth, planning to take up permanent residence.

There are a number of types of herpes. One is the common cold sore, which usually occurs before another, more aggressive virus, such as a cold, is going to take hold in the body. That's why it is called a cold sore. Cold sores on the lips are usually referred to as fever blisters. A cold sore is classified as herpes simplex virus 1 (HSV-1). A more serious kind of herpes is genital, sexually transmitted herpes, called herpes simplex virus 2 (HSV-2). There is also herpes zoster, which used to be called shingles. Finally, Epstein-Barr virus is the form of herpes that causes mononucleosis.

Michele Picozzi, a health writer who specializes in natural medicine and the author of *Controlling Herpes Naturally*, points out that there is some controversy about the relationship between the two HSVs. There is no agreement on the status of "herpes simplex 1, which occurs, technically, above the waist, most often on the face or the lips, and simplex 2, which occurs below the waist. There is a body of evidence that they are actually different viruses, and they are classified as such. However, some researchers think they are both the same virus, which acts differently in different parts of the body. This would indicate that there is merely a herpes simplex 1 that is appearing at different sites."

Herpes can be pervasive, persistent, painful, and embarrassing. It also represents a fairly serious health risk both to the individual and to the community because many people who have herpes, particularly genital herpes—that is, anywhere from 20 to 25 percent—don't know they have the disease, since they don't experience symptoms. Even without symptoms, they can transmit the disease. Herpes is very contagious, and it has no cure.

As Picozzi notes, "Herpes has remarkable staying power. Once you contract it, you have it for life. It never leaves the body. It lies dormant in the nerve endings at the base of the spine. Thus the possibility of infecting people over a lifetime is considerable if there are recurrent outbreaks."

Aside from the facial and genital areas, herpes can affect the eyes and the brain, with more serious health consequences. Herpes sores can also increase a person's risk of contracting AIDS. In addition, for the numerous people who already have a diminished or compromised immune system, recurrent outbreaks of herpes can put a further strain on their immune reserves.

There is, however, some evidence that contracting facial herpes as a child lowers the risk of contracting genital herpes or even AIDS as an adult.

CAUSES

Some factors involving both food and emotional and physical states can cause herpes to recur, although the exact mechanism by which this happens remains a medical mystery.

According to Picozzi, "Stress is considered to be the number-one precursor to a herpes outbreak, and this applies to all types of stress: emotional, mental, or physical. Physical stress would include such things as overexertion, exercising too long, exercising in the sun, and doing a type of exercise for which your body is not ready. For example, you may be lifting weights and trying to increase your weight load. That may put a strain on the body. Stress inhibits the production of interferon, the body's antiviral agent. That's important, because herpes is a virus. Stress also inhibits the body from creating antibodies to fight off infection."

Certain foods have been found to cause herpes recurrences. These are primarily foods high in the amino acid arginine, including chocolate, peanuts, sunflower seeds, soy, and coconut. There are also some foods that raise the acidity of the blood. A high blood acidity level can irritate soft tissues, which is usually where herpes appears. These foods are sugar—that is, processed sugar—white flour, and red meats.

Exposure to strong sunlight—ultraviolet B (UVB)—has been shown to be a major factor in causing facial herpes, that which occurs on the lips, around the nose, or on other parts of the face.

Some people have a recurrence of facial herpes because there has been a trauma to the skin, for example, when they have dental work. Some people have a sensitive mouth, so just the friction of the dentist working in that area can cause the virus to recur.

Also implicated are seasonal changes, particularly the transitions from winter to spring and summer to fall, when the body goes through certain adjustments and detoxifying periods. This can also cause herpes to recur, depending on how well you are taking care of yourself at that particular time.

Genital herpes can be sexually transmitted, and pregnant women can transmit the virus to their unborn children. Moreover, prescription drugs that lower immunity, such as antibiotics, steroids, and antidepressants, can set off an attack.

SYMPTOMS

About 50 percent of people who have recurrent infections of herpes virus experience warning signs. Medically, these signs are known as a prodrome. These sensations are usually experienced in the area where a previous infection has occurred.

Picozzi explains: "The most common of these is a tingling or an itching, twitching sensation. Some people feel heat or a crawling beneath the skin, or "pins and needles." Some feel as if they are coming down with the flu. They feel fatigued. Their lymph glands are swollen, and they have other muscular aches and pains throughout the body. These signals from the brain can last anywhere from a few seconds to a few days."

She describes some recent work on the emotional triggers of an outbreak: "The most interesting thing I have found in researching herpes is the mind-body connection. Most people with genital herpes will tell you that for them, stress is the biggest precursor for an outbreak. I have found that this connection goes even deeper. I call it the overlooked psychological connection."

Genital herpes causes surface sores on the skin and the lining of the genital area. In women, sores can appear on the cervix, vagina, or perineum and may be accompanied by a discharge or vaginal blisters. There is often a burning sensation, especially at the onset of an outbreak. Other symptoms may include urinary problems, fever, and lymphatic swelling. Intercourse is painful and should be avoided during an outbreak to prevent transmission. HSV-2 occurs intermittently and usually lasts five to seven days.

As the name implies, facial or oral herpes tends to attack the skin and mucous membranes on the face, particularly around the mouth and nose. These cold sores tend to appear as pearllike blisters. Although they don't last very long, they can be irritating and painful. Herpes zoster, the result of the varicella zoster virus, causes agonizing blisters on one side of the body, usually on the chest or abdomen. Pain is usually felt before effects are seen, the result of overly sensitive skin covering the affected nerve. The symptoms may last from a few days to several weeks.

Conventional Treatment

There is no conventional medical cure for herpes, although drugs are commonly given to lessen symptoms. The most often prescribed of these is drugs acyclovir (Zovirax), which supposedly reduces the rate of growth of the herpes virus. Herpes medications have many potential side effects, including dizziness, headaches, diarrhea, nausea, vomiting, general weakness, fatigue, ill health, sore throat, fever, insomnia, swelling, tenderness, and bleeding of the gums. In addition, acyclovir ointment can cause allergic skin reactions.

Natural Remedies

Herpes sufferers will be glad to learn that natural remedies are often highly effective in shortening the length of outbreaks and diminishing their frequency. Here are some of the important ones to know about.

NUTRITION AND LIFESTYLE CHANGES

When herpes strikes, it is always a good idea to rest and eat lightly. Short fruit fasts, with plenty of pure water and cleansing herbal teas, can be very helpful. Good herbs to include are sage, rosemary, cayenne, echinacea, goldenseal, red clover, astragalus, and burdock root. Beneficial bacteria, such as those found in nondairy yogurt and in supplements containing lactobacillus and acidophilus, support the digestive processes necessary for the maintenance of the immune system. Other nutrients that directly enhance the immune system include garlic, quercetin, zinc gluconate, buffered vitamin C, and beta carotene. Bee propolis is anti-inflammatory, while B vitamins combat stress. Also good are bee pollen, blue-green algae, and pycnogenol.

Dr. Steven Whiting, author of *The Complete Guide to Optimal Wellness*, has spent a great deal of time looking at the value of lysine. "Lysine is an isolated form of an amino acid. Herpes, like so many viruses, requires complete protein in which to replicate. The lysine molecule mimics the virus's favorite protein structure, yet it is missing several bonds that are vitally important to the virus's lifestyle. When you increase lysine in the blood, the herpes virus attaches itself quite quickly to the molecule, and then it is too late. It is unable to replicate. You can shorten the outbreak of herpes down to a matter of a few hours with this treatment. In fact, if you catch it soon enough, you can keep the outbreak from occurring."

Dr. Whiting recommends a full-spectrum program for the management of herpes: "First take vitamin C, which is a powerful antioxidant and should be used in the presence of all viral infections. Take 2,000 milligrams as a minimum per day. Vitamin E used topically, for example, on the lips, will relieve pressure and irritation quite rapidly. It is also a powerful antioxidant and helps prevent cross-linkage at the outbreak. Take zinc, 100 milligrams per day, and copper, 2 milligrams per day. Acidophilus is certainly very important in any viral condition because of the die-off of the viral material, which eventually has to be processed in the colon. Take four to six capsules once or twice a day. Finally, and most important, is L-lysine, which can be purchased at your health food store in isolated form. In order to achieve saturation at the cellular level, you'll need 1 to 3 grams a day, but take that only for an actual outbreak."

However, as Picozzi notes, lysine is not useful for everyone. "Some people don't do as well as others using lysine alone to control herpes. Some dietary supplement manufacturers have come out with formulas containing lysine with some supporting herbs and vitamins that some people may find more effective."

Nervous system stressors, such as caffeine, alcohol, and hard-to-digest foods such as meat, should be avoided, especially at the onset of an attack. Foods high in the amino acid arginine, such as chocolate, peanut butter, nuts, and onions, are also associated with higher incidences of outbreaks.

Since stress promotes outbreaks, it is important to make time for activities that alleviate tension. Among the many possibilities are biofeedback, yoga, meditation, deep breathing, and exercise.

Toothbrushes should be changed frequently and completely dried before reuse to prevent reinfection. Soaking them in baking soda also fights germs.

HERBS

Picozzi also sees herbs as an important part of the treatment. "Some herbs are very good for building and maintaining immunity. They include echinacea and licorice root, both of which have been shown to have interferonlike properties. Echinacea also has some antiseptic qualities. It helps the body regulate the glandular system."

Also recommended is goldenseal, which is very important because it regulates liver function and in addition is reported to cleanse and dry the mucous membranes, the site where herpes often appears.

Siberian and American ginseng are invaluable in helping the body boost its resistance to stress and infection because they support the adrenal glands and the nervous system.

Tarragon is good because it contains caffeic acid, which has been found to prevent herpes. Tarragon has been shown to be beneficial for fatigue, particularly when taken in combination with lemon balm. Lemon balm has become very popular for both internal and topical use. It's best taken as a tea, two to four cups a day.

Herbs should only be taken for short periods, say one or two weeks, and under the supervision of a health care practitioner.

HOMEOPATHY

According to Dr. Erika Price, a practitioner of classical homeopathy and holistic healing, the following remedies may prove extremely helpful for cold sores:

NATRUM MURIATICUM—When sores are on the lips, especially in the middle of the lips, the 30c potency of this remedy should be taken twice a day.

PHOSPHORUS—Cold sores that manifest above the lips, accompanied by itching, cutting, and sharp pain, should be treated with the 30c potency of Phosphorus twice a day.

PETROLEUM—For cold sores that erupt in patches and become crusty and loose around the lips and mouth, Petroleum is indicated. A 9c potency is needed three times a day.

APIS—Apis helps cold sores around the mouth and lips that are accompanied by stinging; it also helps painful blisters that itch and burn. A 6c potency is needed three to four times daily.

The following remedies may be helpful for female genital herpes:

NATRUM MURIATICUM—This remedy is indicated when the herpetic lesions are pearllike blisters and the genital area feels puffy, hot, and very dry. A 6c potency, four times a day, may be beneficial.

DULCAMARA (BITTERSWEET)—Women who tend to get a herpes outbreak in clusters on the vulva or the hair follicles around the labia and vulva every time they catch a cold or get their period probably need Dulcamara in a 12c potency two to three times a day.

PETROLEUM—Petroleum may be beneficial if herpes eruptions form in patches and the sores become deep red and feel tender and moist. Outbreaks usually occur during menstrual periods, and most often affect the perineum, anus, labia, or vulva. A 9c potency should be taken three times a day.

The following remedies may be helpful for shingles:

ARSENICUM ALBUM—This remedy benefits most cases of shingles, especially when the individual feels worse in the cold, worse after midnight, and better with warmth. If taken at the onset of an attack, it is best in a 30c potency twice a day for two to three days. After the first three days, it is indicated if there is a burning sensation in the areas that were affected by the zoster eruptions (typically the chest and abdomen). At this point 12c, taken two to three times a day, is best. This remedy is excellent for getting rid of the burning sensation that is often present.

HYPERICUM PERFORATUM (ST. JOHN'S WORT)—This is a wonderful remedy for any kind of nerve pain. It is indicated whenever there is intense neuritis and neuralgia with burning, tingling, and numbness along the course of the affected nerves. Take this remedy in a 30c potency, two to three times a day, as needed.

AROMATHERAPY

The use of essential oils has recently gained popularity in the United States, where they are used widely in skin and body care products. However, the medicinal value of certain oils has long been accepted in other countries, particularly France, where in many instances, their antimicrobial properties make them an acceptable replacement for drug therapy.

Aromatherapist Valerie Cooksley, author of *Aromatherapy: A Lifetime Guide to Healing with Essential Oils*, says that pure essential oils, properly used, can heal cold and canker sores. One mouthwash she recommends combines 5 drops each of peppermint, bergamot, and tea tree oil with raw honey, which is used as a carrier. This is important, as oils do not mix with water. The mixture is then added to a strong sage or rosemary tea. Rinsing with the formula several times a day balances the pH of the mouth and helps heal infections. Using this daily may even prevent outbreaks.

Additional spot treatments alleviate pain and restore health. One that Cooksley recommends involves dabbing a cotton swab with myrrh oil and applying it directly onto cold and canker sores. Another aromatherapist, Sharon Olson, dabs a cotton swab with diluted tea tree oil and places it on the cold sore to kill the virus. She follows this up later with lavender, which soothes the sore and stimulates the growth of new skin. The addition of fresh aloe vera gel further promotes healing. A side benefit of the therapy is its ability to lift the spirits. "When I get a cold sore, I get depressed," reveals Olson, "so I usually inhale some rosemary or basil to lift my spirits and clear my mind."

CHAPTER 18

HORMONAL
IMBALANCE

D isturbance of a woman's hormonal cycle can play a major role in the development of various medical conditions. Women are affected both by their monthly hormonal cycle and by the hormonal phases associated with the life cycle of adolescence, maturity, pregnancy and childbirth, and menopause, so an understanding of these natural cycles is invaluable in understanding and treating a multitude of symptoms.

CAUSES

Sherrill Sellman, a psychotherapist and writer on women's health, author of the best-selling book *Hormone Heresy,* tells us that for the body to function properly, estrogen and progesterone have to be in balance. Progesterone and estrogen stimulate each other and help balance each other. One function of estrogen is to stimulate estrogen-sensitive tissues, which include cells in the breast, ovaries, and uterus. Estrogen helps develop the curviness of women. It produces their secondary sex characteristics. It is a very powerful stimulant of these tissues. Progesterone, on the other hand, helps slow down the growth of cells and stabilizes mature cells so that their growth doesn't get out of hand. The proper relationship, as Nature designed it, is one of checks and balances.

"We are seeing a predominance of estrogen in relation to just a little progesterone," Sellman says. "That's caused by the drugs and food we eat and the disharmony in our own bodies. It's been noted that 50 percent of women over the age of thirty-five are not ovulating each month. Now, only if women are ovulating, releasing an egg, can a little endocrine gland called the corpus luteum, which is the primary source of progesterone, be formed on the surface of the ovary. If a woman doesn't ovulate due to stress or bad diet, she can go a whole month without producing the progesterone to balance the estrogen. As a result, women are progesterone-deficient."

Diet and Lifestyle Factors

Dolores Perri, a nutritionist from New York City, lists factors that can interfere with normal hormonal production and balance:

ALCOHOL—Alcohol blocks the body's gamma linolenic acid (GLA) production, preventing the manufacture of natural hormones. This quickens the aging process. Alcohol creates deficiencies in B vitamins, magnesium, and calcium, which upset hormone balance. Further, alcohol damages the liver, which in turn interferes with hormone metabolism.

ANIMAL PROTEINS—Animal proteins are loaded with hormones and synthetic antibiotics that throw our own hormone levels out of balance.

BIRTH CONTROL PILLS—Birth control pills deplete the body's B vitamins, which are needed for natural hormone production; increase susceptibility to allergies; and may cause liver damage, which can affect hormonal balance.

CAFFEINE—Caffeine is found in coffee, tea, chocolate, soft drinks, and certain medications. Like alcohol, it blocks GLA production. Chocolate inhibits the liver's breakdown of hormones. Tea interferes with the absorption of iron and zinc, particularly if drunk with meals. Caffeine also raises adrenaline levels and increases stress.

EXERCISE—Professional athletes and women who train vigorously may use up so many vitamins and minerals that the body has insufficient means to maintain normal hormonal production. This can lead to an abnormal menstrual cycle and even the absence of menstruation altogether.

PHOSPHATES AND POLYPHOSPHATES—The phosphates and polyphosphates found in many food products—such as soft drinks, processed meats, and cheese—can interfere with the absorption of nutrients.

SMOKING—Cigarettes contribute to hormonal problems by increasing the need for vitamins and minerals to detoxify the poisons in tobacco smoke. This reduces the amount of nutrients available for hormone production.

STRESS—Stress is a major contributor to hormonal imbalance. Any type of adverse stimulus that requires the body to change and adapt, such as day-to-day hassles, psychological trauma, financial problems, and environmental pollution, can cause stress. External stress can cause hormones to decline, which puts stress on internal body systems. This further diminishes hormonal production and can interfere with immune function, which can lead to the development of allergies and autoimmune illnesses such as thyroiditis and lupus. Conversely, stress can create problems by causing the body to secrete too many hormones.

SUGAR—Sugar interferes with nutrient absorption, particularly B vitamins. It also interferes with the circulation of hormones throughout the body.

WEIGHT PROBLEMS—Excess weight adversely affects hormonal balance. The ratio of fat-to-lean body mass is critical in the initiation and continuation of the ovarian cycle. Being too thin is equally undesirable. If you fall below a certain weight, the pituitary hormone stops sending messages to the ovaries, and ovulation and menstruation stop.

OTHER FACTORS—Other conditions that contribute to hormonal imbalance include food sensitivity, allergy, chronic illness, candidiasis, menstrual and gynecological problems, drugs taken over long periods of time, and low levels of thyroid hormone.

SYMPTOMS

Dr. Elizabeth Vleit is founder of the Women's Center for Health Enhancement and Renewal at All Saints' Hospital in Fort Worth, Texas, and author of *Screaming to Be Heard: Hormonal Connections Women Suspect and Doctors Ignore.* She describes some of the conditions that hormonal imbalance can trigger and tells when they are likely to occur: "Women's bodies are cyclic in their response to hormones. They have a monthly rhythm of hormonal changes from puberty to menopause, which have a critical bearing on many dimensions of health. Men's bodies, on the other hand, have a tonic pattern of secretion, which means that the same amounts of key hormones are produced every day. They vary within twenty-four hours in terms of their hormone production. But basically each day is similar to the day before and the day after.

"For women, the first half of the menstrual cycle is dominated by a rise in ovarian estradiol. This is the primary estrogen that is active at receptor sites on all the cells in the brain and body, from puberty to menopause. This rise in estrogen allows the ovary to prepare the follicle that will become the egg released at ovulation.

"At ovulation, when the egg is released, the estradiol level drops briefly. The egg then takes over and produces progesterone for the second half of the cycle. Progesterone levels rise, and estrogen levels rise again, though not as high as in the first half of the menstrual cycle. Progesterone and estrogen drop prior to bleeding, when the egg is not fertilized. The body sheds the lining of the uterus and starts over.

"When hormones fall, right before bleeding, a drop in certain critical brain neurotransmitters, such as serotonin and endorphins, is triggered. This is associated with mood changes women describe—feelings of irritability, insomnia, depression, or anxiety. This may be a time in the cycle when women get migraines. The drop in estrogen that triggers changes in serotonin, norepinephrine, and endorphins sets off a cascade of blood vessel spasms that are involved in migraine headaches. That also affects chemical messengers involved in regulating the immune system, the gastrointestinal tract, the heart, heart rate, blood vessels, and as many as four hundred other functions.

"We also see hormonal connections in women who have the diffuse muscle aches of fibromyalgia. These women often develop aches, pains, and tender points after some type of hormonal change, such as postpartum or post–tubal ligation, or following a hysterectomy, even if the ovaries are left in place. We see this in menopause too. If we look at the patterns of this type of pain in women, we see that 80 percent of fibromyalgia patients are female, and that the average age when fibromyalgia appears is about forty-four or forty-five."

Sherrill Sellman notes that infertility and miscarriage are both directly related to hormonal imbalance: an excess of estrogen and a deficiency of progesterone.

CLINICAL EXPERIENCE

Tests

Dr. Vleit says women need to be aware of the relationship between hormonal cycles and medical conditions: "One of the ways to do that is to track patterns relative to cycles, and to test the blood for various hormones that women's bodies produce. I've developed an approach to doing that by measuring the hormonal levels at the right time of the menstrual cycle. This helps women know what is happening to their hormone levels at the time that they are having symptoms. I become frustrated when doctors tell me that we don't need to measure the female hormones because they vary. I respond that that's the whole point. They do vary, and how they vary, relative to women experiencing problems, is what we must find out in order to offer them the most constructive options."

It is also important to check thyroid function. Thyroid hormone controls progesterone, cholesterol, and the ovaries. It acts as a cascading system. When not functioning properly, other hormones get out of balance.

Nutrition

The typical American diet is high in fat, protein, caffeine, simple sugars, and salt, ingredients that interfere with optimal hormonal balance. These foods create a vicious cycle. They fuel premenstrual cravings for sweets and chocolate, and giving in to them worsens the cravings.

Perri advises us not to reach for a prescription drug for hormonal problems. It is better to eat high-quality organic foods and avoid foods that throw the system off balance. Beans and legumes are better sources of protein than meats, which are loaded with hormones. In addition, Perri recommends cold-processed oils, nuts, seeds, fatty fish, and beans. "These foods are all very high in GLAs," she notes. "The GLAs help us make natural estrogen in our own bodies."

Supplements

Wild yam and DHEA promote production of natural estrogens in the body, if the body needs them. If estrogen is not needed, these supplements are eliminated by the body, making them completely safe to use. Magnesium and calcium may also be beneficial, since most women do not get enough of these nutrients.

Herbs

Blue cohosh, black cohosh, yarrow, and chaste tree help balance hormone production. Other balance-promoting herbs include raspberry leaf, dong quai, wild yam, and passion flower.

Janet Zand, a naturopath, doctor of Oriental medicine, and acupuncturist, uses programs that rotate the herbs being used in accordance with the four weeks of the menstrual cycle. Herbs used during the first two weeks nourish blood and balance hormones; those used during the second two weeks clear the liver, which tends to become congested during these last two weeks.

In an article on the HealthWorld Online website (www.healthy.net), Zand recommends the following general herbal program for balancing the hormonal system and building general resistance. (If you have severe PMS, see chapter 29, which discusses her programs for PMS.)

FIRST TWO WEEKS—Combination of red raspberry leaf and dong quai, as a tablet, capsule, tea, or tincture, three times a day.

THIRD WEEK—Astragalus, American ginseng, or Chinese ginseng. These adaptogenic herbs tone the deep immune system. Take as a tablet, capsule, tea, or tincture, three times a day.

FOURTH WEEK—Combination of goldenseal and echinacea. These herbs have antiviral, antibacterial, and anti-inflammatory properties. Take as a tablet, capsule, tincture, or tea, three times a day.

Sherrill Sellman would add a Peruvian herb called maca. "It is wonderfully supportive of adrenal function, thyroid function, and ovarian function," she says. "It helps with bones, and with a variety of health deficiencies."

CHAPTER 19

INFERTILITY

A pproximately two and a half million American couples are unable to conceive. The question of what can and should be done to conquer infertility is not only a complex medical issue but, with the advent of more and more advanced techniques for getting around nature's roadblocks to conception, it is at times a thorny ethical dilemma as well, with high emotional stakes.

After ten years of fertility tests and treatments, Carla Harkness, frustrated by the lack of consumer-oriented literature on the subject, consulted over a hundred medical specialists and put together *The Fertility Book*. Harkness sees infertility as an emotional life crisis that is largely unacknowledged by society: "Reactions include grief and mourning, loss of self-esteem, and impaired self-image. Couples often have difficulties communicating with each other. Their sexual relationship is tested and damaged. All in all, it is a traumatic experience."

She adds that an early end to pregnancy, due to miscarriage, produces the same frustrations: "The failure of a fertilized egg to implant is amazingly common. Often up to 50 percent of fertilized eggs do not make it past the initial two-week period to implantation. Up to 20 percent of confirmed pregnancies are miscarried in the first trimester in women under thirty-five years old. As a woman approaches forty, that number can exceed 25 percent, and by the age of forty-five, the miscarriage rate is almost 50 percent. The emotional impact of miscarriage is similar to the emotional impact of infertility. There is often grief and mourning that are not accepted as genuine mourning in our society. Couples often hear things like, 'I guess it was meant to be,' 'Something was wrong,' or 'You'll have another.' That is often of little solace to someone feeling this kind of loss."

Reasons for infertility in women include endometriosis, a condition in which the glands and tissues that line the inside of the uterus grow outside the uterus; poor diet; deficiencies in folic acid, vitamin B6, vitamin B12, and iron; heavy metal toxicity; obesity; immature sex organs; abnormalities of the reproductive system; hormonal imbalances; and genetic damage from electromagnetic radiation.

It may surprise you to learn that the birth control pill and other sources of estrogen can add to the problem. Barbara Seaman, advocate for women's health issues, author of *The Doctors' Case Against the Pill* and coauthor with me of *For Women Only!*, concludes that the chemicals in the Pill may increase infertility in three ways: by suppressing the natural productions of hormones; by increasing the risk of sexually transmitted diseases (STDs), especially chlamydia; and by upsetting the assimilation of nutrients.

Abnormal Menstrual Cycles

As Seaman reports, "Fertility experts confirm that many women who have been on the Pill for a long time have problems reestablishing their monthly cycles." Robin Wald, a nutritionist and health care writer who specializes in infertility, explains further how birth control pills can cause hormonal imbalances that affect fertility.

"The hypothalamus is the gland that produces gonadotropin-releasing hormone, the hormone that triggers the pituitary gland to secrete other hormones that are important for fertility. These hormones, follicle-stimulating hormone, which tells the ovaries to start producing and maturing an egg each month, and luteinizing hormone, which ripens the egg and allows it to be released, signal the ovaries to produce estrogen and progesterone so that you can have a normal menstrual cycle. It's a very complicated and complex system and must be in a very particular balance to function properly; for the egg to ripen and mature; for the egg to be released and travel through the fallopian tubes; and for progesterone to be there to build up the endometrial lining to nourish an egg, so that if it's fertilized it can be implanted and nourished and grow so that it doesn't miscarry. When you have too much estrogen that suppresses pituitary gland function, you disrupt the normal hormone balance."

Chlamydia

"Another reason the Pill is bad for female infertility," notes Barbara Seaman, "is that it promotes the growth of chlamydia. This condition has reached epidemic proportions in the United States, with over half a million new cases yearly. Chlamydia causes pelvic inflammatory disease, which can then cause sterility. Usually, the first time it strikes, chlamydia does not render a woman sterile. Women who get the condition once should give up the Pill right away."

Nutritional Deficiency

Seaman says there are a lot of nutritional issues involved with taking the Pill. "If a woman has been on the Pill for a long time, she may be very low in folic acid; vitamins B1, B2, B6, B12, C, and E; and trace minerals zinc and magnesium, all essential to normal fertility. Sometimes just getting on a really good diet with really good supplements can get her back into a fertile cycle without needing heavy-duty drugs. It should be noted, however, that any dietary supplements used should be low in vitamin A, niacin, copper, and iron, which tend to be elevated in Pill users."

CLINICAL EXPERIENCE

Assisted Reproductive Technology

"The laboratory options have just exploded in the past decade for infertile couples," Carla Harkness reports. "In 1978, the first 'test tube' baby was born in England through a process called in vitro fertilization. Since then, the process has been instituted worldwide. There are now over 260 clinics practicing some form of that kind of laboratory fertilization, which is now called assisted reproductive technology or ART.

"Now the boundaries have even exceeded menopause. Before, you had the practice of donor sperm for artificial insemination. Now there is the ability to fertilize donor eggs from younger women with the husband's sperm and to implant those eggs in an infertile woman who is over forty-five or fifty. She is able to carry a child to term that is not genetically related to her. These kinds of options have all become available, and they offer a great deal of hope to many couples."

ETHICAL ISSUES

While modern advances in fertility treatments offer a wealth of new possibilities, they also raise new ethical concerns. "A number of religious groups have raised questions about the intervention of technology in the natural process of reproduction," Harkness explains. "There is also a theme of pronatalism at any cost here, emphasizing that to be complete as couples or as women, people absolutely must birth a biological child."

Another big issue revolves around extending maternal age past nature's deadline of menopause. Before, women in their mid-forties probably weren't able to get pregnant because their bodies would stop that function. Now it is possible for women in their fifties and sixties to become pregnant. This raises a number of questions: Is that putting too much demand on their bodies? What about the age difference between them and their children? What about obligations to aging parents while having little ones in your midlife? Additionally, there is a legal and moral question revolving around the status of unused, frozen embryos in the event of death and divorce.

"There are further questions surrounding the availability of this expensive technology to those without the means or the medical insurance. Unfortunately, these treatments are quite expensive. From the moment you walk into a specialist's office asking for an evaluation, you start incurring costs in the hundreds of dollars for examinations and tests, all the way to thousands of dollars for the in vitro techniques. It's about ten thousand dollars per cycle for a straight in vitro lab procedure, all the way up to fifteen thousand dollars if egg-donor in vitro fertilization is utilized."

Many women distrust scientific intervention in general. Problems with intrauterine devices (IUDs) have caused pelvic inflammatory disease resulting in infertility. Diethystilbestrol (DES), an estrogen replacement often used as a "morning after" pill in the United States even after it was linked to cancer and anomalies of the vagina and cervix, has been another big problem, as has thalidomide. Now there is a concern about using female hormones to stimulate ovulation. With most infertility treatments, whether the problem is due to the man or woman, it is mainly the women who undergo the drug treatments, the surgeries, and so forth. What are the long-term effects of exposing women to these drugs?

Natural Options

Dr. Marjorie Ordene, a gynecologist from Brooklyn, New York, believes that while there is a place for technology in fertility, women are too quick to seek out these methods, and she suggests trying various natural options first.

PINPOINTING TIME OF OVULATION

Women should learn to recognize their time of ovulation by taking their temperature first thing in the morning, before getting out of bed. Says Dr. Ordene, "Usually, temperature rises in the second half of the cycle, two weeks before menstruation. The mucus that is produced around the time of ovulation has a clear, slippery quality. This is the kind of mucus that is needed for the sperm to penetrate the cervix."

WHAT TO AVOID

Robin Wald cautions that women trying to conceive should avoid exposure to toxic substances that not only may interfere with conception but have also been linked to miscarriage and birth defects.

"The first thing I tell people to avoid is tobacco smoke. If you're a cigarette smoker and you plan on getting pregnant, quit smoking. Tobacco is very high in chemicals, including cadmium, which is a toxic heavy metal that accumulates in the reproductive organs of both men and women. It interferes with sperm production in men and hormone production in women. Secondhand smoke can cause similar problems.

"I also encourage people to stop drinking, even if they only drink moderately. Alcohol interferes with fertility by causing liver toxicity. The liver is the primary organ for building up cholesterol to form the steroid hormones that are important to reproductive health. Marijuana and other drugs can also cause liver toxicity and should be avoided.

"In addition, I suggest that people eliminate caffeine, both in coffee and in sodas; switch to decaf coffee or herbal teas; and increase water intake. Although the subject of caffeine and fertility is controversial, studies have shown that as few as two cups of coffee a day or two cans of caffeinated soda can increase your chance of a miscarriage by four times and your infertility by 50 percent."

Wald further cautions women to avoid taking some over-the-counter medications. "A lot of women who experience menstrual discomfort think nothing of taking an aspirin or ibuprofen. But nonsteroidal anti-inflammatory drugs are also harmful to the reproductive system.

"One thing to avoid that cannot be overemphasized is pesticides—both pesticides that have been sprayed in your garden and pesticide residue from food that you buy. Pesticides are very toxic to the reproductive system. This is because pesticides are in a class of chemicals called xenoestrogens, synthetic chemicals that act like estrogen on the body. Overexposure to xenoestrogens can result in a condition called estrogen dominance. In estrogen dominance there is too much estrogen circulating in the body, which throws off the balance and production of other hormones that are essential for fertility."

Other sources of xenoestrogens are food additives, preservatives, and meat from animals that have been fed hormones. Dairy products also contain xenoestrogens, both from the cows' own hormones and from hormones given to them to promote milk production.

DIET AND LIFESTYLE

Women should maintain a healthy diet and follow a basic exercise program. Fertility specialists Dr. Talha Sawaf, Dr. Yehudi Gordon, and Marilyn Glenville, writing in *Positive Health* magazine, recommend eating organic foods as much as possible and avoiding food additives, coffee, and tea. They advise eliminating nonessential medications and avoiding exposure to radiation, hazardous substances in the workplace, pesticides, and pollutants such as toxic metals. They point out that becoming as healthy as possible before conception improves the quality of the egg and sperm, thereby maximizing fertility and reducing the risk of miscarriage. Conversely, fertility is decreased by poor nutrition, vitamin or mineral deficiencies, and too much alcohol, cigarettes, and stimulants.

Robin Wald, who suggests that the very first step in optimizing fertility is to examine your diet, says that the standard American diet does not promote either health or fertility. She recommends an organic, whole, live-foods diet. "The advantage of eating live food is that the nutritional value and the quality are that much higher. Good nutrition is vital when you're trying to get pregnant. Vitamins, minerals, fats, amino acids, and other nutritional components from our foods are essential for keeping the reproductive system healthy. Eat fresh fruit and vegetables, especially leafy green vegetables like collard greens, kale, Swiss chard, red chard, and beet greens, which are very high in folic acids and loaded with calcium. Folic acid is essential for preventing birth defects such as spina bifida, and calcium will aid in building your baby's skeleton as well as keeping your own bones healthy."

She suggests minimizing your intake of processed flour, bread, baked goods, and pasta, and incorporating more whole grains into your diet. She recommends brown rice, millet, quinoa, oats, and buckwheat. "Whole grains are loaded with fiber and have very high nutritional quality. Raw nuts and seeds are also good, as are chickpeas, lentils, black beans, and pinto beans, which are both high in fiber and a good source of nonanimal protein.

"Fiber is important in promoting the excretion of toxins and bound-up estrogens from the gut. If you have insufficient fiber to move things through your intestines in a timely way, these estrogens sit in the gut and get reabsorbed into the body. So instead of having environmental estrogens or estrogens your body has created circulating through your body once, they're now going through a second, third, or fourth time, which contributes to estrogen dominance."

Wald advises eating soy products, such as tempeh and miso. "Soy is a good source of phytoestrogens, which have a chemical structure similar to estrogen. Phytoestrogen tricks your body into thinking that it's getting estrogen, but the advantage of phytoestrogens is that they tell your body to lower its own estrogen production, which helps balance your estrogen levels. As well, phytoestrogens block the absorption of xenoestrogens."

EMOTIONAL AND SPIRITUAL ISSUES

Often, a woman has apprehensions that need to be addressed about becoming pregnant. It may be reassuring to talk to the inner child and let her know that even though there will be another child, the little girl in her will still get the attention she needs. This kind of spiritual work is often important in achieving pregnancy.

Feelings of blame, guilt, anger, and frustration that infertile couples often experience will have a negative effect on their fertility. Discussing such issues, perhaps with a counselor, can resolve these negative feelings and improve the chances of conception.

Infertility is a very stressful, major life event, and stress can itself adversely affect fertility. Robin Wald describes how stress affects reproductive function. "Every time there is a stress response in your body, the adrenal glands secrete a group of hormones that have an inhibitory effect on the hypothalamus, which is the master gland that signals the production of the hormones needed for reproduction. When you have excessive stress, the hypothalamus does not function properly.

"Stress can also cause a condition called hypoprolactin anemia. Prolactin is another hormone that prepares the breasts for milk production. If a non-pregnant woman has high levels of prolactin, it will make conception difficult because it can shut down ovulation.

"If you're under a lot of stress, do whatever you can to reduce it," Wald suggests. She recommends yoga, meditation, breathing exercises, spiritual work and prayer, visualization and imagery, bodywork, and massage as ways to lower stress levels.

Nutritional supplements can also help. Wald recommends vitamins C and E, beta carotene, alpha carotene, coenzyme Q10, and antioxidants to protect against stress-induced free radical damage.

Asian Naturopathic Approach

The traditional Eastern approach to fertility depends less on modern technology and more on time-tested knowledge. Dr. Roger Hirsch, a naturopathic physician from California, explains Chinese philosophy and infertility treatments based on this point of view: "We look at making the abdomen happy. This is an aphorism for correcting the digestion, menstruation, and hormones, so that women can conceive. Of course, raising the man's sperm count and sperm motility is important as well, because it is not just the woman who is infertile in an infertility situation. A key to this is the way the blood flows in the pelvic cavity."

Chinese medicine uses acupuncture, massage, heat, or crystals applied at points along the energy pathways, or meridians, to balance the flow of energy in the body. Changing the diet, decreasing emotional tension, and balancing heat and cold will increase the effectiveness of the basic treatment. Thus, acupuncture is more effective when used together with herbs to regulate the menstrual cycle, promote ovulation, and increase general vitality, all of which enhance fertility. Chinese medicine can be combined with assisted reproductive technology to minimize stress and help women tolerate drugs and surgery.

HERBS

"In Chinese medicine," says Dr. Hirsch, "herbs are used to tone renal/adrenal function because reproductive function is related to the kidney and to functions related to the kidney. The actual viability of the eggs for a woman over forty is related to kidney *yang* function."

HERBA EPIMETI—One herb that is very good for kidney *yang* is an aphrodisiac called herba epimeti, which translates as "horny goat weed." The Chinese noticed that goats become sexually active after eating this particular plant. They put the plant into the herbal formula for women who are kidney *yang*–deficient, and they noted that it increased sexual desire.

LUTAIGOU—Lutaigou, the gelatin that comes from boiling the antlers of deer, is used by the Chinese to help women over forty who are trying to extend their egg-producing years. It helps slow down the biological clock.

WORMWOOD—In the European system, we have wormwood, which creates more circulation in the pelvic cavity. The Chinese use this along with daughter seed and fructose litchi, a little red berry.

DONG QUAI AND CORTEX CINNAMOMI—Both of these help the circulation in the pelvic cavity. Cortex cinnamomi is not the cinnamon you put in your mulled cider, but a cinnamon with a very thick bark.

ACUPUNCTURE

In China, acupuncture has been used in the treatment of infertility for centuries. The Chinese look at five principal organ systems—the liver/gallbladder, spleen/stomach, heart/small intestine, lung/large intestine, and kidney/bladder—and use acupuncture to release blockages from these systems so that energy, or *chi*, can move freely. This helps the body return to good health. Promoting fertility is one benefit that can be obtained.

Acupuncture to kidney points releases psychological blocks that interfere with reproduction. Dr. Hirsch uses the treatment to help patients overcome deep-rooted fears connected to sexual abuse and low self-esteem. "In treating self-esteem issues, I work on the heart and kidney points. The acupuncture points that seem extremely valuable for this are Pericardium 5 and 6. If a practitioner is having a problem with understanding whether or not a psychological issue is involved in the infertility, and the patient does not know what the issue is, Pericardium 5 can be needled. If something is holding the person back, that will bring an event or dream to memory, and the patient will understand why she is stuck. In treating self-esteem issues, we may also release stress by needling the Heart 7 point, Heart 9, and sometimes Heart 7 to Heart 5.

"We also address Conception Vessel 17, which is between the breasts. This is a very important place for women because it opens their energy. It also helps relieve liver *chi* congestion or stuckness. Remember, the liver and the liver hormones, both in Chinese and in Western medicine, govern the flow of blood in the pelvic cavity."

Western Naturopathic Approach

Dr. Joseph Pizzorno says that as a naturopath and midwife he saw numerous infertile couples and discovered two causes of the condition that were not generally recognized by the orthodox medical profession: "The first was pituitary insufficiency. The pituitary gland was not secreting enough of the hormones needed to stimulate the ovaries to mature, ripen, and produce a viable ovum. Most of these women had been on birth control pills for long periods of time. Even though they had been off the pills for several years, their pituitary never functioned fully again.

"With these women I did two things. I gave them an herbal concoction using herbs that are commonly used for women's health problems, which are supposed to stimulate proper pituitary functioning. I also gave them raw pituitary gland from an animal. There were surprisingly good results with this treatment. A urine test beforehand measured the level of hormones from the pituitary. If a patient had low hormone levels, I would then use this protocol with them. A surprising number became pregnant once their urinary hormone levels returned to normal.

"The second major cause was pelvic inflammatory disease, where there were infections in the fallopian tubes, the little tubes that go from the uterus to the ovaries. Infections leave scars. Then the ovum cannot penetrate the tube and get into the uterus for fertilization.

"An age-old hydrotherapy procedure, called the sitz bath, helps end this problem. A woman gets two big pots of water. (We use washtubs that are about 3 feet in diameter.) One tub gets filled with hot water (as hot as she can stand it). When a woman sits in it with her arms and legs out of the tub, the water level reaches her umbilicus. The other tub gets filled with ice-cold water. That tub is filled to the point just below the umbilicus. In other words, there is more hot water than cold water. The woman sits in the hot water for five minutes, and then in the cold water for one minute. She alternates back and forth three times.

"The first time a woman does this, she will find it startling. But after a while she will actually start to like it. She does this every day. After a few treatments, she starts getting a discharge. As near as we can make out, this discharge is the body throwing off scar tissue and toxic material in the ovaries. This is a particularly dangerous time for a woman to have intercourse. The ovaries are starting to open up, and there is a high probability of an ectopic pregnancy. The egg will only be able to go partway down the tube since the tube is not yet open enough for it to get all the way into the uterus. We therefore tell women to have no unprotected intercourse for at least three months while doing these treatments every day. Again, a surprising number of them become pregnant."

RESTORING THYROID BALANCE

Even as far back as the 1930s, alleviating low thyroid conditions was found effective against infertility. Dr. Ray Peat says, "To keep thyroid levels up, women should snack frequently and eliminate unsaturated fats. Although unsaturated fats are often touted as beneficial, recent studies show them to inhibit thyroid secretion. More high-quality protein may be needed, especially by women following a weight-loss program or a vegetarian diet. "A daily minimum of 40 grams is recommended. Taking a thyroid supplement for a short period of time can greatly help. "People whose thyroid function is suppressed can benefit from a week or two of thyroid supplementation," Dr. Peat advises. "They don't need to take this indefinitely." (See chapter 33 for more information on thyroid problems.)

NATURAL HYGIENE

Dr. Anthony John Penepent follows the principles of natural hygiene when treating any medical condition: "Over the years, I have seen many wonderful things happen with natural hygiene that would not have been possible with allopathic medicine." Explaining infertility, Dr. Penepent says there are many causes, but that all of them can be treated similarly: "There are many mechanisms that can come into play. You can have basic amenorrhea or failure to ovulate. You can have any variety of hormonal imbalances or fallopian tube obstruction. In 40 percent of the cases it is not the woman's fault, although she may take the blame to save her husband's ego. The man may have a low sperm count, depressed sperm motility, or abnormal sperm morphology. These are all possibilities. Then again, conception may occur, but the egg or ovum may not have sufficient nutrients for the embryo to develop. What happens then is you have unrecognized spontaneous abortions that make it appear as if the woman is infertile, when in actuality she just has a nutritional deficiency.

"In many cases, an infertile woman can conceive and go on to have a successful pregnancy with a minor amount of dietary change. In the case of the fallopian tube obstruction, it may be necessary for her to fast for several days.

I remember one patient, a rabbi's wife, who was childless. Because of their religious beliefs, it was absolutely essential for her to bear children. In her particular case, I put her on a fast for several days and followed that up with a nutritional regimen. She was able to conceive within six months."

CONSUMER ADVOCACY GROUPS

Carla Harkness recommends becoming part of a consumer advocacy group that can provide individuals and couples with support and information. One group, called Resolve, has its national office in Somerville, Massachusetts, and a string of chapters across the country: "Resolve is a great ally that provides literature, referrals, and legal advocacy to the infertile. Chances are, wherever you live, there's a chapter by you."

CHAPTER 20

LUPUS

L upus, or systemic lupus erythematosis, is an autoimmune disorder of the connective tissues that affects eight times more women than men. *Lupus* is the Latin word for "wolf," and *erythema* means "redness." The typical red skin sores caused by the disorder are said to resemble a wolf's bite. Lupus can be mild or life-threatening; it affects 1 out of 130 women between the ages of twenty and forty. Females of African, Native American, and Asian descent develop the condition more frequently than do those of European ancestry.

CAUSES

Lupus occurs when antigen-antibody cell complexes circulating through the body are deposited in various body tissues such as the kidney and skin, causing inflammation. Symptoms may be exacerbated by infections, extreme stress, antibiotics, and certain other drugs. Although the exact cause of this disease is unknown, hormones are believed to aggravate it, particularly estrogen, which is why so many women are affected. According to an article by Anthony di Fabio of the Arthritis Trust of America, which is posted on my website (www.garynull.com), lupus seems to be related to the use of estrogen therapy, indicating that it may be to some extent hormone-dependent.

SYMPTOMS

Initial signs include arthritis, a red "butterfly" rash across the bridge of the nose and on the cheeks, weakness, prolonged and extreme fatigue, and weight loss. There may also be fever over one hundred degrees, light sensitivity, skin sores on the neck, hair loss, chest pain, Raynaud's disease (a constriction of circulation in the extremities that causes fingers to turn white or blue in the cold), joint pain, muscle inflammation, anger, depression, and anemia. If the central nervous system is involved, seizures may occur.

Additional symptoms include mouth or nose ulcers and a nail fungus, which is an outgrowth of infection by *Candida albicans*. Often lupus sufferers have headaches. The characteristic skin sores are raised reddish patches that become scaly and crusted. When they fall off, they leave white scars. If these sores spread to other tissues in the body, tissue wasting may occur.

Lupus may begin abruptly with a fever, or slowly, with infrequent flare-ups. Those whose symptoms appear only in the skin have a better prognosis, while those whose kidneys and brains are affected have a poorer prognosis. In some patients, many different organs—lungs, heart, kidneys—are affected.

CLINICAL EXPERIENCE

Traditional Treatment

Mild cases of lupus are treated with nonsteroidal anti-inflammatory and analgesic drugs such as aspirin, ibuprofen, indomethacin, and sometimes phenylbutazone. Prednisone, a form of cortisone, may be given for arthritis and muscle aches. In severe cases of lupus, steroidal drugs are prescribed for internal and external use. However, long-term use of these medications can damage the liver and weaken the bones. Steroids depress the immune system, leaving the body vulnerable to infection.

For both mild and severe forms of lupus, says Anthony di Fabio, traditional treatments only relieve symptoms; they do not get at its causes.

Natural Therapies

Alternative practitioners have successfully treated lupus with a variety of therapies, generally based on changes in diet and appropriate supplementation.

HERBS AND SUPPLEMENTS

To lessen inflammation, use pycnogenol, cat's claw, black walnut, omega-3 fatty acids, and flaxseed oil. Pau d'arco and aloe vera juice act as blood cleansers. A good nervous system tonic is gotu kola. Colloidal silver is antibacterial, antifungal, and antiarthritic.

According to Dr. Jonathan Wright, a physician and nutritionist from Washington, writing in *Nutrition and Healing*, vitamin B6, up to 500 milligrams three times a day, will help relieve symptoms. People with lupus also need supplementation with hydrochloric acid. He adds, "All lupus patients have food allergies, and will improve when this condition is handled." In addition, over half of women have low levels of DHEA and testosterone and need to take these hormones as supplements.

INTRAVENOUS THERAPIES

According to di Fabio, Dr. Ronald M. Davis of Texas reports success treating lupus patients using EDTA (ethylenediaminae tetracetic acid) chelation therapy with the antioxidant DMSO (dimethyl sulfoxide), and intravenous hydrogen peroxide. Dr. Davis initiates treatment of lupus and other autoimmune diseases by giving antifungal drugs such as metronidazole, since it appears that some antibodies related to autoimmune disease are produced in response to fungal microorganisms found to be present in such diseases.

ACUPUNCTURE

Acupuncturist and massage therapist Gina Michaels of New York City explains that she individualizes her acupuncture treatments according to each patient's unique profile: "The Chinese recognize that there are different kinds of arthritis. One type is from heat and wind, another from cold and damp. Western pharmacopeia treat them all the same, but we make a differentiation according to the symptoms the client is displaying. Then a strategy is formed.

"Each decision an acupuncturist makes looks at the large picture. For example, if the person has a headache, along which meridian is that headache located? Is it the gallbladder channel? The stomach channel? Are they having other symptoms, such as fever or sweat? Is the central nervous system affected? All of this is very, very important in deciding what treatment protocol to choose.

"There are eight meridians formed during conception that go to a very deep constitutional level. Treating these is very useful for illnesses that are systemic or of a much deeper nature."

DIET

The Arthritis Trust of America recommends that women with lupus avoid overeating; minimize intake of cow's milk and beef; eat more green, yellow, and orange vegetables; eat nonfarmed cold-water fish several times a week; avoid alfalfa sprouts and tablets containing L-canavanine sulfate, a substance that can worsen lupus; and avoid taking L-tryptophan, which can exacerbate the autoimmune reaction.

The diet should be high in vegetables and low in grains. Wheat grass is excellent for reducing inflammation. Foods detrimental to healing include peanuts, bread, corn, soybeans, and other foods that can produce fungi and molds. In addition, alcohol, spinach, and carrots may aggravate the condition. Acid-producing foods, such as orange juice, meat, and dairy products, can also be harmful.

FASTING

Di Fabio quotes Dr. Joel Fuhrman, who says, "Having fasted over a thousand patients with various diseases, I can say without hesitation that fasting is very often the only avenue that a patient can use to establish a complete remission.

"This is especially true with autoimmune illnesses such as lupus, where it is almost impossible to shut off the hyperactive immune system with nutritional modifications alone, without total fasting." Fasting, he explains, is not merely a method of detoxifying. "The body clearly has the mechanism to adequately handle the removal of endogenous wastes generated in the fasting state. In fact, fasting has been shown to improve or normalize abnormal liver function." No drugs of any sort should be taken while fasting.

OTHER METHODS

Regular exercise is important, because it helps to keep the joints moving. Lupus can flare up during times of extreme stress. Working at a job one dislikes can be a contributing factor, for example. It is important for people to examine their lives and to create circumstances that promote health and happiness. Aromatherapy may also be beneficial. Essential oils can help calm the emotions and eliminate flare-ups. Rubbing tree oils such as pine and cedar directly onto the joints can diminish swelling. A drop of chamomile, lavender, lilac, or neroli can be placed on the palms and breathed in for relaxation. When there is chest congestion, eucalyptus is excellent for clearing the nasal passages and lungs.

CHAPTER 21

MENOPAUSE

M enopause marks the end of the female reproductive cycle, which typically occurs between the ages of forty-five and fifty but can happen anywhere from forty to sixty, or even earlier as a result of surgery or illness.
Menopause is said to begin when a woman goes through one complete year
without a period. The stage before menopause, called perimenopause, may
last as long as ten years. Many women harbor misconceptions about the nature and effects of menopause. Yet in cultures where menopause is less
feared, symptoms are virtually nonexistent, and in fact menopause is antici-
pated as a rite of passage into a stronger, wiser time of life.

CAUSES

"It is a myth to imagine that the ovaries fail at menopause," says Sherrill Sellman, international seminar leader, psychotherapist, and author of numerous
articles on women's health and of the best-selling book *Hormone Heresy*. "During perimenopause, the ovaries go through a last hurrah. The body is making very high levels of estrogen, trying to kick-start the ovaries so that they
can keep going. There is no winding down, but rather very high levels at this
time, though they tend to fluctuate quite erratically, causing hot flashes.

"Nature produced the ovaries, which are endocrine glands, to keep working throughout a woman's life. There will be a reduction in hormone levels
because during this period she is shifting out of her reproductive nature into
a new stage of life. She does not need to be producing the hormones required for ovulation. At menopause her body shifts just enough so that she is
no longer able to produce eggs, but she is still producing adequate levels of
estrogen to maintain the functions of her body. The two main estrogens are

estradiol and estrone. The estradiol drops only about 15 percent from what it would be during perimenopause, and the estrone drops about 40 to 50 percent. But the body does continue to produce hormones.

"At menopause the outer part of the ovaries, which has been more responsible for producing eggs, begins to shrink because eggs are no longer being created, but the inner part, called the inner stroma, actually gets switched on for the first time. It produces hormones that look after the heart, blood vessels, skin, and libido, protecting the woman's body and her well-being.

"Furthermore, when estrogen production by the ovaries declines, other parts of the body are switched on, such as the adrenals, which help turn body fat into estrogen. So even women who have had hysterectomies, if they are healthy, are able to create enough estrogen to keep themselves vital without needing supplementation."

Sellman adds that progesterone levels do seem to be low at perimenopause, and low progesterone affects a woman more at this stage than does low estrogen. These levels can be assessed through saliva assay tests—which, she asserts, should be the gold standard for assessing hormone levels, not blood assay tests, which are now widely used. "Saliva tests are widely available in the United States and give accurate readings. Blood tests generally show only 1 percent to 9 percent of the hormones circulating in a woman's body, which will lead doctors to think women are deficient. It's this type of misdiagnosis that leads to mistreatment."

SYMPTOMS

One of the first changes perimenopausal women experience is in the frequency of their menstrual cycle. The time between cycles may increase or decrease, or they may skip a month. Usually blood flow is reduced, but women may also experience heavy, irregular bleeding. Other common symptoms associated with menopause are hot flashes, dry skin, mood swings, depression, irritability, vaginal dryness, night sweats, bladder infection, fatigue, and sleep disturbances.

"Many changes appear in perimenopausal women, but the negative ones usually arise from stress, bad diet, pharmaceutical drugs, exhausted adrenal glands, and other things—not from lowered estrogen levels," says Sellman. "I believe, based on my own experience, that the symptoms of menopause—and also those of PMS, which are produced by the same imbalances—are really the result of poor health. When we can correct these imbalances, our hormones automatically go back into balance and we receive all the benefits. Women need to understand that a healthy liver, a healthy digestive system, a healthy adrenal system, and getting the colon working are the factors that contribute to healthy hormone production."

It is well known that there are cultures that do not associate the cessation of menstruation with negative consequences. Sellman explains, "The Japanese, for example, don't have a word for menopause or hot flashes. They look at it as just a transition period, but not one with a significant effect on a woman's life. So the symptoms we are told are inevitable, that all women must endure, are actually symptoms of imbalance. I've found that to be true in my own case. When I notice symptoms appearing, such as night sweats or cramp or fatigue, I get immediate relief when I work with natural healing methods."

CLINICAL EXPERIENCE

Misconceptions about Menopause

According to clinical psychologist Dr. Janice Stefanacci, society expects menopausal women to lose their sex drive, but this does not have to happen. "Many women fear that they are going to lose their passion and sexuality. Really, only a small portion of women who go through menopause have their sex drive adversely affected. For those women who lose their sexual desire or have difficulty becoming and staying aroused, help is available. But most women do not experience sexual arousal problems, and many report feeling more sexual because the risk of pregnancy is gone."

Dr. Linda Ojeda, author of *Menopause Without Medicine*, says many women see menopause as the beginning of the end. "They believe that life is going to be downhill from this point on. They no longer think of themselves as youthful, as able to contribute to society. They fear that their behavior will become erratic, hysterical, and out of control. This is not true. When we reach fifty, we do not turn into raging maniacs, and we are not more susceptible to clinical depression. In some women, however, lowered levels of estrogen, endorphins, and serotonin, substances that affect mood, can create mood swings. Levels can be raised naturally in these women.

"We know that beliefs and attitudes affect the transition. In Asian countries, symptoms are virtually nonexistent. In these countries, menopause is looked at as an important event in a woman's life. She now has more prestige and is viewed as a wise, older woman. Women anticipate this time of life with relish. If you are approaching menopause with fear and trepidation, you need to examine your attitude."

Our medical community has created the belief that menopause is a disease by stressing the need for hormone replacement therapy. In reality, menopause is not a disease but a natural transition that should be dealt with naturally.

Dangers of Hormone Replacement Therapy

"Hormone replacement therapy is based on deceit," asserts Sherrill Sellman. In the 1970s, women turned their backs on supplementation with estrogen alone because it had been found to cause endometrial cancer. So the drug companies came up with hormone replacement therapy (HRT), which used a combination of estrogen and a synthetic progestin such as Provera. They used a synthetic because natural progesterone, which has no toxic side effects, cannot be patented. To sell HRT to women, who were scared of hormones after the revelations of the 1970s, the companies claimed that HRT reduced the risk of a condition most women were unaware of: osteoporosis. In the early 1990s, a new reason for healthy women to take this powerful carcinogenic steroid was introduced. HRT was said to be a way to protect the heart. So doctors began using HRT, originally supposed to be only a short-term treatment for relief of menopausal symptoms, as a long-term treatment to prevent other conditions, conditions that only might occur. A review of the research, however, even that which was used to back the use of HRT initially, has revealed that instead of being beneficial, HRT can actually increase the risk of serious complications and even death. (See chapter 16, Heart Disease, for further discussion of hormone replacement therapy in women with heart problems.)

"The estrogen and synthetic progestin used in HRT are not natural substances, but powerful steroid drugs," Sellman explains. "About 120 risks and side effects are associated with this combination, some of which are life-threatening, including not just heart problems but cancers of the reproductive organs, breast cancer, increased risk of diabetes, asthma, thyroid imbalance, and immune dysfunction."

Progestin also contributes to birth deformities. That is why women on the Pill are told not to get pregnant. It also impairs the liver and the gallbladder, and may contribute to depression and headaches. It promotes increased facial hair, fluid retention, infertility, and miscarriage. A large number of women now have endometriosis, which is at least exacerbated, if not caused, by synthetic estrogens and progestins. Progestin interferes with blood sugar, increasing the risk of diabetes. Progestins are just as dangerous as estrogens in causing a range of serious health problems.

Another important point is that estrogen and progesterone are not just sex hormones. They regulate and influence all the systems of a woman's body, including the digestive, immune, circulatory, and nervous systems. Because tampering with these hormones has grave consequences for a woman's physiological and psychological health, it must be done with great awareness and concern. Instead, what happens is that HRT plays havoc with her physiology.

First off, she gains weight, since taking estrogen leads the body to convert food into fat and store it. This is Nature's way of helping women survive famine. Furthermore, dieting and exercising alone will not take HRT-caused weight off.

Other consequences of estrogen dominance are fibrocystic breasts, depression, mood swings, anger, fluid retention and bloating, fatigue, migraines, and headaches. Estrogen lowers the libido—it does not increase it. There is foggy thinking and memory loss. Fibroids, which are the number-one reason women have hysterectomies, are fed by excess estrogen. There are also aches and pains (fibromyalgia), infertility, miscarriage. Too much estrogen can block the uptake of thyroid hormones, so women develop thyroid problems. Estrogen excess also weakens muscle tone and makes the skin sag.

One of the more serious consequences of a prolonged excess of estrogen, as mentioned, is an increase in cancer. The Boston nurses study, which has been going on for twenty years, has found that women on HRT who have been taking synthetic estrogens and progestins for ten years or more have a 100 percent increased risk of breast cancer. The combination of progestin with estrogen was even more deadly than taking estrogen alone, for progestin, as mentioned, is also carcinogenic, associated with a higher incidence of reproductive cancers: breast, endometrial, and ovarian.

Sellman describes two recent studies, conducted by the American Cancer Society and the National Cancer Institute, which confirmed earlier research linking estrogen and ovarian cancer. "The first study said that women who use estrogen for ten years or more will double their risk of ovarian cancer. And even though a woman may stop using estrogen, the risk will continue for twenty-nine years after she has stopped. The second study said that only four years of use can induce the risk of ovarian cancer.

"Since the 1980s we have known that four years of estrogen use will increase the risk of ovarian cancer by 30 percent. Seven years of use will increase it to 70 percent. These new studies are just reiterating that. But people still say, 'We need more studies.' Women are dying and being maimed by these drugs, and 'We need more studies' is their answer."

With respect to osteoporosis, Dr. Bruce Hedendal of Boca Raton, Florida, comments, "Most people are told that estrogen prevents osteoporosis. This is true to some degree. Around menopause, synthetic estrogen replacement therapy is effective for five to seven years only. It slows down the bone loss, but it does not reverse it in any way, shape, or form. The studies have shown that eight to ten years after menopause is finished, there are no benefits to estrogen replacement therapy on bone loss."

Natural Therapies

Natural therapies can make HRT unnecessary. I completed an eighteen-month study of people who went on a strict program of cleansing and detoxifying, eating no animal proteins, no sugar, no caffeine, no processed food. They exercised 6 days a week for an hour. They drank lots of fresh organic juices, sometimes as much as a gallon a day, and certain herbs.

Three women in that group who had been postmenopausal—one who had been so for eighteen years and had had a hysterectomy—returned to a premenopausal state of health. Skin wrinkles were gone, energy restored, human growth hormone was back, and hormones were balanced. The gray, thinning hair of one seventy-one-year-old woman grew back brown and thick. Another woman had had a low libido, and her mucus membranes had been dry, as was her skin. Her skin and mucus membranes regained moisture, and she enjoyed a level of health and energy that she hadn't experienced for years. Her toenails and fingernails, which had been brittle, yellow, and cracked, became pink and fresh. This was all without medication or any hormone replacement therapy. We just gave her body a chance to rebalance itself; we honored it by not giving it anything that would have led to an imbalance.

DIET

Dr. Jane Guiltinan, a naturopathic physician from Washington, says, "A lot of women don't know that there may be alternatives to estrogen replacement therapy. There are some very good plant sources of estrogens in some of our foods. In fact, you can get significant amounts of plant estrogens. They have been shown in several research studies to improve menopausal symptoms. "The food that has the highest content of estrogen is soy. Soybeans, tofu, tempeh—anything made with soy—will contain plant estrogens. Oats, cashews, almonds, alfalfa, apples, and flaxseeds contain smaller amounts of estrogen. A woman emphasizing those foods in the diet can experience significant decreases in her hot flashes." Studies suggest that too little magnesium in the diet is one cause of hot flashes. Magnesium can be found in whole grains, beans, and soy products.

Sugar, which can cause hot flashes and other menopausal symptoms, should be avoided. Sugar, coffee, and alcohol adversely affect the blood sugar and can disturb the emotions.

Ann Louise Gittelman, author of *Before the Change: Take Charge of Your Perimenopause*, notes that weight gain, a common problem in perimenopausal and menopausal women, can be minimized by eating the right kinds of foods. These foods are incorporated in Gittelman's Changing Diet Plan. "Low-glycemic, or slow-acting, carbohydrates will supply lots of energy for their calories. My favorites are those that are lower on the glycemic index, which is a list of carbohydrates ranked as to how they develop into blood sugar in your system. I like yams rather than white potatoes, and I like whole rye meal rather than wheat. I choose unprocessed carbohydrates that are moderate to low on the index, which also provide high-quality fiber to help eliminate excess estrogen from the system by lowering blood levels of this hormone.

"In addition, a number of fruits and vegetables are particularly high in phytochemicals and phytohormones. These include apples, grapefruits, lemons, pears, peaches, and a wide variety of vegetables that are also high in fiber.

"I have found that a diet with the right amount of proteins, fats, and low-glycemic carbohydrates not only helps regulate sexual hormone production but also helps to balance the hormonal response to food, which I think is critical in keeping blood sugar levels stable. A level blood sugar helps to prevent perimenopausal symptoms such as depression, mood swings, and hot flashes, and it leads to weight loss without any effort.

"Fats are important on the Changing Diet Plan. We need to add essential and beneficial fats, not take them away. These come in the form of the high-lignan flaxseed oil, olive oil, toasted nut seeds, and avocado. These fats stabilize blood sugar levels.

"So we're getting our blood sugar stable, we're assisting in long-term energy, and more importantly, we're providing the raw material for hormones, particularly progesterone, which is the key hormone in perimenopause."

Another natural source of phytohormones is the natural thickening agent kuzu. Several natural-foods recipes incorporate kuzu into sauces in place of flour, making this a way to both enjoy healthy foods and alleviate symptoms.

VITAMINS AND MINERALS

The following nutrients provide an additional boost to good health in the menopausal years:

MULTIVITAMINS—Women need a natural multivitamin/mineral supplement containing higher amounts of magnesium than calcium and high amounts of B and C vitamins. A good multiple vitamin helps build the adrenal glands, which lessens emotional symptoms.

VITAMIN E—This vitamin is known for its ability to rejuvenate the reproductive system and alleviate hot flashes. It also helps lessen vaginal thinning and dryness. Mixed (beta-, delta-, and gamma-) tocopherols are best, as they are found together in nature. D-alpha tocopherol is also preferred over synthetic vitamin E. Generally, 400 units per day should be taken in the beginning. The dosage can be gradually increased to 600 units, although some women may need up to 800 units.

ZINC—This mineral supports ovarian function. A good source is zinc picolinate. It can also be taken as an amino acid chelate or as zinc methionine. The recommended dosage is 25 to 50 milligrams per day.

B COMPLEX—B-complex vitamins are important throughout life, but there is an extra need for these during menopause. They can be obtained from whole grains and green vegetables. B1 and B2 (25 mg/day), B5 (300–400 mg/day) and B6 (150 mg/day), and B12 (1,000 mcg/day) are especially helpful during menopause. Folic acid, 800 micrograms per day, is also recommended.

ESSENTIAL FATTY ACIDS (EFAS)—EFAs, which are precursors to the natural hormones in the body, are very important for both men and women. People on low-fat diets should pay special attention to this. A diet too low in fats can lead to an increased risk of cancer and aging. Omega-6 fatty acids can be found in flaxseed, sesame, pumpkin, and safflower oils. Omega-3 fatty acids are found in fish oil capsules or fish. Both are needed. EFAs help prevent or treat vaginal dryness.

VITAMIN D—The best source of vitamin D is sunlight. It can also be taken in supplementation (400–600 IU/day), although caution should be taken not to get too much of this vitamin. Another source of vitamin D is salmon oil. People living in polluted environments need more vitamin D.

CALCIUM—Calcium is essential to prevent osteoporosis; supplementation should begin before the onset of menopause. There are many forms to choose from. Dairy is a poor source because many people have an intolerance to it. Calcium citrate is easy to digest, as it is already in an acidic medium. Calcium carbonates are alkaline and therefore more difficult to digest. Amino acid chelate is an excellent source of calcium. Calcium lactate is another good source. Calcium gluconate can be made into a powder and mixed into drinks. The recommended dosage is 1,200 to 1,500 milligrams per day.

GAMMA LINOLENIC ACID (GLA)—This is available as evening primrose oil, borage oil, or blackcurrant seed oil; 1,000 milligrams per day is recommended.

BORON—Research shows boron to be a precursor of both female and male hormones. You only need 5 milligrams a day.

SUPPLEMENTS THAT HELP CREATE HORMONES

Sherrill Sellman advocates natural progesterone, which is an identical match to what the body makes, as opposed to the synthetic progestins, such as Provera, which are molecularly altered and thus don't fit exactly with the body's hormone receptors. Instead, these synthetics give instructions that are out of harmony with a woman's physiology. By increasing progesterone levels with natural progesterone, women can eliminate and reverse many of the conditions resulting from estrogen dominance, such as hot flashes, depression, low libido, breast tenderness, fluid retention, and digestive problems. Progesterone helps normalize thyroid function and blood clotting. Progesterone is the hormone that is predominant right after ovulation, and it increases women's libido. Finally, progesterone oxygenates the cells.

PREGNENOLONE—Taking 25 to 30 milligrams a day helps the body create female hormones.

DHEA—Natural DHEA, found in wild yam extract preparations, rejuvenates the body.

PROGESTERONE CREAM OR SERUM—Progesterone is a woman's rejuvenating hormone; it protects against cancer and fibrocystic breasts and increases the beneficial effects of thyroid hormone. In addition, it guards against osteoporosis by putting calcium back into the bones. After menopause, progesterone can be taken three or four weeks out of the month. Wild yam cream contains progesterone and can be purchased over the counter. Natural progesterone can also be taken orally.

ESTRIOL—This natural, friendly estrogen has been shown to inhibit breast tumors in animals. Some gynecologists are beginning to recommend estriol for menopausal women because it is safer and more effective than synthetics.

TRIPLE ESTROGEN—This formula is 80 percent estriol and 20 percent estrone plus estradiol. Estriol affords protection against breast tumors. Together, estrone and estradiol help reduce the risk of osteoporosis and cardiovascular problems. There are no negative side effects.

HERBS

A number of herbs on the market help relieve perimenopausal and menopausal symptoms by restoring the progesterone-estrogen balance. They include alfalfa, black cohosh, blue cohosh, damiana, fennel, licorice root, motherwort, red clover, red raspberry leaves, sarsparilla, and certain forms of wild yam. Flaxseed contains lignan, a phytohormone fiber that removes excess estrogen from the system. This is particularly important, since too much estrogen is believed to fuel breast cancer. Whole flaxseeds can be ground up or can be taken as flaxseed oil.

Vitex, or chaste berry, is commonly referred to as the menopausal herb because it alleviates many symptoms, including hot flashes, vaginal dryness, and mood swings. It works by raising the progesterone level. Ginkgo biloba has been shown to be effective in leveling mood swings.

The Chinese have been using herbs to treat women's problems for five thousand years. Acupuncturist Roberta Certner says that Chinese medicine sees a woman as giving birth to herself at menopause, since she no longer has an obligation to her children. This philosophy thinks in terms of cycles of seven years. When a woman is forty-nine—often the age when menopause begins—it sees her lifespan as half finished. "The next half of the lifespan is for self-growth."

Certner explains that "Chinese medicine is adamant that women should-n't be suffering from night sweats, insomnia, mood changes, and other symptoms, and herbal formulas are good for this purpose. They help to rebalance the energies of the body so that a woman doesn't feel at the mercy of these tremendous moods and powerless over bodily changes."

According to Certner, one virtue of Chinese medicine is gentleness: "People aren't forced to take medications that reduce libido function and that set up terrain for heart conditions. It really addresses the mechanism itself and not just the symptoms. The reason Chinese medicine works is that it goes to the root of the problem. If progesterone is low, you enhance the progesterone, using something like dioscorea or leonorus, whose name itself means 'mother root.'" Many different herbs are available to the practitioner, who chooses the ones to use in a given case according to the nature of the particular person involved. As Certner says, "Chinese medicine doesn't really treat conditions—it treats people."

Important tonic herbs in Chinese medicine include astragalus, dong quai, her shou wu, ginseng, and licorice root.

HOMEOPATHY

The homeopathic remedy chosen should correspond to the symptoms described. According to Ken Korins, a classically trained homeopathic physician in New York City, only one should be used for best results. Sometimes it's a matter of trial and error; if one does not work, another can be tried. Here are some of the remedies Dr. Korins recommends for menopause.

The following remedies are recommended for hot flashes:

LACHESIS—Heat is felt all day long, while cold flashes may be experienced at night. Once the menstrual flow begins, all the symptoms disappear. Symptoms are worse with pressure and heat, and better with the onset of discharges or flows. Increased sexual desire is also associated with a need for Lachesis.

BELLADONNA—There are many hot flashes. The face looks red and feels hot, and there is hot perspiration coming from the face and a pounding, throbbing, congested feeling in the head. Often there is dryness. Condition improves with resting quietly in the dark. Symptoms worsen with light, cold air, and sudden jolts. The emotional state can border on hysteria with rages.

GLONOINE—Hot flashes are focused, with pressure in the head and feelings of congestion. There may be an associated rise in blood pressure at the time of the flashes. Symptoms are worse with heat and better with cold air. Emotionally, there is a fear of death; there is mental agitation.

AMYL NITRATE—Flashes of heat are accompanied by headaches, often associated with anxiety and heart palpitations.

MANGANUM—Hot flashes are associated with nervous system depression. The body does not want to move. Symptoms improve when patient is lying down. Emotional state is peevish and fretful. There is a loss of pleasure in joyful music, but a profound reaction to sad music.

The term *flooding* refers to irregular periods that stop for a while but are very heavy when they return. The following remedies may also help younger women with extremely heavy periods:

CHINA—There is heavy bleeding, with dark, clotted blood, leading to debilitating fatigue. Symptoms get worse with drafts and light pressure, but better with strong pressure and heat. Emotional symptoms are apathy with a strong disposition toward hurting other people's feelings (not the normal state).

SABINA—The period is characterized by heavy, bright red, clotted blood. Expelling the clots is painful, and pain radiates from the sacrum to the pubis. Emotional symptoms are irritability and a dislike for music.

SECALE—Periods are profuse and prolonged. Blood is almost black. Symptoms worsen with heat and improve with cold.

PHOSPHORUS—There is easy, frequent bleeding of bright red blood, often with no clots. The patient is low-spirited, with multiple fears. Also, memory may decrease. Another symptom is constant chilliness.

Remedies for vaginal dryness and thinning include:

SEPIA—The vaginal area is itchy and dry. There is a sense that the uterus is falling out of the vagina. There is also a loss of libido. Symptoms tend to be worse with standing, cold, rest, anything that causes venous congestion. Symptoms are improved with anything that increases venous flow, such as motion. Emotionally, there is an indifference to loved ones, sadness, and a tendency to weep easily.

NATRUM MURIATICUM—Vaginal dryness makes sexual intercourse very painful. Discharges tend to be acrid and burning. There is often a loss of pubic hair. Emotional state is one of depression and irritability, which is worse with consolation. Symptoms also tend to worsen around ten o'clock in the morning.

BRYONIA—Vaginal dryness is accompanied by severe headaches. Any motion is painful and distressing. Condition improves with rest.

NITRIC ACID—Vaginal dryness reaches the point where the mucosa fissures, causing splinterlike sensations in the vaginal area.

EXERCISE

Regular exercise can reduce the frequency and severity of hot flashes. For best results, it is a good idea to begin exercising before menopause begins. Otherwise, exercise may trigger hot flashes. Exercise also alleviates mood swings and depression by naturally raising serotonin and endorphin levels in the brain. The best exercises to engage in are dancing, brisk walking, running, swimming, biking, and tai chi. Additional benefit is derived from cross-training, doing different exercises on different days. This prevents any one part of the body from becoming overdeveloped or overstressed.

AROMATHERAPY

"Aromatherapy is truly holistic because it is a mind-body treatment," states Ann Berwick, author of *Holistic Aromatherapy and Women's Health.* "I think this is part of the secret of its power." Berwick uses essential oils to help alleviate a number of conditions, including hormonal imbalance in women going through menopause. "Cyprus, fennel, and clary sage are believed to have estrogenlike effects. For overall balancing, I recommend that my clients use these oils in a lotion or body oil, and apply it to their body two or three times a day. When women are experiencing hot flashes, I also suggest that they breathe in peppermint or basil on a tissue throughout the day. I find that a great help for most of my clients."

AYURVEDIC MEDICINE

Menopausal women report relief and rejuvenation from Ayurvedic formulas using herbal phytoestrogens and phytoprogesterones. Ayurveda believes that balance is the key to perfect health. It basically determines which mind-body type a person is and helps people choose the type of foods they should eat and the type of exercise that is best for them. (Chapter 8, "Chronic Fatigue Syndrome," discusses some Ayurvedic principles in detail. You can also read *Perfect Health* and *Ageless Body, Timeless Mind* by Deepak Chopra.)

REFLEXOLOGY

Laura Norman, a certified reflexologist from New York City, says, "For menopause, in addition to working the reproductive organs, I would also encourage you to work your thyroid gland, as this will help take over when the ovaries produce less estrogen. This is how to find this point: the base of the toes reflects the neck area where the thyroid is located. Press your thumbs into the base of your toes and thumb-walk across that ridge, particularly in the base of the big toe.

"Another area to massage is the adrenal gland reflex point. You are on the big toe side of the foot. Go about a third of the way down your foot. You are under the ball of the foot, in line with the big toe. If you press your thumb into that area, it will provide energy when you feel fatigued.

"Also, the pituitary gland, which helps all the other glands to work, is located in the center of the big toe. Pressure applied there helps stimulate that area. Both feet should be massaged equally."

CHAPTER 22

MENSTRUAL CRAMPS AND IRREGULAR MENSTRUATION

P ainful and difficult periods are so commonplace in our society that some women have come to think of them as normal. However, they are not normal at all. Many experts feel that the symptoms of menstrual cramps (dysmenorrhea) are related to dietary practices as well as to unresolved emotional difficulties.

CAUSES

What factors may contribute to menstrual cramps? Dr. Pat Gorman, an acupuncturist and educator from New York City, explains: "In addition to toxins found in foods with preservatives, additives, and caffeine, they are due to putrid proteins found in dairy and red meat. These foods contain a lot of hormones that upset the system. In addition, foods fried in heavy oils cause problems and should be cut out immediately by any woman interested in getting rid of dysmenorrhea."

Dr. Gorman adds that the Chinese attribute this condition in part to pent-up anger and frustration: "If you are not happy with your life, if you are angry with people, you must work this out. The liver, which stores blood and prepares it for the period, is also responsible for anger. That's not a Western concept, but with my patients I find that working out anger helps the liver relax. As a result, there is far less of a problem with dysmenorrhea."

Dr. Marjorie Ordene, a gynecologist in Brooklyn, New York, agrees that hormonal and psychological factors cause painful periods and explains the underlying factors: "What causes dysmenorrhea is exaggerated uterine contractions. These contractions are mediated by receptors in the uterine lining that are stimulated by hormonal and psychological factors. Hormonal factors that stimulate the uterine receptors have actually been isolated. They are chemical messengers called prostaglandins. Two things are clear: People with menstrual cramps have an excess of prostaglandins, and there is an imbalance in the types of prostaglandins they produce."

She adds that eating foods we are allergic to can increase prostaglandin production: "For example, many women are sensitive to yeast, and eating baked foods, breads, pastries, and processed fruit juices can cause an increase in prostaglandin production."

CLINICAL EXPERIENCE

Conventional Treatment

Medical doctors often prescribe medications such as ibuprofen to inhibit prostaglandins. While these agents work to relieve menstrual cramps and the accompanying symptoms, problems occur when drugs are taken month after month. The side effects can include gastrointestinal bleeding, decreased blood flow to the kidneys, and leaky gut syndrome, a condition that allows undigested food particles to enter the blood.

Naturopathic Treatment

DIET

Changes in diet can decrease overproduction of prostaglandins and restore normal balance. Cool green foods help reduce hot, stabbing pains and inflammation. It is good to eat foods such as organic grains, legumes, oatmeal, and steamed green vegetables. Deep-sea fish such as salmon, tuna, and mackerel can be included, as well as flaxseed oil. Hot spices should be avoided, along with fried greasy foods, sugar, salt, alcohol, and stimulating foods such as garlic and onions. Foods that produce allergies should be eliminated as well.

Women who have nerve-related menstrual pain can benefit from tofu but should stay away from too many cold raw salads, hot spicy foods, and even white potatoes. Herbalist Letha Hadady suggests this soothing recipe: warm tofu cooked with sweet spices such as pumpkin pie spices and nutmeg. This quiets the nerves and helps a woman feel nurtured and relaxed.

Dr. Anthony Penepent, a physician who practices natural hygiene, helps patients with painful menses by placing them on a strict hygienic regimen: "I put them on a fast a day before the onset of their period. In serious conditions, I might have them fast one day and then prescribe juices or juice blended with salad and fruit for the following days until they complete their menses."

SUPPLEMENTS

Taken throughout the month as a daily supplement, evening primrose oil prevents headaches and blemishes that occur just before the period. Magnesium deficiencies are common and result in the release of prostaglandins that cause spasm and pain. Magnesium citrate is antispasmodic and helps relieve the problem. You can take 300 to 500 milligrams daily and work up to bowel tolerance.

HERBS

The following herbs may help alleviate menstrual problems:

GARDENIA AND PHILODENDRON—These are popular in Chinese medicine and can be obtained by prescription from an herbalist.

CORN SILK TEA—This tea helps get rid of the bloating that comes from too many hormones stored in the blood. Women's Rhythm also eliminates bloating.

XIAO YAO WAN—This is a wonderful remedy that can be purchased at pharmacies in Chinatowns in major cities. It helps digestive processes. Not only does this formula relieve painful periods, it also alleviates anger.

GREEN TEA—Green tea is cooling and satisfying, and has very little caffeine. A pinch of tea can be added to a pot of boiled water, steeped for five minutes, and sipped throughout the day. People experience an energy pickup from the digestion being activated, not from the nerves being stimulated. Green tea helps soothe sharp, stabbing pains.

ALOE VERA JUICE OR GEL—Aloe can eliminate headache, irritability, fever, stabbing pain, blemishes, and bad breath associated with menstrual cramps. Aloe also reduces acid from the stomach and liver and is slightly laxative. Just add to juice, tea, or water.

DANDELION—Dandelion helps break apart impurities in the system. It can be bought as capsules or tea.

SARSAPARILLA—Sarsaparilla helps hot, stabbing pains brought on by inflammation. It is anti-inflammatory, antiseptic, diuretic, and soothing.

VALERIAN—Valerian is a sedative herb that makes a woman feel quieter, more relaxed, and grounded. It is especially good for nervous women who experience insomnia, anxiety, crying jags and emotional upsets, and other nervous problems. Valerian quiets the nerves that go to the uterus.

YUNNAN PAI YAO—This combination of herbs helps reduce heavy bleeding and stabbing pain. Because it increases the circulation, internal bleeding is healed and swelling and pain are reduced.

HOMEOPATHY

Homeopathy was developed in Germany more than two hundred years ago by Dr. Samuel Hahnemann. The word *homeopathy* means "like cures like." The same substances that cause a disease in a healthy individual can heal an ailment in a sick person when they are diluted and given in minute proportions.

Homeopathic physician Dr. Ken Korins explains that the dilution process is what makes homeopathic remedies so safe: "Homeopathy is a vibrational medicine. We are dealing with very subtle energies. Substances are given in extremely small doses that cannot possibly have any toxic effects. In fact, if you were to analyze these substances, you would not find a trace of the original material in the final dilution."

The correct homeopathic remedy is the one that most closely matches the symptoms that manifest themselves. Dr. Korins recommends that dysmenorrhea sufferers choose from among the following:

COLOCYNTHIS—Colocynthis is a frequently indicated remedy that is useful when you have a severe onset of sudden cramps, particularly on the first day of menstruation. Emotionally, intense irritability and anger are associated with the menstrual cramps. A key indication is that you feel better when your knees are pulled up toward the stomach and held with firm pressure.

MAGNESIA PHOSPHORICA—Magnesia phoshorica helps spasmodic cramps with bloating. The key indication for this remedy is that you feel better from warmth. Magnesia phosphorica and Colocynthis help alleviate the symptoms in 85 percent of cases.

PULSATILLA—A key indication for Pulsatilla is variation; the cramps and the flow of bleeding are changeable. The pains themselves are typically cutting and tearing and may be felt in the lower back or kidney region. Generally, you feel worse in warm, stuffy rooms and better in the fresh open air. Emotionally, you tend to be mild, gentle, and weepy when entering the menstrual state and prefer the company of other people to being alone.

VIBURNUM—Viburnum is indicated when the menses are very scanty and often late. In fact, they may last only a few hours. When you get cramps, the flow of blood stops. Cramps tend to radiate to the sacrum and the thighs. You may feel faint or feel like passing out.

CIMICIFUGA—Cimicifuga is indicated for spasmodic, cramping pains. The pain radiates across the pelvis from one thigh to the other. It is often associated with a premenstrual headache. Increased flow results in more pain. Emotionally, you may feel nervous to the point of being scattered and are often somewhat depressed.

CHAMOMILLA—Chamomilla is helpful if you are either hypersensitive or insensitive to pain. Emotionally, you tend to be irritable and contrary. Someone brings you something that you ask for, and then you don't want it. During intense periods, you may become dependent on coffee and other stimulants and sedatives. Another symptom is anger. When you become angry, your symptoms become worse.

AROMATHERAPY

Marjoram, clary sage, and lavender are wonderful analgesics. Eighteen to 20 drops of oil added to a lotion or oil and massaged into the abdomen and lower back will help relieve menstrual pain. Breathing in the cooling fragrances of rose, lavender, or sandalwood can alleviate sharp, stabbing pain.

STRESS MANAGEMENT

Deep abdominal breathing, meditation, tai chi, and other mind-body disciplines can help eliminate frustrations and anger that bring on pain. Additionally, it is helpful to slow down the pace of life from the time of ovulation to the period.

AMENORRHEA AND MENORRHAGIA

Amenorrhea and menorrhagia are medical terms for abnormal blood flow. Amenorrhea refers to the cessation of bleeding or very light and infrequent periods, most often caused by an abnormally functioning hypothalamus, pituitary gland, ovary, or uterus as a result of drugs or surgery that removes the ovaries or uterus. "Bulimics and anorectics also exhibit this pattern," notes Dr. Pat Gorman. "Sometimes this is caused by excessive dieting and overexercise. Not accepting who she is, a woman thinks, 'I've got to make myself thin, beautiful, and perfect.' If this is going on at the end of the cycle, when toxins are being released into the system, the woman is aggravating her body to the point of saying, 'We're not going to give up this blood. We desperately need it. Forget ovulation, forget periods.'"

Dr. Ruth Bar-Shalom and Dr. John Soileau, naturopaths from Alaska, in an article on the website of the American Association of Naturopathic Physicians (www.naturopathic.org), list several other causes of amenorrhea. First, it happens normally after a woman stops using birth control pills, during pregnancy, and during all or most of the breast-feeding period. It is important to establish that pregnancy is not the reason for amenorrhea, since some of the remedies for this condition may harm the woman and her child while she is pregnant or nursing.

Malnutrition, crash diets, obesity, stress, intensive exercising, extreme obesity, abuse of antidepressants and amphetamines, and mental illness are other causes of amenorrhea, say Drs. Bar-Shalom and Soileau. When a young woman of sixteen has not yet begun to develop sexually, when weight fluctuates dramatically, and when amenorrhea is accompanied by severe depression, drug use, or pain, consult a qualified health-care professional.

With menorrhagia the opposite scenario occurs, and there is profuse bleeding. The condition can be debilitating, sometimes bad enough to warrant immediate attention in a hospital's emergency ward. "The Chinese say menorrhagia is caused by excess toxins and heat in the blood from foods containing preservatives, additives, and caffeine, especially coffee. It's like water in your car radiator becoming low," Dr. Gorman says. "The engine will overheat and explode. Alcohol adds more toxicity because it constantly removes water from the blood. As water diminishes, it heats up the blood. When the blood is what we call 'hot,' or fast-moving, it's very hard for the body to hold it in. It can't stop the bleeding."

The emotional profile of a menorrhagic individual is someone who sees herself as a victim. Dr. Gorman explains: "This person feels the need to serve everybody. She does not know how to set boundaries. Whatever anybody wants, they get. She keeps pouring out her energy and pouring out her blood."

Dr. Vicki Hufnagel, a gynecological surgeon and activist for women's health rights, adds that heavy bleeding is often a sign of an underlying problem in the female system, especially when it is accompanied by pain. The problem is frequently because of a hormonal imbalance. "Anything can throw off a cycle," she says, "including emotional stress, insomnia, too much estrogen in the system, or too little light, as in the winter. Other physical problems that can cause menorrhagia are fibroids, polyps, and a malfunctioning thyroid gland."

Before you can restore the blood flow in patients with amenorrhea or menorrhagia, you must discover the reason for the problem. Once the cause is addressed, periods should return to normal.

Asian medicine can diagnose amenorrhea and menorrhagia by examining the skin. Amenorrhea manifests as pale, sallow, slightly yellowish skin from a deep lack of blood and nutrients. Often this is accompanied by a great deal of emotional anxiety. With menorrhagia, the tongue has a red tip and tiny red dots. When the condition is long term, a woman can become anemic.

Clinical Experience

HORMONAL BALANCING FOR MENORRHAGIA

Dr. Hufnagel says that hormonal dysfunctions in women with menorrhagia can be corrected with oral doses of natural progesterone. "Often the creams women use are not adequate because they don't cause a rise in the blood level. We often have to give what we call oral physiological levels of progesterone. I give women natural hormones in a cyclic manner, the way the body should be getting them."

Hormone balancing can also be accomplished through the diet. Fatty diets cause higher levels of estrogen in the system, which in turn can cause menorrhagia. Lean diets and exercising with weights produce more testosterone, which in turn helps balance hormones and put an end to menorrhagia.

DIETARY REMEDIES

Dr. Anthony Penepent says that amenorrhea is one of the easiest conditions to correct. He recommends a diet that includes two green salads daily, using romaine lettuce, fresh lemon juice, olive oil, and some brewer's yeast. You should also include two pieces of fresh fruit and two soft-boiled eggs in the daily menu. When amenorrhea is caused by a thyroid condition, a thyroid supplement is needed. Additionally, if stress is in the picture, the stressful situation must be remedied. For more serious cases, additional dietary intervention is necessary.

Usually, small changes in diet are all that are needed. Dr. Penepent says, "Even if the woman doesn't follow a completely natural hygienic regimen and is not vegetarian, she can still get tremendous results simply by increasing the amount of green leafy vegetables in the diet and providing concentrated nutritional sources, such as eggs and unsalted raw-milk cheese."

Drs. Bar-Shalom and Soileau add that women with amenorrhea need adequate protein, which means eating a number of grams per day equal to half your weight in pounds. They advocate fish and chicken instead of red meat, as well as nuts, seeds, and beans. Second, they advocate eating seaweed of all kinds.

SUPPLEMENTS

Drs. Bar-Shalom and Soileau recommend the following supplements: 400 international units (IU) of vitamin E a day; 25 milligrams of B-complex vitamins a day, 1,000 milligrams of vitamin C twice a day, and 1,200 milligrams of calcium a day.

HERBS

The following herbs are good for amenorrhea, say Drs. Bar-Shalom and Soileau:

GINGER TEA—Drink one to four cups of ginger tea each day (made from powder or grated fresh ginger).

BLAZING STAR, FALSE UNICORN, BLUE COHOSH, CHASTE TREE, AND ANGELICA
—Mix together equal parts of these herbs and steep 1 tablespoon of the mixture in a cup of boiling water for twenty minutes. Drink three cups a day. You can also combine tinctures of these herbs. Drink 1 teaspoon of the mixed tinctures added to 1/4 cup of water three times a day.

The following Chinese herbs have specific effects on the blood and are needed at different times of the monthly cycle. Dr. Gorman recommends working with a health practitioner to create an individual protocol and monitor progress but offers these general guidelines.

At the beginning of the cycle:

DONG QUAI—High in vitamins A, E, and B12, this blood builder can be taken most days of the month, up to the point of menstruation, or just before it begins if there are strong premenstrual symptoms. "You don't want to be building blood if you are having trouble moving that blood," Dr. Gorman warns.

WOMEN'S PRECIOUS—This formula is a tremendous blood builder that is taken for about three weeks after the period ends. Women's Rhythm is then used the following week.

At the end of the cycle:

GARDENIA—Gardenia is taken when the symptoms of premenstrual syndrome (PMS) arise. By moving blood that is stuck, gardenia helps relieve that heavy, bloated feeling.

WOMEN'S RHYTHM—Women's Rhythm helps release a woman's blood. It is usually taken a week before the period to help move toxins out of the organs. (Women's Precious and Women's Rhythm are Ted Kapchik formulas that can be found in some health food stores and ordered directly from Kahn Herbs.)

Can be taken every day:

FLORADIX WITH IRON—This wonderful product is available in most health care stores. Liquid Floradix is superior to the dry form because it contains more live nutrients.

PHYSICAL MEASURES

Drs. Bar-Shalom and Soileau stress the importance of focusing on deep breathing, consciously giving yourself periods of relaxation, and getting sufficient exercise to reduce stress as much as possible. Other suggestions include:

SITZ BATH—Make an infusion of a pound of oatstraw boiled for a half hour in 2 quarts of water and add it to warm bath water. Sit in the water, which should reach your navel, with your feet propped on a chair outside the tub. Cover your top so that you stay warm. Soak like this for ten to fifteen minutes once or twice a week.

CLAY COMPRESS—Sterilize clay by heating it in a low oven for an hour and then grind it and make a paste with water, or use the powdered French healing clay that you can buy in health food stores. Apply the paste to your abdomen, cover with a cloth, and leave until the paste dries.

CASTOR OIL PACK—Put a cloth soaked in castor oil on your abdomen, then cover with plastic and then a dry cloth. Rest for an hour.

HOMEOPATHY

Two homeopathic remedies are good for amenorrhea, according to Drs. Bar-Shalom and Soileau:

NATRUM MURIATICUM is for amenorrhea that occurs after extreme mental strain in women who have trouble expressing emotion. Use the 12c potency.

PULSATILLA is for a woman who misses her periods after stressful and emotional situations. Take it in the 6c potency three times a day for three weeks or until the period begins.

TOXIC SHOCK SYNDROME

Toxic shock syndrome (TSS) is a rare but serious and sometimes fatal disease. The victims tend to be tampon users under the age of thirty, especially those between fifteen and nineteen.

Causes

This sudden and serious disease affects persons with severely compromised immune systems who are poisoned by a strain of bacteria called *Staphylococcus aureus*, phage group I. This type of staph produces a substance called enterotoxin F, which can overpower and destroy a weak body.

Toxic shock syndrome is linked to the introduction of tampons with four new ingredients in the early 1980s. Before then tampons were made primarily of cotton. In the 1980s, though, highly absorbent polyester cellulose, carboxymethyl cellulose, polyacrylate rayon, and viscose rayon came into use. Three of these new ingredients were soon taken off the market; today only one of the new ingredients, viscose rayon, is in use. Today's tampons are either entirely viscose rayon or a blend of cotton and viscose rayon. In addition, the tampons on the market today may contain an assortment of chemicals, including pesticides used in growing cotton, chemicals used in the manufacture of viscose rayon (lye, sodium sulfate, and sodium hydroxide), and dyes (some of which have been considered carcinogenic since the 1950s).

One theory about the cause of TSS is that the vagina is normally an oxygen-free environment that limits the growth of dangerous bacteria. However, air is trapped between the fibers that make up tampons. When that air is inserted in the vagina along with the tampon, the possibility of toxin production increases. Even after the tampon is removed, some of its fibers may remain.

TSS was originally thought to affect only women who wore high-absorbency tampons, but now it is known to affect newborns, children, and men as well. The initial indications can include a high fever, headache, sore throat, diarrhea, nausea, and red skin blotches. These signs can be followed by confusion, low blood pressure, acute kidney failure, abnormal liver function, and even death.

A severe case of TSS is a medical emergency that may necessitate hospitalization. However, there are many natural ways to support the system once a crisis is over for quick recovery and prevention of recurrence.

Clinical Experience

NATUROPATHIC PROTOCOL

Dr. Linda Page, author of *Healthy Healing: An Alternative Healing Reference*, developed a protocol for healing from TSS out of necessity: "I actually came close to death on an operating table from TSS. I had to bring my body back, and I did it herbally. It took a couple of years, and now I can speak from experience."

HERBS

Dr. Page's personal ordeal gave her a great deal of confidence in the power of natural remedies. The following herbs helped her overcome toxicity, restore immunity, and return to health:

GINSENG—Both Panax ginseng and Panax quinquefolius (American ginseng) varieties are general tonics that balance and tone all body systems as well as improving the circulation. Ginseng should not be used when there is a high fever.

CAYENNE AND GINGER—These nervous system stimulants can help the body recover from shock. They can be taken internally or applied to the skin in compresses.

HAWTHORN EXTRACT—Hawthorn speeds up and normalizes the circulation and restores a sense of well-being.

DIET

In addition to herbs, Dr. Page ate supernutritious foods that could be easily digested and quickly utilized by her failing system. These foods included high-potency royal jelly, bee pollen, wheat germ, brewer's yeast, and unsulfured molasses. The addition of green drinks, including chlorella, barley grass, spirulina, and wheatgrass, supplied her with high potencies of vital minerals. "All these go into the body very quickly and help it recover even from a near-death situation," explains Dr. Page. "By going on a program of concentrated nutrients, I was eventually able to create a state of health that was better than before."

PREVENTION

Alternatives to tampons have included sea sponges. However, sea sponges are no longer sold as menstrual products. A 1981 report alleged risks from embedded sand, chemical pollutants, bacteria, and fungi. No additional studies were done, but the U.S. Food and Drug Administration (FDA) halted menstrual-sponge sales. Another alternative is called the Keeper, a rubber cup that sits in the lower vagina. The Keeper may hold an ounce of menstrual blood and should be emptied several times a day. This device does not promote the growth of bacteria in the vagina. However, the Keeper is not widely available. Tampons that are 100 percent cotton and thus present less risk than do modern superabsorbent tampons that may also contain added chemicals are available in many health food and natural goods stores.

CHAPTER 23

MENTAL
HEALTH
CONCERNS

DEPRESSION

Depression is a major health problem that can leave an otherwise healthy woman unable to cope with the even the simplest of everyday situations. It affects nearly 20 million Americans. This does not include the many individuals who function normally for the most part despite frequently finding themselves in low moods. Two-thirds of those who suffer from true depression are never treated and live their lives in misery without being recognized as sufferers of a mental illness. The American Psychiatric Association estimates that 80 percent of depressed people will recover with appropriate diagnosis and treatment.

Types of Depression

Several types of clinical depression have been identified:

MAJOR DEPRESSION interferes with normal, everyday life. It is characterized by sleep disturbances, agitation, appetite and weight changes, feelings of guilt and worthlessness, and an inability to work and concentrate. Suicidal thoughts may occur. These symptoms may last several months or more.

DYSTHYMIA is milder than major depression, but it lasts longer. It prevents people from functioning at their full capacity. Some people with dysthymia also have major depressive episodes.

BIPOLAR DISORDER OR MANIC DEPRESSION, which affects about 1 percent of Americans who are depressed, manifests as serious cycles of depression and mania. In the depressed phase, the person may be sluggish, sad, hopeless, and withdrawn. In the manic phase, the person swings to the opposite extreme: hyperactive, energetic, impatient, easily distracted, and too "busy" to sleep. Most often the changes are gradual, but some people, known as "rapid cyclers," may change moods several times a day. Bipolar disorder is usually chronic and generally begins in the teenage and young adult years.

Causes

BIOCHEMICAL FACTORS

For the past thirty years psychiatry has been aware that certain biochemical changes that take place in the brain can both influence and reflect fluctuations in people's moods. A change in the delicate biochemistry of the brain is capable of governing how a person feels at any given moment. A deficiency in any of the chemicals responsible for maintaining "good moods" may lead to depression, just as a psychologically stressing factor in a person's life may manifest itself in the body by altering the sensitive chemical balance in the brain, also causing depression or low moods.

While psychiatry has recognized this mind-body connection in general terms for the past three decades, it is only in the last ten to fifteen years that it has actually isolated some of the specific brain chemicals involved. Especially important among these chemicals are substances called neurotransmitters, which are released at nerve endings in the brain and allow messages to be relayed throughout the rest of the brain and the body. Perhaps the most commonly known neurotransmitters are the endorphins. They are responsible for pain relief within the body and are thought to be responsible for the "high" that runners experience after exercise.

Mood swings can be traced to a similar mind-body relationship. Scientists have found that a large number of depressed people have significant deficiencies of the neurotransmitters norepinephrine and serotonin. These neurotransmitters belong to a chemical group called the amines, which are responsible for the control of emotions, sleep, pain, and involuntary bodily functions such as digestion. Almost 90 percent of these amines are found deep in the brain; because of their importance, the normally functioning body has developed a recycling system, called reuptake, by which the nerve cell takes back 85 percent of a neurotransmitter for future use once the chemical reaction has been completed. Only the remaining 15 percent is destroyed by enzymes.

The metabolism of the neurotransmitters is intricate, and deficiencies can occur for many reasons. Dr. Priscilla Slagle, a board-certified orthomolecular psychiatrist who practices in southern California, states that age or genetics may cause one person to use up amines more rapidly than someone else. She also points out that a defective receiving cell or reuptake mechanism, or a deficiency of the amino acids, vitamins, and minerals that make up amines may be the culprit here. The nutrient deficiencies involved may result from excessive intake of caffeine, sugar, alcohol, or tobacco. Sugar and coffee can destroy the B vitamins and the minerals magnesium and iron, all of which figure significantly in neurotransmitter formation. Alcohol and tobacco also deplete almost all the B vitamins, vitamin C, zinc, magnesium, manganese, and tyrosine. These nutrients are essential to maintaining a good mood.

STRESS

Stress is another factor that can contribute to depression. Most people tend to associate depression with what are called major stressors, such as the loss of a loved one, being fired from a job, or another circumstance that upsets one's life in a significant way. However, even the stress associated with everyday living can directly deplete the vitamins, minerals, and amino acids that are so important in maintaining a good mood.

Dr. Slagle explains, "We have found very high levels of the hormone cortisol, which is secreted by the adrenal glands, in severely depressed patients. Indeed, scientists have devised a test that measures the levels of this hormone in the body to determine the degree of depression. When people are depressed and highly stressed, their adrenal glands may secrete higher levels of cortisol, triggering certain enzymes in the body that destroy tyrosine and tryptophan. One would think that under extreme stress the body would compensate for this breakdown by facilitating the survival of these important amino acids. Instead, for whatever reason, these amino acids are used up. I believe that high cortisol levels induce depression in certain people."

SIDE EFFECTS OF MEDICATIONS

Dr. Slagle also points out that depression is a common side effect of many prescription medications. The list of medications that can cause depression is quite extensive; it includes antibiotics, antiarthritis pills, antihistamines, blood pressure medication, birth control pills, tranquilizers, and even aspirin. When people are given these medications, they are often not warned that they may experience depression as a side effect. Most orthomolecular psychiatrists believe that drugs for which the *Physician's Desk Reference* (PDR) lists depression as a side effect should include a nutritional program with the prescription in order to replenish the vitamins and amino acids that may be depleted by the medication.

ENVIRONMENTAL FACTORS

It is common for depressed people to have a family history of depression. In addition to the genetic factor, such family histories may also be due to common environmental factors, shared experiences in depressed families, and poor eating habits that are passed on from one generation to the next.

Environmental factors may play multiple roles as causes of depression. For example, being raised in a family in which one or more people are depressed may often be associated with poor nutrition. As Dr. William J. Goldwag reminds us, "Just being exposed to depressed people can be an influence, since children learn how to behave by imitation. Also, family members are eating the same food, and if, for instance, the mother is depressed and is cooking for and serving her family, that food is apt to be sparse in nutrients since she is interested in just getting the meal over with and has difficulty finding enough energy to prepare it."

The children of depressed parents may be abused physically or verbally. As a way of handling abuse, a child may withdraw and become depressed and inactive as a defense against harsh treatment from the parent.

Dr. Doris Rapp, a board-certified pediatric allergist and specialist in environmental medicine, adds that mood disorders often lead to battering of family members and intimates: "Husbands batter wives, wives batter husbands, they both batter the children, and boyfriends batter their girlfriends. Mother battering, I might add, is very common. Many of the children I treat beat, kick, bruise, bite, and pinch their mothers. When some individuals have typical allergies and environmental illness, if they have a mood problem, they can become nasty and irritable and angry. All I ask is, 'What did you eat, touch, and smell?'

"To help find the cause, I try to discover whether the change in behavior occurs inside or outside, after eating, or after smelling a chemical. It might be a food, dust, mold, pollens, or chemicals, which affect not only the brain as a whole but also discrete areas of the brain. As a result, the allergen or food or chemical exposure may make you tired or, if it affects the frontal lobes, make you behave in an inappropriate way. It could affect the speech center of the brain so that you speak too rapidly or unclearly, or stutter, or don't speak intelligently. It's just potluck as to what area of the brain or body will be affected when you are exposed to something to which you are allergic."

MAGNESIUM DEFICIENCY

According to Dr. Lendon Smith, a specialist in nutrition-based therapies and the author of many books on that topic, including *Feed Your Body Right: Understanding Your Individual Body Chemistry for Proper Nutrition Without Guesswork,* craving chocolate may also be a sign of depression. It usually means that people need magnesium, because there's magnesium in chocolate.

"I often had the delightful experience of giving an intravenous mixture of vitamin C, calcium, magnesium, and B vitamins," Dr. Smith says. "Usually it has more magnesium than calcium. Afterward I asked patients whether they would like some chocolate and they told me they didn't need it. It really is connected."

Dr. Smith explains that once food has been processed, magnesium is one of the first minerals to disappear. "Magnesium is also one of the first minerals to leave the body when there is stress, which accounts for how many women behave a day or so before their periods. They feel stressed because they're losing their magnesium.

"We need to supply magnesium to these people. We can determine who needs it by a blood test and by the sense of smell. If people smell a bottle of pure magnesium salt—magnesium chloride is a good one—and it smells good or if there's no smell, then the person needs it. The blood test we usually use is the 24-chem. screen, the standard blood test.

"Many symptoms of depression, hyperactivity, headaches, loss of weight, and other conditions are related to genetic tendencies. If there is a tendency to be depressed in the family, a magnesium deficiency will allow that tendency to show up. If there's alcoholism, diabetes, or obesity in the family, low magnesium may allow those things to show up in a person. There are reasons for all these things, and nutrition is basic. These patients don't have an antidepressant pill deficiency; they usually have a magnesium deficiency."

TOBACCO

Orthomolecular psychiatrist Dr. Abram Hoffer tells the story of a classic case of a misdiagnosis corrected, enabling one man to start anew after his life had seemingly been ruined. "A high school teacher and principal about forty-five years old developed a severe depression. In fact, I believe he was misdiagnosed as a schizophrenic. He exhibited what we call a straightforward, deep-seated, endogenous depression. He was in a mental hospital for about a year or two and was then discharged. He was so depressed that no one could live with him. His wife divorced him and eventually he was living with his aunt, who looked after him as if he were a child. As a last resort, he was referred to me.

"When he came to see me, which was many years ago, I had just started looking into the question of allergies. At that time, I wasn't very familiar with food allergies, but I thought he was a very interesting case and I said to myself, 'He is a classic case of a depression, maybe schizophrenic. He'd be the last person in the world who would respond to this antiallergy approach.' At that time I was using—and I still do—a four-day water fast. This is a way of determining whether or not these allergies are present. He agreed that he would do the fast, which also involved refraining from any smoking or consuming of alcohol; he had to drink about eight glasses of water a day and nothing else. His aunt said she would help make sure he complied. When he came back to see me two weeks later, he and his aunt explained that at the end of the four-day fast, he was normal. All the depression was gone.

"This man then began to get tested for food allergies, and he found that not a single food made him sick. But now he began to smoke again. Within a day after he resumed smoking, he was back in his deep depression. The ironic thing was that he had a brother who was a tobacco company executive, who kept sending him free cartons of cigarettes. When we made the connection to his cigarette smoking, he stopped smoking. Thirty days later, after he had been depressed for four years and hadn't been able to work, he was back in school teaching. I remember this clearly because the insurance company that was paying his monthly pension was so astounded at this dramatic response that it sent one of its agents to see me, to find out what the magic wand was that I had waved to get this patient off their rolls. This is a classic case of an allergy to tobacco that was causing this man's depression."

Clinical Experience

DIAGNOSIS

Traditional psychiatrists diagnose depression according to the criteria set forth in the DSM-IV (*Diagnostic and Statistical Manual of Mental Disorders*, 4th edition), which essentially defines major depression as a condition that includes at least five of the following symptoms during the same two-week period:

1. Depressed mood
2. Markedly diminished interest or pleasure in all or almost all activities
3. Significant weight loss or gain (when not dieting)
4. Insomnia (a constant inability to sleep) or hypersomnia
5. Psychomotor agitation (a hyperanxious state) or retardation
6. Fatigue or loss of energy
7. Feelings of worthlessness or excessive or inappropriate guilt
8. Diminished ability to think or concentrate or indecisiveness
9. Recurrent thoughts of death

While orthomolecular psychiatrists may use this definition as a starting point, they do not confine the diagnosis to these criteria. Orthomolecular psychiatry views depression or any other illness as a unique and individual condition. While there may be certain guidelines, such as those set forth in the DSM-IV, a diagnosis that rigidly adheres to these criteria can arrive at a wrong conclusion either by missing the diagnosis altogether, because the person's symptoms are not those normally associated with depression, or by falsely diagnosing a person as being depressed simply because he or she has the textbook symptoms.

Often a depressed patient is not aware of the condition, especially when it is complicated by associated physical symptoms. If you suffered from chronic back pain, indigestion, or neck stiffness, would you immediately think that you might be manifesting symptoms of depression? Probably not. You might go to several doctors in search of relief, and there would be a very good chance that none of them would ever consider depression as the root of your problem. Even if someone were to ask whether you were depressed, you might quickly protest if, as Dr. Priscilla Slagle puts it, you "have 'somatized,' that is, put [your] emotional feelings into the body, thereby inducing bodily symptoms."

Sometimes a patient may develop responses to medication that are misinterpreted as purely physical. "For example," Dr. Slagle says, "an acquaintance of mine who lost her daughter through death a year ago became so anxious that her doctor started her on tranquilizers. Although she was on tranquilizers for six months, she got worse and worse. When I visited her, it was readily apparent to me that she had severe depression. It was difficult to convince her of this because she could relate only to the anxiety and the insomnia she was having. I started her on a nutrient program, and she improved dramatically in two to three weeks. Of course, I tapered her off the tranquilizers, because if they are stopped abruptly, one can have withdrawal symptoms that can aggravate the anxiety."

TRADITIONAL TREATMENTS

Orthodox treatments for depression range from counseling and psychotherapy to medication and electroshock therapy. However, when a traditional psychiatrist arrives at a diagnosis of depression, more likely than not the next step will be to put the patient on antidepressant medication. Some of the most common of these medications are the selective serotonin reuptake inhibitors (SSRIs) such as Prozac (fluoxetine), Zoloft (sertraline), Paxil (paroxetine), and Luvox (fluvoxamine). They are all designed to increase the concentration of the neurotransmitter serotonin. Other types of antidepressants include the older tricyclics, monoamine oxidase inhibitors, and new inhibitors that act on the brain chemicals norepinephrine and dopamine.

For bipolar disorder, lithium, Depakote (divalproex), and Tegretol (carbamazepine) are used to stabilize moods. If the mania is severe, antipsychotic drugs such as Risperdal (risperidone) may be prescribed. In the depressive phase Wellbutrin (bupropion) and the SSRIs are often used. Some patients receive monoamine oxidase inhibitors or tricyclic antidepressants.

Although the manufacturers claim that there is no evidence of addiction to most of these drugs, they are not without side effects. The *Physician's Desk Reference* (PDR) entry for the monamine oxidase inhibitor Elavil (amitriptyline), for instance, mentions many contraindications, warnings, precautions, and adverse reactions, including severe convulsions and possibly death if this drug is used improperly with other drugs, complications in patients with impaired liver function, hypertension, stroke, disorientation, delusions, hallucinations, excitement, tremors, seizures, blurred vision, dizziness, fatigue, baldness, and elevation and lowering of blood sugar levels.

Because suicidal tendencies are a common characteristic of depression, perhaps one of the most serious problems associated with antidepressants is the potential for drug overdose. The potential for suicide caused by the very medication prescribed to prevent it is further enhanced by the synergistic interaction of antidepressants with alcohol, barbiturates, and other central nervous system depressants. A glance through the PDR indicates that the quantity and magnitude of the dangers associated with Elavil are equally present with the other antidepressants.

ALTERNATIVE THERAPIES

Diet and Nutrition

It is surprising how often diet and nutrition are factors in depression and how effective enhanced or improved nutrition can be in helping someone suffering from depression to improve her mood. According to Dr. William J. Goldwag, "Often the quality of the diet suffers in depressed people. If the depression is profound, the individual doesn't even feel like eating. Depressed people who live alone or who are major providers or cooks in the home may not feel like preparing meals or even shopping. They're apt to restrict their nutrition to fast food or anything just to get eating over with." In many cases, weight loss is a symptom of severe depression. In others, there is substantial weight gain.

Dr. Goldwag notes that significant weight loss is likely to bring about "marked deprivation of the essential nutrients, including the amino acids needed to manufacture the proper proteins, as well as a deficiency in many vitamins and minerals. That in itself can aggravate the depression."

Dr. Goldwag suggests straightforward solutions to at least some of the challenges associated with depression. "There are some simple ways to prepare food in advance so that the food has to be prepared less often. I recommend preparing a raw salad once a week. Certain fresh vegetables keep well for quite a while in a refrigerator. There are a whole variety to choose from: carrots, celery, radishes, cauliflower, broccoli, peppers, red cabbage, green onions, snow peas, string beans. They can all be cut up and mixed together. They can be stored in a plastic bag or sealed container. When mealtime comes, a person can take a handful of these vegetables and then perhaps add some other ones that don't keep as well, such as tomatoes and sprouts. You then have a fresh salad that is already prepared with a lot of important nutrients. This is just one way of having food prepared in advance. It's good for people who are depressed and don't have the energy to make a whole meal."

Dr. Goldwag believes that the B-complex vitamins are especially important. "One of the major groups of vitamins to incorporate is the B-complex family. Years and years ago, when people suffered from severe vitamin deficiencies, some of the resultant diseases, such as pellagra, were characterized by accompanying psychotic reactions. That is, the thinking process was the most obvious one to be affected by the vitamin deficiency. Simply providing the proper vitamin, in this case vitamin B3, or niacin, was the treatment. It cleared up the psychosis.

"There's no doubt that brain function is very dependent on nutrients such niacin and others, because when they're absent there is apt to be some very disturbed thinking. Depression is one of the symptoms that can occur with this."

All of the B complex vitamins are important, but niacin is especially so. As Dr. Goldwag explains, "Niacin is often used in much higher doses than the others to accomplish some of these changes. Niacin is a ubiquitous vitamin. It is being used to improve cholesterol levels, to increase the good cholesterol and reduce the bad. The doses being used are much greater than those used to simply overcome a deficiency."

At the same time, there are plenty of foods that should be avoided. Fast foods can affect mental symptoms by causing blood sugar abnormalities. Women who have tendencies toward hypoglycemia, or low blood sugar, should avoid eating too many simple carbohydrates, such as candy bars, which are converted very rapidly to sugar in the blood. As Dr. Goldwag says, "Simple carbohydrate foods temporarily raise the blood sugar, but then they drop it to a very low level several hours later, resulting in depression. This encourages the individual to repeat the cycle of taking sugar or some simple carbohydrate that's converted to sugar in order to feel that high again. This constant seesaw from a high to a low mood can account for many episodes of depression in individuals."

Both alcoholics and chronic dieters often have depressive tendencies. Alcoholics often suffer from symptoms of low mood. Although alcohol may appear at first as a stimulant and mood enhancer, it is in fact a depressant and substantially decreases the ability of the body to extract nutrients from the food we eat. Dieters tend to eat very few B-complex-containing foods, and they often suffer from depression as well.

Amino Acids: Tyrosine and Tryptophan

A leading authority on the treatment of depression with amino acids and nutritional therapy, Dr. Priscilla Slagle became interested in the treatment of mood disorders as a result of her own depression, which lasted for many years and did not respond to traditional psychoanalysis or psychotherapeutic treatment. Disinclined to use antidepressant medications because of the adverse reactions that so commonly accompany them, Dr. Slagle discovered that "there are natural food substances that will create the same end effects, that is, elevate mood in the same way without causing side effects or toxicity. I started myself on [a program using certain single amino acids to control mood] and achieved very dramatic results. Although I have had tremendous stress over the past ten years, particularly the past year, I have not had one day of a low mood. This has been a marvelous reprieve, since I have had, and therefore understand, the pain that low moods can create for many people."

In her book *The Way Up from Down*, Dr. Slagle outlines a safe and easily implemented program of treatment for depression using amino acids and other precursors required for the production of norepinephrine and serotonin. She is careful to emphasize that people should follow the program under the supervision of a physician. For those already on antidepressant medication, it is not advisable to stop abruptly because of the potential for withdrawal symptoms.

Dr. Slagle explains the basis of the program: "It consists of taking an amino acid called tyrosine, which in the presence of certain B-complex vitamins, minerals, and vitamin C will convert into norepinephrine in the brain. This neurotransmitter not only sustains positive moods but also helps our concentration, learning, memory, drive, ambition, motivation, and other equally important qualities. Additionally, it helps to regulate food and sexual appetite functions. Thus it is a very important chemical. The other amino acid used in the program is tryptophan, which forms serotonin in the brain if the requisite cofactors–the B vitamins, minerals, and vitamin C—are present. In addition to sustaining mood, tryptophan has other functions, such as controlling sleep and levels of aggression. People who are quite aggressive, irritable, or angry are often suffering from a marked deficiency in serotonin. Indeed, very low levels of serotonin have been found in the brain of suicide victims at autopsy.

"With these two amino acids, a good multivitamin-mineral preparation is taken to provide all the nutrients necessary to catalyze or promote the conversion of the amino acids into the neurotransmitters."

Dr. Slagle suggests the following dosages for the two amino acids: about 500 to 3,000 milligrams of tyrosine taken twice daily and about 500 to 2,000 milligrams of tryptophan. Public sale of tryptophan was banned by the Food and Drug Administration in 1990, but the supplement is now available by prescription through most compounding pharmacies. Dr. Slagle recommends that tyrosine be taken first thing in the morning on an empty stomach and then also sometime in the midmorning or midafternoon. Tryptophan, because of its sleep-inducing effects, is taken before bed. Any amino acids used therapeutically must be taken separately from other protein foods, because protein interferes with their utilization. Dr. Slagle also specifies that the amino acids be taken in capsules (tablets can pass through the body undigested) or in the "free form," a preparation in which the amino acids are ready for immediate absorption by the body.

Other Supplements

Other nutrients that can improve mental and emotional states are listed below:

OMEGA-3 FATTY ACIDS—A study from Harvard Medical School published in the May 1999 *Archives of General Psychiatry* found that omega-3 (fish oil-type) fatty acids may be important mood stabilizers. Thirty people with bipolar disorder received either fish oil or a placebo (olive oil) along with their standard medications for four months. Sixty-five percent of those who got the omega-3s improved during this period, compared with only 19 percent of the placebo group. The omega-3s were associated with longer remissions and fewer symptoms.

SAMe—S-adenosyl-l-methionine (SAMe), available commercially in Europe since 1975, recently became available in the United States. The SAMe molecule is a methionine, an amino acid.

ACETYL-L-CARNITINE—This nutrient crosses the blood-brain barrier and provides the brain with more energy. The energy it provides is a gentle, not jittery, type of energy, and it is especially important for older people, who tend to lose brain cells due to a lack of energy. Between 500 and 1,500 milligrams should be taken on an empty stomach.

LIQUID ZINC—Dr. Alexander Schauss, clinical psychologist, certified eating-disorder specialist, and author of *Anorexia & Bulimia*, describes his studies with liquid zinc: "In our eating-disorder studies, we used a multidimensional design and evaluated the affective or mood state of our patients for five years. One of the first things to improve in patients treated with liquid zinc was the degree of depression that they were experiencing based on psychometric instruments such as the Beck Depression Scale, the Profile of Mood Scales, and other indexes of depression. This suggests that we might consider using zinc as an antidepressant. There is a growing concern among many patients, and even therapists, that antidepressant drugs, such as Prozac, may not be safe, and we are looking at viable alternatives. We have discovered this antidepressive effect and have documented it in patients under blind conditions."

PHOSPHATIDYL SERINE—This nutrient is produced by the body but lessens with age. Taking 200 to 500 milligrams improves the ability of brain cell membranes to receive signals and improves their function. That, in turn, can elevate mood levels, help overcome winter depression, and enhance short-term memory.

Herbs

ST. JOHN'S WORT (*Hypericum perforatum*) is an herbal remedy for depression that has become popular in recent years. It contains a number of compounds that have documented biological activity. Studies have shown that it is most effective for mild to moderate depression. Recommended dosage is 300 milligrams three times daily. You'll need to take the herb for about two to three weeks before you feel any real therapeutic effects.

Other plants containing chemicals with antidepressant properties include the following:

> *Pastinaca sativa* (parsnip)
> *Myrciaria dubia* (camu-camu)
> *Malpighia glabra* (acerola)
> *Lactuca sativa* (lettuce)
> *Amaranthus* spp. (pigweed)
> *Portulaca oleracea* (purslane)
> *Nasturtium officinale* (berro)
> *Chenopodium album* (lambs'-quarter)
> *Cichorium endivia* (endive)
> *Spinacia oleracea* (spinach)
> *Brassica chinensis* (Chinese cabbage)
> *Brassica oleracea* (broccoli)
> *Lycopersicon esculentum* (tomato)
> *Avena sativa* (oats)
> *Raphanus sativus* (radish)
> *Anethum graveolens* (dill)
> *Phaseolus vulgaris* (black bean)
> *Cucurbita foetidissima* (buffalo gourd)
> *Corchorus olitorius* (Jew's mallow)

Homeopathy

Homeopathic remedies can be quite effective in lifting depression. Dr. Gennaro Locurcioas, a homeopathic physician, says that while money does not create happiness, the king of remedies for treating depression is gold, also known as Aurum metallicum. Here he describes this and other remedies for treating depression in women; men can benefit as well.

AURUM METALLICUM—Gold is for a perfectionist woman who has set high goals for herself but is unable to meet them. At first she will become irritable, a state that can last for several months. She feels as if she has lost the love of those around her and that it is her fault. This leads to feelings of frustration, accompanied by a strong sense of guilt, which may push her to suicide in extreme cases. Dr. Locurcioas observes, "At first sight, this woman appears perfect and polished. When we start talking to her, we get the idea that there is an abnormal focus on career and achievement. Being a workaholic just covers up the emptiness inside."

ARSENICUM—This remedy is for depression accompanied by anxiety. The woman is restless day and night. She fears being alone and is constantly calling her friends. She wakes up at night and walks around the room thinking about her fears and anxieties. She is afraid of a poverty-filled future and of death. "Arsenicum is from arsenic," says Dr. Locurcioas. "If we give that to a person, the person dies. But giving homeopathic Arsenic to a person is completely safe and better than Xanax."

IGNATIA—This helps depression associated with grief. A woman has lost her child or her mother, or has been disappointed by a romantic relationship. The patient may exhibit physical characteristics such as a tic on the face, numbness, a lump in the throat, and sighing. "According to the homeopathic literature, if the patient says that she gets aggravated when she eats sweets and she improves by traveling, these are signs that Ignatia is indicated," notes Dr. Locurcioas.

SEPIA—Sepia is a good example of how homeopathic healing uses substances that relate to a person's symptoms. According to Dr. Locurcioas, "This remedy is made from a black mollusk that emits a black ink. Black is the ink from which the remedy is prepared, and black is the color the depressed woman sees around herself. She sees black in her future. This little sea creature, at some point in its life, will deposit about three hundred eggs, which are incredibly big for the size of this little animal, and then it will die. This is the housewife who has had a job and has also had to come home and prepare dinner for the husband and children. For years, she has given the best of her energy to her family and children. Now she is forty, forty-five, or fifty. The children are gone, and she feels as if her mission in life is over. She sees no purpose in her life anymore. She does not hate her husband, but feels indifferent toward him. She does not want to be touched sexually, and cries many times during the day without knowing why. Inside she feels despair and isolation. Physically, she has a dull, inexpressive face, and the muscles of the body have lost their tone. The woman has varicose veins; she is constipated. Sepia is a remedy for the exhausted housewife."

Acupuncture

Acupuncture frees blocked energy, and in so doing naturally lifts depression. Look at what one woman has to say about her experience: "When I was in my twenties, just after finishing college, I would go into a depression whenever I was about to get my period. It came on so suddenly that it was frightening. I went to see a doctor about it and was given a referral to an acupuncturist.

"After I was in treatment for six months, my practitioner and I sat down to talk about how I was feeling. I realized then that the depression was gone.

"That was twelve years ago. I've stayed in treatment, although not as regularly as when I first started. It's my primary form of health care. My eating habits and sleeping patterns have become totally regulated. I have been able to lose forty pounds and maintain my weight without dieting. I also quit smoking without ever trying. I never get sick anymore. I never get colds or flus. In general, I'm much more balanced.

"The whole experience of being brought into harmony keeps me from going to extremes. I don't work too hard, I don't play too hard, I don't rest too hard. I manage to stay pretty much in the center of my life. It's a huge improvement. I often wonder how people live without going through a treatment process like I did."

Exercise

Physical exercise is another key to lifting depression, especially when accompanied by a nutritious diet, meditation, and vitamin and mineral supplementation. According to Dr. William J. Goldwag, exercise is one of the most profound aids in the treatment of depression: "One of the major errors in the thinking of patients and therapists is the notion that in order to be active, you have to feel better. This is exactly contrary to our approach.

"We recommend that you do first, and the feeling comes later. In other words, you must do what you have to do regardless of how you feel. This aids in feeling better. You can't wait until you feel good to do something, because in depression that may take days, weeks, months, or even years. You want to accelerate the process."

Dr. Goldwag explains that people who exercise regularly will have days when they just don't feel like doing it. "That's the way depressed people feel about everything. They just don't feel like it. They don't have the energy, the motivation, the stimulation to do even the ordinary things. When it's severe, you may not even have the will or desire to get out of bed in the morning.

"The exercise may consist of very, very simple things, such as just getting out and walking, getting up and doing some simple movements, some mild calisthenics, any kind of physical movement that gets the body in action. For some people just getting out of bed and getting dressed is a big accomplishment. That may be the first step."

Exercise has many benefits. Dr. Goldwag adds, "Even doing a little bit of exercise will make you feel more energized later on. Finishing an exercise routine, even one that's fatiguing, after a brief period of rest will give you a feeling of revitalization, energy, and a psychological feeling of accomplishment. It gives a feeling of 'I've done it. It's completed.'"

Yoga and Meditation

Dr. Michele Galante, a complementary physician in Suffern, New York, overcame depression in adolescence by learning how to center energy with yoga and meditation: "When I was in my late teens, I went through a period of depression where my energy was low. My whole being was unhappy. My parents and others I loved thought I should try seeing a psychiatrist for a while. I went a few times, but that wasn't satisfying to me. I thought nutrition might help, so I started drinking raw vegetable juices and became a vegetarian. I started eating to detoxify myself and to get myself back to feeling stronger again.

"Then I got into meditation and kundalini yoga. I learned about energy centers and started to learn how inner energy flows through the system. I began to sense blockages and to identify emotions and limiting thoughts that were holding me back. Through practice, I was able to center energy into the emotional center in the chest and abdomen, where stabilizing rootedness can occur. That started to awaken inner energies and to strengthen me."

Dr. Galante says that depression is not limited to the mind. "The important thing is to not get too hung up in the head, where we have all these conflicts. Our center is the lower abdomen, where a baby grows in a woman. The Japanese call this the *hara.* In Zen we concentrate the mind and the whole being there. That's the hub of the wheel. The mind can be clearer when you do that, and you don't get hung up living in the realm of thought.

"Set aside ten to twenty minutes daily to quiet the mind, let tensions drain, open up, and resonate with the environment. Everyone does it in a different way. You can do it with meditation or biofeedback. You can do it with music, yoga, a hobby, it doesn't matter what. Anything that takes you to a creative, quiet place and allows you to recharge. Learn to take the time to express your inner needs.

"I like to ask my patients the question, 'Why do we have a physical body?' My answer is always that we exist as a physical entity to carry around our minds and our hearts, in a sense our spirits, so that we can fulfill ourselves. We can then learn and grow and do what we need to do in life. We are nothing without our emotions. Yet we neglect and suppress our feelings. We don't consider nourishing ourselves in a spiritual way. We need some sort of daily practice."

Dr. Galante adds, "We have a lot of outward pressures. We have rules made by corporations that are fulfilling needs for profits and ruining resources. There is a huge lack of wisdom across the board. The only thing that can make you happy is looking inward. Bring your mind and energies inside.

Sometimes, when you start out, all you see is unhappiness and tension. But if you keep at it, sitting down, breathing quietly, not moving, and slowly bringing the mind inside, you will start to feel a sense of peace, relaxation, and buoyancy. That is recharging your battery. That is the most profound thing you can do to bring your energy up."

ANXIETY DISORDERS

Nearly twenty million Americans suffer from anxiety disorders. Traditional medicine seeks to alleviate anxiety by calming the nervous system. Unfortunately, as Dr. John Douillard, Ayurvedic physician and author of *Body, Mind and Sport,* explains, "Giving a sedative in this situation will only suppress symptoms and may deplete the nervous system further, making the situation chronic." Instead of being depleted, "the nervous system must be built up and rejuvenated so that it can put itself to sleep, stabilize its energy and moods, and stay that way."

Causes

Anxiety can have many different causes. Psychiatrist Helen Derosis, author of *Women and Anxiety,* points to external pressures on people who lead busy lives and have never learned to plan properly and set priorities: "Practically everyone I encounter in this country is anxious to some extent. One can be slightly anxious or very anxious, anxious occasionally or continuously. The most devastating type involves being anxious all the time over the little things we have to do everyday. People worry that somehow things will not turn out right for them."

Dr. Derosis continues, "A woman about twenty-five years old came to me who was very bright and educated and was working for a large TV company. She wanted to be a producer, but was only a gofer, though at a very good salary. She was very upset, disappointed, and angry. She would cry to her husband every night when he got home. Yet as soon as she realized it wasn't possible to achieve that goal so quickly and saw that life was not as easy as she thought, she calmed down.

"Earlier, a doctor or psychiatrist would have treated her with Valium and said her problems were not real, all in her head. Remembering those older treatments, a patient will come in today asking for medication, which is not a solution. Getting over anxiety involves growing. If you can keep growing, you will have problems, but the constant activity of being alive, thinking about what you want to do next, and planning how to achieve it will keep you from being bogged down in anxiety."

How Metabolism Affects Anxiety

From the perspective of orthomolecular psychiatry, practically any nutritional deficiency that affects the mind—and almost all do in one way or another—can cause anxiety as a symptom.

A glucose tolerance test is important in determining whether sugar is being properly metabolized. Anxiety attacks can occur when sugar levels get too low, as in hypoglycemia. Hypoglycemia can also cause a rebound effect when adrenaline is secreted to raise blood sugar levels. This adrenaline rush also causes anxiety. Orthomolecular psychiatrist Dr. Michael Lesser checks out sugar tolerance "rather than getting involved immediately in looking for Oedipal or pre-Oedipal fantasies," because in a recent review of his cases he found that 92 percent of people with neuroses had abnormalities in the glucose tolerance test.

Dietary recommendations based on the results of a glucose tolerance test may help a patient far more effectively, quickly, and safely than either psychotherapy or drug treatment will. The main objective is to create stability so that sugar levels neither drop nor rise too sharply or rapidly. For a person with hypoglycemia, a high-protein diet is recommended by Dr. Lesser because it digests very slowly, sending just a small trickle of sugar into the bloodstream so that the blood sugar is kept stable for a long period of time. Then, when the patient eats frequently, the blood sugar remains stable. "I have these patients eat six or seven times a day, small snacks so as not to put on weight," he reports. "Actually, they can handle more calories than they could if they were eating one, two, or three large meals a day because the body is set up to metabolize the small meals frequently. When you have a large meal, you cannot metabolize all that nutrition, and the body turns a portion of that into fat."

THE ROLE OF DIGESTION

Dr. Walt Stoll, a board-certified family practitioner who combines his traditional Western (allopathic) training with holistic healing practices, has found that anxiety disorders are often linked to an inability to completely break down proteins during the digestive process into their amino acids.

"Just three or four amino acids still hooked together (peptides), if they get through the intestinal lining, can stimulate the immune system to make antibodies against them. Since the body is also made up of peptides hooked together to make proteins, these antibodies can attack us. To an antibody, a peptide is a peptide. It frequently doesn't matter whether the peptide came from outside the body or is a part of the body. It is now being found that many of the chronic diseases that are so baffling to the allopathic disease philosophy of conventional Western medicine are related to autoimmune processes.

"In addition, some of these peptides have been found to be identical to certain brain hormones (endorphins) that are associated with panic attacks, depression, manic depression, schizophrenia, and other conditions. In these cases—with more certain to be discovered—there is no need for the immune system to be involved; the effect is direct. The two first examples to be discovered were peptides from imperfectly digested casein (milk protein) and gluten (wheat protein). Of course, these are the two most commonly eaten foods in our culture."

Dr. Stoll usually sees patients after they have tried a number of different therapies. "These patients come with stacks and stacks of records documenting that nothing seems to have worked in spite of every imaginable test having been done and every imaginable treatment having been tried. Psychoactive drugs either have worked poorly or have even caused the problem to worsen because the side effects exceeded the benefits.

"Since every other conceivable cause has been ruled out by the time I get to see them, I am free to look for the things that have not been evaluated. One of the first things I look for is how well the lining of their intestinal tract protects them from their environment. I frequently find that either they don't have the normal bacterial balance in the colon or they have gone beyond that stage to having candidiasis. Candida can escape from our control only if the normal bacteria are not under control. If candida has converted from the yeast form, which is a normal part of the intestinal flora, into the disease-causing fungal form, it further damages the lining so that the leakage of peptides is much greater.

"The greater the amount of peptide leakage, the more likely it is that the brain will interpret these protein particles as being identical to the endorphins it produces during panic attacks, depression, and the like. This leakage is responsible for the increasing sensitivities we see in patients who are sensitive to environmental substances other than foods. In most cases, it is much simpler to correct the leakage than it is to eliminate the substance. But why not do both?"

According to Dr. Stoll, dramatic improvement is often seen once the reason for the leakage is corrected. "The antibodies involved last only for seventy-two hours. Once the leakage is stopped completely, symptoms lessen substantially in just a few days; even a reduction of the leakage helps. There are many patients today who have had that kind of experience. Not everyone's mental symptoms are caused by poorly digested food playing tricks on the brain. However, in my experience it is the most commonly missed diagnosis and one that is relatively easy to resolve."

Clinical Experience

IDENTIFYING CAUSES OF ANXIETY

In Dr. Derosis's plan for reducing anxiety, the first step is to identify one thing that causes anxiety or creates tension, guilt, anger, and so on. One of the main problems in anxiety is that the person cannot discriminate between "distracting and anxiety-producing components" of life.

"For example, one of my patients had a teenage son who was troubling her a great deal. She said her son was coming to the dinner table that summer without any shoes, in his underwear, and with dirty, unkempt hair. She would yell at him, then they would argue, and he would get up and stomp out. Then she'd feel bad because she was kicking him out. In other words, those little details of life. So I asked, 'What is it that bothers you the most?'

"She responded, 'It's his wearing underwear to the dinner table.' Then she added, 'But he does so many things to get me mad.'

"I stopped her and said I wanted only one thing. Then I asked, 'What could you do about that one thing?' This was the second step. Once you have isolated a problem, you have to plan what you are going to do about it.

"I also suggested that she behave in a low-key way, for she had been carrying on just as her son did, and it never got her anywhere. In fact, it made things worse.

"She was able to keep quiet for quite a while and then she thought, 'What if I got him some summer shorts. Maybe he might wear them.'

"So she asked him if he might like them and he said, 'Yes.' She did that, and he wore them all summer. Every once in a while, she would grab them and put them in the washing machine. As a result, their whole relationship changed. But this change involved one of the little details that can make life easy or anxiety-filled."

DIET AND NUTRITIONAL REMEDIES

Orthomolecular treatment of anxiety involves approaches that would rarely be thought of in traditional psychiatry. These include metabolic studies, digestive analyses, diet modifications, and stress-reduction techniques.

Dr. Lesser stresses that good nutrition is also important, since junk foods can spur anxiety. Simple, processed carbohydrates such as white sugar and white flour products may give a quick lift to the a person with hypoglycemia, but this is followed by excessive insulin secretion that drives the blood sugar down again, only to be pumped up once again by an adrenaline rush. This episode leaves a person with cold hands, jitters, anxiety, and panic.

Special nutrients can help alleviate this problem, especially chromium— also called the glucose tolerance factor–which helps normalize blood sugar.

Zinc and the B vitamins, especially thiamine and vitamin B1, are also beneficial. Niacin, has also been identified as an antistress factor. It lowers cholesterol and triglyceride levels, which are increased by anxiety, and affects the brain in ways that are similar to the effects of tranquilizers. Dr. Lesser is convinced of the efficacy of this nutritional approach, but emphasizes the need to be patient when looking for results.

It may take months for the condition to begin to clear because "the body has often been run-down for a number of months or years, and you have to gradually repair all the cells in the body. The old cells have to die off and be replaced by new ones that are better nourished. The natural life span of cells varies throughout the body. Some, such as blood cells, live 120 days, so you cannot really expect sudden, dramatic improvement unless the condition has come on suddenly and you have caught it early."

According to Dr. Allan Spreen, a specialist in nutrition-based medicine, anxiety disorders respond to treatment with certain natural substances. The advantages of treatment with natural substances can be numerous and substantial: by freeing people from having to take more toxic medication, the holistic approach can spare the patient the medication's side effects as well as the extra expense.

"Some amino acids, when given individually," says Dr. Spreen, "can be very effective in calming down the symptoms of anxiety disorders and panic attacks." For example, tryptophan, which has been banned from public sale as a nutritional supplement, "was used as a sleeping agent until there was a problem with some batches of it being contaminated, which caused a syndrome that was related not to the tryptophan but to the contaminant. Some doctors use tyrosine for depression and anxiety. The 'DL' form of phenylalanine is often used on a short-term basis for depression and can be very effective if given correctly. It can lessen anxiety and depression in people by giving them more of an 'up' mood. Phenylalanine is also an appetite suppressant for many people. If they're given correctly, there seems to be no toxicity associated with amino acids, and they're much cheaper than antidepressants or antianxiety prescription medications."

Another nutritional approach is advocated by Dr. Steven Whiting, author of *The Complete Guide to Optimal Wellness*. He argues, "Once we have addressed the question of whether you are eating the proper foods, then you need to take certain supplements."

For Dr. Whiting, key supplements are calcium and magnesium. "We have been told that the B complex is centrally important. Although this is true, the importance of calcium and magnesium should not be underestimated. Remember, at periods of high stress, calcium and magnesium as well as vitamins C, B1, B12, and pantothenic acid are consumed by the body at a phenomenal rate. One recent clinical study showed that up to 1,200 milligrams of pantothenic acid can be consumed in a twenty-four-hour period of severe anxiety. With the recommended dietary intake of those nutrients well below that, we can see it is not sufficient for high-stress periods.

"So in addition to these supplements that are commonly given for stress, calcium and magnesium are probably the best weapons we have because of their action on the central nervous system. I would recommend 800 milligrams of calcium and 400 milligrams of magnesium every four to six hours, as well as at bedtime. By accelerating that, you can create what I designate 'a natural tranquilizer replacement.' While it should be used only for short periods of time, it certainly can be used for three to five days with no side effects whatsoever."

Dr. Whiting also believes in using vitamin and mineral supplementation to replace tranquilizers. He notes, "A combination that I have used successfully to replace such harmful drugs as Valium and Librium goes as follows: calcium at 600 milligrams, magnesium at 400 milligrams, vitamin B6 at 200 milligrams, potassium at 1,600 milligrams, and vitamin B12 at 500 micrograms every four hours under the tongue. This is used every four to six hours. We have had a phenomenal response with this, in terms of removing people's need for these highly habit-forming drugs."

HERBS

A number of herbs have been found to help reduce anxiety. These include:

Piper methysticum (kava kava root)
Scutellaria lateriflora (skullcap)
Valeriana officinalis (valerian)
Eschscholzia (California poppy)
Passiflora incarnata (passionflower)
Matricaria chamomilla (chamomile)
Artemesia vulgaris (mugwort)

STRESS REDUCTION

In addition to dietary modifications and nutritional supplements, anxiety may be ameliorated by relaxation techniques, yoga, massage, exercise, and stress management. An orthomolecular psychiatrist will often suggest these approaches before turning to drugs. Drugs, unlike nutrients or stress-reduction techniques, often become addictive. If you suffer from anxiety and then develop an addiction to drugs that were intended to help that problem, you will only have augmented the agony you were trying to eliminate. In addition, the direct side effects that drugs often have may leave you less capable of living a normal, healthy life than you were when you first underwent treatment.

Orthomolecular psychiatry also puts psychotherapy on the back burner. The shortcoming of psychotherapy, according to Dr. Michael Lesser, "is that most people who suffer from anxiety have only a limited capacity to deal with it through insight psychotherapy. There is a real risk and danger that an individual, by concentrating on her pathology—phobias and anxiety—and by delving deep into her childhood and looking for trauma, will become 'fixed' on the idea of her pathology. Rather than becoming more able and competent, she will become fixed in her neurosis and in some cases will become even more anxious as a result of exploring the so-called unconscious. I have seen many cases—I am not saying this occurs in every case; perhaps I am seeing only the failed cases—of individuals who have been in psychotherapy for four, six, eight, or even twelve years with no apparent improvement. It seems to me that when a case goes on that long, someone should think about the possibility of using another approach."

OBSESSIVE-COMPULSIVE DISORDERS

Obsessive-compulsive disorders affect an estimated six million Americans. They are characterized by repetitive thinking and the inability to control or put a stop to this thinking process. As orthomolecular psychiatrist Dr. José Yaryura-Tobias explains, these thoughts become urges that are so demanding that it appears to the person who has them that they *must* be carried out. Two of the main compulsions are double-checking and hand washing.

Causes

According to Dr. Yaryura-Tobias, "As to why this condition exists at all, we don't have a sure answer to that question. The behavior may result from a learning process that takes hold during childhood…. It may relate to changes in neurotransmitters—the chemical substances in the brain that build bridges between nerve cells so that they can transmit signals from the outside into our system or, in the reverse direction, direct us to act to affect the outside world. The key neurotransmitter that is being studied in this regard is serotonin."

Symptoms

Dr. Yaryura-Tobias talks about some of the peculiar characteristics of obsessive-compulsive behavior: "It usually takes about seven years or so for a patient to come in for a consultation, which tells us that the condition tends to occur gradually, becoming part of the patient's behavioral system in a very, very slow manner. It occurs with equal frequency in males and females. Fifty percent of obsessive-compulsive patients manifest their sickness during childhood or adolescence. Later on—primarily after the age of forty—it fades away, and it becomes very rare after age fifty.

Clinical Experience

CONVENTIONAL TREATMENT

According to Dr. Robert Atkins, there is some common ground here between conventional and alternative medicine. "Both orthodox medicine and complementary medicine, which is the nutrition-based alternative to orthodox medicine, recognize that if a certain neurotransmitter is in short supply, certain syndromes will result. A classic example is that a serotonin-deficient person will often be an obsessive-compulsive. These are the people who can't get out of the house because they've got to make sure the light switches are off or the gas jet isn't on, the people who have to wash their hands twenty times a day, and the people whose desks have to be perfectly neat. These people are serotonin-deficient."

The difference between the conventional and the alternative medical communities lies in how they address the problem. Dr. Atkins describes the conventional approach: "Now there are drugs that block the degradation of serotonin and allow the serotonin level to lift, but those drugs do a lot of other things: They poison a lot of enzyme systems, and that's why so many people got into trouble with Prozac and drugs like that." In addition to Prozac, other drugs used to treat obsessive-compulsive disorders are Anafranil, Luvox, and Paxil.

ALTERNATIVE THERAPIES

To treat obsessive-compulsive disorders, Dr. Yaryura-Tobias uses conventional behavioral therapy and an amino acid approach, along with some other nutrients.

"We basically treat with behavioral therapy. We try to use thought-stopping, exposure (flooding), and response prevention to prevent the brain from repeating the same thought. That is difficult, so we also use cognitive therapy to explain the reasons we think the things we do and try to modify the thoughts."

Behavioral therapy is most effective in dealing with compulsions. Dr. Yaryura-Tobias explains that it's important to expose the patient in some way to her fears. "If you have fears of AIDS or of blood, you are exposed to blood or taken to the hospital where there might be patients with AIDS. Or you will read articles on the condition.

"If it is contamination from dirt the patient is afraid of, we teach that person how to touch objects and not be afraid of them. Then we prevent the patient from washing her hands; in other words, she must remain unclean for a while. I'm talking about patients who, when they are seriously ill, might completely use up one or two bars of soap per day. They might engage in rituals of washing for many hours. They may wash their hands sometimes a hundred or more times a day. Some of these patients will also clean their hands with alcohol or other substances. Sometimes their skin becomes extremely raw. I've seen cases where patients require plastic surgery.

"Overall, the treatment takes about six months. With medication there is improvement up to 60 or 70 percent of the time."

People with obsessive-compulsive and anxiety disorders often improve on the amino acid tryptophan. But, as Dr. Robert Atkins explains, "Since the FDA [Food and Drug Administration] ban on tryptophan, pure tryptophan has not been available in the United States, even by prescription. However, some pharmacies will compound capsules of 5-hydroxytryptophan. This compound is an intermediary between tryptophan and 5-hydroxytryptamine, which is serotonin, the neurotransmitter you are trying to build up. The whole idea of supplying a precursor to build up a neurotransmitter that is in short supply is a fruitful approach to treating psychiatric disorders and should, in my opinion, be considered before the use of nonphysiological psychotropic drugs, which have more potential for toxicity."

Dr. Yaryura-Tobias adds, "My colleagues and I were the first to use tryptophan, and with it we were able to reduce and almost eliminate completely the use of drugs for this condition, and we obtained very good results. We were using between 3,000 and 9,000 milligrams per day.

"Then we used vitamin B6, 100 milligrams, three times a day. Vitamin B6, pyridoxine phosphate, is a vitamin that is very important for the breakdown of tryptophan into serotonin. The idea behind this was that these patients didn't have enough serotonin in their brains or were very dependent on serotonin or that the normal conversion of tryptophan into serotonin was not occurring.

"When we found by measuring that there was a lack of serotonin, this could be reversed by the administration of L-tryptophan with niacin and vitamin B6. Some medications also accomplish this result, but with medications we face many types of side effects.

"About 30 percent of patients do not respond to any form of therapy. But it is not a closed chapter for these patients either. An investigation has to be conducted. Now that we have brain imaging, we are able to visualize the brain. We can measure, for instance, the metabolism of sugar in the brain. We find, for instance, that the frontal and temporal lobes and the basal ganglia, which are related to Parkinson's disease, are disrupted. We see the metabolism of the breakdown of sugar and also images of an abnormal brain. The same can be seen with some electrophysiological measurements of brain wave tests and so forth.

"Interestingly, work has been going on using pure behavioral therapy before and after measuring serotonin. With just behavioral therapy, we were able to modify the levels of serotonin in the body. In other words, we may not need medication to change or challenge the presence of a neurotransmitter such as serotonin. Behavioral techniques alone may have an effect."

ADDICTION

General Considerations

There are a number of alternative approaches to beating addiction, including detoxification and hypnotherapy. Let's start by talking about detoxification, a process whereby the body is cleansed of the toxins created by the addictive substance.

DETOXIFICATION

Dr. Elson Haas is a practicing integrated medical physician and the director of the Preventive Medical Center in San Rafael, California. He is the author of several best-selling books on health and nutrition, including *The Detox Diet*. Dr. Haas describes the best times to detox: "Right now, I'm on day six of my twenty-fifth annual spring cleanse, so I've been doing juices and broth. I usually cleanse in spring. That's one of the best times. Seasonal change times are usually fraught with problems, and a cleanse can help a person. Going into autumn is another good time.

"I live on the West Coast, and even though it's a rainy and lightly cool March day here, back East it's probably colder. Probably a good time out there would be as it warms up into mid-April. Then you can count on a little warmer weather. Because when you do cleansing programs, your body gets a little cooler, so you need to take a little more protection from the cold, and dress warmer. Exercise, keep your body warm and all those things."

Of course, in embarking on a detox program, there are other considerations besides the seasonal. It may be a good idea to begin when you experience congestive problems or are having regular headaches or sluggish intestines. Dr. Haas adds, "Other good times to start are when allergies are kicking up, when blood pressure is getting too high and the cholesterol is rising. Those are times when I, as a physician, would use detoxification as one of my medical treatments. When I see people who have problems of toxicity and congestion, and other things stemming from or related to addictions, I see that detoxification works better therapeutically than almost anything I can do for them. So we have both the time of the year and also the individual time for people when it's appropriate."

Dr. Haas adds, "Anytime you decide to go off any of these substances, you have to get your mind set first. When we are using any of these substances, we are hooked in emotionally. Mentally, we think we need them, and physically, we are slightly dependent on them. This varies with the substance. Nicotine is probably the most addictive, alcohol next, caffeine after that. Sugar is probably the least physically addictive, but emotionally people are really hooked into it."

Types of Programs

Various levels of detoxification can be used. Juice cleanses, dietary changes, drinking more water, getting more exercise and doing steams or saunas may all help in the detoxification process.

Dr. Haas's prescription for the type of detox regimen to follow depends on how advanced the person's level of toxicity is. "If you treat somebody too extremely," he explains, "and she has too much toxicity, then she'll have more symptoms come up and more problems. In any kind of diet change—and the detox diet particularly—there's usually a couple of days of transition during which, as you're starting the diet, you may feel headachy, a cold, irritable. Usually by the third day, you start to click in. It's much like aerobic exercise. The first few minutes are difficult, but as soon as you get into that aerobic state, you think, 'Wow, this feels good. I'm moving forward.'"

Note, however, that people who are pregnant, convalescing from illness, or taking medications, as well as those who have diabetes, hypoglycemia, mental problems, or metabolic imbalances should not undertake any type of cleansing program unsupervised. First they must determine that any proposed supplements or juices are not contraindicated by their medical program. During the program, if the person becomes weak, faint, or dizzy, she should have a protein drink made of high-quality soy- or rice-based protein containing anywhere from 20 to 35 grams of protein. Grains such as brown rice, millet, or barley, beans, or a serving of fish may help while cleansing to maintain blood sugar. Eating these foods does not detract from the cleansing program.

Dr. Haas says detox is broadly helpful. "Anybody," he says, "can benefit from a detox program if it is done in the right way at the right time. That's why I wrote *The Detox Diet*, to show people how they can take very simple steps that most anybody can handle. The detox diet provides nutrition for people with fruits and grains and vegetables, which provide many vitamins and minerals. With this diet, you are being nourished while you are detoxing."

HYPNOTHERAPY

Another health practitioner with experience in dealing with addictions is Michael Ellner, a medical hynotherapist with a private practice at the Chelsea Healing Center and co-author, with Dr. Richard Jamison, of *Quantum Force.*

Ellner begins by explaining that anyone a healer works with is an individual who has her own story about why she does something. Ellner says, for example, that there are many underlying reasons why a person might use food as the addiction of choice. "Some use food to fill up the empty feeling they have. Other people have social issues with eating. Such a person might eat wisely when at home, but in social situations, just to be part of the crowd, may indulge in food that ordinarily would not be appealing. If the person is very active socially, then suddenly it becomes habitual, almost a license to eat junk food.

"Some people use food as a shield. Very often when a relationship ends, a woman puts on ten to fifteen pounds. It provides a cushion, because people are unlikely to hit on her. The woman gets a little bit of space. Very often when she begins to feel better about herself and is ready to go back into the world, it occurs to the woman that it is time to let go of the extra pounds. I can help the person do that very quickly."

Explaining his treatment for addiction, Ellner uses tobacco addiction to illustrate. "To deal with any addiction, I use one of two ways. For people with combined physical and psychological addictions, in the case of cigarettes, for instance, I work as an adjunct to an acupuncturist. She helps the person resolve the physical addiction, while I am working to help resolve the psychological addiction."

The treatment begins when the addict decides she wants a change of behavior. The next step is to develop the self-confidence and self-esteem necessary to move forward, which means stopping the addictive behavior.

"I use hypnotic conditioning to help the person create a shift. The shift would make the desire to be smoke-free much more important to the person than any impulse to smoke. Ordinarily, the impulse to smoke is much stronger. The hypnosis enables the person to make choices rather than responding to preconditioned reflexes."

To some people, the very word *hypnosis* has a stigma attached to it. Ellner comments: "If you ask fifty of the leading experts in the world about what hypnosis is, then you'd probably get fifty different answers. When I use the word *hypnosis*, I'm talking about a way to help a person change neurological patterns. This is done through imagery, metaphor, and the power of suggestion."

Hypnosis is actually a communication tool. "There are a number of practices that are quite popular and are in fact hypnosis, but the practitioners avoid using the word. An example would be guided meditation. Guided imagery and visualization are also forms of hypnosis. Many meditation practices are forms of self-hypnosis. I myself am working very hard to educate the public to understand the word and to appreciate that hypnosis is one of the most powerful self-help tools available."

Ellner's clients who are dealing with smoking addiction often find relief in just one session, especially if they also have some adjunct sessions with an acupuncturist. "These two systems work very well together to help a person stop smoking very quickly and with little or no withdrawal.

"With food issues, it could take between four and eight sessions. There are a lot of additional areas that have to be worked with that involve building self-esteem, building a better self-image, helping a person gain confidence."

For people with alcohol and drug addictions, Ellner tries to get the person involved in another rehab program and to act as an adjunct. "I will recommend different programs for helping a person stop using drugs and stop drinking. Then the hypnosis would take the edge off. It would give the client a higher quality of motivation."

A substance abuser may find that it's not so difficult to stay off drugs in the rehab environment, but going back home is a different story. When the person goes home, all of the things that contributed to the problem in the first place may still be there. Ellner says he could help the person address this hypnotically in such a way as to "create space and disassociate from those triggers that ordinarily lead back to the addiction."

He mentions some triggers that may start a person drinking. "We live in a country where the founding principle is freedom of speech. Yet the greatest phobia in America is public speaking. You'd be amazed at how many people develop drinking problems because they have a drink or two before they have to speak. It becomes a ritual. Very often, it diminishes the quality of whatever they're saying, but they can't appreciate that. The speaker feels helpless without that drink or two.

"The situational triggers produce anxiety and the anxiety says, 'Hey, I need a drink. Maybe I need a drink and a cigarette.' With the hypnosis, the same stimuli can now create a relaxation response. Instead of anxiety overwhelming the person in that situation, suddenly the person feels calm and peaceful. Suddenly, speaking to the people in front of her is as natural as taking a deep breath. The person is in the same situation, but the triggers don't provoke the same response, don't produce the old unwanted behavior. In that respect, in conjunction with a program and a support system, most people can turn these behaviors around rather quickly and dramatically."

Another adjunct to his counseling is nutrition. "When I am working as an adjunct to the acupuncturist, I have the acupuncturist also do nutritional counseling. If I am not working with her, I would refer the client to a nutritionist. One of the more popular programs I recommend is to join one of Gary Null's study groups, which provides peer support and a firm education about nutritional issues and gives people something to do that is a good use of their time. This is very important in making this kind of change."

Ellner speaks passionately about how thought processes can have a negative impact. "To me, the biggest and most dangerous addiction is toxic thinking. People are very often addicted to negative beliefs, negative opinions about themselves and the world they live in. This addiction really diminishes one's quality of life. Instead of having fun, life is always a drag. Very often, that primary addiction gives rise to all the secondary addictions that people put all their time and energy into. One of the first things I do is make people aware of the nature of toxic thinking. Then I help them do a mental detox and change the way they think.

"As part of that I use meditation, creative visualization, and other forms of hypnosis. One of the most engaging forms of hypnosis comes about when a person has some kind of creative pursuit, whether it's strumming a guitar and going into an enhanced state of consciousness, or reading a very exciting book, or taking a walk and having contact with nature. All those things are hypnotic experiences. All those things involve moving from one state of consciousness to another. I encourage a person to get very active in everyday life."

Alcohol Addiction

One out of every thirteen Americans ages twenty-one and older has an addiction to alcohol. Four million American women have alcohol problems, and the number is expected to grow. Surveys conducted in 2000 found that teenage girls are catching up with boys when it comes to binge drinking. Alcoholism can affect all aspects of a woman's life, including health, career, and relationships. According to the National Institute of Alcohol Abuse and Alcoholism, symptoms of alcoholism include a craving for alcohol, loss of control, increased tolerance, and physical dependency.

Excessive drinking of alcohol has serious negative nutritional consequences. "Alcohol doesn't have a lot of nutrients in it," Dr. Haas explains. "People will say wine has a little bit of vitamin C and some nutrients from grapes. Beer has some B vitamins. Yet the levels aren't really that significant. Alcohol is also a diuretic. It causes loss of nutrients through the urine."

Dr. Haas does not espouse teetotaling, however. "When people have a drink here or there and they are eating a healthy diet, it will not cause a problem. In fact, a recent study showed that people who drink wine tend to have a better, more Mediterranean-like diet" and the associated better health, "whereas people who drink beer and other kinds of alcohol tend not to eat as conscientiously."

He adds, "One thing I've seen over the years is that bad habits tend to multiply. People who tend to abuse any substance, whether sugar, alcohol, nicotine, or caffeine, tend to also be less conscientious about how they take care of their bodies. They have other habits that are undermining their health."

Alcohol also irritates the liver, and people who drink more tend to consume more calories. Dr. Haas explains, "Alcohol is a sugar that gets absorbed relatively directly into the body and causes an overstimulation of insulin.

Then you are dealing with problems in the whole sugar metabolism. These heavy drinkers then tend to consume less nutrient-rich foods. They get depleted that way. Those are some of the ways that alcohol endangers the body."

What is the best detox program for getting off alcohol? "For alcohol," Dr. Haas advises, "you want a nutrient-rich program. If you have been taking a lot of alcohol, you will definitely need professional guidance and intervention to help get through the period of withdrawal." Dr. Haas finds that the best daily combination of supplements for getting off alcohol is vitamin B, vitamin C, and a combination of calcium and magnesium, which helps alleviate the agitation that accompanies withdrawal. Chromium is another substance that can help in sugar metabolism. He advises a person to take either chromium picolinate or another form of chromium. "You'll need at least 200 micrograms, which is the way they usually come in capsules. Take these a couple times a day to help with processing the sugar."

Another amino acid that can really help is L-glutamine, which affects brain chemistry. "Remember, a lot of the addictions we have are related to the opiate receptors, which oversee addiction in the brain. L-glutamine seems to help feed the brain the nourishment it needs. It appears to reduce both sugar cravings and alcohol cravings. It's been used successfully in several alcohol clinics for people with more serious problems. The amount of glutamine that people might use is 500 to 1,000 milligrams, two to three times a day. If you have cravings, you can take more. It's safe. I never see problems with it."

Dr. Haas does suggest that "with any amino acid or any B vitamin, you don't want to use one substance for a long time by itself because you can throw the body off balance a little bit. So if you are using the amino acid or B vitamin for more than a few weeks, you may want to use a whole complex."

Orthomolecular psychiatrist Dr. Abram Hoffer has this advice: "For alcoholism the basic treatment starts with Alcoholics Anonymous. Bill W., the co-founder of Alcoholics Anonymous, first showed that when you added niacin to the treatment of alcoholism, you got a major response that you did not see before." Today, there are a large number of very good alcoholism treatment programs in the United States that combine AA's twelve-step approach, various social aids, good nutrition, and the right supplements.

Caffeine Addiction

How can detox help you escape the clutches of caffeine addiction? First, let's make it clear how bad for the body caffeine is and how people come to ignore its negative effects. "If you do something for the first time, such as drink alcohol, smoke a cigarette, or have a cup of coffee," Dr. Haas says, "you will be aware of the irritating, stimulating, or sedating effects of the substance." When people start to use any of these substances regularly, however, they tend to overlook those initial effects. They now have an addiction and take the substance not so much to feel the original sensations as to counteract the withdrawal symptoms."

Caffeine is bad for you, particularly over time. In the short term, it raises your blood pressure. It can also make you hyperagitated, increase anxiety, and affect sleep. Over time, because caffeine is a diuretic, it causes the loss of many minerals, such as calcium, magnesium, and potassium, particularly through the urine. The result of these losses is a more permanent increase in blood pressure. Two other long-term effects of caffeine are to weaken bones and to create mineral deficiencies, both of which can lead to a variety of other problems.

In women, Dr. Haas notes, caffeine seems to increase the incidence of all kinds of cystic problems, such as fibrocystic breast tumors and uterine fibroids. Studies on the relationship between caffeine use and cancer have produced conflicting results. However, a number of studies suggest that caffeine does increase the risk of certain types of cancer. Dr. Haas observes that "most people, when they go off caffeine, will have some secondary effects, usually a headache, at least for twenty-four hours. Sometimes they will feel agitated or fatigued. They are going through a short-term withdrawal. If they have a very large habit, it may last forty-eight hours, but usually it's only twenty-four hours." Dr. Haas says that some people can mitigate the withdrawal headache by taking an over-the-counter aspirin, but he thinks it's better to avoid that chemical medication if possible.

Dr. Haas recommends that you begin a detox diet the day before you start getting off caffeine. You can either go cold turkey or try to reduce your intake so that over a week you get down to maybe half a cup a day or less. If you do it gradually in this way, you will have fewer symptoms. According to Dr. Haas, "Many of the withdrawal symptoms happen because of elimination of acid from the foods and chemicals that we're cutting out.

"Doing the detox diet will reduce the withdrawal. I advise that you take additional nutrients, as follows: 2,000 to 10,000 milligrams of vitamin C from calcium ascorbate, 1,200 milligrams calcium and magnesium from citrate, 400 milligrams potassium, 400 milligrams alpha lypoic acid, 200 milligrams ginkgo, 1,500 milligrams essential fatty acids, a 20-milligram capsule of cayenne pepper, 200 milligrams ginseng, 400 international units (IU) vitamin E, 500 micrograms vitamin B12, and 200 milligrams nonflush niacin.

"Drinking lots of water helps. Also make sure the bowels move. Some people like caffeine because it gets their bowels to move in the morning. It stimulates the intestine's peristaltic activities. For these people caffeine withdrawal may cause constipation. Now, not moving your bowels enough can cause more toxins to back up, and you will feel worse. So it's really important to do what you can about this. Even a day or two after you go off caffeine, you might get something from the natural food store such as laxative tea or laxative tablets or find other means of cleansing the bowels."

Sugar Addiction

Many people may debate whether sugar is addictive in the same way nicotine and alcohol are addictive, but it is definitely a hard habit to break. Dr. Haas notes: "When I talk to people about cleaning up sugar because there are so many books out now recommending lowering sugar intake and mentioning the problems with refined sugar, I find that it is an emotional problem above all. People were trained so early on that sugar is a reward. Sugar is sweet. All the love-talk words involve sugar. You're 'sweet on someone,' the person is your 'honey' or 'sweetie.' Sugar is associated with love and reward. So it's hard to break that emotional pattern."

Yet getting rid of sugar improves health. "When women who have problems with their menstrual cycle, who are irregular, who have pain, who have PMS clean that sugar out of their diets, often within a couple of months they are feeling a lot better, as long as they are taking some other nutrients," says Dr. Haas.

Not only does sugar affect behavior and moods, it is responsible for quite a few health problems. As Dr. Haas tells it, "Although some studies have refuted these findings—studies sponsored by the industry, I might add—researchers have found that sugar causes problems in kids in their focus and behavior. I think it causes increases in candida and parasites. It causes weakness in the digestive tract. Clearly, it's a cause of tooth decay. It has some causal relation to obesity, diabetes, and chronic digestion problems, as well as menstrual irregularities. It also hooks into alcohol abuse."

He has seen psychological problems that he believes had strong roots in the patient's sugar intake. "I've had a number of young women patients who came in. They were on medicine for depression and other low moods. When I interviewed them about their diet, which their psychiatrist never did, it turns out they were drinking a quart of Coke or Pepsi or one of those heavily sweetened beverages a day. So they were getting in the neighborhood of 40 to 50 teaspoons of sugar a day. Those intakes were really influencing their moods. The women whom I've gotten to pay attention to their diets and get off sugar have been able to reduce their medicines and be more stable without these psychoactive drugs."

He echoes a theme that recurs throughout this book: "I think there's a lot to be said about how lifestyle and these habits affect our health and sanity. One of the key overall views is that when people don't feel well, they need to look at their lifestyle first and see if there are factors in the way they are living that may be contributing to their decline. Then they should look at natural remedies. Lastly, I would tell them to turn to medicines, which I still use in my practice because I think that's part of being an integrated doctor. I use any system that I think is going to be of benefit to my patients. Sometimes people do need prescription medicines to help them get out of trouble. If they lived better, however, they wouldn't be getting into that trouble in the first place."

To really eliminate sugar, he encourages people to read labels and work on cleaning up their diet as a whole. He commonly sees people who have some form of yeast infection, or candidiasis. They also have problems with moods, energy, and brain function, secondary to the yeast fermentation process in their intestinal tract, which causes toxins to get into their bodies. A key to recovery for such a person is to eliminate alcohols and sugars to stop feeding the yeast.

"Usually, within three or four days of cutting out the sugar, the person will feel a change. She doesn't have any symptoms in the way she would from alcohol withdrawal, but for the first couple of days she may feel headachy and moody. This will only last a day or two.

"Again, if you drink more water and you take your extra Bs and other supplements, you'll have a smoother transition. Typically, by the third day and definitely within the week, you'll notice smoother and more balanced energy and better brain function."

Dr. Haas is not against sweets per se. Breaking sugar addiction, he says, "doesn't mean we can never eat anything sweet. Fruits are sweet, and they are some of the purest foods we have. Most sweet foods are based on extracts from either grains, such as corn syrups, or from other plants that are naturally sweet. Overall, we just want to balance out the diet."

Food Cravings and Addictions

Jerry Dorsman makes the unusual point that food addictions are harder to kick than drug or alcohol addictions. He's a certified addiction counselor from Oakton, Maryland, and the author of *How to Quit Drinking Without AA* and *How to Quit Drugs for Good*.

"Let me begin by saying that in my clinical experience, it is harder to get people to change their diet than to break an addiction to drugs and alcohol," Dorsman says. "I've seen statistics on this recently that show we have a 30 to 40 percent success rate for people breaking addictions to substances; but there is only about a 5 percent success rate for people who are trying to change diet and get away from bad food habits.

"The reason for this, I think, is that we have deeply ingrained addictions to food. Our body has come to expect certain foods in our diets. We have a metabolic expectation. If we don't get those foods, we begin to crave them. If you take a look at it, we've been eating foods since we've been one year old, whereas, typically, drugs or alcohol aren't started until we are in our teens or early twenties. So they have had a shorter period in which to change the body. I think it's a longer-term, more deeply ingrained pattern that creates the difficulty in changing diet."

To break food addictions, one has to get a handle on cravings. According to Dorsman, "The more balanced we can make our diet, the healthier it becomes. The addiction causes a certain imbalance in the body. The body has to be constantly prepared to metabolize this substance that it's experiencing over and over again. This creates a severe imbalance. Our natural response is to balance it. The place to start is dealing with this physical part of cravings. By changing the diet based on the contractive/expansive as well as the acid/alkaline balances, we can really begin to settle our metabolism and find greater peace based on diet alone. In fact, in my opinion, changing diet is the number-one stress-reduction technique available.

"A second way to handle cravings is to just wait it out. Most cravings, according to scientific studies, last for only about five to ten minutes. Once we know that up front, that particular piece of knowledge can help us beat the cravings. You can think to yourself, 'Hey, I just have a few minutes here to wait this out and manage it.'"

The basic difficulties in resisting cravings—and this applies to any type of addiction, from food to drugs to alcohol—can, in Dorsman's opinion, "be broken into two categories: problems that substance use caused and problems it concealed. The most common problems that substance use causes are the physical problems, because of the biological effects of the drug or alcohol or food on the body, which are very devastating at the cellular level and to the nerve cells. The problems that are concealed are emotional ones. Those are problems that, when a person drank or used drugs or binged on food, tended to go away, because the person could ignore such things as depression, anxiety, and anger. Those emotional difficulties a person ignored when drinking or drugging or bingeing will come back up when the person puts down the addictive substances."

Using Addictions to Battle Depression

If you are taking a substance because you are depressed, your depression may be physiologically induced, perhaps due to some form of brain imbalance. You might have an underactive thyroid, for example, or a blood-sugar imbalance—whether high or low blood sugar. Either of these conditions can be manifested as depression. In order to get away from the chronic feeling of emptiness that frequently accompanies depression, people will start to drink.

One of the reasons people drink is that it takes away the feelings: both the highs and the lows. It gives the drinker a sense of being in a never-never land. The same is true of many drugs. People take drugs because it gives them a euphoria they wouldn't have achieved on their own or that they may have had but could not sustain. So they keep going back to it. Once you get used to that, it's quick and easy to just stick a needle in your arm or put some form of narcotic up your nose. You drink it or ingest it. None of this helps us resolve the underlying conflict, which may be biological, psychological, or a combination of the two.

I have found that the best way to approach this is to get the person into a systematic cleansing program—and there are many—where the person actually breaks all physical addictions, and not just to one thing like sugar, but also every other thing they could be allergic to. That seems to be a major first step. The person's energy comes back. A very big thing about any addiction withdrawal is the lack of energy. So when you substitute for the energy they had been getting from the drug by giving it to the person naturally, through the body's own process of metabolism, the person feels better.

Then you start to rebuild the center of the brain with phosphatidyl serine, 500 milligrams; acetyl L-carnitine, 500 milligrams; phosphatidyl choline, 500 milligrams; and with certain herbs that are known to have an impact, such as feverfew and green tea. Also flood the body with flavonoids. The person should also juice, juice, juice, taking anywhere from four to six glasses of fresh-made organic vegetable juice a day. Within six months to a year, I have seen people who have been totally addicted clear up about 80 percent, stay off, and not come back.

CHAPTER 24

MIGRAINES

Twenty-three million Americans suffer from migraines. One in five women is affected, compared to only one in twenty men, making women four times more susceptible to this widespread health problem.

CAUSES

It is now believed that migraine headaches occur when a sudden dilation of the blood vessels creates pressure on the brain. There are numerous triggers for migraines. Dr. Mary Olsen, a chiropractor from Huntington, New York, who specializes in craniosacral adjustments and applied kinesiology, tells about the eight most common reasons for their occurrence.

Allergic Reactions

Allergies can be dietary or environmental. "Dietary triggers can be foods, food combinations, or additives in foods," Dr. Olsen says. "Alcoholic beverages, particularly red wine and beer, are among the most common causes of migraines. Tyramine, a chemical found in cheese, smoked fish, yogurt, and yeast extracts, may be involved. Monosodium glutamate (MSG), which is found in some preparations of Chinese cuisine and most processed foods, is often implicated, as is sodium nitrate, found in cold cuts and hot dogs. Aspartame, a commonly used artificial sweetener, may lower serotonin levels in the body. Some researchers believe that this contributes to severe headaches. Chocolate and other foods containing caffeine can also be dietary triggers.

In addition, people can have allergies to such common foods as wheat, dairy products, corn, and eggs. A person can also have environmental allergies to toxic fumes emitted from modern products found in the home."

Hormonal Fluctuations

Women suffer from migraines to a much greater extent than do men. Dr. Olsen explains: "Among women who suffer from migraines, approximately 60 percent correlate headaches to their menstrual cycle. The major contributing factor is the hormone estrogen. We know that women who take oral contraceptives are more susceptible to severe migraines and that women experience a lower frequency and severity of headaches after menopause, when there is a sharp reduction of estrogen. Unfortunately, the widespread use of estrogen replacement therapy has resulted in many women having a return of these headaches. Although the exact relationship between migraines and estrogen is unknown at this time, we do know that estrogen affects the central nervous system, including the systems involving serotonin, which can be involved in the development of migraines."

Cranial Faults

"Malposition in cranial bones, or cranial faults, is another factor contributing to migraines," says Dr. Olsen. "Trauma to the head, such as striking the head on a car door or birth trauma, may be enough to lock a bone into a particular position. A whiplash injury may also result in cranial faults."

Meridian Imbalance

Applied kinesiologists and acupuncturists check for a meridian imbalance. "Meridians are twelve bilateral electromagnetic channels of energy in the body identified within the Chinese science of acupuncture," says Dr. Olsen. "Blocked energy, or *chi*, within a meridian causes dysfunction, including migraine headaches."

Upper Cervical Subluxation

Cervical subluxation (partial dislocation) in the upper part of the neck is another common cause of migraine. Dr. Olsen says, "This is especially prevalent among people who use the telephone as a regular part of their work. The tendency to hold the phone between the neck and the shoulder forces the vertebrae in the opposite direction. You also see this with people who tend to read in bed. Propping the head up in one direction causes the vertebrae to shift, which puts stress on the nerves and contributes to the migraine."

Low Magnesium Levels

"A number of studies have noted that many people suffering from migraines have low levels of magnesium in their blood," Dr. Olsen says. "This is also true of people who suffer from fibromyalgia, a myofascial condition that can cause severe pain to the head, mimicking a migraine."

Drugs

Medications may also cause migraines. Dr. Olsen explains: "If you use aspirin, acetaminophen, mixed analgesics, or other acute care medications to get rid of your headaches, you may actually be causing them. The use of these painkillers is the single most common reason for migraines. They are called rebound headaches, and this is why they occur: When you take a painkiller often, the body gets used to having a certain amount of that drug in the bloodstream. When the level falls below that threshold, the body begins to experience withdrawal symptoms. One of these symptoms is a headache. If this situation exists, any preventive treatment for migraine will be undermined."

Stress

Finally, Dr. Olsen cites stress as a factor in migraines: "Although stress is not a cause in itself, it can exacerbate the effects of a headache or cause an increase in the frequency of headaches."

SYMPTOMS

Migraines differ from regular headaches in that they usually occur on one side of the head. They can be accompanied by nausea, vomiting, sensitivity to light and sound, fatigue, weakness, irritability, and vision problems. An aura sometimes precedes a migraine. Usually, this is a visual phenomenon that may appear as flashes of light or visual distortions. However, other sensory systems can be disturbed, causing the aura to manifest as numbness, tingling, odor hallucinations, language difficulties, confusion, or disorientation.

CLINICAL EXPERIENCE

Alternative Treatment Approaches

Although the exact treatment depends on a patient's individual needs, Dr. Olsen suggests general guidelines for treating migraines brought on by different factors. Of course, combination approaches are often indicated as well.

Addressing the Causes of Migraine

FOOD ALLERGIES

As Dr. Olsen explains, "Since migraines don't necessarily follow immediately after ingesting a food, it may be difficult to make a connection between a particular food and the resultant headache. We often have patients keep a food diary to record what is eaten and their physical reactions. That makes it easier to correlate foods with delayed reactions. If we suspect that a particular food is troublesome, the patient is asked to place a sample of that food under the tongue. If there is a sensitivity, a muscle that tested strong previously will weaken. The pulse is also evaluated for such changes as increases in intensity or frequency. Treatment can be as simple as removing the offending food from the diet."

ENVIRONMENTAL ALLERGIES

Dr. Olsen states, "If the migraines appear to be caused by environmental allergies, the British Migraine Association recommends keeping houseplants. Different plants have the ability to absorb different toxins. For example, spider plants absorb the formaldehyde released from particleboard, plywood, synthetic carpeting, and new upholstery, while chrysanthemum protects against the toxic effects of lacquers, varnishes, and glues. If you don't feel like keeping a lot of chrysanthemums around the house, the same effect comes from drinking an herbal tea made with this flower."

HORMONAL IMBALANCE

Dr. Olsen suggests that supplementing the diet with vitamin B6 and evening primrose oil around the time of a woman's menstrual period may help restore hormonal balance enough to forestall migraine attacks.

Cranial Faults

Dr. Olsen says, "Since migraines involve the cranial nerves, patients suffering from migraines should always be examined for cranial faults. These faults are extremely difficult to evaluate, due to the subtle movement of bones, but correcting them can be key to healing.

"One of my patients responded only partially to treatment after we corrected other findings that contributed to her headaches. Although the frequency decreased, she still reported migraines. At first, she had a general examination for cranial faults; there were no positive findings. Finally, after examining every single sutral point (or area of articulation) along the frontal bone in the forehead, we found the problem and corrected it. Her headaches stopped. In this case, the patient had an internally rotated frontal bone. Applied kinesiologists find this to be the most common cause of migraines from a cranial fault. This is particularly true if the patient reports eye pain with the migraine.

"The correction for this is done in three steps. First, pressure is applied to the posterior aspect of the palate on the side of internal rotation. Then light pressure is applied on the lateral pterygoid muscle, located behind the upper molar in the mouth. Next, pressure is applied to the medial pterygoid on the opposite side. That completes the treatment."

Meridian Imbalance

Dr. Olsen states, "The task of the practitioner is to balance the energy by stimulating the meridians. There are various ways of accomplishing this. Acupuncturists use needles, while applied kinesiologists prefer to stimulate the meridians with a finger.

"Three acupressure or acupuncture points are helpful in treating migraines. Lung 7 is located about two finger widths from the crease in the wrist, on the thumb side of the anterior part of the arm. Bladder 67 is found at the nail point of the little toe, and Gallbladder 20 is located between the mastoid and the occipital protuberance in the skull. These points are stimulated in a circular or tapping motion until there is an effective change."

UPPER CERVICAL SUBLUXATION

Dr. Olsen suggests that migraines caused by upper cervical subluxation will cease with chiropractic adjustment to the proper area.

LOW MAGNESIUM

Dr. Olsen says that for migraines caused by low magnesium, "I have found a combination of magnesium and malic acid to be helpful. A health care practitioner should be consulted because the dose varies with each patient."

Medications

Dr. Olsen says that people whose migraines are triggered by medications "must gradually wean themselves away from drugs, with the help of their doctor. When they are no longer dependent on these medications, treatment can begin."

Stress

According to Dr. Olsen, "Studies in England suggest that the herbal remedy feverfew can reduce the frequency of migraines. Feverfew has sedative qualities and can be taken as a tea. One cup per day is usually effective. In addition, relaxation techniques such as meditation, progressive muscle relaxation, and yoga can help to reduce stress. Regular moderate exercise, such as swimming or walking, also lowers tension and creates a psychological sense of well-being."

Dr. Jennifer Brett, of Stratford, Connecticut, also comments on the benefits of feverfew: "An important study reported by the *British Medical Journal* back in 1983 found that one to two capsules of a freeze-dried extract of feverfew would prevent most migraines from occurring."

Supplements

In addition to feverfew, Dr. Brett makes the following recommendations: "When feverfew is taken with magnesium in doses of 250 to 500 milligrams daily, as well as with ginkgo biloba, most people notice a significant reduction in the number of migraines, even to the point of disappearance. This includes people who suffer daily migraines. Many people come to me who have had no success with more conventional treatments. After I start them on feverfew and magnesium, they get a significant reduction in the number of headaches and the severity of pain. Even when they have headaches, they tend to be less frequent and less painful. In my experience, this combination will work for more than 70 percent of migraine sufferers.

"Some people find that they need to add the nutrient niacin. Niacin causes flushing in many people, and it is exactly this flushing that stops the migraine headache. When the blood moves out of the head and into the skin in the form of a flush, the migraine can be aborted before it even starts."

Biofeedback

Using thermal control, a biofeedback technique, people may be able to control migraines by learning to raise their finger temperatures with a digital-temperature device. They learned the technique in the practitioner's office and from manuals and audiotapes at home. Generally people need about two months to learn the technique. It appears to work by increasing blood flow, which is decreased by nervous tension.

Another biofeedback technique places sensors on the temples, over the temporal arteries. People learn to change their pulse rates in order to diminish their migraines.

Other Therapies

A variety of other therapies can help relieve or prevent migraines, says naturopath Dr. Emily Kane, in an article on the website of the American Association of Naturopathic Physicians (www.naturopathic.org). She cautions, however, that people with severe or frequent migraines should first have a physician rule out serious conditions that may be causing their headaches, including diseases that cause seizures, brain tumor, aneurysm of a carotid artery, Meniere's disease (which affects the inner ear), and hemangioma (a tumor composed of new blood vessels).

PHYSICAL MEDICINE

Aerobic exercise, says Dr. Kane, can lessen the frequency of migraines if it is performed regularly, three times a week for a minimum of twenty minutes.

There are many inventive forms of hydrotherapy that involve applying cold to the head and heat to the feet. For example, cold wet packs on the forehead, back of the neck, and head will constrict the blood vessels so that less blood flows into the head. Soaking the feet in a hot footbath in which peppermint and apple cider vinegar are added to the water will bring the blood away from the head and into the feet, and also cool and cleanse the blood. A hot hip bath will also bring the blood away from the head. When the headache is severe, try alternating hot and cold, using towels that are soaked and then wrung out and applied to the face and head. The last application should be cold. You can also alternate hot and cold hip baths.

An enema with cool water may give relief, since migraines are frequently related to wastes remaining in the colon.

HERBS

If you are interested in taking herbs, Dr. Kane recommends that you consult a qualified professional, especially since different herbs are effective for migraines with different causes. Some nontoxic recommendations are as follows: For migraines associated with poor digestion or depression, lavender, which calms the nervous system, can be added to your bath water or rubbed into your temples. Feverfew works for the kind of migraine that is relieved by applications of heat. Eating three leaves a day has been known to prevent migraines. Willow relieves pain and reduces inflammation.

Dr. Kane suggests that the following herbal tea, by cleansing the system, can prevent or decrease migraines:

1 part hops
1 part chamomile

1/2 part oatstraw
1/2 part catnip
1/2 part skullcap
1/4 part peppermint leaf

You can make this formula yourself or order it from Frontier Herbs (800-669-3275). Add a heaping tablespoon to a cup of water that has just boiled and steep for three to five minutes. You can add honey to sweeten. Drink this tea two to three times a day.

DIET

One strategy is to fast for a few days to detoxify the body. A glass of water to which lemon juice and a half teaspoon of baking soda have been added can help eliminate waste in the digestive tract.

Certain foods, says Dr. Kane, tend to promote migraines and should be avoided. These include spicy foods; stimulating foods such as chocolate, tea, and coffee; alcohol; and fried food. Obviously, any food to which you personally have a bad reaction should be avoided.

HOMEOPATHY

Many homeopathic remedies can help relieve migraines; the remedy must be matched to the particular symptoms. Some of those mentioned by Dr. Kane include the following:

ARNICA MONTANA—Arnica montana is for treating migraines that feel as though the head is burning but the rest of the body is cool. There is aching above the eyes that radiates to the temples. Sneezing and coughing cause shooting pains. Arnica is also used for migraines caused by head injuries such as concussion.

LACHESIS—Lachesis is for a severe congestive migraine, usually on the left side, that involves vomiting and loss of sight. There is throbbing and a sense of bursting. The headache is induced by sun (chronic). It is relieved by pressure on the top of the head and gets worse if discharges are suppressed (e.g., with antihistamines).

NATRUM MURIATICUM—Natrum muriaticum (table salt) is particularly effective for chronic headaches that involve intense pain accompanied by a feeling of bursting or of compression, as if in a vice.

NUX VOMICA—Nux vomica relieves migraines associated with stomach, liver, abdominal, and hemorrhoidal conditions. The migraine comes on when the person awakes or gets up, after eating, in the open air, or when the eyes are moved.

PHOSPHORUS—Phosphorus is used to treat congestive migraines in which the head throbs. These headaches are made worse by motion, light, noise, lying down, hunger, and heat; they improve with rest. The person feels cold but likes cold applied to the head.

PULSATILLA—Pulsatilla is used for congestive migraines in which the head throbs and is hot. The headache improves with applications of cold or walking slowly outside. It may be associated with overeating and menstruation.

RHUS TOXICODENDRON—Rhus toxicodendron is used in cases where the person feels intoxicated or stupefied, as though the head were being weighted down. When the person wakes and opens her eyes, a violent migraine comes on. Children may get this type of migraine when they get cold or damp or have wet the bed.

SEPIA—Sepia is used for migraines, especially in women, that are related to nervousness, indigestion, or heartburn, and may be violent or periodic and improve when the person lies quietly. This type is often cured by sleep, by strenuous activity such as dancing, or by long walks outdoors.

SILICA—Silica relieves chronic migraines involving nausea and vomiting that begin at the nape of the neck and move over the crown of the head to the eyes. The headache improves with pressure, lying down, heat, and urination.

THUJA OCCIDENTALIS—Thuja occidentalis is used for the person who feels as though a nail were being driven into the top of the head and who has severe stitches in the area of the left temple and pulsation in both temples. Thuja is effective for severe headaches that follow vaccination.

ACUPRESSURE

Dr. Kane describes acupressure points that can be used to relieve different types of migraines. A point known as Wind Gate is effective for migraines related to the change of seasons. It is actually two points located at the highest point of the neck just below the hairline on either side of the muscles that run up the spine. You can press these points or put two tennis balls in a sock and lie on your back so that the balls press into these two points.

Another point is in the fleshy area between the thumb and forefinger. Squeezing it can reduce migraine pain and also stimulate a bowel movement, which itself often relieves the headache. A point below the bottom of the big toe can relieve migraines that affect the upper part of the face and the eyes.

A PSYCHOLOGICAL APPROACH

Dr. Kane suggests pondering some themes that make connections between migraines and a person's emotional or mental condition. Insight into hidden stresses that manifest physically as migraines may help you release the tensions that lead to the migraine. For example, Dr. Kane explains, some experts believe that migraines represent an attempt to live out one's sexuality through the head. On a physiological level, the pattern of tension manifested as constricted blood vessels releasing into relaxation when the vessels finally dilate and the pain is relieved can be compared to an orgasm. This type of migraine can frequently be relieved by masturbation, although it may require more than one orgasm to bring relief. Dr. Kane notes further that constipation and problems with digestion are often associated with migraines. This indicates a "closed-up" condition in the lower body.

COLORS

Dr. Kane describes the use of color to relieve migraines as well as other ills. You can wear certain colors or use gels placed over lamps or other light sources. The colors most effective during a migraine, she says, are purple and scarlet. Purple increases the ability to tolerate pain and makes a person drowsy when a purple light is shined on the chest, throat, and face. Scarlet can be shined on the face to raise blood pressure, though only for migraines caused by decreased blood flow. For migraines that affect the right side of the head, shine blue on the face or the liver for five minutes.

In between migraine attacks, use lemon (said to dissolve blood clots) and yellow (which works on the lymphatic system and motor nerves) for two weeks. Then use lemon and orange, which act as decongestants, for four weeks. Repeat this pattern for as long a period as required.

REFLEXOLOGY

Applying pressure to the feet can alleviate migraines because specific reflex points correspond to the head area. Reflexologist Gerri Brill says that the greatest benefit comes from a routine that encompasses all body systems. Here she gives a detailed description of her program:

CREATING A COMFORTABLE ENVIRONMENT—"I start off by getting you to feel relaxed. Sometimes I use a foot basin to soften and warm up the feet. Then I have you lie down on my massage table while I explain the anatomy of the foot and the idea that each part corresponds to an area of the body. The big toe relates to the head, and the little toes relate to the head and sinuses. Under the toes is a ridge that corresponds to the neck and shoulders. The chest-lung area corresponds to the ball of the foot. The narrow part is the waist area, and at the heel you have the small and large intestines, the sciatic nerves, and the lower back."

RELAXING BREATHING—"There is a special place on the foot that corresponds to the solar plexus. This is a little notch just below the ball of the foot. The solar plexus is the seat of the emotions. By placing my thumb in this little notch as you inhale and releasing as you exhale, I help you to let go of a lot of stuck feelings held inside. It helps promote relaxation and is good to do at the end of the session as well."

WRINGING THE FOOT—"As you lie down, I wring out your foot three times or so, as if I were wringing out a washcloth. That helps the foot relax."

LUNG PRESS—"This is where I press the fist of my right hand into your chest-lung reflex while holding your foot with my left hand. This area is on the pad of your foot, directly beneath the ridge of the toes. As I press, I slowly bring the flat of my fist down to the heel. I repeat this action three times. It is another relaxation technique."

FOOT-AND-TOE BOOGIE—"Next I do what is called the foot boogie. That means rocking your foot back and forth to loosen it up. Then I do the same with your toes. I place my hands around each toe as I shake your toes back and forth. It sounds silly, but it feels great."

ZONE WALKING—"Zone walking is performed with the outer aspect of the thumb. If you place your thumb on your lap, it is the area that rests on your lap. It's important to keep the fingernails short to avoid digging into anyone. Using the outer aspect of my thumb, I start way down at the heel. I mentally divide the foot into five zones, with each zone leading to a different toe. Starting at the outside portion of the foot, the fleshier part, I bend the working thumb at a 45-degree angle and apply pressure as I creep up the foot ever so slightly. Each move is no more than a sixteenth of an inch. There are a lot of nerve endings in the feet, and I want to hit all of them. Applying steady pressure, I work my thumb upward all the way to the tip of the toe. When I reach the top of the toes, I go back down to the heel again to repeat the process. These steps are repeated for all five zones. By covering the whole body in this way, I help to create an equilibrium."

SPINE REFLEX—"Now I am at the inside aspect of the foot. That's the spine reflex, and it is very important because the spine supports you and holds you erect. I start at the bottom by your heel with my thumb. Again, I work with the outside corner of my thumb held at a 45-degree angle and walk up your spine. I go all the way up to the big toe. Then I turn around and thumb-walk down, using little steps and steady pressure. I don't want to hurt you, but I do want to exert a good amount of pressure since this is pressure therapy."

SHOULDER AND NECK REFLEX—"Now I move to the ridge underneath the toes. This corresponds to the neck and shoulder line, and it is important for headache relief because when people have tension and headaches, their neck and shoulders are usually tense. Again, I use the thumb-walk. I start at the outside of the big toe and thumb-walk to the ridge. I bend the toes back slightly to get inside. This is repeated until I get to the little toe. Then I turn around and thumb-walk back."

HEAD AREA—"The big toe relates to the head, so of course I want to work this area. I place the fingers of my right hand over my left hand and thumb-walk down the fleshy part of the big toe. I divide the big toe into five zones and work down each area using very, very tiny bites or steps. My aim is for twenty-five bites on that big toe. That covers the whole area. I do that five times. This is very important."

BRAIN REFLEX—"Rolling my index finger over the top of the big toe stimulates the brain and relieves aches caused by migraines. Often this area feels sensitive because of crystal deposits that accumulate. These deposits need to be broken up."

HEAD AND SINUSES—"After finishing the big toe, I move to the little toes. Again, using my thumb, I divide each toe into three zones and thumb-walk, using little bites. This is repeated three times on each toe. This is another place where I feel tiny grains of sand. Breaking them up is the main way to relieve migraines."

CLOSING THE SESSION—"Just to make the session complete, I go back to the top of the foot while supporting the heel with the fist. I finger-walk with the right hand between the little bones on the top of the feet. This area helps the lymphatics, chest, breast, and part of the back. Massaging here helps you to achieve a state of balance. Then I work around the ankle areas. The ankles relate to the reproductive organs and alleviate headaches caused by PMS. That's just one foot. Now I wrap up the foot that was worked on and start over on the other side. Afterward, I massage both feet at the same time, which is very soothing. At this point, you know that the session is coming to an end. Once again, I massage your solar plexus area and have you take a deep breath. Finally, I do a nerve stroke to soothe the feet. This is where I ask you to imagine taking in peace and balance with each breath. This promotes a profound sense of relaxation. At this point the session is over, but you should rest a few moments instead of getting up quickly. Just relax and acknowledge how great you feel. Be sure to drink some water after the session to flush out the deposits."

CHAPTER 25

MUSCULOSKELETAL INJURIES

REPETITIVE STRAIN INJURIES

In all the hoopla that has accompanied the manifestations of the computer revolution—from the original PCs to the World Wide Web—not much attention has been paid to how the installation of computers in offices has physically affected their users. What is talked about is how jobs that were grimy, dirty, and physically grueling, such as those in steel mills and automobile plants, are being replaced by jobs in service industries—for the less educated, flipping burgers and for the more educated, sitting in offices at terminals processing and moving information.

Those who are infatuated with the world of computers see this exchange—back-breaking labor in the mills traded for work in sanitary, air-conditioned offices—as all to the good. However, although there are undeniably benefits to workers from this exchange, they do not necessarily fall in the area of occupational health and safety. It is undeniable that the owners and managers of plants that manufactured heavy industrial equipment were notorious for disregarding toxic chemicals and other dangers in the workplace, but it is also true that the managers of many light industries have exposed people to years of looking into computer screens and rattling out numbers on keyboards without ever taking a look at the possible health effects of this labor.

One of the better books to profile these effects on both physical and mental health is Barbara Garson's *The Electronic Sweatshop*. She moves up the job ladder, starting with data-entry clerks and moving up to Wall Street traders and Pentagon officials, in order to show how their lives are impacted negatively by working with computers. In her interviews, she hears consistently about loss of autonomy and ill health. This chapter will look at a common type of health problem experienced by people whose jobs involve a lot of time at a computer terminal: repetitive strain injuries, and particularly carpal tunnel syndrome.

Symptoms

Dr. Timothy Jameson, author *of Repetitive Strain Injuries: Alternative Treatments and Prevention,* is a graduate of Los Angeles Chiropractic College and a certified chiropractic sports physician. He notes that many people today have repetitive strain injuries. These injuries, he points out, "can affect every structure of the body, which is what sometimes makes them so hard to treat. Most people will start off with simple muscle fatigue, such as affects people who work on computers or on assembly lines. The muscles fatigue because of the overexertion, that cumulative trauma."

To continue to put stress on an already fatigued muscle will eventually lead to problems with the connective tissue, or fascia, that forms a sheath around muscle. The fascia responds to repeated stress on the muscle by becoming harder and thicker. It can start getting "sticky" and begin to bind to the muscle and other neighboring tissues. The muscles and fascia become tight and restricted. Eventually, the nervous system gets involved.

A recent study in Great Britain showed that the sensory nerves, the nerves that pick up perceptions from the hands, the skin, and so on, are affected by repetitive strain. They are damaged by cumulative trauma. Cumulative trauma can also affect the tendons that connect muscles to bones. When this happens, the tendon and the sheath that holds the tendon may become inflamed. (When this occurs in the wrist, you have carpal tunnel syndrome.) This condition may lead to problems with the bursas, sacs that protect the joints.

These problems may even involve the spine, according to Dr. Jameson. "People with this type of injury tend to have a lot of pinched nerves that lead down to the arms. The process is very complex."

Dr. Jameson adds that repetitive strain injuries can be extremely serious. "You become very limited in your ability to do any type of work, especially repetitive work. In severe cases, people cannot work at all, cannot even get dressed in the morning. They cannot do the things they normally would do."

Clinical Experience

DIETARY FACTORS

If you are doing things that can lead to repetitive strain injury or are already suffering from this disability, there are foods you should cut out of your diet. The number-one items to avoid, which are major precursors of joint pain, are refined sugars, particularly high-fructose corn syrups. These increase sugar within the body, which sets off the whole process of the insulin reaction, with release of prostaglandins, which starts the inflammatory reaction.

Dr. Jameson recommends the book *Enter the Zone* by Barry Sears as a good source of information on proper nutrition. The book "goes into depth on how to prevent an inflammatory reaction. If you look through the aisles of the grocery store, you'll see that something like 50 percent of the products sold there use high-fructose corn syrup as an ingredient. The body has a lot of trouble digesting that. I know of cases where people cut it totally out of their diet, and their repetitive injury subsided within a few days."

Processed meats, such as corned beef, salami, and hot dogs, are very tough for the body to digest and can trigger an inflammatory reaction. Some of the more saturated oils, such as corn oil, palm oil, safflower oil, and butter, should also be avoided. Margarine, too, is bad. Many people think margarine is better than butter. However, margarine, because of its trans-fatty acids, is actually worse for the body than butter.

VITAMINS AND MINERALS

Dr. Jameson recommends a number of supplements. "I would recommend vitamin C, which is very important for tissue healing, starting out with about 1 gram and going up to about 3 grams a day. Also very important are the B-complex vitamins. These are used for nerve regeneration and nerve healing."

Minerals are another important supplement that can help in cases of repetitive strain injuries. As Dr. Jameson puts it, "You should never underestimate the power of minerals to rejuvenate cellular tissue." He puts his patients on a complete mineral regimen, with either colloidal or chelated minerals.

"A lot of people—especially people in jobs that involve heat, a lot of sweating, in the summer—are sweating out many of the minerals in their body. So if they are doing a lot of cumulative work and sweating, they are depleting their body's mineral's resources." A list of the minerals and vitamins that Dr. Jameson finds useful for preventing and treating repetitive strain injuries follows. "I usually prescribe these substances in pill form," he notes, "but you can also get all these things in food."

CALCIUM—Calcium is very important for muscle activity and for bone growth; it is also a muscle relaxant. Take about 800 mg a day of calcium, a little more if you are pregnant or postmenopausal.

MAGNESIUM—Magnesium is also important for muscle relaxation and for coenzymes. It is required for the functioning of about 80 percent of the enzymes in the body. Good sources of magnesium are vegetables and whole grains. Dr. Jameson recommends starting out with about 200–300 mg of magnesium a day. He says. "That's a small amount, considering that magnesium is not well absorbed. However, I always like to start my patients out with small amounts to see how they react."

MANGANESE AND ZINC—Dr. Jameson says that zinc, in particular, is really important for enzyme function and for cellular healing. He recommends about 20 or 30 mg a day. Zinc is found in fish, meat, and poultry.

SELENIUM—Selenium, another valuable substance, is found in fish, wheat germ, and garlic. Take 50–200 mcg a day in the pill form.

VITAMIN E—Vitamin E is a very important antioxidant; Dr. Jameson recommends 200–400 IU a day.

BETA CAROTENE—"Beta carotene," Dr. Jameson remarks, "is a compound found in vegetables of a yellow-orange or dark green color. Carrot juice is a great source of beta carotene. I recommend that patients drink carrot juice to get a natural, fresh form of the compound."

COENZYME Q10—Dr. Jameson says coenzyme Q10 is particularly important for patients with underlying heart disease. It's also important to maintain cellular energy, which is vital in cases of repetitive strain injuries.

PROTEOLYTIC ENZYMES—These enzymes "scavenge around the cells and rake up any cellular debris, aiding the healing process." Dr. Jameson explains.

CARTILAGE GROWTH FACTORS—Dr. Jameson adds, "There is also some good research now on the cartilage growth factors glucosamine sulfate and chondroitin sulfate. I recommend them for patients who have a great deal of joint discomfort—joint pains, irritation of the elbow, the spine, or the hands and fingers."

HERBAL REMEDIES

Certain herbs help the body relax, which is important in overcoming some repetitive strain injuries. Although Dr. Jameson doesn't have specific dosage recommendations, he offers the following ideas:

"Valerian root can be used for reducing muscle spasms. It should be taken toward the end of the day, because it's a relaxant. You wouldn't want to take it throughout the day, because it might affect your ability to perform. Garlic is a natural antibiotic as well as antifungal. Some of these muscular problems can stem from an underlying fungal problem, something we also see in fibromyalgia. A third valuable herb is ginkgo biloba, which increases circulatory function and brain function and enhances memory. It helps the blood flow get down to the extremities. Cayenne has also been found to help increase circulation. And ginseng is great for stress relief."

HOMEOPATHY

In addition to vitamins, minerals, and herbs, homeopathic remedies can be of service. Try the ones you find in health food stores that are recommended for muscle and joint injuries and for rheumatoid arthritis.

Carpal Tunnel Syndrome

Carpal tunnel syndrome, a widely recognized type of repetitive strain injury, is a common disability affecting office workers who sit at computer terminals. It is important that workers at risk for carpal tunnel syndrome not only follow the suggestions we make here but also learn to sit and type with the correct posture and to use ergonomically designed chairs and keyboards.

CAUSES

The direct cause of carpal tunnel syndrome is the effect on the tendons of the lower arms of day-in, day-out use of the same muscles and nerves to perform a repetitive task. The result is numbness, tingling, and pain that worsens at night. It's a miserable disorder.

Dr. Ray Wunderlich, who is board-certified by the American Academy of Pediatrics and the College for the Advancement of Medicine, practices preventive medicine in St. Petersburg, Florida, and is the author of many books, including *The Natural Treatment for Carpal Tunnel Syndrome.* When treating a case of carpal tunnel syndrome, he starts by looking for contributing factors. For women, he asks immediately, "Is she taking birth control pills?" The Pill, in essence, "puts you in a simulated state of pregnancy, and we know that pregnancy is one of the risk factors for carpal tunnel syndrome. Birth control pills also diminish the nutrients in the body, some of the water-soluble vitamins. Moreover, many women who take them become bloated. They develop minor degrees of fluid retention." The carpal tunnel is a narrow space in the arm, which becomes too narrow if the tissues are swollen. Women who are taking birth control pills and who perform tasks likely to lead to carpal tunnel syndrome should consider some other form of birth control.

Two other contributing factors, says Dr. Wunderlich, are hormone replacement therapy (HRT) and thyroid deficiencies. With regard to HRT, Dr. Wunderlich says, "If the estrogen preparations are not in balance with the progesterones, this can cause problems."

Dr. Wunderlich finds that 75 to 80 percent of his patients have some kind of thyroid disorder. He says, "On top of the repetitive movement of their jobs, many people have thyroid disorders, which contribute to the syndrome and may be hard to diagnose. To pin this down, look for a pale, puffy person, edematous, which is to say retaining fluid. When there is swelling, especially in connective tissue and in the nine tendons that run through that carpal tunnel, that medial nerve in the tunnel is often screaming for more room."

Another background factor may be low adrenal states, which may occur for a variety of reasons. People who overwork themselves, who take caffeine and/or sugar, who have bombarded their body with these substances and are now faced with repetitive tasks and sedentary living, may wind up with low-functioning adrenals. In the workplace, they develop various allergies, sometimes combined with low blood pressure. These people often have swollen tissues, which contributes to the problem.

Then, of course, there is diabetes. Type II diabetes in particular is often accompanied by edematous conditions. This may not be readily observed, Dr. Wunderlich cautions. "It may be microedema rather than pure edema. The ankles may not be swollen, for example, or the lungs congested, but the tissues may be slightly swollen.

"When the blood sugar is too high—which is almost a definition of diabetes—osmotic pressure rises. As we know from high school, osmosis is what controls the body's fluid pressure. The fluid should be in the blood vessels and in the lymph tissues. When it's outside in the body tissues, as happens in high blood sugar states or after we eat a lot of candy or, sometimes, fruits or juices in excessive quantities, the tissue may become water-logged. This, too, can cause problems in that narrow carpal tunnel. The medial nerve is screaming with numbness and irritability and pain every time we move our fingers."

Food allergies are another potential contributing factor to the development of carpal tunnel syndrome—and many other disorders. The repetitive, monotonous diets that so many people consume, especially with high-protein antigens—such as milk, cheese, and sometimes eggs—often produce food allergies. And a hallmark of the allergic response is swelling. Although the swelling is on the microlevel, the little cramped carpal tunnel reacts to the swelling, causing pain.

But even if you are not allergic to what you're eating, if you're on a typical American diet, you may have problems. "The 140 pounds of sugar per person, per year, that the average American still eats is one problem," Dr. Wunderlich says. "We're not talking about a long time ago. It's still happening. And there are also the salt-laden diets, which could be improving as people are counseled by alternative nutritionists to take high-potassium foods over high-sodium foods. There are also animal foods, which are high on the inflammatory scale—they tend to accentuate the inflammatory cascade, or series of chemical reactions through which inflammation develops. Animals are on top of the food chain, and that is where all the refuse accumulates, all the toxic chemicals that get into the animals' fat. This is especially true if the animals are domesticated and not wild, which is the case with most of our animal food sources." Thus if you are not following a pristine, organic diet, which the majority of people are not, you may be contributing to the risk of carpal tunnel syndrome or worsening an already existing condition.

Finally, Dr. Wunderlich says, there are "the chemicals in the workplace. When you are sitting at your computer, you may be bombarded with pesticides they have sprayed around your place—every month they come in and do that, or every two weeks if they see a lot of roaches. All of this adds to the toxic load as background factors."

CONVENTIONAL TREATMENT

By the time a person with carpal tunnel syndrome consults a physician, the condition is often in a quite advanced stage. According to Dr. Wunderlich, "The person often has atrophy of the muscles and irreversible or nearly irreversible nerve damage. The doctors operate, often with excellent results. So it's very appealing." However, this is a drastic therapy and will result in a life with further impaired function.

For less severe cases, conventional medicine's procedure is less felicitous. "What ordinary medicine does is give pain relievers—aspirin, Tylenol, ibuprofen, and other nonsteroidal anti-inflammatory drugs, which in the long term are all counterproductive, damaging the gastrointestinal system, producing leaky gut, as well as actually destroying cartilage. But those are the standard therapies that are offered."

ALTERNATIVE TREATMENTS

Dr. Wunderlich's program is short, sweet, and sensible. "The number-one approach in treating this problem," he states, "is detoxification. We do a vitamin C bowel flush. That's the first step for bowel tolerance." The vitamin C flush gets accumulated toxins out of the body. Follow this up with the second step, taking your favorite bulking agent, rice powder or psyllium, for example. "Number three," he mentions, "is to support the liver. I like artichoke and thistle compounds. Maybe 100 milligrams of thistle, three times a day, and 500 milligrams of artichoke leaf three times a day. Those are basics, plus water.

"I also use infrared heat to have people sweat, carefully monitored, of course, so there is exchange of body fluids. Also, exercise is important. I do running."

In his program, then, he emphasizes detoxification of the body, shifting to a sensible vegetarian diet, exercising, and improving stress management.

It is a question of priorities, Dr. Wunderlich concludes. "Many people have kids, two jobs, and so forth, so they think they do not have time. But you have to sort out the priorities, which we are not doing. You have to have good air and an appropriate amount of sleep. You need to avoid toxic foods. It is also important to have regular bowel movements, and you have to use your body appropriately for you, hopefully in some sweating way."

The advice that Dr. Wunderlich gives about carpal tunnel syndrome also applies to people who have any type of repetitive stress syndrome. Ultimately, we need to make our workplaces more livable. This will involve the improvement of human interaction and of the machines we surround ourselves with. If we upgraded our environments as obsessively as we upgrade our computers, we might have very few occupational disorders with which to cope.

TEMPOROMANDIBULAR JOINT (TMJ) DYSFUNCTION

The temporomandibular joint (TMJ) is a hinged joint that opens and closes the jaw. There are two such joints at either side of the head. The jaw is part of a wider system, the craniosacral system, which extends from the skull to the lowest segment of the spine. Disruption at any level of the craniosacral system can result in TMJ dysfunction.

Causes

The two most common causes of TMJ problems are poor bite and stress. Poor bite may be the result of new dental work that affects tooth alignment. Sometimes braces shift the palate, which affects the jaw.

TMJ dysfunction affects larger numbers of women than men due to stresses brought on by hormonal changes. Dr. Deborah Kleinman, a chiropractor who works with TMJ patients, explains, "There are various stress factors we can talk about that are specific to women. First, we have premenstrual tension. This further weakens an already weakened system. I know women who only have a problem with their jaw three days before their period. As soon as their period comes, their pain goes away. This tells me that there is a weakness in the system and that hormones push the body past the point of being able to compensate for it.

Hormonal changes also occur during pregnancy. "Hormones loosen the pelvis so that the woman is more flexible during delivery. And pregnancy creates structural changes through weight gain and the loosening of ligaments. These changes can further aggravate TMJ dysfunction.

"With nursing, postural changes can play a big role. Nursing places stress on the upper back muscles, especially if the woman doesn't use the proper pillows or if she gets lazy and slumps over while feeding her baby. These upper back muscles insert into the occiput, which is part of this craniosacral system. The occiput is the bone at the bottom of the skull. Tightening or pulling on the occiput can affect the head, neck, and TMJ."

The hormonal changes that occur during menopause also play a role in TMJ dysfunction.

Symptoms

Pain can be isolated in the joint itself or it can radiate to the face, neck, ear, and shoulder. Headaches may be a part of the picture. There may be a nagging toothache, even though the tooth is healthy. A person with TMJ problems may find it difficult to open the mouth all the way. Inflammation of the muscles around the joint may cause a spasm in those muscles, locking them open. Clicking, grinding, or popping noises may accompany chewing or movement of the joint.

Clinical Experience

CRANIOSACRAL THERAPY

Cranio means "skull" and *sacral* refers to the sacrum, which consists of the lowest five vertebrae of the spine. Craniosacral therapy is founded on an understanding of the relationship between these structures and several points in between, including the TMJ. Dr. Kleinman, who uses a specific form of craniosacral therapy called the sacro-occipital technique, explains: "A chiropractor like myself who uses this technique understands that there is a balance between the nervous system and the musculoskeletal system, and a relationship between the pelvis and the sacrum and then the head and the cranium. Between both structures rests the spine, the shoulders, the neck. All of these structures react to shifts in the pelvis and the cranium. The TMJ is part of that." She adds that a stable pelvis balances the body and works in harmony with the cranium. This allows information to flow to the brain smoothly.

Dr. Kleinman says that with TMJ the first step is to have a doctor perform a series of tests to determine whether structural stresses exist, and, if so, where. Once the structural stresses are identified, treatment can begin. Dr. Kleinman explains: "We place wedges or blocks under the pelvis. The muscles will relax and contract around these levers in an unforced way, based upon what these levers tell the brain. Then we incorporate breathing techniques to assist the brain in making musculoskeletal changes. This reestablishes the proper craniosacral flow." Sometimes secondary manipulations are necessary to readjust parts of the spine that lie between the pelvis and cranium that get knotted up as a result of compensating for the pelvis and the cranium. Cranial adjustments, made specifically to the temporomandibular joint, also help to reestablish proper balance.

OTHER PHYSICAL THERAPIES

Isotonic exercise, done regularly, can help some cases of TMJ dysfunction. In addition to jaw exercise, self-treatment for TMJ problems may include jaw awareness, in which the patient tries to notice and avoid clenching and grinding the teeth, as well as biting on gum, ice, or fingernails. Eating soft foods and avoiding resting or sleeping on the stomach can also help, as can learning to rest the jaw and to adopt proper jaw posture. Other potentially helpful techniques include self-massage; relaxed rhythmic opening and closing of the jaw; alternating moist heat (fifteen minutes) with ice (two to three minutes) to increase circulation; cool sprays and cryotherapy; bite guards; and splints. Surgery should be a last resort when dealing with TMJ problems.

Another physical therapy that can help relieve TMJ problems is Body Rolling, a technique developed by bodyworker Yamuna Zake, author of *Body Rolling: An Experiential Approach to Complete Muscle Release.* "Many of the muscles that run up the back and insert in the skull, as well as the muscles in the front of the neck, have attachments between the head and the chest. Thus the amount of tension in the muscles of the back, front, and sides of the neck can affect the level of contraction of the sutures (joints) and muscles of the cranium, and specifically the TMJ," she explains.

In Body Rolling, a 6-inch-diameter ball is used to apply traction that lengthens and releases muscles. "The degree of tension in the TMJ is controlled by the tension maintained in the neck," Zake explains. "By working the neck muscles with the ball to keep them at maximum length and minimum tension level, you can help reduce the buildup of tension in the TMJ." Zake has designed specific routines that use the ball to release the front and back of the neck, as well as an around-the-neck routine that helps break the holding pattern of tension that distorts head and neck alignment.

NUTRITION

Nutritional supplements may help in treating TMJ problems. Some of the most useful are listed here:

CALCIUM AND MAGNESIUM—These minerals are essential for proper muscular function and have a sedative effect.
B-COMPLEX VITAMINS—Take 100 milligrams of B-complex vitamins three times a day. B-complex vitamins are essential for combating stress.

PANTOTHENIC ACID—The appropriate amount of pantothenic acid to take is 100 milligrams, twice daily. B-complex vitamins, such pantothenic acid, are for combatting stress.

COENZYME Q10—Coenzyme Q10 is another stress fighter.

OTHER SUPPLEMENTS—L-tyrosine and vitamins B6 and C will improve sleep quality and alleviate anxiety and depression. It is also important to take a multivitamin and mineral complex.

PAIN MANAGEMENT

A Gallup survey released in 2000 revealed that nearly 90 percent of American adults experience pain at least once a month. Every day millions of people wake up knowing they are going to contend with pain, whether it be from repetitive strain, TMJ dysfunction, back injury, arthritis, or a host of other conditions. Many believe they just have to live with the pain. Unfortunately they do not realize that there are varied ways of treating pain naturally.

In this country we need a different approach to acute and chronic pain. We need to go from treating just the symptoms to treating the sufferer holistically. As mentioned in the sections above, getting the proper nutrition through sensible eating and ingesting natural supplements, including minerals and herbs, are key ways of treating pain. Other methods such as chiropractic, shiatsu, acupuncture, and the Trager and Alexander techniques also have a part to play.

One Physician's Personal Experience with Back Pain

Dr. Art Brownstein, author of *Healing Back Pain Naturally*, is a clinical instructor of medicine at the University of Hawaii who also teaches yoga. He was a back pain patient himself for twenty years. Like many of the fifty million Americans who have chronic back pain, he ended up on an operating table in a futile attempt to relieve his suffering. He describes his experience and how it bolstered his views on alternative healing:

"I've got two vertebrae that are only halfway there, and I was getting worse after the surgery to the point where I couldn't work for three years as a physician. I got hooked on the narcotic pain pills, and I was depressed and suicidal. At the end of the three-year period I was offered another operation, at which point I remembered my professors in medical school saying, 'Physician heal thyself.' To make a long story short, I ended up traveling around the world several times during the next three- to seven-year period and discovered some very simple, ancient mind-body healing techniques, including yoga, which allowed me not only to heal my own back pain naturally but also to help thousands of others."

Dr. Brownstein's back pain protocol emphasizes the importance of the muscles in supporting the health of the back. "When people have back pain, they automatically assume, because it is so painful, that there must be a problem with the discs or the bones. And that is what conventional medicine focuses on with its diagnostic tests such as MRIs and X rays. Muscles don't show up on MRIs or X rays, so in performing these tests, physicians are simply bypassing the most important system."

Often, Dr. Brownstein says, the back problem relates to the condition of the muscles. "If you look at other cultures that have very little furniture and very low-tech kind of societies, they have virtually no back pain. We spend so much time sitting down, sitting at our jobs, sitting while we are driving, that these muscles in our back just don't get used….We have to really tone our muscles in our backs and stretch them….Yoga is an effective strategy for this."

Stress management is part of his program. When people are under mental stress, the nerves are overstimulated. This can cause the muscles, including those of the back, to tighten and contract. If you have pain in your back, it will get worse. "If you don't have pain," Dr. Brownstein says, "you are an accident waiting to happen. Just bending forward and picking a paperclip off the floor can send your back into tremendous spasms." Among the stress management techniques Dr. Brownstein uses are breathing, relaxation, meditation, and visualization.

Diet is also part of Dr. Brownstein's program. He explains: "I've discovered a very strong connection between what you put in your body and not only every cell and tissue of your body but particularly your back."

Take coffee, for example. "I had a patient who had been to the top specialists all over the country—the Mayo Clinic, Johns Hopkins, Harvard," Dr. Brownstein says. "[T]hey were all recommending surgery for him. I asked him about his diet and it turned out he was drinking eight to ten cups of coffee a day. I asked him if he would be willing to quit, and reluctantly he agreed. Of course he had the caffeine-withdrawal headaches, but after two to three days he got over that. Within three weeks his back pain was totally cleared up. So it can be something that simple."

Diet

As Dr. Brownstein's example shows, one of the most important ways of combatting back and other types of pain is by guiding your diet to avoid abrasive foods and concentrate on those that build up the body's biochemistry. You should eat the same way you should drive—defensively.

It seems that people are really taking a new look at diet, especially people who used to think that relief from aches and pains could come only from a jar or bottle or from even more drastic remedies such as surgery. Not in every case, but in many cases, we're finding that diet can be the most powerful medicine.

One physician who has been looking is Dr. Neal Barnard, author *of Food That Fights Pain* and president of the Physicians' Committee for Responsible Medicine, a nationwide group that promotes preventive medicine and addresses controversies in modern medicine. As he sees it, there are four ways pain is manifested in the usual course of an illness. He uses arthritis as an example. First, there is some type of injury. Second, there is inflammation with redness, swelling, and stiffness. Third, there is irritation of the nerves that transmit the pain signals to the brain. Fourth, the brain receives the signals.

Dr. Barnard explains that there are three steps that must be taken in using diet to help with health problems. First, it is necessary to look for possible trigger foods. These are foods that commonly set off pain: dairy products, wheat or citrus for some people, tomatoes, meat, and eggs. "We want to do a little detective work and see which one is a trigger for an individual, because the triggers may be different for each person," Dr. Barnard counsels.

The second step is to find out which foods are safe to eat. "We focus on the pain-safe foods, which is fairly simple to do."

The third step, which Dr. Barnard believes is especially necessary for women, is to use foods to balance hormones. Because low-fat, vegetarian diets reduce hormone swings, they can dramatically reduce pain.

FOODS THAT WEAKEN RESISTANCE TO PAIN

In contrast to normally innocuous foods such as strawberries, which may trigger a pain reaction in certain people, some foods may reduce pain but also weaken the body's ability to resist pain. Coffee is one of those foods.

Dr. Barnard mentions sugar as another substance that lowers a person's pain tolerance. "Sugar never gets good press, and I'm sorry I have to add to the list of its problems. In a research study, people have taken volunteers and put a little metal clip on the web of skin between the fingers. Then this clip is hooked up to an electrical generator. The participants are given a little bit of electrical energy, which is gradually increased, and asked when they can feel it and when it becomes intolerable. Those numbers are written down. Then they are given sugar and the progression is repeated. These studies find that after ingesting the sugar, they feel the pain sooner and it becomes intolerable sooner.

"I've been so struck by the fact that people would start their breakfast with a cup of coffee, which, as a vaso- and cerebrodilator, temporarily reduces pain, then add a little sugar, which will increase pain sensitivity. It goes on for the rest of the day, where we are mixing up foods that cause and reduce pain."

PAIN-SAFE FOODS

Pain-safe foods include rice—any kind of rice, but especially brown rice—and cooked green vegetables such as broccoli, Swiss chard, and spinach. If you get an upset stomach from broccoli, cook it a little longer; this knocks out some of the vitamins, but the proteins in the broccoli are what cause stomach irritation in some people. Also, cooked orange vegetables such as sweet potatoes and carrots are pain-safe. Cooked yellow vegetables such as squash are also good. For fruits, pick the noncitrus ones, especially dried or cooked.

PAIN-REDUCING FOODS

Dr. Barnard has also found that some overlooked foods are especially good for dealing with pain. "One of the things we like to use is hot peppers, jalapeño peppers. The zing in the jalapeño is from a chemical called capsaicin. This doesn't just make your mouth hot, it actually changes what happens in the nerves. It stops the nerves from being able to conduct pain. Pharmaceutical manufacturers have taken this capsaicin straight out of the pepper and mixed it into a cream, which is applied externally. Two brands of capsaicin cream in the United States are Capsin and Zostrix.

"At first when you put on the capsaicin, it tingles and may even burn a little just as a hot pepper would. Do it day after day, and gradually the pain will diminish. You will still feel touch and pressure, but you won't feel pain. Give it a couple of weeks to work."

VITAMINS, MINERALS, AND OTHER SUPPLEMENTS

Most people know that minerals are essential for building up the body, maintaining the body's fluid balance, and helping with many chemical reactions. Let us look specifically at how minerals and vitamins have proved effective in treating pain.

Magnesium salts are useful for those with pain from the torso or joint aches. Many people are already deficient in magnesium. This calmative mineral is obtained from nuts and seeds that are raw and not roasted. Nuts are also beneficial in that they contain essential oils, including the omega-3 fatty acids, which also have mild anti-inflammatory properties that help reduce pain. For torso and joint problems, intake of magnesium citrate salts should be 400 milligrams per day, divided into doses of 100 to 200 milligrams.

Sound sleep is an essential part of good health. For people who have trouble sleeping due to headaches or other pains, there are a number of useful supplements. Valerian, hops (the same element found in beer), skullcap, or passionflower can be used. These supplements, which can be mixed, should be taken a half hour before going to sleep, in either capsule (one or two) or tincture form. You might also try taking 1 milligram of melatonin before sleep.

General musculoskeletal pain can be relieved by a number of substances. L-carnitine allows the body to burn fats and soak up excess lactate, which may be causing pain. Also helpful with muscle aches are the methyl donors, such as DMG (dimethyl glycine) and TMG (trimethyl glycerin), taken in doses of 100 milligrams per day.

To reduce the soreness after exercise, one should take vitamin E (400 to 800 IU/day), which prevents the leakage of enzymes from the muscles.

A final way to approach pain is to modify the way the brain perceives it. DL-phenylalanine (DLPA), which is a synthetic amino acid, slows down endorphins, making the ones you have work better. Taken in a dosage of 500 milligrams three times a day, it reduces chronic pain while getting the sufferer off analgesics.

Chiropractic

Chiropractic treatment involves the manual manipulation of vertebrae that become misaligned, causing nerve pressure and energy blocks to various organs. This manipulation is called an adjustment. It involves the chiropractor's gentle application of direct pressure to the spine and joints. The chiropractor may squeeze or twist the torso, pull or twist the limbs, or wrench the head or back. What the chiropractor is doing is readjusting the spinal column to restore the normal vertebral relationship. This eliminates the body's energy blocks and keeps life-sustaining energy flowing freely to the vital organs.

Chiropractic is effective in dealing with pain and as a preventive treatment because it relieves nerve pressure. The buildup of this pressure is cumulative in its erosion of the health and integrity of specific body organs or regions. If one vertebra is out of relationship to the one next to it, a state of disrelationship is said to exist. This disrelationship throws off that vertebra's environment, that is, the blood supply and detoxifying lymphatic drainage surrounding it. When this occurs, a congestion of blood, toxins, and energy creates pressure that upsets both local and systemic homeostasis, or balance.

Tissues all need normal nerve functioning in order to transport required nutrients to the cells. Insofar as the vertebrae are misaligned, the blood becomes congested and slow in its delivery, creating the absence of this nutrient supply. The cell's normal activity is thereby hindered, and it becomes irritated. Moreover, once the cell's metabolic processing is interfered with, its waste-removing lymphatic servicing to that area is diminished. This leads to toxic buildup that causes further irritation and inflammation. The chiropractor is concerned with alleviating all these problems.

Acupuncture

Acupuncture sees pain as being derived from blocked energy or *qi (chi)*. In treating this blockage, the practitioner has to determine whether it stems from an overabundance or a deficiency in energy, so that treatment can be adjusted depending on whether it is necessary to strengthen or decrease *qi.*

The acupuncturist first records the patient's medical history in the manner of a conventional doctor. Then, with the patient lying down or seated, depending on the area to be treated, fine-gauge, stainless steel needles are inserted into significant points and meridians to exert different physiological effects on the body and induce both relaxation and energization. The patient will remain in this position for twenty to thirty minutes, though an appointment with an acupuncturist may last up to an hour, since part of the time will be spent consulting about the employment of other traditional and herbal treatments that might be recommended. Bodywork and massage may also be included in the session.

Dr. Christopher Trahan notes that the treatment will have analgesic and anesthetic effects, block pain, and accelerate recovery from motor nerve injury. Moreover, it enhances the immune system, which has a sedative effect; helps with muscular spasms or neurological problems; has a homeostatic effect in that it helps balance blood pressure; and has positive psychological effects, acting directly on brain chemistry.

Many patients with chronic low back pain find that acupuncture will not only help break the pain cycle, it will also allow them to reduce pain medications and participate more vigorously in physical therapy. Dr. Emily Kane, a naturopath who practices in Juneau, Alaska, says in an article on the website of the American Association of Naturopathic Physicians (www.naturopathic.org) that experiments have shown that acupuncture stimulates the nervous system to release endorphins as well as other chemical pain relievers in the body. Some people get immediate relief from low back pain after the first acupuncture session, but she recommends having six or eight sessions within a short period of time before assessing whether or not it is working for you.

Bodywork

SHIATSU

Shiatsu is based on the principle that a vital energy, called *qi* (*chi*), flows through the body. The primary cause of pain is an imbalance of this energy. The goal of the healer is to balance the client's energy so that pain and discomfort do not manifest or, if they do appear, will be relieved.

As bodywork practitioner Thomas Claire explains it, thumbs, fingers, palms, forearms, elbows, and even knees are used to apply pressure to specified points in the body to modulate the flow of energy. During a shiatsu treatment, the client lies on the floor on a comfortable padded surface, such as a futon, fully clothed or undressed to her level of comfort. What the client feels is pressure, which can be gentle or deeper at the places where the practitioner is working. As the pressure continues, the patient generally feels relaxed and energized at the same time.

Shiatsu is good for treating a variety of different pains. It is especially beneficial in combating chronic pain in the back, neck, or shoulders, but it has also proved effective in treating whiplash, herniated discs, and problems affecting the nervous system, such as Bell's palsy.

A shiatsu healer concentrates on certain pressure points that have metaphoric names that tell us something about what they do or how they are to be worked with. The first point of interest is on the ankle and called Spleen 6. It is at the meeting of three yin meridians and is the most powerful point for tonifying the feminine energy in the body. It can be located by placing the little finger on the border of the inside ankle and counting up four fingers. At the very top of these fingers, and at the center, is Spleen 6. To modulate the energy, you can put pressure on this point with your thumb, pushing three times in succession for seven to ten seconds each time. This pressure will also help a woman control PMS and irregular cycles.

The corresponding point for male tonification is called Stomach 36. To locate this point, find the indentation just outside the kneecap. Put one finger at this indentation and go down four fingers. There you'll find Stomach 36, which is also known as Leg 3 Mile. This second name is given since, it is said, if you have a strong Stomach 36, you will have enough stamina to walk three miles with no trouble. For women, this point can be used to ease childbirth and labor pains.

A third important point, located at the middle of the web of the hand, is Large Intestine 4, also called Meeting Mountains. The latter name is derived from the "mountain of flesh" found jutting up between the thumb and index finger when you close your hand. To locate this point, find the highest point on that protruding flesh and then open your hand. This point should be pressed three times running for seven to ten seconds to tonify the upper body. Pressing this point can also help with nausea, vomiting, colds, and constipation.

TRAGER TECHNIQUE

The Trager technique is a way of working with the mind and body simultaneously. According to the philosophy behind this technique, pain comes from the accumulated action of the patient frequently tightening her movements and posture. To correct it, the practitioner uses gentle motions to increase the patient's pleasure in the quality of the tissues and decrease the restriction and the sense of holding. The practice works by reaching into the functional subconscious with particular qualities of movement, posture, and sensation. Gentleness is emphasized so that no message will be sent to the body alerting it that pain is on the way or causing the patient to tighten up. The movement reaches into the central nervous system with a motion at once pleasurable, lengthening, softening, and opening, conveying this sensation to the tissues and joints. The movements can be very small and internal or can be done at the periphery of the body in the limbs. In the latter case, the limbs are used as handles to reach the core.

Roger Tolle, a Trager practitioner, says that some clients will feel results immediately, as the touching allows them to release pain. In other cases, it takes a repetition of the information into the body and mind, which will gradually allow the client to relearn how to go about daily activity with a different quality of motion.

The Trager method works particularly well against pain in the temporomandibular joint (TMJ), neck, back, pelvis, and carpal tunnel.

ALEXANDER TECHNIQUE

Jane Kosminsky, an Alexander technique teacher, describes this modality: "The Alexander technique is an educational tool that teaches us first how to balance our heads well at the top of the spine. It teaches the correct use and relationship of the head to the spine and the spine to the limbs. We deal with the problems of the lower back, the arm, or the leg by focusing first on the balance of the head and its relationship to the spine."

Actual exercise is not part of the Alexander program. "In Alexander we don't do exercise, we don't try to fix ourselves," Kosminsky says. "We notice what we are doing and then we make the decision to say no to a habit that is not good for us. For example, we note excessive tension, crunching in the spine, pulling in the shoulders, and then we use the technique of visualization to effect change."

ROLFING

According to the practitioners of Rolfing, pain is due to chronic shortenings in the tissue. Correction of this pain can be accomplished through soft-tissue manipulation. This manipulation acts to create order in the body so that the client stands tall and free of restriction.

David Frome, a physical therapist, states that Rolfing is done in a ten-session series designed to address all the shortenings in the structure systematically. Each session works in a different area. In the first hour, for instance, concentration is on the trunk, shoulders, and hips. In the second hour, work is done on the back and lower leg. Going through the complete series allows the therapist to work through all the body's shortenings. During a session, a patient may experience a tingling sensation and a sense of release. The patient should strive to draw the deepest possible breath to aid in treatment.

The major goal of the treatment is not pain relief per se, but it has been found to help with TMJ pain, frozen shoulder, tennis elbow, carpal tunnel syndrome, chronic hip problems, sciatica, cervical neuropathies, and knee, foot, and ankle problems.

CRANIOSACRAL THERAPY

The sacral region is at the bottom of the spine. Between it and the cranium (skull), there should be a balanced rhythmic motion maintained for the health of the organism. When pain arises, it may be due to a restriction that disturbs the harmony between these two regions or between them and the rest of the body.

In craniosacral therapy, the practitioner places his or her hands on the client's body in such a way as to try to bring the cranium and sacrum back into alignment, reestablishing a natural rhythm. Charles A. Kaplan, the founder and director of the Center for Pain Management, points out that this hands-on technique usually centers on touching the head or lower back but can be done anywhere, such as on the fingers or toes. Some patients will go through a first treatment and not feel anything, but most will leave the treatment table feeling very relaxed and stress-free.

Craniosacral therapy is recommended for dealing with muscular and skeletal pain, headaches, pains in the back and neck, sports injuries, sciatica, and nerve pain. It can also be beneficial to those recovering from pneumonia or bronchitis, helping by loosening the rib cage. Craniosacral therapy is a tremendous stress reducer.

Magnet Therapy

With an ancestry as old as that of acupuncture and shiatsu, magnet therapy also acts to influence the body's energy. Dr. Jim Joseph mentions that the healing power of magnets was known in China over four thousand years ago. Such ancient fathers of medicine as Galen and Aristotle discussed magnets, as did Paracelsus, one of the founders of chemistry. Mesmer and others in the nineteenth century also elaborated on the value of magnet therapy, and it is still being developed and practiced today.

Down through history, magnets have been used to deal with the causes of various ailments. As Dr. Joseph remarks, "Pain is a messenger. We don't want to kill the messenger but find the cause."

Pain in the body can be caused by positive energy being drawn to the site of injury. To bring about this transfer, the brain sends out a negative signal. Using the negative side of a magnet can augment and assist that reaction. Furthermore, around an injury there will be an acidic buildup. The negative side of the magnet is an alkalizing force that can help alleviate the pain accompanying this acidity.

A second source of pain arises when a person is overworked or suffering from undue stress, causing that person's cells to be overly positively charged. Putting a negative magnet on a weakened area will repolarize the cells, restoring the balance between positive and negative charge.

The distortion of the cells' polarity and resultant pain may also be caused by our technological environment. We are swamped with positive electromagnetic pulses coming from televisions, radios, electric clocks, and all the other electrical devices around us. The pulses of their fields are not congruent with the one found in our body and can throw us into disharmony and disease.

Magnets can be obtained in a plastiform case that can be molded and shaped for a particular area. They last indefinitely and are low priced. A medium-sized magnet may cost twenty dollars. Healing magnets are color-coded with the negative pole green and the positive red. The positive side of the magnet is active and sun-oriented; the negative side is relaxing and earth-oriented. All the treatments discussed here utilize the negative pole. One must be careful with the positive pole, since positive magnetism causes growth in any biological system, even cancer. Treatment should last from twenty minutes to overnight. The magnet's power should be from 1,000 to 6,000 gauss.

A magnet can be wrapped with Velcro on the area to be covered. Special wraps in which the magnets are inlaid in Velcro are available. These wraps can be placed on most parts of the body, though they should not be used on the eyes. Negative magnetism attracts fluids and gases, and a negative magnet placed near the eye would draw out its fluids. If work is to be done on the eyes, the magnet can be placed off to the side. From this position, magnetism can be exerted on cataracts to reduce oxidation and free-radical development. The magnet's value in reducing oxidation is due to the fact that oxygen is paramagnetic. When you breathe, you are pulling negative energy from the earth into your body.

At night, it is useful to lie on a magnetic bed pad and put magnets behind the head, where they will bathe the pineal gland in energy. This will induce a restful night's sleep. By using a magnet, one can feel rested even after sleeping fewer hours than one normally does. Magnets have also been known to increase sexual abilities.

Magnets can help with shoulder pain, pain in the rotator cuff, and aches in the lumbar region of the back. They can be attached to the head or neck to deal with hypothyroidism, depression, migraine headaches, and problems with the vestibular system. For depression, the magnet should be placed near the occipital lobe.

The Mind-Body Connection

Some therapists such as Dr. Art Brownstein, mentioned earlier, recommend a more eclectic approach, one that looks for and relies on the often-overlooked synergies that flow between the mind and the body. Dr. Ron Dushkin brings up a number of points to consider in dealing with pain. He notes, first, the importance of relaxation, which will quiet and calm the nervous system. Remember that when we feel pain, we are also feeling a layer of stress on top of that pain. If the layer of stress is relieved, the pain will diminish significantly.

Human touch can also play a part in relieving pain. As babies we like to be touched and as adults we still find this important.

A third overlooked factor in healing is humor. The writer Norman Cousins tells the story of how he was hospitalized with a critical health problem. As he saw it, a lot of his physical deterioration was due to stress and negative thoughts from that stress. He reasoned that if we can create disease with stress, then by alleviating stress through means such as humor, we can cure disease. He had a movie projector brought into his hospital room and·began showing Marx brothers films and other comedies. Soon his room became a place of congregation for other patients who wanted to enjoy the shows. It got rather chaotic because so many people were coming into his room and laughing. You're not supposed to laugh in a hospital. Some people were scandalized. Cousins said that the doctors would give him blood tests before and after he had been laughing at a humorous film and would find an improvement after the film. He also had less pain after laughing.

Guided imagery is also an element of the mind-body connection. With this technique, a sufferer places a hand over the injured area and invites the other cells in the body to go to the aid of the damaged area. After all, the body's cells always work together, and this is one way to encourage their interplay.

All the methods mentioned as part of the mind-body connection get the patient to take charge of personal recovery. Many people are strong in many areas of life—pursuing a career, forming good relationships, playing sports—but when it comes to their own health, they turn over all control to a doctor. To really escape pain, the patient must play a big role in the recovery process.

CHAPTER 26

NERVOUS SYSTEM DISORDERS

MULTIPLE SCLEROSIS

Multiple sclerosis (MS) is a progressive and deteriorating muscular disability in which there is a loss of the protective covering of nerves in the brain and spinal cord. MS affects some 350,000 Americans, twice as many women as men.

Dr. Michael Wald, who holds degrees in nutrition and chiropractic, and has authored five books about health, explains, "Multiple sclerosis is a syndrome of progressive nerve disturbances. What we have is a gradual loss in myelin, which is part of the outer covering of the nervous system. The nervous system breaks down."

MS is a condition that can present itself quite suddenly, Dr. Wald says. A young woman could be quite healthy and then one day have problems moving the limbs. Muscle weakness, dizziness, and problems with perception and touch may appear. Vision may be blurred.

"Generally the person will go to a neurologist and the neurologist will take an MRI," Dr. Wald continues. "Maybe he will take some of the patient's cerebrospinal fluid and look for things. Then the doctor says, 'You've got the disease.' Then the person is put on one of several steroids and that is the end of that.

"That's really not enough. There is enough nutritional and medical literature to support the use of a whole host of dietary and nutritional changes in the lives of these people. What we want to do in natural medicine is slow down and reverse the degeneration of myelin. When myelin breaks down, it's called demyelinization. In about two-thirds of the cases of MS, the onset is between twenty and forty. We are talking about the most fit people in the prime of their lives being struck with this condition."

Possible Causes

No one pretends to know the causes of MS. Some postulate that it is due to a virus. Often, a woman will have a viral problem and will get MS shortly thereafter. So that may be a cause or a trigger. Yet, Dr. Wald cautions, "Human beings are complicated, as we well know, so even if we knew the cause, we would still want to approach it from a natural medicine perspective by giving the body whatever it needs to help whatever it wants to correct. Whether it's MS or a headache or some other problem, the natural healer strives to give the body what it needs."

The theory that MS is caused by a virus is based on animal studies. "Certain viruses can be given to certain animals, for example, which will cause every single symptom of MS," Dr. Wald says. "So it's not unreasonable. The common viruses they think might be involved in causing MS are the rabies virus, herpes simplex virus, and the parainfluenza virus. So natural approaches should be antiviral in nature. We want to think of echinacea, astragalus, goldenseal."

Multiple sclerosis is classified as an autoimmune disease. An autoimmune disease is one in which the immune system fails to recognize a component of the body's systems as "self" and mounts an attack on that component. For example, says Dr. Wald, "The body may be breaking down the myelin, causing symptoms of MS. So anything we do to slow that down or reverse it should theoretically help."

He adds, "In autoimmunity, the problem with immune breakdown occurs eventually to everyone as aging happens, so we are really talking about a situation that will affect everyone."

Clinical Experience

NATURAL TREATMENTS

Diet

In terms of diet, the first thing is to identify and eliminate food allergies. Dr. Wald remarks that allergies also indicate problems with the immune system. "An allergy means that the immune system becomes hyperresponsive. We already have that going on in MS, so we don't want to create any other hyperresponsiveness with foods."

A number of foods commonly cause allergies, including gluten-containing foods such as barley, rye, oats, and wheat. "These are common offenders.

Milk products also fit this category. In fact, the intake of milk in adolescents is correlated with a far higher MS incidence. That much has been proven."

How would a person determine if she were allergic? Dr. Wald says, "You can do what is called an IgG4/IgG1 combination test for allergy, which is a blood test. Ninety foods can be checked, and you can determine quite quickly how your immune system hyperresponds to some of them. Then you eliminate the foods and use substitutes. Another way to approach this would be to look at your diet for the top ten or fifteen foods that you eat most often or that are your favorite and eliminate them, because those best-loved foods tend to be the allergy foods. Even allergists recognize this."

Dr. Wald adds, "Most people find it strange that their favorite foods are what are getting them into trouble. A person will say, "But I eat the food all the time." Yes, but you are also causing some disruption of the immune function by doing that, particularly if you have a weak immune system to begin with." By eliminating these foods, "you will reduce overall stress on the immune system. That means healing has a chance to take place." (See chapter 15 for more on food allergies.)

Aside from allergens, other foods to be avoided in relation to this disease are animal fats. "A high intake of saturated fats in the diet, animal fats, is definitely linked to MS."

Dr. Wald notes that some studies have supported vegetarianism as a positive path for MS sufferers. "Dr. Roy Swank, professor of neurology at the University of Oregon Medical School, did one of the longest studies of MS ever done, which was about twenty-six years in duration. People who had MS symptoms were put on an essentially vegan diet, cod liver oil, and several other similar things. Over time he noticed that those on this diet who had initially had symptoms had fewer exacerbations and less worsening of their condition over the years or had no exacerbations, and did very well or better in comparison to those who had had an initial MS diagnosis and were given the standard drugs."

Supplements

Another important avenue to explore is supplementation. Dr. Wald told me about an unusual supplementation therapy developed at Harvard. "One practical suggestion is something called myelin basic protein. This is something that you or anyone can buy in the health food store. Harvard has investigated reactions with MS patients, using oral myelin from a cow, actually. Basically, if you eat myelin, the stuff in the nervous system will attack the myelin you are eating, leaving your nervous system alone and giving it a chance to repair. The technical term for that is molecular mimicry. You are mimicking your myelin, so it's a distraction technique. That's very important."

Less experimentally, there are certain supplements of proven effectiveness, particularly the omega-3 and omega-6 fatty acids. Dr. Wald notes, "Most of the readers probably know something about these. Evening primrose oil is an example of an omega-6. We get that from grains and seeds. The omega-3s can be obtained from such things as flaxseed oil and fish oil. There are dozens of other types of fats that are important. I do recommend that those with MS have what is called an essential fatty acid blood test done, so that you can find out exactly what oils you need and then simply put them back."

These oils control inflammation in the body and immune function. They are also needed for vascular function—in other words, all the things we need for healing MS. Dr. Wald says that even if you don't have these special tests done, you certainly would want to at least purchase a supplement that contains a reasonable balance of omega-3 and omega-6 oils. Probably, you should look for one that is heavier on the omega-3 oils, the flax and fish oils.

"I myself find that MS patients have difficulty metabolically breaking flaxseed oil down into what they need. So, rather than flax, I tend to recommend what is called ephedra, a supplement. For dosage, you should follow the directions on the bottle unless you are seeing a health care practitioner who can individually tailor the dose."

Another very important nutrient for MS is glutathione. This amino acid is the major immune booster in the body. If you are going to help your health, regardless of what the concern is, you have to somehow raise glutathione levels. Dr. Wald recommends anywhere from 250 to 500 milligrams orally.

Selenium helps the body utilize the glutathione. The recommended dose would be in the 200 to 400 micrograms range.

Vitamin B12 is also extremely important. Dr. Wald says, "Alcoholics, for example, can have the shakes, which are caused by degeneration of their myelin, due to a B12 deficiency. This seems very similar to the problems of MS. So, though a B12 deficiency is probably not the cause of MS, many MS sufferers have a B12 imbalance, one that doesn't necessarily show up on a blood test. So every MS patient we see gets a B12 shot. Oral supplements might do it, but it really depends on the level of disability."

Enzymes are also extremely important. As Dr. Wald puts it, "Any conversation about autoimmune disease would not be complete without speaking about them. Bromelain and papain are plant-derived enzymes. They are pancreatic enzyme supports."

Dr. Wald notes that these enzymes are key to defending the body against autoimmune chemicals in the blood, which irritate and break down tissues. Enzymes that you eat, such as bromelain, papain, and others found in fresh fruits or vegetables, as well as pancreatic enzymes, get into the blood and literally digest some of these irritating chemicals. It's a must to include lots of those enzymes.

"Lastly," Dr. Wald says, "some other supplements should be mentioned. One is N-acetyl-cysteine (NAC). Cysteine and methionine are sulfur-containing amino acids that help liver detoxification and overall body detoxification.

So any anti-autoimmune approach should contain generous amounts of NAC, between 250 to 1,000 milligrams orally. It works really well orally. The NAC increases glutathione levels. As we said earlier, glutathione is the single most important immune-boosting chemical in the body."

Herbs

Dr. Wald also uses extracts of herbs that are standardized, meaning they have been assayed for the active ingredient. "In other words," he says, "what the bottle says is in there, is in there." The herbs goldenseal, astragalus, and echinacea are the ones most often recommended for autoimmune disorders.

He mentions a common criticism of herb use. "I do want to recall a question I often field about herbs. A person will ask, 'If MS is a case of the ultrasensitization of the immune system, would you want to take herbs that would bolster the immune system?'

"Well, the wonderful thing about how nature has worked this out is that these supplements will not enhance immunity. They are what are called biologic response modifiers. They work to balance what is wrong. If your immunity is too high, they will work to bring it low. If your immunity is low, they will bring it up. Of course, you can abuse these things to a certain point. But almost no one, if she follows the general directions on the bottles, will be caused any harm. The most the person will experience is a little gastrointestinal upset, and once she experiences that, she will naturally decrease the dose." In taking herbs, no matter which ones, Dr. Wald recommends a four-day on, four-day off cycle so that the body doesn't become insensitive to the herbs, which could result in the herbs losing some of their effectiveness.

Oxygen

Dr. Wald also notes that work has been done with oxygen in aiding sufferers from this illness. "Something not commonly talked about in MS is hyperbaric oxygen. It is possible—and there are many studies on this with MS—for a person to get into a chamber and be exposed to clean, purified oxygen under pressure for health reasons. The purpose of the pressure is to increase oxygen levels in the blood so that healing can take place. As we age—and you can think of MS as accelerated aging of the immune and nervous system—we do not use oxygen well, so tissues break down, producing lots of free radicals. Anything that helps prevent or reverse that has to be healthy just in general. So for those with less severe cases of MS, hyperbaric oxygen will be quite valuable."

Exercise

In Dr. Wald's experience, the effectiveness of exercise for those with MS depends very much on the individual. "Sometimes exercise worsens MS and sometimes it helps it. I think the reason is that if someone's nutritional status is lousy, and the person is exercising, she is only increasing her stress. So you want to have a complete holistic program where supplements, diet, exercise, and stress reduction are all combined intelligently."

PARKINSON'S DISEASE

Michael J. Fox, the television and film actor, has had his career cut short by Parkinson's disease. He seemed to be a young, healthy, happy, and active person. How could this have happened to him? It raises all kinds of questions as to what is Parkinson's disease and how we can prevent it. He is devoting his life now to raising awareness of Parkinson's disease.

Dr. Michael Wald describes the condition, also known as PD: "It is characterized by tremors and muscular tightness and problems with posture and reflexes. It is one of the most frequently encountered disorders and is a predominant cause of disability in those older than fifty years of age. Its prevalence is estimated at one million to two million cases in the United States, and the incidence increases with age. There are different types of Parkinson's, primary and secondary.

"Particular to PD is a loss of cells in the area of the brain known as the substantia nigra, locus cerleus, and substantia innominata, and a formation of abnormal bodies called Lewy bodies. Basically we don't know the cause, but the most likely mechanism of the cellular damage is oxidation by toxic free radicals. In particular, this oxidation might break down a certain amino acid we need for normal health and normal motor function that leads to dopamine depletion.

"Someone with PD has what is called a 'resting' tremor or 'pill-rolling' tremor, as if they were rolling something between their thumb and their first finger and their hands are moving. During sleep it fades away. If you try to move their arms and legs, the muscles are very rigid, called 'lead pipe' rigidity, and the muscles move with a 'cogwheel phenomenon.' These individuals walk very slowly and often shoot forward and fall down and hurt themselves because their motor function is skewed. Infrequency of blinking is one of the early signs and a loss of overall facial expression, a loss of voice volume, with a poverty of body movement. Reflexes are diminished."

This lack of movement is called bradykinesia, and the shuffling gait with poor arm swing is very characteristic of Parkinson's patients. One key is that the incessant tremor disappears with intentional movement and then returns as soon as the arm is at rest. There is also a very strong association between PD and depression and eventual dementia.

These clinical signs are due to the nerves in the brain starting to degenerate and are a strong clue in the diagnosis. MRIs sometimes show atrophy, or wasting, in advanced cases, but mostly the CT scan and MRIs of the brain do not show anything. The diagnosis is usually made based on the clinical picture.

Parkinson's is mostly a disease of the elderly, but it can sometimes be seen in younger people, such as Michael J. Fox. Younger people tend to develop the motor and muscle problems first. In the older population there is a much higher incidence of dementia. Other kinds of dementias can also have features that look like Parkinson's disease, and many times there is an overlap of different causes for the dementia.

Potential Causes

The cause is unknown, but there is a lot of speculation. A current theory is that PD may be caused by a toxic environmental agent or chemical compound. This is because there were reports of greater prevalence in rural areas. The herbicide Parquat is a likely culprit. Dieldrin and DDT have also been implicated. Another study by Scheider and colleagues in 1997 found that the antioxidant lycopene (found primarily in tomatoes and related products) was not associated with higher PD risk, but intake of sweet foods, including fruit, was. They theorized that pesticide residues in the fruits and vegetables may have contributed to the development of PD.

"There have been a number of studies of pesticides and insecticides," Dr. Wald says. "If you are genetically susceptible and are exposed to toxins in the soil or air, they can break down or oxidize the dopamine. In the *Journal of Neurology* they reported causing PD with pesticides, and they were able to reverse it. It is our liver that detoxifies toxins. They also say that ongoing exposure to manganese and copper of greater than twenty years will cause PD. A diet higher in mono and disaccharides, the simple sugars, is associated with a higher risk of PD."

Dr. Jay Lombard is chief of neurology at Westchester Square Medical Center and assistant professor at Cornell University Medical College. He has seen and treated many Parkinson's patients. He has this to add about the causes of Parkinson's: "Environmental toxins have been implicated in the etiology of Parkinson's disease, particularly pesticides. It appears that patients who have Parkinson's disease have an inability to detoxify these very common pesticides found in the environment because they lack a particular enzyme."

It is also known that certain drugs can cause a reversible form of PD. These drugs are the phenothiazines and butyrophenones, drugs that affect the central nervous system. Carbon monoxide poisoning has been known to induce a Parkinsonism.

Clinical Experience

CONVENTIONAL TREATMENT

Levodopa (L-dopa) has been the standard Parkison's treatment since it was introduced in the 1960s. Medical doctors usually prescribe a drug called Sinemet, which is a combination of carbidopa and levodopa. Other drugs are also used in combination with or as an adjunct to L-dopa, including seleggline (Eldepryl) and amantadine (Symadine). Side effects are not uncommon. None of these drugs can cure the disease or stop its progress.

ALTERNATIVE APPROACHES

Dr. Jay Lombard is also the author of *Brain Wellness Plan.* He talks about some of the things we can do to prevent PD: "It is known that glutathione is diminished in the brains of Parkinson's patients. One of the major strategies in preventing the progression of Parkinson's disease is to boost up the natural glutathione levels in the brain. There are various compounds that do that, for instance, antioxidants such as lypoic acid. It is worth further study to see if indeed giving dihydrolypoic acid prevents progression of the disease.

"Gangliosides are a type of lipid or fat membrane that is found in high degrees in our nervous system. Gangliosides have also been studied to help prevent progression in Parkinson's. Administering medications that increase dopamine production are beneficial for symptomatic improvement, but the underlying process in Parkinson's patients has to do with our antioxidant defense systems being deficient. Anything we can do to raise those defense systems certainly would help with the underlying disease.

"What I tell patients with Parkinson's disease is that the medication they have been given will help them feel better, and the natural products or antioxidants that I prescribe may not really make them feel much different, but these are addressing the underlying cause of Parkinson's disease. It is possible that those two things don't always match."

Dr. Lombard follows three general strategies in attempting to prevent progression of the disease. He remarks, "These strategies are useful for other neurodegenerative conditions as well. We know the immune system is overactive in particular ways that is destructive to the brains of Parkinson's patients. We know that patients with Parkinson's have an inability to handle a particular metal found in our diets called iron and we know that Parkinson's patients may have a deficiency of a part of the cell called the mitochondria that is responsible for the manufacture of ATP [adenosine triphosphate, which is involved in the storage and transfer of cellular energy]. Using these three evidences, a comprehensive program can be drawn up that addresses each of these issues separately.

"In regard to excessive inflammation, certain types of white blood cells make a compound called nitrous oxide, which is a free radical. It is very destructive to areas of the brain in Parkinson's disease. There are certain antioxidants that are effective in quenching or inhibiting the effects of this free radical. These include an extract of green tea that has profound antioxidant properties. Dihydrolypoic acid, which is a glutathione precursor, increases brain glutathione levels and is very effective as an antioxidant. Lycopenol is another antioxidant that crosses the blood-brain barrier and inhibits excessive free radical activity.

"Second, we know Parkinson's patients have too much iron in their brains, and iron acts as a free-radical inducer. So we try buffering the effects of increased iron with a protein called lactoferrin. This prevents excessive iron absorption from the intestinal tract into the bloodstream.

"Finally the mitochondria, the energy-producing units of the cell that make ATP, are also deficient in Parkinson's patients. Ways of increasing the mitochondria include coenzyme Q10, serotonin, and two other compounds —NADH, which is also called ignatia, and ubiquinone, which is a coenzyme Q10 analog. They dramatically increase brain ATP levels. These three things are a very worthwhile strategy for treating a Parkinson's patient."

Dr. Wald has devised a detoxification program that he feels is worthwhile for PD. "Beta carotene has been fairly well studied in PD. It is an antioxidant, and I use about 50,000 units. It helps protect the liver and other cells and the nervous system from premature degeneration. Vitamin C helps protect dopamine, an important neurotransmitter that is low in those with PD."

"Essential fatty acids, such as omega-3 and omega-6, are important for protecting the nervous system. Toxins in our environment known as zenobiotics are fat soluble, meaning they love to hang out in the nervous system. We need to take all the antioxidants I already spoke of with essential fatty acids such as omega-3 and omega-6. So we want to get vitamin E, 400 to 800 IU a day, and vitamin C to balance tolerance. Some of the studies show PD patients have low levels of vitamin B3, niacin. There is a nonflushing form called hexaniacinite, 250 milligrams a day. Melatonin is a very important hormone not just for sleep and repair but also as an important antioxidant in the nervous system. It slows down the breakdown of dopamine. Another important amino acid is N-acetyl cysteine or NAC. It is used by the liver to convert fat-soluble toxins into water-soluble toxins so that we can excrete them in the urine. The body must be able to eliminate toxins once they are mobilized. Any detoxification program needs to focus on the liver and intestine and the lymphatic system and so on to get these things out."

Dr. Wald adds, "Glutathione has been found to be low in PD. The most effective way to increase it is with Vitamin C. Glutathione is not only an immune booster but helps fight degenerative changes. It tends to become lower as we age."

ALZHEIMER'S DISEASE

Alzheimer's disease is the leading cause of senile dementia in this country. It is a degenerative disease of the nervous system, meaning that the nerve cells in the brain start to malfunction and then degenerate and die. Alzheimer's disease is slow but progressive and wipes out many functions of the brain, especially memory. The heartbreaking tragedy of Alzheimer's disease is that it steals the person by taking away who they are. Over time, they do not know themselves or remember anything familiar from their past—not their family, their homes, their careers, or their life histories.

In the last ten years, there has been an explosion of Alzheimer's disease in this country—up to a ten-fold increase. We know Alzheimer's dementia is a disease of old age, as many as 30 percent of those over the age of eighty-five are suffering from this dementia. And we can anticipate Alzheimer's disease to reach epidemic proportions in the twenty-first century as more and more people reach their seventies, eighties, and nineties, and even their hundreds.

Signs and Symptoms

How can you know if someone is starting to suffer from Alzheimer's dementia? It can be tricky because there is such a *gradual* decline. The decline in cognitive function usually starts with memory loss. First, the ability to learn new material and recent, short-term memory start to go. There may be some language paucity, mild impairment in drawing or puzzles, and difficulty with higher functions such as planning and problem solving. The personality starts to change, with occasional irritable outbursts and sometimes apathy. But you can think to yourself that Grandma or Grandpa is just getting on in years and getting more forgetful or crankier.

As the disease progresses, memory becomes worse and the personality more flat. Constant restlessness and wandering without direction can start. If the doctor orders a CT scan of the brain at this later stage, there is fifty-fifty chance that it will start to show brain atrophy.

In the end, there is no memory, no trace of former personality, difficulty talking—in fact, difficulty making any sense with language. Intelligence is gone. Limbs become rigid. People at this stage develop poor sphincter control and become incontinent of urine and stool.

Diagnosis is made on clinical grounds. There is a short test doctors give called the Mini-Mental Status Exam (MMSE) that can provide some clues. It tests functions such as short-term memory, language skills, and perception. It is useful information for the doctor, but cannot be used to make a firm diagnosis of Alzheimer's. The head CT scan shows more definite atrophy, but only at the late stages of the disease. The definitive diagnosis is only by brain biopsy after death, although there is a lot of research now under way to find some way to make the diagnosis before death.

There is another disease that looks just like Alzheimer's disease on clinical grounds. It is called Lewy body disease, and researchers are finding that this disease is much more common than previously thought. The differences from Alzheimer's disease—and these are subtle distinctions—are that Lewy body disease patients are more psychotic with visual hallucinations and severe depression, and also have some features of Parkinson's disease.

At autopsy what the doctors see when they examine the brains are neurofibrillary tangles, senile plaques, cell loss, and impaired synaptic function. They find that cholinergic, noradrenergic, and dopaminergic cells in the brain are lost. It is believed that oxidative stress and the accumulation of free radicals leads to this nerve cell degeneration. Excessive lipid peroxidation seen in the brain is the cause of the nerve cell death.

Causes

According to Dr. Michael Wald, "There have been extensive studies of this condition, and certainly genetics plays some role." However, he remarks, "even though genetics plays a significant role in determining susceptibility to the condition, like most chronic degenerative diseases, environmental factors also play an extremely significant role."

In talking about causes of dementia, Dr. Wald mentions metabolic disorders such as vitamin B12 deficiency, folate deficiency, hypoglycemia (low blood sugar), and thyroid disease. He also enumerates environmental causes such as trauma, aluminum or silicon ingestion, and exposure to known neurotoxins such as pesticides, insecticides, and other chemicals from the environment in water, food, and air. All of these things cause free radical damage. Free radicals are highly reactive molecules that interfere with normal function of the body. Dr. Wald says, "As we age normally, free radicals increase that actually cause the aging, but in certain susceptible individuals, either genetically or environmentally, they've got too much aging in specific areas that result in these kinds of symptoms [of dementia]. In medicine they call it Alzheimer's or Parkinson's."

Dr. Wald explains his concern with aluminum ingestion. "With Alzheimer's disease, we really must focus on aluminum and metals in general. Aluminum specifically concentrates in an area of the brainstem causing neurofibrillary tangles. This is a type of defect that is characterized by Alzheimer's disease. Whether aluminum causes it or results from the formation of these neurofibrillary tangles no one quite knows, but in either case we want to make sure aluminum is removed. Basically this aluminum has a very strong affinity for the nervous system. The fact is that as we grow older, blood levels of aluminum increase, and studies of Alzheimer's patients show that they have higher aluminum levels than normal people without dementia or symptoms. It doesn't have to be high doses of aluminum. It could be very low, trace doses over a long period of time that cause oxidation in the brain, which in turn causes neurofibrillary tangles and all the symptoms."

So what are sources of aluminum that we want to eliminate? "Antacids commonly have aluminum. Drinking water has trace amounts of aluminum. Researchers have shown that trace amounts of aluminum from water—just that single source—immediately enter brain tissue. The frightening news is really that aluminum in water not only occurs naturally but is added to some water supplies. There is aluminum in deodorants, cooking pots and pans, aluminum foil. Certain nondairy creamers have aluminum, as does baking powder to keep the powder from becoming very lumpy when you mix it with fluid."

Dr. Wald explains that there are ways to decrease the body's aluminum absorption. "It can be chelated or removed with either intravenous chelation or oral chelating supplements," he says. "Calcium citrate prevents the absorption of aluminum. Aluminum absorption can be decreased, not just with calcium but with its partner magnesium. Magnesium, like calcium, competes with the aluminum for absorption. Probably people with Alzheimer's disease need much higher levels of calcium and magnesium. It's very important to supplement these on a daily basis. So if we are juicing every day, if we are taking our natural antioxidants and our natural chelaters, we will offset this accumulation over a lifetime."

Clinical Experience

CONVENTIONAL TREATMENT

There is currently very little that can be done by Western medicine to stop the progression of Alzheimer's disease. Several drugs are being used, mostly to treat the symptoms in mild to moderate cases. One drug given regularly is Aricept (donepezil). It has been shown to slow the rate of decline in early Alzheimer's disease. It is an acetylcholinesterase inhibitor. Its side effects are nausea, vomiting, and diarrhea, all because it increases cholinergic activity. A study published in 1997 in the *New England Journal of Medicine* showed that megadoses of vitamin E together with the drug Segeline slowed the progression of moderate Alzheimer's disease. A decade ago they gave a drug called Tacrine, but it caused so much liver toxicity that they had to stop.

ALTERNATIVE THERAPIES

Dr. Jay Lombard outlines a four-pronged approach for the treatment of Alzheimer's disease: "The broad headings for treating Alzheimer's have to do [number one] with reducing excessive inflammation. Number two is raising a neurotransmitter called acetylcholine, which is very vital to memory. Number three is reducing antioxidant activity. Free radicals appear to be very involved in Alzheimer's disease. Fourth is boosting the mitochondria. The mitochondria are the energy-producing units of the cell that make ATP [adenosine triphosphate, which is involved in the storage and transfer of cellular energy]." Dr. Lombard feels the mitochondria play an important role in neurological diseases such as Alzheimer's disease and Parkinson's disease, and that "increasing mitochondrial activity is a common theme in treating these diseases."

So what specifically does Dr. Lombard suggest? He says, "In regard to raising brain acetylcholine levels, there is a natural product that is currently available called hypericin A, which acts to block the enzyme that breaks down acetylcholine and therefore raises our brain acetylcholine levels. [It is] very effective in improving memory, and preliminary data in Alzheimer's will hopefully be available soon." Dr. Lombard also recommends ginkgo biloba, vitamin E, and melatonin. In addition, there is an analog of coenzyme Q10 and the amino acid acetyl-L-carnitine. Ignatia has also been shown in preliminary studies to be effective in raising brain ATP levels in Alzheimer's.

"Finally the last thing in Alzheimer's is looking at hormones, particularly estrogen and DHEA," Dr. Lombard says. "Estrogen is very effective in inhibiting an enzyme that is detrimental to Alzheimer's patients. Estrogen blocks that enzyme and therefore inhibits the production of these pathological proteins found in the brains of Alzheimer's patients. DHEA, a natural adrenal steroid, again may be effective in Alzheimer's disease."

Dr. Wald offers the following additional nutritional advice for Alzheimer's disease and dementia in general. Start by avoiding processed foods, milk and dairy products, and increasing consumption of vegetables, grains, nuts and seeds from organic sources. Avoid aluminum and the metals. Then, he says, "Take a high-potency mulitvitamin. Supplement that with vitamin C, between 500 and 3,000 milligrams three or more times a day; vitamin E, between 400 and 1,000 IU; and flaxseed oil. Flaxseed oil is needed for overall cell membrane health and nervous system repair, about a tablespoon a day. I also recommend thiamine (vitamin B1) 3 to 8 grams a day; phosphatidyl serine, about 100 milligrams three times a day; acetyl-L-carnitine, about 500 milligrams three times a day; vitamin B12, about 1,000 micrograms twice daily; and ginkgo biloba."

"The importance of thiamine or vitamin B1 in Alzheimer's disease," Dr. Wald says, "is that it has a profound effects on the brain. It actually mimics an important transmitter in the brain known as acetylcholine, which tends to be low in Alzheimer's patients."

He continues, "B12 deficiency is one of the more common deficiencies in the elderly to begin with. Up to 42 percent of people over age sixty-five are absolutely deficient in B12. A deficiency of that will cause every symptom of Alzheimer's disease—neurological and motor or muscular symptoms, plus impairing mental function."

Zinc deficiency is another common deficiency seen in the elderly. Dr. Wald suggests, "It could be a major factor in the development of Alzheimer's disease. There are many zinc-containing enzymes involved in cellular repair and DNA repair. Ineffective DNA and error-prone DNA can cause mental diseases. Zinc supplementation has been used with as little as 27 milligrams in a study of ten Alzheimer's patients, and only two failed to show remarkable improvements. I think that is pretty good."

Dr. Wald also recommends phosphatidyl choline. "To date there have been eleven double-blind, published studies that all reported success using phosphatidyl choline in Alzheimer's disease. People with anywhere from mild to moderate dementia using a very high quality phosphatidyl choline can expect some improvement. The doses are between 15 and 25 grams. If you don't see improvements within two weeks, it probably isn't going to work."

What role do hormones play? Dr. Wald remarks, "There have been twelve population-based studies indicating that women on hormone replacement therapy have a lower rate of Alzheimer's disease. If we need to do hormone balancing, we want to use natural hormones whenever possible and see what happens. Even these studies admit that these people were much healthier to begin with."

Dr. Wald has used DHEA, an adrenal hormone. "DHEA has been found to be low in the blood and brain of Alzheimer's patients. I have used between 25 and 50 milligrams per day in men and 15 to 25 in women with benefit."

In the October 1997 issue of the *Journal of American Medical Association,* a study concluded that ginkgo biloba stabilized and in some cases improved cognitive performance and social function for six months to a year. LeBars and colleagues, the authors of the study, stated that ginkgo may be as effective as any drug, hormone, or vitamin used to treat Alzheimer's. It is safe and inexpensive.

CHAPTER 27

OSTEOPOROSIS

M ore than 10 million Americans have osteoporosis. The disease is responsible for more than 1.5 million fractures a year. Osteoporosis (the word means "porous bones") is a serious problem in which the skeletal system weakens and fractures easily. It may be accompanied by pain, especially lower back pain, loss in height, and body deformity.

More females than males become afflicted, with postmenopausal women being at greatest risk. Osteoporosis is attributed to the gradual loss of calcium. In women, this loss begins in the mid-thirties at a rate of 1 to 2 percent a year, and can increase during menopause to a rate of 4 to 5 percent a year.

In the past, osteoporosis was thought to be an inevitable part of the aging process, particularly in women. Now most of us know that it is treatable and, more important, preventable.

CAUSES

According to naturopathic physician Dr. Jane Guiltinan, the most likely candidates for osteoporosis share a number of characteristics:

Northern European ethnic origin
Small frame
Family history of osteoporosis
Diet high in meat, caffeine, sugar, refined carbohydrates,
and phosphates (found in sodas and processed foods)
Cigarette smoking
Alcohol use
Sedentary lifestyle

It may surprise some people to learn that dairy foods, while rich sources of calcium, can also contribute to the condition of osteoporosis. Registered nurse and acupuncturist Abigail Rist-Podrecca notes, "When I was in China, we noticed that no dairy was used. We expected to see a high incidence of osteoporosis, rickets, and other bone problems. In fact, we saw the lowest incidence. In the West, dairy is used a lot and osteoporosis is rampant. Something is not quite right here." Three main factors responsible for the Chinese not getting osteoporosis, she learned, are diet, weight-bearing exercise, and acupuncture.

DIAGNOSIS

In the past, osteoporosis was not diagnosed until the condition was so advanced that patients began to break their bones. Today, however, bone mineral density testing is being used to detect the disease and those at risk for developing it. The National Osteoporosis Foundation recommends that every woman over the age of sixty-five have a bone density test. For people under sixty-five, the test is recommended if there are risk factors for fracture, such as excessive thinness, cigarette smoking, a previous fracture in adulthood, or a family history of fractures.

Bone density testing is noninvasive and takes only a few minutes to perform. It provides a measurement known as a T-score. T-scores can indicate normal bone density, low bone density, or osteoporosis.

CLINICAL EXPERIENCE

Conventional Approach

For people with T-scores below specific levels, conventional treatment involves the use of prescription medications. Synthetic estrogen is the traditional drug of choice for postmenopausal osteoporosis and its prevention, but controversy surrounds its safety and effectiveness.

Naturopathic Prevention and Treatment

The first step in osteoporosis prevention is noting whether or not you are at high risk for the condition, says Dr. Guiltinan. Obviously, certain risk factors cannot be changed, but many can be addressed, and will prevent the destructive effects of the disease.

DIET

A diet that is low in animal products and high in plant foods promotes bone growth and repair. Green, leafy vegetables contain vitamin K, beta carotene, vitamin C, fiber, calcium, and magnesium, which enhance the bones. Other calcium-rich foods include broccoli, milk, nuts, and seeds. Sesame seeds have high calcium content. The Chinese, who as mentioned earlier have low rates of osteoporosis, use sesame often in their foods, and cook with sesame seed oil.

Foods to avoid include sugar, caffeine, carbonated sodas, and alcohol, as these contribute to bone loss. Chicken, fish, eggs, and meat are also contraindicated. These are high in the amino acid methionine, which the body converts into homocysteine, a substance that causes both osteoporosis and atherosclerosis.

The official recommended dietary requirement for calcium for people at risk of osteoporosis is 1,000 to 1,300 milligrams per day. I recommend that women over twenty-five take in approximately 1,000 milligrams in supplement form and an additional 500 to 1,000 milligrams from the diet. For those over forty, supplements of 1,500 to 2,000 milligrams are needed. Women on estrogen replacement therapy require between 1,200 and 1,500 milligrams.

In addition to calcium, the following nutrients are critical for keeping bones strong:

> Magnesium (800–1,200 mg in citrate form)
> Vitamin D (400 IU)
> Vitamin C (1,000 mg)
> Vitamin K (100 mcg)
> Beta carotene
> Selenium (75–150 mcg)
> Boron (3 mg)
> Manganese (5 mg)
> Strontium
> Folic acid (1 mg)
> Silica
> Copper
> Zinc

A balanced vitamin/mineral supplement will provide most of these nutrients. It is best to take zinc separately, however. Otherwise, it can have an adverse effect on vitamin and mineral absorption.

NATURAL HORMONES

Research indicates that natural progesterone from wild yams is safer and more effective than estrogen in that it builds strong bones and has no harmful side effects. Dr. Jane Guiltinan notes, "Estrogen minimizes calcium loss from bones, but progesterone can actually put calcium back into bones." Natural progesterone can be taken in pill form. It also comes in a cream form.

Half a teaspoon should be rubbed into the skin over soft tissue and the spine, twice a day, for two weeks out of every month.

DHEA, a precursor to estrogen and testosterone, is important in the prevention of numerous chronic conditions associated with aging. As we get older, there is often a drop in DHEA. If blood levels are low, 5 milligrams a day can safely be taken as a supplement.

HERBS

Herbalist Susun Weed recommends horsetail, taken as a tea every day, to restore bone strength and density. She adds that dandelion root tincture will promote absorption of calcium. The micronutrients important for bone flexibility and strength are found in the greatest abundance in seaweeds, dandelion, and nettles, and in organic vegetables and grains.

EXERCISE

Dr. Howard Robins, former director of the Healing Center in New York City and coauthor of *Ultimate Training* and *How to Keep Your Feet & Legs Healthy for a Lifetime*, stresses the importance of weight-bearing aerobic and weight-lifting exercises for osteoporosis prevention.

Aerobic exercises use major muscle groups in a rhythmic, continuous manner. Weight-bearing aerobic exercises such as brisk walking, jogging, stair climbing, and dancing produce mechanical stress on the skeletal system, which drives calcium into the long bones. Non–weight-bearing aerobic exercises such as biking, rowing, and swimming are not as helpful in osteoporosis prevention, but they do promote flexibility, which is useful for people prone to arthritis.

People "need to perform aerobic exercises anywhere from three to five or six times a week," says Dr. Robins. "You need a day off every third or fourth day so that the body can heal and reenergize."

"Most women stay away from weight training because they are afraid of developing, huge muscles like Arnold Schwarzenegger," says Dr. Robins. "The good news is, that won't happen. No matter how hard she trains, a woman will never get huge muscles unless she takes steroids to alter her body's metabolism."

Not only is weight training safe, it is important for preventing osteoporosis. As muscles are pulled directly against the bone, with gravity working against it, calcium is driven back into the bones. It also stimulates the manufacture of new bone. This adds up to a decrease in the effects of osteoporosis by 50 to 80 percent. People need to do weight training two to three times per week for fifteen to thirty minutes. All the different muscle groups should be worked on. Twenty-four hours should lapse between sessions to rest muscles. For women, an exercise program should be started long before the onset of menopause.

A complete routine is more than aerobic and weight-training exercises only. It incorporates warm-ups at the beginning and cool-downs at the end of a routine. Warm-ups are not to be confused with stretches. Rather, they are gentle exercises that produce heat by getting blood to flow into the muscles. To warm up leg muscles, for example, one could lie down on one's back and move the legs like a bicycle, or walk gently in place. Moving the arms and joints gently in all their ranges of motion will warm up the upper body. Warming up the body helps prevent injuries.

After exercise, when the body is loosest, stretching is performed. Stretches are long, continuous pulls, not bounces. Bouncing only tightens the muscles and can lead to injury. Dr. Robins's book *Ultimate Training* describes a holistic workout in detail. Aromatherapist Ann Berwick adds that essential oils enhance a warm-up and cool-down routine. "Before exercise, use warming and stimulating oils, such as black pepper, rosemary, ginger, and sage. Additionally, eucalyptus helps to deepen breathing. After exercise, you can apply a blend of lemon, rosemary, and juniper. These help to carry away waste products and ease any stiffness."

YOGA

Yoga prevents osteoporosis by building and fortifying bone mass, keeping muscles strong and flexible, improving posture, and helping balance and coordination. Physical therapist and yoga teacher Bonnie Millen explains why this is important: "With yoga, the old adage 'Use it or lose it' applies. Building and maintaining bone mass is most important for preventing osteoporosis. Remember, bone is alive. Yoga is unique in that it incorporates weight bearing on the upper extremities. This is important because many wrist, forearm, and upper arm fractures occur when people reach forward with outstretched arms as they are falling.

"Also important is building and maintaining muscle strength and flexibility. Let's keep the muscles strong so that they can receive the stress before the fracture happens. Also if the body is strong and flexible, it can cushion falls when they occur."

What about posture? "Good posture improves overall functioning and prevents osteoporotic fractures of the spine," Millen says. "I teach yoga to a lot of older women who tell me they are afraid of getting a dowager's hump. This is where the body slouches forward and there is a hump on the back. Just take a moment to get into that posture where your chest caves in and your shoulders slump forward, with your head looking down toward the floor. Try to raise one arm up as if you wanted to touch the ceiling, and see how high the arm comes up. Now let the arm down and come into a nice seated posture, as if someone were going to take your picture. Sitting very tall, raise your arm up and see how high it goes. You can see from that little exercise that the slouched posture really decreases your range of motion. That makes it difficult to function. This is why you want to keep a good posture."

The dowager's hump can create additional problems. Millen explains: "By placing great pressure on the spinal vertebrae, the dowager's hump often leads to compression fractures of the spinal column. This is very painful, as you can well imagine, and you do not have to do anything special for it to happen. Just going up and down stairs or taking a step can cause breakage."

Yoga also helps to improve balance and coordination. "When you are balanced and coordinated, there is less chance of your falling in the first place," Millen says. "You are quicker to respond. And that can help prevent fractures."

Millen points out that there are several styles of yoga, but that all systems have foundation poses that address the above needs. Here she outlines a few basic postures:

DOWNWARD-FACING DOG—This posture strengthens bone mass in the wrists and arms. In this pose, you stand and bring your hands to the floor so that the space beneath you is triangular. One part of the triangle is from your hands to your hips, and the other part is from your hips to your heels. The space on the floor between your hands and your feet is the third part. As you hold the position, you will feel that you are bearing weight on your arms.

WARRIOR POSES—These poses increase muscle strength and flexibility as well as balance. Here you are standing with your legs 3 to 4 feet apart, depending on your height. With your legs apart, you work at the hip to turn one leg out to the side. The other leg is turned slightly inward. That really works the hip muscles, which is important in helping to prevent the all-too-common osteoporotic hip fracture. The arms are either held out to the side or up over the head, depending upon which warrior posture it is.

COBRA—This is a back-bending pose that helps posture and gives flexibility and strength to the paraspinals, the muscles of the back of the spine. To begin, lie facedown on the floor. Using the back muscles, sequentially lift the head and chest away from the floor.

SIMPLE STRETCH FOR CHEST MUSCLES—This is another exercise for improving posture that is especially helpful for women who tend to slouch forward. Take a blanket and fold it to resemble a box of long-stemmed roses. Lie down on this bolster, making sure that your head and your entire spine are completely supported. Place your arms out to the side or up to form a V-shaped position with the palms facing up toward the ceiling. Just allow gravity to relax the shoulders down to the floor. Shoulders should not be on the blanket. Breathe deeply. That will expand the intercostals, the muscles between the ribs. This is important because the intercostals become constricted with slouching. That, in turn, decreases lung capacity and causes all the organs to become compressed. This is a wonderful pose where you don't have to actually do anything. You just allow gravity to work for you and your breath to move through you.

Millen says that the best time to begin yoga is before osteoporosis sets in. "The time to begin a yoga practice, or any exercise, is not when you've gotten to menopause, and all of a sudden you realize, 'Oh my gosh! I'm at risk for osteoporosis.' You need to build bone mass throughout your whole life so that you have bone stored up. It's like preparing for retirement. You build up bone mass through exercise, you eat right, you maintain a healthy lifestyle. Then, when you reach your menopausal years, you've got a good store of bone mass to help protect you."

BODY ROLLING

This technique, developed by Yamuna Zake, a bodyworker in New York City, uses a 6- to 10-inch ball in a series of routines designed to elongate muscles and increase blood flow in all parts of the body. As you relax your body weight onto the ball, the ball applies pressure onto bone, stimulating even bone that has begun to ossify to "wake up." "To me," says Zake, "bone is like dried fruit. Just as a raisin plumps up after you put it in water, when bone is stimulated and becomes alive, it undergoes a subtle change, acquiring a supple quality.

"Studies have found that, by stimulating bone, weight-bearing exercise can prevent and possibly reverse osteoporosis. Weight bearing is nothing more than pressure exerted on bone. Body Rolling is actually a mild form of weight-bearing exercise in which the pressure is never more than the person's own body weight."

ACUPUNCTURE

As mentioned earlier in this chapter, in China, osteoporosis is the exception rather than the norm. When it is present, acupuncture is used. Acupuncturist Abigail Rist-Podrecca explains how this works: "The Chinese use an electrical stimulus along the spine. The electrical impulse actually helps the bone-stem cells, which are the reproductive cells of the bone, to reproduce, thereby strengthening the bone mass. It was very exciting to see this because we have some Western studies proving that peripheral stimulation by electricity, especially in the long bones in the leg, help this process also." She adds that women low in calcium need to take this supplement so that the body has the raw materials for making bones denser. When weight-bearing exercises are added, the benefits are remarkable.

HOMEOPATHY

Homeopathy can be used as an adjunct to the nutritional and lifestyle factors discussed above. Among the remedies to consider are the following:

CALCAREA PHOSPHORICA—This may help where the bones are weak, soft, curved, and brittle. It can be given for a long period of time.

CORTICOID—Homeopathic Corticoid is for painful posttraumatic osteoporosis, especially when it affects the hip. Consider this remedy for an elderly person who has fractured her hip because of osteoporosis.

PARATHYROID—For diffuse pain in the bones, especially the long bones. Walking is very painful. Often, there is pain in the ankles, hips, and knees.

Regarding the appropriate potencies for these substances, homeopathic physician Dr. Ken Korins says, "For acute conditions, meaning they come on suddenly, and they are very intense, use a 200c potency. That is a very dilute potency, but energetically speaking, it is very powerful. For more chronic conditions, where you will be giving the remedy for a longer period of time, you might want to start with 12c or 30c. In general, the remedies should be taken as three to four pellets placed under the tongue. Take them on an empty stomach. Wait fifteen to twenty minutes before or after eating. Avoid coffee and aromatic substances, such as mints, perfumes, and camphors, which can interfere with the remedies' effectiveness. Also, it is a good idea not to touch remedies with your hands because any residues from perfumes or other substances can interfere with their energetic properties."

CHAPTER 28

PREGNANCY

W hat we in the United States accept as the safest, most acceptable way to give birth is a historical anomaly—something that has existed for only seventy-five to a hundred years and is not practiced in the rest of the world. Suzanne Arms, an independent researcher and activist who has published seven books on pregnancy and women's health, including *Immaculate Deception, Breast Feeding,* and *Seasons of Change,* explains.

"In other parts of the world," she says, "childbirth is seen as a natural process. The only exceptions are areas where American obstetrics and neonatal approaches have been aggressively promoted and marketed. Many European countries and a growing number of Third World countries are gradually adopting these practices as they buy our wares, such as neonatal monitoring devices."

In the United States, the vast preponderance of women give birth in hospitals. They are led to believe, Arms explains, that the larger the hospital, the better the care. They are told that the more narrow the subspecialization training of their doctors, the safer the birth will be. So women don't want to go to a general practitioner (GP), but instead go to a perinatologist with a subspecialty in obstetrics. Says Arms, "Our home-birth rate in 1998 was 2.5 percent, the lowest in our history. Although we do have midwives in hospitals and birthing centers outside hospitals, and we do legally permit home births, fewer than 5 percent of births are done with these resources, even if we count births done with midwives in hospitals."

Most of the world—the United States being a large exception—sees the natural way of giving birth as the sanest and healthiest way to bring a child into the world. After examining the issue of natural childbirth and American attitudes toward it, this chapter will turn to the stages of pregnancy, certain things you must avoid to have a safe pregnancy, and the many things you can do to make pregnancy as healthy and uncomplicated as possible.

NATURAL CHILDBIRTH

One reason for the greater American preference for hospital births as compared to the rest of the world is that Americans have been led to believe you are risking the baby and the mother if you choose not to have a hospital birth. But, Arms points out, "If we look at the facts, we see this is not true." In the United States, there has been very little comparative study of the benefits of home delivery versus hospital births. "Therefore, to actually compare the safety of hospital and home births," she says, "we have to go to a place like England, where they have very good national statistics on births and they have commissioned studies to see which are the safer methods."

Back in the 1970s, a controversial study appeared called the Peel Report. It was used to support a belief among politicians that home birth should be outlawed. At the time, Marjorie Tew, a statistician who was not involved in the controversy but happened to be analyzing statistics in a number of epidemiological areas, noted flaws in the report. She restudied the statistics on home births and found these births were as safe as hospital births. This was true not only for low-risk women—those who enter the process in a healthy state—but even for those with problems.

As a result of these findings, England has reversed its policy, which had been focused on eliminating home births and getting rid of midwifery. The country has gone back to supporting midwives, birthing centers, and local home births. They are finding that hospitals are not the best place to give birth. "In fact," Arms concludes, "there is no study that shows a hospital is a safer place than alternative venues for giving birth."

One aspect of women's fear of birth is that they think it will be unendurably painful. So, in many cases, they fill themselves with painkillers before the process even begins.

Arms recognizes this tendency. She says, "Those who advocate natural childbirth are often asked, 'Why should modern women experience painful childbirth rather than benefit from the painkillers modern medicine provides?'"

The issue of pain is a complex one, in her view. "Our media tell us that we should be free of any pain and discomfort in our lives. If you look at TV advertising, billboards, and so on, you see there are a tremendous number of products geared to the elimination of the pain that occurs in pathological conditions. We are taught we shouldn't have to experience pain. Since we are used to taking drugs for everything else, why not for labor? But childbirth is not a pathology and the cause of pain during birth is not a disease."

In addition, the potential problems caused by drugs and anesthesia need to be addressed. Drugs and anesthesia can distort and warp the birth process and make it harder for the baby to do the work he or she is supposed to do. They can complicate labor and make birth a pathological problem, something that we do, in fact, need to treat in the hospital.

WHAT IS MIDWIFERY?

The most important difference between midwifery and traditional medicine is that medicine treats disease, whereas midwifery is about preventing complications while going through a natural process. Obstetrics, a subspecialty of medicine, seems to consider birth "too unwieldy." Doctors need to get in and out of the hospital quickly, so they want to control the length of time a woman is in labor and how long it takes to give birth. However, the natural variability of giving birth does not conform to their standard. Each human body is unique, as is each human psyche. A four-hour labor may be normal. A thirty-six-hour labor may also be normal. But under a physician's management, a day and a half is too long.

Medicine focuses on giving drugs and doing surgery. Midwifery concentrates on following through the process normally, spotting problems as they arise and treating them as simply as possible before they become complications, while teaching people how to handle contingencies.

Midwife Jeanette Breen is a great enthusiast of using water during labor: "It has a wonderful analgesic quality, which is much better than an epidural. Being immersed in water provides tremendous relaxation. It does not take the pain away, but women do report feeling less pain in the water. They feel less effect from the pull of gravity. Their movements are very easy, and there is much better tissue relaxation, which means there is almost no tearing in a water birth. It is also easier for the baby because the mother is more relaxed and moving freely. She is not stuck in one position. It is easier for the baby to negotiate the pelvis and to slip out into a warm, moist environment that is quite familiar.

"Two keys to a normal healthy pregnancy and birth are a healthy diet and good social support," says Breen. "Those seem to be overlooked, especially in traditional maternity care in this country. The focus is on diagnostic testing, but not a lot of emphasis is placed on healthy diets, other than prescribing prenatal vitamins and iron. There is no question that a high-quality diet rich in all the nutrients can make a woman's whole body work more efficiently and effectively.

"Social support creates an environment of love that is all-important, but too often overlooked in hospital birthing environments, which focus solely on technology. No one can have the baby for the pregnant woman; she has to do it herself. But if she is surrounded by love and support rather than fear and technology, she is able to give birth in a very intuitive, instinctual way which is satisfying and safe."

STAGES OF PREGNANCY

A woman's body undergoes numerous changes during each stage of pregnancy. These physiological changes are described by nurse practitioner and massage therapist Susan Lacina.

First Trimester

"The fetus grows rapidly, and the mother's body changes to support this swift development. Hormonal balance changes. Human chorionic gonadotropin hormone (HCG) is needed for development. As it is released, it causes many discomforts, such as breast tenderness, digestive problems, nausea, and vomiting. Progesterone levels increase and may cause mild hyperventilation, heartburn, indigestion, and constipation. Increased blood flow and its change in composition contribute to fatigue, overheating, and sinus congestion."

Second Trimester

"The placenta takes over the hormone production, and the levels of HCG drop. Along with that, the discomforts of nausea and vomiting ease up. Physical growth of the fetus crowds the abdomen, and a woman's body expands to accommodate the growth. Fetal production of thyroid stimulating hormone (TSH) begins in the fourteenth week and causes the mother's thyroid level to increase. This can lead to irritability, mood swings, mild depression, increased pulse rate, and hot flashes. Adrenal hormones become elevated and remain that way until delivery. This may cause impaired glucose tolerance and swelling.

"Skeletal structure becomes softer and more flexible to allow for expansion. If a woman doesn't have enough muscle flexibility, she will have some pain, for tight muscles do not allow for these adjustments. She may experience sciatic nerve pain from the lower back down the back of her legs due to the extension of the pelvis, especially at the joint of the sacrum and the pelvic bone. The growing baby puts pressure on the inferior vena cava, which can cause light-headedness, nausea, drowsiness, and clamminess. Prolonged reduction of blood flow can cause backaches and hemorrhoids. Lying on the side decreases this problem.

"From the twentieth week on, the uterus expands by stretching muscle fibers. Abdominal muscles and ligaments stretch to support the uterus, and there may be abdominal pain. There is an increase in melanin production, causing darkening of the nipples and a line called the linea nigra down the abdomen. If the lymph drainage system is not functioning well, an excess of melanin in the skin can cause brown spots. A well-functioning lymph drainage system is believed to keep melanin levels down so that brown spots do not occur. Increased progesterone causes sinus congestion, postnasal drip, and bleeding gums. Increased capillary permeability may cause the hands and feet to swell."

Third Trimester

"As the baby continues to grow, the expectant mother changes her posture to shift her center of gravity. Heavier breasts can cause shoulders to slump forward. The spine is pulled out of alignment, and this commonly causes backaches. The growing fetus also compresses the veins and the lymphatic system. That can cause ankle edema and varicose veins. There is increased pressure on the intestines and bladder, causing frequent urination and constipation. Pressure on the sciatic nerve can cause more lower back and leg pain. As the diaphragm starts to rise, breathing becomes more difficult. Insomnia is common."

MISCARRIAGE

Surprisingly, two-thirds of all pregnancies end up as miscarriages. One reason is that many women miscarry before they even know they are pregnant. Most commonly, genetic abnormalities precipitate the problem. The embryo develops wrongly, and the woman's body naturally aborts the fetus. Endocrine system imbalances are also associated with miscarriages. Women in their late forties have an especially difficult time carrying to term because of hormonal changes that accompany aging. Poor thyroid gland functioning can also interfere with pregnancy, as can intercourse during pregnancy.

Another cause of miscarriages is low-grade infections, which are often the result of sexually transmitted diseases. The woman is not conscious that a problem exists, but the body knows, and rejects the fetus. Bladder infections are also common; as the uterus enlarges, it places great pressure on this organ. Miscarriages may also occur when women are too hard on their bodies. Women who push themselves to the limit by overexercising and undereating to the point of anorexia are risking miscarriage. They are not getting enough nutrition for their own bodies, much less for the fetus.

When a miscarriage occurs more than once, a woman needs to have a thorough medical workup. Once the problem is understood, it is often correctable. If a woman is having intercourse during pregnancy, for example, she may simply need to take precautions. Using a condom during intercourse can prevent a miscarriage because it keeps male prostaglandins out of the female system, which, in turn, prevents premature uterine contractions. Low-grade infections must be cleared up, and increasing the intake of liquids and vitamin C can sometimes do the trick. Mixing 4 ounces of strawberry juice with 4 ounces of water is an especially good source of vitamin C, which acidifies the urine and helps prevent bladder infections. More serious infections should be cultured and treated appropriately. Sometimes, this means taking antibiotics. Older women who are having a difficult time holding on to a pregnancy due to hormonal changes may need low doses of progesterone, about 25 milligrams, in suppository form.

Some herbs seem to prevent miscarriage. Midwife Jeanine Parvati Baker uses the following formula. She mixes together 1 ounce wild yam root, 1 ounce Mitchella repens (also called partridgeberry, twinberry, squawvine or partridge root). Baker also adds 1/2 ounce false unicorn root and 1/2 ounce cramp bark. She puts them together in a half-gallon jar, fills it to the top with boiling water, and lets it sit for about four hours. You can sip this brew slowly until you are over the symptoms of miscarriage or, if you are just worried about your pregnancy, drink a half cup each day.

HEALTHY PREGNANCY THE NATURAL WAY

What to Avoid During Pregnancy

Before describing the positive steps you can take to make your pregnancy, labor, and time after delivery as healthy as possible, I want to note some things, a few of which are normally benign, that you should avoid.

Susun Weed is an herbalist and teacher with more than thirty years of experience. She has written four books on herbal medicine, including *Wise Woman Herbal for the Childbearing Year*. According to Weed, it is well known that the health of a baby's parents affects the health of the baby. If the mother has an overgrowth of candida, so may the child. If the father is a heavy drinker, this may cause liver problems for the child. During the first two months after conception, women and their fetuses are the most sensitive to toxins, hair dyes, aspirin, and so on. Thus it is of paramount importance that a woman be aware of what things can have a detrimental effect on her growing fetus.

HIGH HEAT

Drawing from her store of knowledge of American Indian lore, Weed tells us, "First of all, we need to be very aware of something that may come up before a woman is even aware that she is pregnant—because, of course, we are pregnant for two weeks before we miss that first period—which is that high heat during these first few weeks can permanently damage the fetus." This heat may come from a hot bath, a sauna, or even a sweat lodge. This is one reason why, she elaborates, "in many native American traditions, women in their fertile years do not go into the sweat lodge."

CERTAIN VITAMIN SUPPLEMENTS

Women must also be careful about taking vitamin supplements. Women who take 10,000 units of vitamin A during the first six weeks of pregnancy are five times more likely to have a child with birth defects than women who don't take the vitamin. "I believe that during her fertile years a woman should be quite cautious about taking supplements," Weed says. "Of course, we want to get those good vitamins, but we want to try to get them from our fruits, our vegetables, our beans, and so on."

It is not only vitamin A that can lead to birth defects; vitamins D and E are also potentially dangerous. "Those three are oil-soluble vitamins," says Weed, "and they tend to be quite detrimental to fetal development when taken in pill form."

CERTAIN MEDICATIONS AND HERBAL THERAPIES

Avoid aspirin and certainly antihistamines. This last is a hard one, especially for women who are dealing with hay fever. Antihistamines have a fairly tarnished record when it comes to causing birth defects, Weed says. "I don't just mean drug antihistamines but herbal ones as well, such as ma huang or ephedra."

Laxatives are not the way to go. Unfortunately many people use them and, even worse, many misguided herbalists even suggest women use them to clean out. Of course, there's nothing to clean out. All laxatives, Weed believes, should be avoided by all people, but especially by women during their fertile years, or at least if they are having a baby or trying to get pregnant. This includes herbal laxatives like senna, aloe, castor oil, rhubarb root, buckthorn, and cascara sagrada. Even a bulk-producing laxative like flaxseed should be taken with some caution. To use it, buy the whole flaxseed, grind it up, and sprinkle a small amount into foods.

Generally, you should stay away from diuretics. A woman in her fertile years usually doesn't take them anyway, but anyone inclined to take diuretics should be aware that they could cause problems. Herbal diuretics such as juniper berries and buchu can also cause problems. Avoid hair dyes, all kinds of chemical stimulants and depressants, antinausea drugs, sulfa drugs, vaccines, and anesthetics, especially at the dentist's office.

Weed notes, "There is some question about what happens if we take steroidlike herbs. The more we look into steroids, the more widely we find them spread across the herbal kingdom. As a matter of fact, carrots, the regular carrots you find in the supermarket, contain so many phytohormones that generous use of carrots may prevent conception. We know that wild carrot seed, in fact all parts of the carrot plant, act to prevent contact between the egg and the sperm and prevent that egg from attaching to the uterine wall. So we often advise pregnant women to avoid drinking any carrot juice at all and to cut back on the amount of carrots they are eating."

There are a few other herbs that you need to avoid only if you have miscarried frequently. "Some women get very concerned about miscarriage," Weed states. "If you are concerned, there are some herbs normally used in cooking that you would do well to avoid during the first trimester of pregnancy. Don't go overboard in worrying about them; they will not harm the fetus, but they might, in a highly susceptible woman, cause uterine contractions." They include many herbs in the mint family, such as basil, thyme, sage, rosemary, marjoram, savory, and peppermint itself. The entire family of herbs in the carrot family, such as celery seed, parsley, cumin, coriander seed, aniseed, and fennel seed may cause problems for the sensitive woman. Ginger, nutmeg, and saffron have been used to cause a fetus to leave the uterus. Of course, to achieve that effect, they must be taken in enormous quantities, but for a very sensitive woman, it is best to avoid even small amounts in foods for the first trimester.

One other herb that Weed thinks is especially important for pregnant women to avoid completely is goldenseal. She tells us, "I've been an herbalist for thirty-five years, and I've never once had the opportunity to use goldenseal. Where I live, the native people used to give it to their enemies in order to torture them."

OTHER THINGS TO AVOID

It won't surprise you to learn that smoking and drinking are not good for your fetus. Radiation is not good, so even a mammogram should be avoided during pregnancy or if you think you are going to get pregnant. Caffeine in any form should be avoided. Coffee and latte, tea, and many soft drinks contain generous amounts of caffeine, and all can cause birth defects. Nutritionist Gracia Perlstein also says to avoid chemical exposure to toxic household cleansers, as well as fumes from paints, thinners, solvents, wood preservatives, varnishes, glues, spray adhesives, benzene, dry cleaning fluid, anything chemically based and questionable.

Perlstein also counsels women to avoid a toxic psychological environment. "As much as possible, avoid stress, negative people, and aggravating situations. Instead, try to spend quality time alone and with loved ones, people who are supportive. Spend time in nature. Read inspiring literature. Listen to beautiful music. This has a beneficial effect on your mental and emotional state. That, in turn, affects your baby's biochemistry."

Diet

The best insurance for a well baby is to follow a highly nutritious whole-foods diet. What you eat now will impact the health of your child later, according to nutritionist Gracia Perlstein. "When a woman is considering pregnancy, it is important that she address her diet to see how healthful it is, as many difficulties have their root in prenatal deficiencies. Scientific studies reveal that birth defects, and even problems that develop much later in life, can be prevented when the mother has excellent nutrition. I would like to include the father there too, because the quality of the sperm is also very important." Since the most crucial stage of embryonic development occurs in the first few weeks, before a woman realizes that she is pregnant, good-quality foods should be eaten all the time.

Eating properly means selecting unprocessed or minimally processed foods. A wide assortment of whole grains, legumes, vegetables, fruits, nuts, and seeds supplies multiple nutrients. "So many people eat the same ten or twenty foods over and over again," Perlstein says. "In traditional cultures, people have much more variety. I would like to emphasize that supplements should only enhance an excellent diet. Make the effort to eat high-quality, nutrient-dense foods. That means whole foods, the way nature produced them."

The body intuitively knows what it needs to support new life, and paying attention to its messages can be a helpful guide. "A woman's body is very wise when she is pregnant. Many women can't stand the look or smell of coffee or cigarettes, even when they used to smoke or drink coffee several times a day," states Perlstein. She adds that worrying about eating the right foods all the time is stressful and can produce more harm than good. But nutrition education can benefit women with highly processed diets, who need to learn about better food choices. "Vegetarian women may crave animal foods or be drawn to dairy when they are pregnant. Usually it is good to pay attention to these cravings, but to respond in the most wholesome way possible."

Wholesome means organically grown. Pesticide-free fare is better for everyone, of course, but vitally important for young children and developing fetuses, according to recent research. Dairy and other animal products should be from creatures naturally raised. One reason for this is that pesticides and other contaminants tend to concentrate in an animal's tissues. The higher up the food chain, the higher the concentration of toxins. Fortunately, many health food stores, and more and more supermarkets, sell the healthful varieties.

Animal products, when a part of the diet, should be eaten in moderation. Although protein needs increase during pregnancy, they can be easily met from vegetarian sources, which are less toxic than their animal counterparts. Excellent vegetarian protein sources include fortified soy milk, tofu, tempeh, beans, nuts, and seeds, for example.

The increased need for calcium is similarly fulfilled in such a diet. "Many women do not realize that there are excellent sources of calcium other than milk and dairy. There are green leafy vegetables, fortified soy milk, tofu, almonds, and many other calcium-containing foods. If you eat a diet rich in fresh vegetables and fruits, you tend to get quite a bit of calcium. If you want a supplement, calcium citrate is easiest on the stomach. Other forms sometimes cause digestive upsets or constipation. Definitely avoid calcium-depleting foods: coffee, chocolate, and sodium."

Perlstein adds that eating several small meals throughout the day offsets common complications: "Hunger, not calorie counting, is the most reliable guide to eating during pregnancy. Five to six small, nutrient-dense meals per day is a sensible ideal. This is a good habit to develop in the last trimester of pregnancy, when the organs in your stomach are somewhat constricted, and good in the early stages to prevent nausea. It keeps the blood sugar from falling, and nausea has a lot to do with low blood sugar."

Water should be pure and taken in adequate amounts. Eight to twelve glasses are recommended to help flush out toxins from the liver and kidneys: "Many people do not drink enough fluids," notes Perlstein. "This is especially important during pregnancy because the woman is filtering the waste for two bodies."

Vitamin Supplements

Perlstein recommends the following daily nutrients for pregnant women: multiple vitamin and mineral supplement, vitamin C, B12, zinc, and folic acid. Folic acid, which is also contained in green leafy vegetable and whole grains, is especially important in pregnancy because science has shown it to prevent neural tube defects. Even when included in the diet, extra folic acid should be taken in supplement form, since it is fragile and easily damaged by heat. Additionally, acidophilus helps prevent constipation and other types of colon problems.

Extra iron may be needed, but a woman should have her hemoglobin tested first, just to be sure it is really needed. Research shows that excess iron in the system can have damaging effects.

Herbs

Susun Weed has a number of herbal recommendations for pregnant women:

RED RASPBERRY TONIC—Tonics are herbal preparations that keep your body in good trim, up and running for optimum performance and healthy living. Weed's recommendations for tonics start with red raspberry. "It is probably the best known, the most widely used, and the safest of all pregnancy tonics."

To prepare red raspberry tonic, buy dried red raspberry leaves in bulk. Weigh 1 ounce in a quart jar, preferably a canning jar. If you don't have a scale, fill your jar about one-third full. Pour boiling water right to the top of the jar, cover it tightly, and let it steep for four hours or longer. Weed says: "Actually what I do is put up a nice infusion before I go to sleep at night. Then the next morning, it's ready for me. I strain the plant material, squeezing it to get the last of the good stuff out. Give that plant material back to the earth. The liquid is what I drink. I can heat it up, drink it at room temperature, or pour it over ice. Whatever I don't drink right then, I refrigerate and drink up within the next thirty-six to forty-eight hours." A quart a day of red raspberry tonic is usually not too much.

This tonic increases fertility in both men and women. It helps prevent miscarriage and hemorrhaging during the birth. It's one of the best herbs to ease morning sickness, and it helps provide a safe, fast birth, reducing pain during labor. It reduces afterbirth pains, helps bring down undelivered placenta, and increases the amount and quality of breast milk. The rich concentration of vitamin C, vitamin E, carotenes, vitamin A, calcium, iron, the B-vitamin complex, and the large amounts of phosphorus and potassium make taking red raspberry well worth it.

STINGING NETTLE TONIC—Another tonic for early pregnancy is stinging nettle, which is one of the most nutrient-rich substances available. It is loaded with carotenes, from which we make vitamin A; vitamins C, E, and D; the B vitamins; vitamin K; and calcium, potassium, phosphorous, and immune-strengthening sulfur.

Make a tonic the same way as for raspberry. Weigh out 1 ounce of the dried herb, put it in a jar, fill the jar with boiling water, then tightly lid it and steep overnight. You can drink it warm, cold, or in between, up to four cups a day. The chlorophyll in this brew is so high that the infusion will actually look black rather than green.

Nettle is tremendously nourishing. It eases leg cramps and any other muscle spasms during pregnancy. Because of nettle's high calcium content, it diminishes labor pains and birth pains. It is such a superb source of vitamin C that it is one of the world's most highly favored herbs for preventing hemorrhaging after birth. It's a wonderful way to reduce hemorrhoids. It can increase the amount and richness of your breast milk. Stinging nettle tonic can also help pregnant women who have fatigue, moodiness, and preeclampsia.

DANDELION AND OTHER HERBS—Dandelion is also good for mood swings. You can take it in any form. You'll probably find dandelion root tincture in any health food store. The usual dosage is 10 to 20 drops, taken before meals, in the morning, and just before you go to bed—a total of five times a day.

Dandelion leaves, especially when eaten as a cooked green, provide tremendous amounts of potassium, calcium, and good-quality vegetable salt. They can even be used as a remedy for a woman who already has preeclampsia.

Here are a few more suggestions about herbs: Ginger is one of the best natural remedies for nausea. Ginger works best when the person taking it eats small, frequent meals and gets plenty of fresh air and rest. Ginger can be taken as a capsule or tea. A washcloth soaked in ginger or comfrey tea and applied to the area where an episiotomy has been performed promotes healing. Rosemary added to bath water relieves tension and back pain. Finally, adding jasmine and clary sage to a bath has an uplifting effect and prevents postpartum depression.

Massage

Susan Lacina tells why a pregnant woman and her unborn child benefit greatly from massage: "We tend to think of a baby in utero as being cut off from the world," she says. "In reality, the child within is a conscious being who responds to sounds, emotions, and the inner environment that its mother creates, either through her sense of well-being or through her lack of it." Here Lacina describes how maternity massage promotes a comfortable and healthy pregnancy:

"Research shows that prolonged stress builds up abnormal levels of toxins and chemicals in the bloodstream. These are passed through the placenta to the baby. Minimizing the buildup of toxins can be achieved by periodic deep relaxation. Relaxation increases the absorption of oxygen and nutrients by the cells of the muscles. When oxygen and nutrition increase, the woman has more energy. Some doctors also believe morning sickness and nausea are eliminated by lowering stress levels.

"Massage assists the lymphatic system in eliminating excessive toxins and hormones. Unlike the heart, the lymphatic system has no pump. It moves freely until muscles tighten up, but when muscles become too tense, either from the fetus or from stress, lymph movement decreases and the concentration of toxins rises. In the lower extremities, the growing uterus can inhibit lymph drainage, leading to swelling, varicose veins, hemorrhoids, and fluid retention. By relaxing the muscles, massage helps stimulate lymphatic drainage of toxins. It decreases the development of varicose veins by its draining effect and helps reduce swelling in the legs."

Massage also helps with overall muscle tone and elasticity. "A woman's body must expand to accommodate the growing fetus," Lacina says. "Hips widen and abdominal, lower back, and shoulder muscles stretch. Legs must accommodate increased weight. Massage promotes flexible muscles, joints, ligaments, and tendons. It also helps decrease muscle spasms and leg cramps by getting rid of lactic acid buildup, and can alleviate the pain caused by sciatic nerve pressure. Added flexibility helps the muscles that are needed for labor."

In addition, massage assists in hormonal balance. "Massage balances the entire glandular system. An overactive thyroid gland becomes less active, thereby decreasing irritability, mood swings, and hot flashes. An underactive thymus gland is stimulated, which increases its ability to fight infection. The alternating relaxation and stimulation that massage provides helps a woman's body function in a more balanced manner."

Lacina describes the benefits of a peroneal massage. "This is a gentle stretch of tissues in the area between the vagina and rectum. Learning peroneal massage increases the mother's awareness of the muscles she needs to relax during the actual delivery and decreases her chances of having an episiotomy, an incision made to enlarge the vaginal opening at the time of birth.

"The actual procedure is as follows: Using warm vitamin E or vegetable oil, the mother places clean, oiled thumbs or index fingers an inch to an inch and a half inside the vagina and applies firm, gentle pressure downward and outward. Stretching continues until a burning sensation is felt. This is held for a few minutes. Performing this once or twice a day, up until the time of delivery, can result in an easier birth."

What about during labor and the postpartum period? "Massage during labor helps to reduce pain and anxiety by offering relief from muscle contractions." Lacina says. "The stimulation of certain acupressure points can speed up labor.

"Postpartum is the name given to the six-week recovery period after birth. During this time, hormones readjust and the uterus involutes (returns to its prepregnancy size). Massaging the abdomen in a circular motion helps the uterus to contract and helps to expel blood. Massage also helps to stimulate milk flow. The following techniques can be applied for this purpose: The pressure point at the base of the sacrum can be held for about fifteen seconds, and then released. Breast massage is another technique that can be used. Using some light oil, a woman circles her breasts with her fingertips. She places the hands flat on the breasts, starting at the nipple, and moves outward and up. That helps the glands to release milk. Additionally, there is an acupressure point at the top and middle of the shoulder. Holding it for fifteen seconds helps milk production. Pressing the point between the sixth and seventh ribs at the nipple level on the breast bone helps to release milk."

Acupressure Points

Thumbs can be applied to the sacrum, at the bottom of the spine, and walked up the spine to the waist. Each point is held for about five seconds.

The point in the center of the buttocks is pressed in as the mother exhales and released as she inhales.

Thumbs can be pressed along the shoulder blades between the spine and the scapula.

On the legs, pressure can be applied to Spleen 6, an acupressure point located approximately 3 inches above the ankle, on the inside of the leg right below the tibia bone. Holding this spot for ten seconds and then releasing it helps to stimulate uterine contractions and speeds up labor.

The uterus point is on the inside of the foot, just under the ankle bone. The ovary point is on the outside of the foot, under the ankles, near the heel. Squeezing these points at the same time for about ten seconds and then releasing them helps to speed up labor.

Breast and nipple stimulation helps create oxytocin, the hormone that helps the uterus to contract.

Alexander Technique

The Alexander technique differs from massage in that the pregnant woman is actively engaged. Kim Jessor, an Alexander teacher, makes an analogy to a piano lesson: "We talk about being Alexander teachers, the people who come to us are students, and the context is a lesson. So while the results are very therapeutic, I don't think of the work as a therapy but rather as a learning process. This is significant in that it empowers students to take charge in changing their movement habits."

The Alexander technique is based on the concept that all of us know how to move comfortably as children, but lose that natural flexibility over time. The method teaches people how to move freely again, which is especially valuable for women undergoing the stresses of pregnancy.

Jessor describes some of the ways the Alexander technique helps women during and after pregnancy: Lower back pressure is relieved, breathing improves, rest is enhanced, labor is eased, stamina increases after delivery, and breast-feeding is easier. In addition, there are less tangible, but equally valuable, benefits from working with the Alexander technique during pregnancy. "Women begin to realize that they can make different kinds of choices about the kind of birth they want to have, where they want to have it, and who they want to use for labor support. In the same way that they begin to find freedom in movement, they find greater options in terms of the choices they make about their pregnancy."

Exercise

The American College of Gynecologists and Obstetricians (ACOG) endorses physical activity during pregnancy and has created specific guidelines for the dos and don'ts of exercise:

Pregnant women derive health benefits from a mild to moderate exercise routine. Exercising sixty minutes, three times per week, is preferable to intermittent activity, but some benefit can be derived from shorter durations as well. Sometimes little oxygen is available for aerobic exercise due to the body's increased oxygen demands. Therefore, a woman should begin an aerobic activity slowly, and gradually build to capacity. She should not push too hard, and certainly not to the point of breathlessness. Pregnant women should not exercise in the faceup position after the first trimester. This position limits blood supply to the baby.

Avoid standing for prolonged periods of time, doing heavy work in the standing position, and exercising at high intensities. These activities are associated with diminished birthweight in newborns. It's better for women to engage in non–weight-bearing activities such as cycling and swimming, rather than exercises like running. Non–weight-bearing exercise minimizes the risk of injury and allows activity levels to remain closer to prepregnancy levels, right up to delivery. A woman should be aware that her center of gravity is different, and that she might lose her balance when exercising. Anything that could involve falling over, or even mild abdominal trauma, should be avoided.

Pregnant women require an extra 300 calories per day in order to maintain their normal metabolic rate. Exercise increases the need for more calories.

A pregnant woman must be careful not to raise her body temperature with vigorous workouts, especially in the first trimester. Excessive body heat in the mother can adversely affect the development of brain tissue in the baby. The threshold for this is a body temperature of about 39.2 degrees Celsius, which is 100 or 101 degrees Fahrenheit.

When should a pregnant woman not exercise? "Basically, every pregnant woman can benefit from starting an exercise program at any point in pregnancy. However, there are certain exceptions to this rule. When any one of the following conditions is present, a pregnant woman should limit or avoid exercise: pregnancy-induced hypertension, premature rupture of membranes, incompetent cervix, persistent second- or third-trimester bleeding, premature labor during the prior or current pregnancy, and intrauterine growth retardation."

Other medical contraindications include thyroid, heart, vascular, or pulmonary conditions. Women with medical problems need a physician's evaluation to determine whether an exercise program is appropriate.

Aromatherapy

Ann Berwick reports that in Europe, where aromatherapy is scientifically studied and widely prescribed, hospital maternity wings utilize essential oils for their soothing and uplifting mind-body effects: "There is a report of one woman who had severe anxiety throughout her pregnancy. They gave her neroli oil, which helped to keep her blood pressure down and allowed her to go into delivery in a more relaxed state. During delivery, she was given lavender and clary sage to relax her uterus. Clary sage is also slightly euphoric, so it helped her to cope mentally with the birth." Here are some formulas to try before, during, and after birth:

As an antidote for nausea and vomiting, peppermint oil is effective when a very dilute amount is rubbed into the stomach or inhaled.

For relaxation, 8 ounces vegetable oil, 13 drops lavender, 2 drops geranium, and 10 drops sandalwood can be massaged into the skin or used as a compress.

To clear nasal congestion, a teaspoon of eucalyptus oil can be added to a cold-air humidifier or pan of hot water. The steam inhaled reduces congestion.

To help heartburn, place 2 to 3 drops of diluted peppermint oil on the back of the tongue.

A good massage oil to use during labor consists of 5 drops rose, 12 drops clary sage, and 5 drops ylang-ylang in 2 to 3 ounces vegetable oil.

To prevent stretch marks, massage 2 ounces wheat germ oil, 20 drops lavender, and 5 drops neroli oil into the thighs.

To soothe sore nipples, mix 1 pint cold water, 1 drop geranium, 1 drop lavender, and 1 drop rose oil.

After an episiotomy, a sitz (shallow) bath is helpful, especially when 2 drops cyprus and 4 drops lavender oil are added. Soak for fifteen to twenty minutes.

To promote milk production, take 2 drops fennel oil with some honey water, every 2 hours.

Hemorrhoids will be helped by 5 drops cyprus oil added to the bath.

The astringent action of cyprus and lemon oil constricts varicose veins. A few drops can be added to a body lotion and applied to the veins morning and evening.

Homeopathy

Homeopathic physician Stephanie Odinov Pukit lists a variety of remedies for all stages of pregnancy. She begins with treatments for morning sickness.

SEPIA—Ambivalence is the key word here. There is a conflict between self-preservation and the urge to procreate, which makes wanting a child questionable. The woman becomes angry and irritable and feels as if a black cloud hovers over her. Although her appetite is insatiable, heavy pains worsen with smells or thoughts of food.

PULSATILLA—This is the opposite scenario. Pulsatilla is an excellent remedy for the woman who is cheerful, sweet, and somewhat helpless. The person is warm and may throw the covers off at night. She becomes worse with emotional excitement. Nausea comes and goes and is characteristically worse in early evening.

NUX VOMICA—This is a wonderful remedy for soothing the nerves after a woman has abused her body with alcohol, drugs, or coffee. She tends to be constipated. She tends to wake up at night to think about business because she is ambitious and driven.

ARSENICUM—The picture here is a person constantly anxious about her state of health. She always runs to the doctor fearing that something is wrong. The woman tends to have burning pains. She has great thirst and takes little sips. Symptoms are usually exacerbated at midnight.

COCCULUS INDICUS—This remedy specifically helps motion sickness. The woman tends to lose sleep and to be constantly exhausted. She may be nursing children or caring for someone. The woman feels dizzy standing and better when lying down. She feels worse in fresh air.

PETROLEUM—Petroleum may be indicated if there is a voracious appetite followed by persistent vomiting.

BRYONIA—The person has strong sensitivity to smells and may have connective tissue and arthritic problems. Nausea becomes worse with motion.

Dr. Odinov Pukit suggests the following remedies for problems that occur in the latter stages of pregnancy:

SEPIA OR PULSATILLA—In the third to sixth month, the fetus presses high up in the abdomen, causing heartburn, shortness of breath, and indigestion. These remedies also help hemorrhoid problems. The one chosen depends on the other symptoms manifested. Sepia is for a gloomy disposition, while pulsatilla is for a sweet nature.

CARBO VEGETABILIS (CARBO VEG)—The woman is slightly heavy and tends to have indigestion and shortness of breath due to poor oxygenation. Although she tends to be chilly, she prefers open windows with the air directly on her.

BELLIS PERENNIS—As the baby drops into the pelvis, pressure is felt on the organs in the lower part of the bladder. Pain and arthritis may occur as a result. Bellis perennis is specific for pain in the uterine area or groin. The woman might be walking when all of a sudden her legs weaken from a sharp nerve pain. After childbirth, once Arnica has done its job (see below) and there are still some lumps remaining in the tissues, Bellis perennis is also excellent.

KALI CARBONICUM—Kali carbonicum is for women with back pain, especially those who tend to wake up between two and four o'clock in the morning.

This individual's personality is somewhat crabby and closed. She is vague and evasive about answering questions. Pains are better with pressure and rubbing. The person tends to be anxious and chilly.

ACONITE—High-potency Aconite is wonderful to use at any point in pregnancy when there has been shock or fright. Arnica and Calendula may be useful for this purpose as well.

Midwife Jeanette Breen finds homeopathy useful during labor and after birth:

ARNICA—Starting a month before delivery, regular application of arnica cream directly to the nipples prevents later tearing and cracking with breast-feeding. After birth, arnica quickens recuperation. Calendula can be used in the same way.

CALIFILUM—Califilum may help a stalled labor. This is specific for a weak uterus or a uterus running out of steam. The woman often experiences weakness, exhaustion, trembling, and shivering. Sharp, brief, unstable, and painful lower uterine contractions fail to completely dilate the cervix and push the baby out.

GELSEMIUM—Gelsemium may be indicated as a follow-up to Califilum. It is also good for neuralgia, rheumatic discomfort, and pains in the bladder and vaginal area. The person tends to be thirsty and chilly.

CIMICIFUGA—Cimicifuga is good for stalled labor, especially when the woman is becoming fearful, hysterical, and exhausted, and the pains are becoming erratic. This tones the uterus, calms it down, and helps it to become more coordinated.

BREAST-FEEDING

For many of today's working mothers, breast-feeding is difficult because they can't be at home enough to be with their infants. However, women are further encouraged to neglect breast-feeding by the growth of fallacies about it, as well as a lack of full knowledge of its benefits.

The first major benefit of breast-feeding is the mother's milk itself: It gives the baby the appropriate nutrients. For the first nine months, Arms notes, the baby doesn't need any other food at all other than from breast milk, which helps establish and nourish the baby's immune system. Feeding the baby from the breast creates in the mother a feeling of calm, relaxation, and deepening love for her child. For the baby, just being there, skin to skin, with the mother, affords immune protection.

The components of breast milk actually change from feed to feed, and, for a mother who has more than one child, the milk changes from child to child. This is why formula can never mimic breast milk. Nor can the container that breast milk comes in ever be duplicated. There's a real difference between providing pumping stations at work and giving working mothers access on their job time to day care where mother and baby can be together when the baby wakes up—not to mention allowing mothers to be home with their babies until the babies are old enough to be without milk for more than four hours at a time.

Breast-feeding does many things for the baby and the mother. It causes the mother's gut to secrete twenty-three hormones (that we know of), which bottle feeding does not do. These hormones cause a woman to lose weight as well as help her sleep better and feel calmer. If a mother is malnourished and underweight, breast-feeding helps her to get as much nutrient value out of her food as possible. More nutrient value is absorbed in her gut than would be if she were not breast-feeding.

Arms tells us, "All babies need to be breast-fed and almost all mothers, even those who have had breast surgery, can breast-feed, if we give them three months to get settled before we even think of having them go back to work. And then we need to create work situations where they can breast-feed during the day."

The following corrections to common fallacies about lactation and breast-feeding are from K. G. Auerbach, "Breast-Feeding Fallacies: Their Relationship to Understanding Lactation," *Birth* 17, no. 1 (March 1990): 44–49:

Nipple soreness is not related to skin color.

The lactating breast is never empty.

All women do not experience pain during each breast-feeding.

Nipples do not get tougher with nursing.

Creams and oils on the breast are not encouraged for nipple soreness; vitamin E toxicity could be a concern because of liberal applications, and pesticide residues are a concern in sheep-fat-derived lanolin.

Engorgement may be experienced by newly breast-feeding mothers but is almost always indicative of inappropriate or infrequent suckling.

The let-down process is not a singular event, but occurs continually during suckling.

Noninfectious mastitis rarely requires antibiotic therapy; infectious mastitis includes temperature elevation and flulike systems as well.

Extra fluid intake is not needed for breast-feeding; drinking to quench one's thirst is sufficient.

The lactating mother's breasts become full usually between one and three days after the infant starts suckling.

Colostrum, which is a highly concentrated source of protein and antibodies, is produced as early as the third month of pregnancy.

Women with inverted nipples can breast-feed.

Healthy babies do not need supplemental feedings before the mother's milk comes in.

Breast milk helps reduce bilirubin concentrations by coating the small intestines, reducing bilirubin recirculation.

Additional water or glucose given to the infant reduces total caloric intake and diminishes the coating action of milk feedings.

Human milk is far superior in all aspects to artificial formula.

CORRECTIVE VAGINAL SURGERY (EPISIOTOMY)

In the United States, about 80 percent of women who give birth have an episiotomy performed. This is an incision that is made during birth when the vaginal opening does not stretch adequately. Of those operations, most are improperly performed. "Doctors are just not instructed in how to do this surgery," says Dr. Vicki Hufnagel. "All you have to do is go to your local medical school, get out the textbook on obstetrics, and look at what an episiotomy is. It will have a drawing and a discussion that says to put one or two sutures here, and one or two there. They are teaching physicians to close an entire organ system in just one or two layers. If you were to close a laceration on your face in one or two layers, your muscles wouldn't work, your face wouldn't work. You'd be a real mess. We are teaching students how to close the vaginal vault area in a manner that is not allowable in other places. That is the standard of care that we have, and it is completely unacceptable."

Incorrectly performed episiotomies result in problems down the road. Without the support of the vaginal muscles, the cervix pushes through the vagina. It appears that the uterus is being forced out, when really it is not. Doctors mistakenly diagnose a prolapsed uterus and commonly recommend a hysterectomy. Tragically, 100,000 to 200,000 women with this misdiagnosis receive this operation each year.

Corrective surgery easily ameliorates the problem. Repairing the vagina is a simple procedure that can be performed in a doctor's office. It takes all of forty-five minutes, and patients can go home the same day.

POSTPARTUM DEPRESSION

Depression after childbirth affects thousands of women each year. Although the exact cause is unknown, hormonal shifts after birth, particularly drops in progesterone, may play a large role. Research also links the condition to low levels of the neurotransmitter serotonin. Emotionally, it is often connected to difficult labor and disappointments after birth.

Symptoms range in degree, but are generally worse than a temporary feeling of the blues immediately following childbirth, according to Dr. Marjorie Ordene, a complementary gynecologist from New York: "Postpartum depression is defined as a gradually increasing sullen mood and a loss of interest and enthusiasm starting around the third postpartum week. This is different from the 'baby blues,' which is a common occurrence in the normal population. The blues happens the first week postpartum, and basically goes away by itself. We are talking about something much more severe." In the worst-case scenario, women can become sick for years and lose touch with reality.

Homeopathic Remedies

Homeopathic physician Dr. Jane Cicchetti recommends that women try the 30c potency of the remedy that best addresses their symptoms. If this does not help, a visit to a homeopathic physician can provide more individual support.

SEPIA—Sepia may be needed after an exhausting delivery, after giving birth to two or more children at once, or after having several children. The woman feels completely worn out and depressed. Physically, she feels as if her uterus might fall out, and finds herself crossing her legs a lot. Often there is an actual prolapse of the uterus. Emotionally, a woman who loves her husband and children suddenly has an aversion to them. In fact, she has an aversion to everyone and wants to be alone. She becomes irritable and angry if anyone bothers her, and has an aversion to sex. The woman cries often but cannot understand what is wrong; in fact this problem is caused by a hormonal disturbance rather than an emotional one.

NATMUR (NATRUM MURIATICUM)—Natmur is for chronic grief. The woman is introverted and dwells on past, unpleasant memories but keeps them to herself. She tries to put on the appearance that everything is fine, and becomes aggravated if someone tries to comfort her.

IGNATIA—Ignatia is for postpartum depression brought on by emotions. It is needed when disappointment follows childbirth. A woman imagines an ideal pregnancy and birthing situation. When that does not work out, she feels extremely let down and depressed. These feelings may occur after a stillbirth or a miscarriage. There is uncontrollable sobbing and sighing, and a rapid change of emotions, which are often contradictory.

ARNICA—This commonly needed remedy is useful for depression, upset, and malaise brought on by bruising, soreness, and pain that lasts a long time. Arnica helps heal the physical trauma and improves the mother's energy and emotional state.

PULSATILLA—Pulsatilla is given when a woman cries a lot and wants to be taken care of. She needs to attend to her newborn baby, but feels as if someone should be attending to her. This individual will eat sweets and other goodies to alleviate overwhelming feelings of sadness and loneliness. The woman is often warm-blooded and enjoys the fresh air. She is happier walking around outside, and much happier if she can be with people.

CIMICIFUGA—This remedy is used less often, but is very important for those who need it. Cimicifuga is derived from black cohosh, a powerful herb for treating hysteria and female complaints. It is needed when a woman feels as if a dark cloud of gloom has settled over her. She fears losing her mind. Often this stems from a very difficult delivery. She may have had a mini-nervous breakdown, feeling at one point as if she was going insane. This leaves her with a great fear of ever having a baby again. Often she alternates between different emotional states. When she is not under this dark cloud of gloom, she becomes excitable and talkative, jumping from one subject to another in an almost hysterical fashion. Cimicifuga heals the nervous system.

KALI CARBONICUM—This deep mineral remedy is indicated for women who become anxious and irritable after a delivery that leaves them feeling weak. Easily startled, they want to be left alone, and have an aversion to being touched. They tend to be chilly and to have insomnia from two to four **A.M.** Further, they are regimented and have trouble going with the flow of caring for a new baby. Often these symptoms follow a delivery that primarily consists of back labor. Sciatica develops to some degree, which can lead to an emotional state like this.

PHOSPHORIC ACID—Homeopathic Phosphoric acid is helpful when a woman is extremely disappointed from physical or emotional shock. She may have lost the baby, or something might be wrong with the baby. A loved one may have died at the time of birth, or she may be affected from the loss of much bodily fluid during delivery. Indifferent to everything, the woman lies in bed with her face to the wall. It is as if her emotions have completely disappeared. She doesn't want to talk, think, or answer questions.

COCCULUS—This is a remedy for fatigue and emotional depression brought on by loss of sleep. The woman feels drunk and may go through the day feeling dizzy and staggering. These feelings are brought on by sleep deprivation.

AURUM METALLICUM—Aurum metallicum is for profound depression characterized by total hopelessness, self-destructive behavior, and a longing for death.

Natural Progesterone

"Studies show that postpartum depression can be prevented by treating women with progesterone," reports Dr. Ordene. "Companies that make natural progesterone cream recommend using a half teaspoon twice daily, starting a month after delivery. Since postpartum depression is supposed to start three weeks after giving birth, it makes sense to begin using natural progesterone at that time."

Vitamin B6

According to research, this vitamin raises serotonin levels. Patients given B6 for twenty-eight days after delivery did not have a recurrence of postpartum depression.

ABORTION AFTERCARE

Although most women who have abortions do not have any serious medical complications from the procedure, the period after an abortion is a time for a woman to focus on herself; she may have a variety of physical and emotional needs that require attention.

It's particularly important to remember that after an abortion your body's hormone levels have to readjust to the sudden change from a pregnant to a nonpregnant state. Dr. Susanna Reid, a naturopathic physician, describes the physical changes in a woman's body after an abortion.

"Hormone levels are elevated dramatically during pregnancy, so the body has to readjust itself to its prepregnancy state," Dr. Reid explains. "One way to help the body to do that is by focusing on dietary factors that would be beneficial in regulating hormone levels. As well, you want to increase the circulation in the lower abdomen so that the body can heal itself. The more circulation in an area and the more nutrients that are in that area, the easier it is for the body to remove the toxic waste products. You'd also want to strengthen liver function, since the liver is essential to the balancing of hormones in the body; it functions to promote excretion of hormones. So if the liver isn't functioning correctly, you can have an imbalance of hormones."

To strengthen liver function, she suggests eating foods that contain fiber, particularly fruits, vegetables, and whole grains. The gut needs fiber to prevent the reabsorption of hormones. "If there isn't enough fiber in the diet, the hormones are reabsorbed through the intrahepatic circulation. So fiber is very important. In the springtime, one can strengthen liver function by eating large amounts of fresh dandelions and other greens such as cleavers. In other seasons, use yellow dock, nettle, dandelion, and cleavers with some red raspberry to make a tea. Red raspberry is a uterine tonic, so it helps to heal the uterus. You can put some peppermint in the tea to make it taste better and aid in digestion."

About two weeks after the abortion, she suggests using cold friction on the lower abdomen for ten minutes at a time before going to bed or first thing in the morning.

Preventing Infection

One of the more common complications from an abortion is infection. It's important not to put anything into the vagina for several weeks after the abortion and to refrain from intercourse. Dr. Reid suggests several natural remedies to help prevent infections.

"If we enhance the immune function, we prevent infection. You can use an immune-enhancing diet that focuses a lot on fruits and vegetables. Fruits in particular are immune-enhancing." She also recommends echinacea, goldenseal, astragalus, and ligustrum to help immune function.

Dr. Allan Warshowsky, a board-certified obstetrician and gynecologist who practices holistic gynecology, recommends taking vitamins C, A, and E and other antioxidants to enhance immune function.

Dr. Reid also emphasizes fluid intake. She explains that an abortion creates many by-products, and one way the body can help eliminate them is through the exchange of fluids, so you should drink a lot of fluids. Although each woman experiences abortion in her own way, it can sometimes create a strong emotional response, either positive or negative. "If it is a desired pregnancy and it's a spontaneous abortion," Dr. Reid says, "then people are dealing with grief. Even if it is a therapeutic abortion, there can be many reasons for the abortion. It may be because the pregnancy isn't viable or wouldn't be viable, or maybe it isn't the right time. So there are just a lot of grief issues for some women around abortion."

Dr. Warshowsky believes it is very important to deal with any negative feelings. He suggests that women who experience grief and other emotional and psychological consequences after an abortion may be helped by using meditation or visualization techniques.

IS CIRCUMCISION NECESSARY?

Sixty percent of babies born in hospitals in the United States are circumcised. Suzanne Arms, an independent researcher and activist who has published books on pregnancy and women's health, including *Immaculate Deception, Breast Feeding,* and *Seasons of Change,* sees this as a wasteful and counterproductive practice. "The difficulty with circumcision," she believes, "is that it touches some of the most sensitive tissue on the human male body and takes a large amount of material from the penis. You are taking away all the natural protection of the penis, the tissue that keeps it from getting infected and getting diseases and that makes sexuality more exquisite."

She also says that in Europe, circumcision has never been routinely performed on infants, as it is in the United States. She believes that the U.S. practice of routine circumcision is one aspect of a cultural attitude that grew, in part, out of seventeenth-century Puritanism, which viewed sexual pleasure, including masturbation, as sinful, and advocated tying babies' hands to their cribs to keep them from touching their genitals, which might provide pleasure. In the 1920s and 1930s, for the same purpose, clitoridectomies were performed on little girls in some parts of the country. She regards circumcision as an outgrowth of such attitudes: it was done to prevent male babies from using their penises as organs of pleasure.

Arms says, "We can contrast this with the reason for circumcision under Judaic law. In that tradition, circumcision was done on the eighth day as part of a convenant with God. Many Jews now believe that circumcision can be done without cutting the boy."

She also argues that the medical reasons once given for this operation— for example that it prevents cancer—have turned out to be false. Circumcision has no medical value at all and has a lot of risks associated with it, including bleeding and other effects of surgery.

She continues: "It exposes newborn babies to what is for them excruciating pain. Some babies feel it less than others, but, by and large, it puts the baby into shock and trauma."

Many advocates of circumcision apparently feel it is a way to harden the boy. In the past, children to be circumcised were tied down on boards, six in a row. A baby would lie there unable to move, listening to the screams of the little boys next to him. This was considered a way of preparing boys to be ready as adults to give up their bodies in war.

Arms concludes: "I think it's very important that we begin to understand the shock and trauma from this process that we have called normal in the United States. And we don't even acknowledge this trauma, so how can we heal it? People are running around with the long-term effects in their nervous system of an unresolved trauma. Believe me, that is what we are seeing in this culture."

CHAPTER 29

PREMENSTRUAL SYNDROME (PMS)

Premenstrual syndrome (PMS) refers to the symptoms that begin during or after ovulation and end with the conclusion of the menstrual flow. Because of diet and lifestyle, PMS is more widespread in Western societies than in Asian and less developed countries. Dr. Jesse Hanley, in an article in *Alternative Medicine* magazine, says that PMS is an indication of imbalance in the body, which can be psychological, nutritional, or hormonal. Dr. Hanley sees PMS as "a wake-up call" signaling us to pay attention to these imbalances and fix them before they turn into a more serious condition.

CAUSES

Dr. Hanley points out that menstruation does not create pain and discomfort when a woman is healthy. However, we live in an environment full of synthetic chemicals, including herbicides and pesticides, which mimic estrogen once they get inside the body, enhancing the effects of natural estrogen and disturbing the hormonal balance. Further, an excess of estrogen in relation to progesterone causes problems of hormonal imbalance.

SYMPTOMS

The effects of PMS range from mild to severe, and they vary from woman to woman. They may include bloating, cramps, headaches, swelling, fluid retention, low back pain, depression, abdominal pressure, insomnia, sugar cravings, anxiety, irritability, breast tenderness, mood swings, and acne.

Dietary Remedies

Dr. Michael Janson, an orthomolecular physician and author of *The Vitamin Revolution*, says, "Sugar, caffeine, and alcohol precipitate or worsen symptoms and should be avoided. This is because a lot of patients with PMS have overt hypoglycemia. Their sugar levels fluctuate up and down. Eating sugar sends blood sugar levels way up, and the body responds by dropping sugar levels way down. Additionally, caffeine, even when taken in small amounts in the morning, can aggravate symptoms such as breast tenderness and sleep disturbances."

According to Dr. Janson, the best diet for lessening the symptoms of PMS is high in fiber and complex carbohydrates; meals should be small, with snacks in between. This helps to regulate blood sugar, and in many cases is enough to reduce or eliminate PMS symptoms. Herbalist Letha Hadady recommends eating a lot of cool green foods such as salads; avoiding hot, spicy, and acidic foods; and eliminating coffee from the diet. Some people, however, need more help and can benefit from vitamin therapy, exercise, and a stress management program.

Dr. Hanley recommends that a woman who suffers from PMS should completely avoid milk and milk products, for milk has a high concentration of pesticides and other estrogen-mimicking chemicals.

Nutritional Supplements

When symptoms are severe, diet alone may not be enough. The following nutrients may prove useful:

VITAMIN B6 (PYRIDOXINE)—Pyridoxine has a number of helpful properties for alleviating PMS. As a smooth muscle relaxant, it can decrease cramps. As a diuretic, it reduces fluid retention, swelling, and breast tenderness. Between 200 and 400 mg should be taken daily, and vitamin B6 can be taken throughout the month, rather than just premenstrually. For the first two weeks of the cycle, take 100 mg a day in a B-complex vitamin; take an additional 250 mg the last two weeks of the cycle. Note that the more B6 you take, the more magnesium you need.

MAGNESIUM—Magnesium calms the nervous system and relieves anxiety, depression, irritability, nervousness, and insomnia. As an antispasmodic, it alleviates cramps and back pain. Magnesium also helps reduce cravings for sweets. Between 500 and 1,000 mg may be needed.

GAMMA-LINOLENIC ACID (GLA)—GLA is a precursor of prostaglandin-E1, a hormonelike substance that helps to regulate neurological and hormonal functions. Prostaglandin-E1 helps reduce muscle spasms, cramping, sugar cravings, mood swings, depression, anxiety, irritability, acne, and to some extent breast tenderness. It also reduces inflammation and decreases the stickiness of the platelets, which prevents blood clotting. One 1,000 mg capsule of borage oil provides a daily dose of 240 mg of GLA.

EICOSAPENTAENOIC ACID (EPA)—EPA, which is found in fish oil and flaxseed oil, produces prostaglandin-E3, which helps to alleviate breast tenderness. Flaxseed oil is fragile and should not be used for frying. It can be used in salad dressings or over cooked foods.

VITAMIN E—Vitamin E, 400–800 IU, can reduce cramps, breast tenderness, and fibrocystic breasts, which often swell up before a woman's menstrual period.

Exercise

Exercise helps to improve mood, reduce cramps, eliminate excess fluid, and control sugar cravings. Aerobic exercises should be performed three to four times per week.

Herbs

Naturopathic physician Dr. Janet Zand, in an article on the HealthWorld Online website (www.healthy.net), suggests the following herbal program, which builds blood and balances hormones during the first two weeks, then decongests the liver during the second two weeks.

For the first and second weeks, or until ovulation occurs, take a combination of red raspberry leaf and dong quai, taken as tablets, capsules, tinctures, or tea, three times a day.

For the third and fourth weeks (starting when ovulation occurs, until the menstrual flow begins), take the following: magnesium and vitamin B6, two to three times a day; choline, methionine, and inositol, two to three times a day; bupleurum and dandelion, taken as tablets, capsules, tinctures, or tea, two or three times a day.

Herbalist Letha Hadady offers the following recommendations for PMS pain. "We must approach the pain of PMS from both the emotional and the physical sides. Emotionally, there are two types of PMS. One is the angry type. Aloe leaf is recommended for this. It cleans the system and cleanses the liver. It may taste a little bitter, but it is easy to take when added to a little apple juice. A stronger gallbladder and liver cleanser that lessens the impact of 'angry' menstrual pains is the Chinese preparation *lung tanxieganwan.* Twenty percent ginseng, it aids digestion and reduces anger. It also calms and quiets headaches and other pains.

"The second type of PMS is weepy. It comes from sadness and excess phlegm brought on by eating foods that are too rich, sweet, and oily or by drinking too much milk. Eating radishes, parsley, or barley soup will cut down on the phlegm. (A homeopathic remedy for this type of pain is Pulsatilla.)"

To treat both types of menstrual pain, Hadady says, warming herbs such as cinnamon and myrrh are invaluable. Capsules or drops taken in tea will increase blood circulation and clean the uterus, inducing a more complete period that does not start too early, stay too long, or finish early only to begin prematurely. A warming and cooling remedy for the pain is as follows: 1/2 cup aloe vera gel, 10 drops or one capsule myrrh, and apple juice. This combines the cleaning action of myrrh with the cooling of aloe.

In addition, xiao yao wan helps relieve PMS symptoms of depression, poor circulation, indigestion, and bloating; and Women's Harmony increases circulation.

Homeopathy

The homeopathic remedy chosen should correspond to the symptoms described; only one should be used for best results. Sometimes it's a matter of trial and error; if one does not work, try another.

Dr. Ken Korins, a classically trained homeopathic physician in New York City, recommends the following remedies for PMS and lists the type of PMS symptom for which they are most useful.

LACHESIS—Lachesis helps most physical and emotional symptoms that accompany PMS, such as headaches, right ovarian pain, and breast tenderness. It may be indicated if PMS symptoms stop once menstrual flow stops. It is also indicated when symptoms get worse with heat and with constricted clothing around the abdomen. Emotional indications are restlessness, paranoia, and a tendency to be talkative.

LACANINUM—Think of Lacaninum when the only symptom is a painful, swollen breast, the pain leaves once the menstrual flow begins, and there is a tendency to be irritable.

BOVISTA—Bovista is indicated when gastrointestinal symptoms, such as diarrhea, occur before the period begins. There may also be traces of blood before the actual flow begins. Subjective and objective feelings of swelling occur throughout the body, even through the hands, resulting in a tendency for the women to feel clumsy.

PULSATILLA—Pulsatilla is good for emotional symptoms of PMS involving a weepy disposition and a need for consolation from others. It helps curb a strong craving for sweets.

NATMUR—Natmur is good when the woman's emotional state is melancholy and sad and worsens when others attempt to console her. Headaches occur before, during, or after the period, and there is a craving for salty foods and an aversion to sex at the time of the period.

SEPIA—Sepia is indicated in the presence of symptoms such as sadness, depression, indifference, and feelings of discontent and discouragement about life. Often a colicky pain is felt before the menses. There may also be a sensation of the uterus dropping, as if it would fall through the vagina due to congestion in that area.

FOLLICULINUM—This is a new French remedy that can be given on the seventh day of the cycle in a 30c–200c potency.

Homeopath Dana Ullman, in an article on the HealthWorld Online website (www.healthy.net), suggests some additional remedies. Take each one in the 6c, 12c, or 30c potency every two hours while symptoms are strong, then every four hours after symptoms diminish. When symptoms become mild, stop the remedy. If you experience no clear improvement within twelve hours, try another remedy.

BELLADONNA—Use Belladonna when the major symptom is "bearing down" pains or cramps that appear and disappear suddenly. It is also useful when cramps are made worse by motion, a draft, or being jarred, and when they are associated with a headache.

MAGNESIA PHOS—Magnesia phos is recommended for cramps made better by warmth, by simply bending over, or by bending over and at the same time firmly massaging the abdomen, and made worse by cold and by being uncovered.

COLOCYNTHIS—Colocynthis is indicated for cramps like those just described when those cramps are accompanied by feelings of extreme restlessness and irritability.

IGNATIA—Ignatia is good for bloating accompanied by strong emotional downs, such as hysteria and grief, and when the woman experiences conflicting feelings.

CIMICIFUGA—Cimicifuga is used for bloating accompanied by sharp, labor-like pains shooting across the body, perhaps accompanied by sciatica or back pain, difficulty tolerating pain, hysteria, talkativeness, and a sense of everything being "just too much to bear."

NUX VOMICA—Nux vomica is used for Type A personalities who are often highly stressed, who experience bloating and nausea along with irritability, and who become quarrelsome and critical.

Progesterone

To restore hormonal balance, Dr. Hanley advocates natural progesterone, preferably in the form of cream made from wild yam, which is rubbed into the skin. This is because only 10 percent of hormones taken by mouth actually reach the bloodstream; the liver filters out the rest, which stresses the liver and gallbladder and increases the risk of gallstones, gallbladder disease, and liver cancer. Progesterone cream is used between ovulation and the day before the menstrual flow starts.

Progesterone promotes youthfulness, and is beneficial against cancer and fibrocystic breast disease. Dr. Michael Janson says additional progesterone is especially important for women exposed to estrogens from pesticides, food additives, drugs, and other chemicals in the environment. These lead to an overload of estrogen and a deficiency of progesterone. Progesterone is extremely helpful for treating PMS symptoms when such an imbalance exists.

Dr. Hanley also cautions that women taking herbs to relieve PMS symptoms should be sure to include herbs that promote progesterone production. Dong quai, alfalfa, licorice root, ginseng, anise seed, garlic, fennel, papaya, red clover, and sage are all estrogenic herbs. They may relieve symptoms, but they may also lead to fibroids, tumors, and cancers. They should be balanced with progesterone-precursor herbs, including wild yam, sarsaparilla, and chaste berry.

Liver Detoxification

According to Dr. Hanley, detoxifying the liver can relieve many female health problems. The first step is to reduce fat in the diet; and the second is to use a detoxifying formula that contains herbs and plant enzymes that work to remove toxins from the liver. The herbs and enzymes must be used together; neither should be used by themselves. Dr. Hanley recommends a liver detoxification program two or three months out of each year; women who suffer from severe PMS can do the program for longer time periods and more frequently.

Reflexology

Reflexology is a science and an art based on the principle that we have reflex areas in our feet that correspond to every part of the body. Massaging specific reflex areas in the feet helps to improve the functioning of specific organs and glands.

Laura Norman, a certified reflexologist from New York City, describes three reflexology techniques:

"Thumb-walking can be used on the bottom, tops, and sides of the feet, although it is most often used on the bottom. The procedure entails bending the thumb at the first joint and inching along the bottom of the foot like a caterpillar, pressing from the heel up to the toe. The right hand is used on the right foot. Taking little tiny bites, press, press, press the whole bottom of the foot.

"Finger-walking is similar to thumb walking, but is done by bending the finger at the first joint and using the tip of the finger on the outside edge.

"Finger-rotation is where you rotate the finger into the foot."

Massaging the feet with thumb-walking, finger-walking, and finger-rotation using a nongreasy, absorbent cream warms the feet and helps promote overall relaxation. For addressing specific problems, reflexology must be applied to specific areas.

Reflexology for PMS helps most when performed three or four days before and then during menstruation. First the right foot is worked on, while resting on the left leg. Then the same actions are repeated on the left side.

A FINAL NOTE: PREMENSTRUAL DYSPHORIC DISORDER (PMDD)

In the early 2000s, pharmaceutical giant Eli Lilly introduced a new drug, claiming it would change the lives of hundreds of thousands of women by treating a condition known as premenstrual dysphoric disorder (PMDD). The symptoms of PMDD, as described by the company, were exactly the same as those of PMS. So why the new name? The story of PMDD and the drug designed to treat it provide yet another cautionary tale about the unholy alliance between the drug companies and the medical world. Sherrill Sellman explains.

"Eli Lily, the maker of Prozac, which has been grossing over $2 billion a year, lost the patent on Prozac. So they can't really make their profits off of Prozac and in fact they expect their profits to plummet to $645 million. That is a pretty big drop. So what they did was convince the FDA to create a new condition for which their drug and their drug only is the solution. This new drug is called Seraphim and it is actually made as a pink and purple pill. It is very sweet and feminine. This drug is designed to take away PMDD. It's Prozac. It is the exact same drug. It has been colored differently. It has been given a name change and it has been increased in price. When I checked with my local pharmacy here, I actually found out that a prescription of Seraphim costs $10 more than Prozac.

"Why is Prozac a problem? Well, we know that Prozac is highly toxic to the liver. It can cause brain damage. It can cause huge mood swings. It can cause greater types of suicidal thinking. It is a drug that puts women at greater risk of breast cancer. Some of the other side effects of Prozac include depression, anxiety, insomnia, loss of libido, and mood swings, which sound pretty much like the very condition it is supposed to treat.

"The massive amount of advertising that is going on through the TV, through women's magazines, doctors seminars and conferences convincing everyone, doctors and women alike, that they have a solution to this new disease is a marketing ploy of the highest degree. It is designed to push a drug that cannot be pushed in the old way. They have created a new disease. They have created a new market. I'm really concerned about the long-term consequences of basically healthy women needing to adjust some of the issues going on in their life to heal their PMS, but why are we putting them on this toxic antidepressant drug? Women need to wake up to the fact that again they are being sold a bill of goods, that this is not the solution, and that the motive behind it is purely profit."

CHAPTER 30

SEXUAL DYSFUNCTION

P sychologist Dr. Janice Stefanacci says that sexual dysfunction stems largely from a society that offers people no models of normal, healthy sexuality. "If we look to the media, we see things that are totally aberrant in terms of frequency and potency. We see relationships portrayed between males and females where there is power and domination, or submission and seduction. Role models of healthy sexual communication and actualization are virtually nonexistent. People need a sense of what is normal.

"They also need time to think about sexuality as an integrated part of their personality. Our culture is very fragmented in this regard. Many, many people, men and women alike, never spend time thinking about their sexuality. In fact, if you were to take an informal survey and ask people, 'What is sexuality?' a good proportion of them would say, 'It's sex. It's something you do, maybe in the bedroom, maybe at night.' Nobody is really sure how often you are supposed to have it or how long it is supposed to last. Most people don't realize that sexuality is a completely integrated part of their personality, as much as actualizing in education or interpersonal relationships. Sexuality is very much a part of who we are, how we present ourselves in the world, what we do, and how we think of ourselves. Our adequacy and our self-esteem are tied up in our sexuality."

CAUSES

Some sex researchers are beginning to question the whole concept of sexual dysfunction, promoting broader and less rigid definitions of sexual response and pleasure. "The Masters and Johnson model of sexual response—excitement, plateau, orgasm, and resolution—is very performance-oriented," says

Rebecca Chalker, a women's health activist whose book, *The Clitoral Truth*, explores ways in which feminists are redefining male standards. "After desire and willingness, the only other compulsory element is pleasure," Chalker points out. "Pleasure and intimacy are the real goals of sexual activity, and if you look at it that way, the concept of sexual dysfunction simply collapses."

Nevertheless, women may worry when they have difficulty achieving orgasm, especially with a partner, and men become concerned if they have difficulty controlling ejaculations and getting or maintaining erections. Both women and men are also distressed when they don't feel sexual attraction. In fact, most people who seek out counseling do so for difficulties with sexual communication and the lack of sexual desire.

Early on, through regular masturbation, boys learn what feels good and how to reliably get orgasms. Girls often wait to begin sexual exploration until they engage in sexual activity with a partner; they miss out on the benefits of self-exploration. "Learning about sex from boys or men isn't the best thing for women," Chalker says.

Many sex therapists recommend that women explore their sexual response through masturbation, using a vibrator, sex toys, and sexy videos to stimulate sexual fantasies. You may also want to experiment with things like aromatherapy, oils, and herbs. After sufficient homework, you can try integrating these changes into sex with your partner. Another important change heterosexual couples can make is to try rewriting the "intercourse script." That is, plan to have sexual sessions where intercourse will not take place.

Chalker points out that there are two powerful aspects of our sexuality—the physiological and the psychological—and that "neither can live without the other." Unfortunately, it is the psychological problems that are the more difficult to deal with. Psychological problems manifest themselves in various ways. "Today, we have enormous resources that we didn't have a few years ago to help with sexual problems," Chalker notes. "I've reviewed some of the herbal aids and remedies here, and I encourage the reader to explore the wide range of resources available in book stores or by mail order."

Of course, sexual dysfunction can also have physical causes. One, Dr. Vicki Hufnagel reminds us, is "improperly performed episiotomies." In *Prevention* magazine, Dr. Tori Hudson lists a number of other factors that can affect the sex drive. She says that sexual problems can be related to menopause, non-menopause-related hormonal changes (often following pregnancy), medications (Prozac, Zoloft, Sertraline, and others), depression, relationship issues, a chronic health problem, fatigue, and others. "In order to diagnose the cause correctly, your health professional would have to ask you many specific questions," she says. Hormonal factors may involve low levels of testosterone or DHEA, although it is not known precisely what effect these hormones have on the libido. If blood tests show that levels are low, supplementation may be in order.

CLINICAL EXPERIENCE

Nutrients, Hormones, and Supplements

Studies show that a heightened libido and orgasmic intensity are related to blood levels of histamine. Women who have low histamine levels tend to experience low sexual excitement, while those with a high level are more able to sustain orgasms. Nutrients that increase histamine levels include vitamin B5 and the bioflavonoid rutin. Broccoli, parsley, cherries, grapes, peppers, melons, and citrus fruits are good food sources of vitamin B5 and rutin.

Dr. Tori Hudson says that oral testosterone (available only by prescription), and/or a testosterone cream applied two to three times a week or rubbed into the external genital area before sex have been used to stimulate sexual responsiveness. DHEA, the B-complex vitamins, adrenal extracts, and the herbs ginseng and damiana may also help improve sexual response. Dr. Hudson notes, however, that remedies that focus on sexual drive without addressing general health and emotional issues will not have a consistent effect.

Dr. Janson offers an example of a general supplement program that can be an initial step in treating sexual dysfunction:

Multivitamin, three capsules twice a day
Vitamin C, two 1,000 mg capsules twice a day
Vitamin E, 400 IU mixed natural, twice a day
Ginkgo biloba tincture, 60 mg twice a day
Gamma-linoleic acid, 240 mg in the form of borage oil, once a day
Magnesium aspartate, 200 mg twice a day
Coenzyme Q10, 100 mg once a day

Aromatherapy

"Aromatherapy is fantastic for helping women regain their sense of sensuality," declares aromatherapist Ann Berwick. Following are her recommendations.

Rose is wonderful for enhancing feminine qualities. It brings out the loving, tender side of us that wants to surrender. Clary sage heightens sensation. It takes you out of your body and into a different realm, allowing you to relax and enjoy the romance. Sandalwood is a wonderful oil for people not in touch with their physical side. It is very earthy and very deep. Jasmine restores self-confidence in people who have been through traumatic sexual experiences. It can help women who have been abused or who are emotionally closed off from damaging relationships.

"By blending different oils, you can create a formula that enhances the sensual side of your nature," says Berwick. She suggests adding them to the bath or using them while massaging a partner or in self-massage. A personal perfume can be made and used daily. "Surrounding yourself with these glorious scents is a wonderful help."

Chinese Medicine

Registered nurse and acupuncturist Abigail Rist-Podrecca explains sexual dysfunction from an Eastern point of view: "Chinese medicine looks to the root of the cause rather than just the symptoms, and the root seems to be the kidney. The kidneys are called the roots of life. Everything stems from the kidney, they say."

Weak kidney function can be diagnosed in Eastern medicine in multiple ways, including facial diagnosis: "Under the eye is the thinnest tissue in the entire body," explains Rist-Podrecca. "You can see through the skin there. If the blood is not being cleared by the kidneys and detoxified, you will see a darkness under the eyes. People will say, 'I haven't had enough sleep,' but it goes beyond that. In Chinese medicine, that darkness signals that the kidneys are not functioning optimally, so the blood isn't being cleansed."

She goes on describe various factors that can drain the kidneys. "Cold can deplete the kidneys. Many people can't tolerate cold. This is so because in the winter, the kidney's function becomes suppressed, much the same way as the sap in a tree runs to the core and into the roots. When people have a compromised kidney situation, where it isn't functioning optimally, they can't stand cold weather.

"Overwork and tension can also weaken kidney function because the kidneys and the adrenal glands (the adrenal sits on top of the kidney) are considered one and the same in Chinese medicine. So too much stress, and too many chemical toxins, deplete kidney functioning." Hundreds of Chinese herbs nourish kidney function. Here Rist-Podrecca names a few:

HAR SHAR WOO—This is an essential herbal formula for nourishing kidney function. It is also said to darken the hair. Hair, bone, teeth, joints, and sexual functions are tied up with the kidney energies. When you energize the kidneys, you affect all these different areas. When combined with dong quai, har shar woo helps the type of kidney dysfunction that causes low back pain.

ROMANIA—Romania is a dark black herb that is high in iron and helps to nourish the blood and improve kidney function.

DONG QUAI—Dong quai resembles a cross-section of the uterus, and has an affinity for this area of the body.

CHAPTER 31

SEXUALLY TRANSMITTED DISEASES

S exually transmitted diseases (STDs) were once a scourge that could bring death or madness. As recently as the 1940s, they were deeply feared. These diseases are now much better understood and more treatable. However, although many people realize that there has been progress in the conventional medical treatment of STDs, what they may not know is that there has also been progress in using alternative, particularly herbal, treatments.

GONORRHEA

Gonorrhea is caused by the bacterium *Neisseria gonorrhoeae*; women are far more likely to become infected than men.

Carol Dalton, a nurse practitioner, says that because gonorrhea can cause pelvic inflammatory disease (PID) and other illnesses, as well as infertility, she believes in treating it by conventional means. "We don't want women who have the infection to pass it on. Gonorrhea can occur without any symptoms for a long time, so that you might be passing it on without being aware of it. We treat this very aggressively."

The first recourse is antibiotics. However, Dr. Allan Warshowsky cautions that antibiotics must be carefully monitored. Dr. Warshowsky is a board-certified obstetrician-gynecologist whose specialty is holistic gynecology. He says, "Most of my treatment of this disease is fairly conventional. I use antibiotics unless patients specifically ask me not to use them. But it is also important to maintain and restore gut bacteria while treating a patient with antibiotics. I use bifidum, acidophilus, and some of the *Saccharomyces* strains of beneficial yeast to maintain normal gut biosis. I think this is paramount."

He combines this with herbal treatment and psychological counseling. "It is also important, especially if a patient is having recurrent problems with STDs, to look at her relationships, because whatever is going on physically is a manifestation of a deeper energy problem in the individual. If the patient is amenable to examining these deeper problems, it can really help lead to a much more lasting cure than just taking antibiotics.

"There are certainly people I see who prefer not to have antibiotics and, then, as long as the patient is a willing partner in her own therapy and not just looking to me to cure the disease, I use some herbal products, such as echinacea and goldenseal, and other herbs and supplements that can be helpful in enhancing immunity and fighting off infection."

Dr. Linda Page, a doctor of naturopathy who is the author of *Healthy Healing*, has found a variety of herbs useful in treating STDs, including gonorrhea. She uses a combination that includes goldenseal, myrrh, pau d'arco, vegetable acidophilus, ginkgo, and dandelion. Another combination she uses is burdock, juniper, squawvine, bayberry, dandelion, gentian, and black walnut.

She adds, "You can see where we are going with these herbs. This is obviously a broad-spectrum approach—antifungal, antiviral, and antibacterial. This is because these categories of STDs seem to exhibit symptoms of all these types of infections: fungal symptoms, such as discharge; bacterial symptoms, such as inflammation; and viral symptoms, in that these infections can migrate to other parts of the body."

CHLAMYDIA

Amanda McQuade Crawford, health expert and author of *Herbal Remedies for Women*, describes chlamydia as one of the most widespread STDs in North America. The infecting organism, *Chlamydia trachomatis*, is a one-celled parasite with a rigid cell wall. Crawford notes that chlamydia is harder to clear up with herbal agents than some other one-celled organisms, such as bacteria and yeast, which respond very well to herbal treatment. "It often goes undiagnosed and can cause an inflammation of the cervix in women. This is why it is one of the leading causes of more serious pelvic diseases, particularly PID."

Symptoms

"Usually the first symptom is a painless bump that goes unnoticed, followed by swollen lymph glands and headaches," Crawford says. "Some women get strange fleeting pains in their joints and muscles, as well as chills, and even weight loss, one to four weeks later.

"There will be a vaginal discharge that feels like mucus but has a bad odor. There may also be pain with sexual intercourse and some spotting after intercourse. If there is spotting between menstrual periods, a woman should see a licensed practitioner to look for signs of redness on the cervix.

"Other signs that women might experience are urinary frequency and painful urination, as well as some lower abdominal pain, although these symptoms may be caused by some other conditions as well."

Dalton emphasizes that chlamydia often leads to PID. "It can go up into the uterus, the fallopian tubes, and the ovarian area and cause very serious infections and scarring and, therefore, infertility." As with so many diseases, early detection is essential. It can also cause problems in pregnancy, including premature or difficult delivery.

Treatment

In conventional drug treatment, antibiotics are used. Crawford explains: "Which antibiotic is chosen, if any, will depend on whether a woman is pregnant or not. There are often secondary infections with bacteria or viruses, and that can complicate the picture. That's another reason why chlamydia is difficult to treat with simple remedies."

In Dalton's practice, she uses antibiotics. "We use antibiotics because of the risk factor. I think in health care you always weigh the risks versus the benefits of treatment. In this case, you see that the risk is great. Even if someone isn't concerned about fertility, you still weigh the risk of damaging the woman's immune system because you have an active infection that could become very serious. So chlamydia is one of the things that we don't really fool around with. We treat it with antibiotics; and we recheck it to make sure it's gone."

Crawford has looked into herbal treatments for chlamydia. One is the anti-inflammatory herb calendula, or marigold—not the garden variety but the medicinal single-flower kind. Demulcents such as plantain are also useful and are often combined with herbs that help normalize the hormones. As she puts it, "Sometimes a hormonal imbalance will have led to a change in the reproductive tissues, so these rectifying herbs are needed to make it possible to clear up this infection."

Herbal douches can also be of some help with reproductive infections, though, according to Crawford, they really can't get to the source of the problem. While the douche is rinsing out the infectious agent, it is also rinsing away the helpful bacteria, which is why you should be cautious about using herbal douches with any kind of infection. Still, the antimicrobial herbs used in the douches can help reduce the infectious organisms. "What we normally do," Crawford explains, "is follow each douche with a rest period, because these douches can dry out the tissue, making the irritated vaginal walls more susceptible to other infections. Even plain water douches will have that effect."

Crawford describes a douche formula that uses 2 ounces of organic grape root, also know as barberry bark root, and 1 ounce of calendula flower. Steep

1 ounce of this mixture in a pint of boiling water for about 45 minutes. Strain it and let the tea cool to a comfortable temperature for vaginal use. To this mixture add about 7 drops of essential oil of tea tree. You can use a wire whisk to help mix them together. Make sure all the containers used are sterilized. Use this as a douche twice a week for up to three weeks. It's not necessary to rinse the herbs out of the vaginal canal afterward, but Crawford says that it feels very comforting to get rid of some of the bad-smelling discharge from chlamydia.

Dr. Page uses vaginal ointments to treat chlamydia. She suggests a combination of berberine-compound herbs: goldenseal, barberry, and Oregon grape. Mix this with vitamin A oil and apply directly to the cervix via a tampon.

PELVIC INFLAMMATORY DISEASE (PID)

Pelvic inflammatory disease generally originates from an infection, such as chlamydia, that spreads out of control. Dalton says that chlamydia is the primary cause of PID. Because PID can be a "silent" infection, someone can have it for years without knowing she is infected. "So, it's easily transmitted. It can fester in the cervical canal, and then, when the immune system is low, can creep up into the other pelvic organs and cause a major infection."

She adds that it was a shift in birth control methods that played a big part in the rise of PID. "We really saw a lot of this disease when IUDs became popular, particularly when the Dalkon Shield was still being used. The Dalkon Shield had a multifiliment string; there were multiple threads within this string, and bacteria could climb up the threads more easily, and into the uterus. The problems with the Dalkon Shield brought about a greater understanding of PID: how to develop cultures for it, how to study it, and what treatment to use knowledge of the damage that PID could do."

Symptoms

PID symptoms vary; some women have very severe symptoms, other women have symptoms so mild that they are unaware they are infected. The most common symptom is pain, which ranges from a dull ache to pain so debilitating that walking is impossible. Other symptoms are bleeding, a foul discharge, cramps, swelling in the abdominal area, fever, and chills.

In addition to damaging the internal organs, PID can also result in scarring, particularly of the fallopian tubes. As Dalton explains, "This is how PID causes infertility. Even after you have cleared the infection, even if it hasn't blocked the tubes completely with scarring, the wavelike, hairlike projections that sweep the sperm through the fallopian tube to the egg and that sweep the egg up into the fallopian tube to meet with the sperm are often damaged and flattened. So that even though you may have a good, clear tube, the system isn't working properly. When this happens, it's a very serious problem, particularly for young, fertile women. It's probably one of the major causes of infertility. That's why we have to be really aggressive in testing for chlamydia and in treating it. We can clear the infection. We can give women antibiotics, but if we don't catch it soon enough, it can do all of this damage and may result in infertility."

Treatment

Dalton explains that once a woman is at the point where PID has really taken hold, there is severe swelling and inflammation in the entire pelvic area. To heal properly, the woman has to rest her body completely, which means bed rest. "Because whenever we are standing or walking, just because of gravity and the weight of the body, the pelvic area is impinged upon and there is a lot of pressure. So we encourage a woman to go to bed and rest while she is being treated. We get a much better response, much better healing, quicker healing, and less recurrence when this is followed.

"The other thing we advise patients to do is to use diet and supplements to encourage healing. We use zinc and vitamins C and E to encourage good oxygenation and tissue repair. We have to remember that the antibiotic just kills the bacteria, it does not cause healing to take place. Those tissues have to heal on their own, and if you give them a little extra encouragement with extra nutrients they are going to do that in a quicker and better fashion."

HUMAN PAPILLOMA VIRUS (HPV)

Different strains of HPV (human papilloma virus) cause either genital warts, warts on other parts of the body, or cervical cancer. HPV is particularly hazardous, says Carol Dalton, because it often goes undetected. "People often have no idea that they have it because it's microscopic, so it's easily transmitted during sexual intercourse. One study showed that 75 percent of a group of women and men who were tested were positive for HPV, and most of them did not realize they were infected." HPV is diagnosed in women most frequently by a Pap smear. The Pap smear results come back as "atypical, suspicious of HPV" or "dysplasia, suspicious of HPV," Dalton explains. She also underlines the possible consequences of getting HPV. "It's the primary cause of dysplasia. Probably over 90 percent of the time, dysplasia of the cervix or, eventually, cervical cancer, is caused by HPV. That's why it's so important to get a proper diagnosis."

The condition of the immune system is related to the health of a woman's vaginal and cervical cells. "Clearly, a woman can be infected with this, and we know it is in her system, but she is not having any problems. It's not invading the cells and growing and changing them into abnormal ones. Whether or not a woman will develop HPV depends on the response of the immune system.

"Once a woman develops abnormal cells, we diagnose it by doing a colposcopy and biopsy of any abnormal cells. A colposcope is an instrument we use to look at the cervix, vagina, and labia. It magnifies these areas so that we can actually see the cells to identify the areas where abnormal cells are present. After we have identified the abnormal cells, we do small biopsies—pinhead size or smaller. The biopsies are sent to a pathology lab where they section them and examine them under a microscope to identify the cells and see what is going on there."

Treatment

There are several treatments for HPV. "The typical treatment can be to do nothing and watch for a while to see if the body can heal itself and reverse the process. Cryotherapy, freezing of the cells, may be used, as well as laser therapy or a procedure called LEEP (loop excisional electrosurgical procedure), which uses an electrical wire to cut out abnormal tissue. All of these destroy the abnormal cells."

The fortunate thing," Dalton continues, "is that the vagina and cervix produce a new surface of cells about every six to eight weeks. So if we can remove the cells that are abnormal, new, healthy cells will hopefully grow in. One reason it is important to remove the abnormal cells is that new cells tend to be like the cells next to them, so if abnormal cells remain in the body, the new cells will grow into abnormal cells too."

The unfortunate thing is that just removing these abnormal cells often does not end the problem. As Dalton notes, "You can't kill off the virus completely, since it is in the surrounding tissue. You can't cauterize or remove the whole lining of the vagina. We only remove the cells that have become abnormal. There is a very high recurrence rate, with HPV causing the same abnormal cell growth all over again, unless you improve the woman's immune system and strengthen those normal cells."

Oral supplements of zinc, vitamin C, beta carotene, folic acid, and general B complex, along with a multivitamin-mineral, may aid in this process. Dalton says, "We recommend larger than usual doses of these because we have found that the new cell growth responds well to these nutrients. Moreover, many of these are antiviral nutrients. They help the woman's body fight the virus more readily and more systematically.

"We also use vitamin A suppositories. There's been a fair amount of work done on how cervical dysplasia can be treated with topical vitamin A. There are also suppositories we use called papillo suppositories that are made to fight the HPV virus topically. With these, we are treating the whole vaginal area and not just the cells that have become abnormal. We also use something called formula W, for wart virus, that contains herbs that help fight the HPV virus."

Her clinic uses both oral and topical treatments. They also examine patients' stress levels, their diet, and their lifestyle issues. This seems to be a successful approach, since, she maintains, "We have about a 1 to 2 percent recurrence rate with HPV, while the national average, when conventional methods are used exclusively, is 10 to 15 percent recurrence. So we feel that treating the whole person has made a huge difference in our ability to prevent recurrence, which is really the issue. HPV is not so hard to treat initially, but it's keeping it from coming back that is really the problem. I would encourage women who have this problem to look at the whole person."

HIV and AIDS have created a further difficulty in treatment." We've had to be very careful about screening for HIV and AIDS and treating those patients," Dalton points out, "because the immune system with HIV is so compromised that if a woman with HIV does contract HPV, it seems to grow at a very rapid rate. The cells can turn into cancerous cells much more easily on the vulva, labia, cervix and vagina. Practitioners treating patients who have HIV and AIDS need to be extremely cautious in doing colposcopies and biopsies. Even more than with the average patient, be aggressive with treatment and in building the immune system. Because having these other problems will greatly increase the risk factor of the abnormal cells turning into cancerous cells."

GENITAL WARTS

Genital warts are caused by HPV. Symptoms of genital warts can take as little as three weeks and as long as eight months to develop after exposure to the virus. Genital warts are contagious, even before they become symptomatic.

Dr. Page treats genital warts successfully with vitamin C therapy. "Up to 10,000 milligrams daily is used to enhance white blood cell activity and boost immune interferon. We use a mix of carotenes up to 200,000 IU daily." She also uses aloe vera gel as a topical application for genital warts. She particularly recommends an aloe vera/garlic mixture. "You steep garlic cloves in the aloe vera gel, so you have a very high sulfur mix. We ask patients to drink two glasses of aloe vera juice daily. We also use a 'vag-pack' for genital warts, which includes goldenseal, burdock, chaparral, and sarsaparilla. Blend the herbs and put them on a tampon and insert into the vagina. This is an internal poultice to draw out the infection. It is very effective, especially when you add B complex with extra folic acid. Both these supplements help normalize those abnormal cells."

She adds, "This is a virus, so you would want to take antiviral herbs. The ones I use regularly are lomatium, St. John's wort, and bupleurum. Occasionally, I also use myrrh. Any combination of these works. It's best to use them in an extract if you want antiviral activity."

Dr. Warshowsky notes that genital warts should be treated creatively and holistically. "When a woman is willing to do an entire body-balancing protocol, where she is looking at what is going on in her life that is making her susceptible to infection, balancing out her gut bacteria, eating a nutrient-rich diet, and employing some of these beneficial herbs and supplements, I think there is good success in restoring order, restoring balance, and getting rid of infection."

CHAPTER 32

STROKE

$\int$ trokes are the third leading cause of death in the United States. Every sixty seconds, someone dies of a stroke. In 2001, an estimated 100,000 women between the ages of thirty and sixty-five suffered a stroke.

CAUSES

There are two different types of strokes: hemorrhagic stroke, which is a rupture in a blood vessel, and ischemic stroke, which is caused by a blockage in the blood vessels. The result of both types of strokes is a lack of blood flow to the brain and consequently insufficient oxygen for brain function.

SYMPTOMS

Symptoms of stroke include dizziness, blurred vision and loss of sensation, slurred speech, loss of bladder control, and partial loss of hearing. A person should seek medical help immediately if she experiences one or more of these symptoms. Often a stroke will be accompanied by paralysis of an arm or leg on one side of the body. Strokes can cause swelling of the brain, stupor, and coma.

Enzyme Therapy

Dr. Anthony Cichoke is a leading medical researcher in the field of enzyme therapy. Dr. Cichoke has taught at the University of Minnesota and the University of Rochester Medical School and is the author of hundreds of articles and seven books, including *The Complete Book of Enzyme Therapy*.

Dr. Chichoke uses enzyme therapy to boost the immune system and detoxify the body. "Enzymes are catalysts," he explains. "Anything that is alive has to have enzymatic activity—whether it is in the grass outside or whether it is in your body. Enzymes are critical for every cell of our body. Nothing can go on in the body without enzymatic activity. Without enzymes there would be no breathing, no digestion, no growth, no blood coagulation, no reproduction. Enzymes, he says, fight strokes by acting "as sort of 'Roto Rooter' that helps break up cholesterol and toxins in your body.

"Strokes can be treated systemically with enzymes. They are used as digestive aids; they improve the absorption of other nutrients, herbs, health foods, whatever, Enzymes aid absorption and metabolism at the cellular level."

Dr. Cichoke has his patients take enzyme supplements orally between meals. He recommends enzymes such as bromelain, papain, trypsin, chymotrypsin, pancreatin, and microbial proteases, all of which have primarily proteolytic enzyme activity. Dr. Cichoke describes how enzyme supplements pass through the gut into the small intestine, where they are absorbed into the circulatory system. "These are all enzymes that work in the bloodstream and the various organs as well as at the cellular level of the body."

Enzymes aid in detoxification at the cellular level in various organs and in the bloodstream and digestive tract. He explains why it is important to have a well-ordered circulatory system: "The blood must get to the cells in order to bring nutrients to the body, and blood needs to help take the waste products away from the cells. Further, enzymes help break up the cholesterol and fibrin in the blood vessels." Dr. Cichoke pictures a blood vessel as a stream or river, with little curves and eddies. These curves fill up with fibrin and cholesterol, which clog blood vessels so that the blood and oxygen can't get through.

"Proteolytic enzymes help to break up the fibrin and cholesterol and allow the body to eliminate these waste products. Enzymes also improve circulation. They help keep the bloodstream normalized." He explains that it is important to have a balance between blood coagulation and blood thinning. "Enzymes help to keep this critical equilibrium in order."

Enzymes also help break up free radicals. "As part of the aging process, and also as a result of stress and illness and injuries, the cells of our body tend to oxidize—they rust. Think of the body's tissue as if it was like a lovely leather jacket. When you first buy that leather jacket, it's soft and pliable. But then, as it gets older, the leather oxidizes and it becomes cracked and hard. As we go through life, our body tends to oxidize. When you take antioxidant enzymes, such as superoxide dismutase, catalase, glutathione, and peroxidase, they fight free radical formation and work as antioxidants."

Enzymes can also dissolve large blood clots, which can cause strokes. Dr. Cichoke says that enzymes are currently being used both in and out of hospitals to break up blood clots and also to break up fibrin formations. "In hospitals, some enzymes used for this purpose are brinase, which comes from *Aspergillus oryzae*; streptokinase, which is of bacterial origin; and urokinase or prourokinase, which is actually from human urine."

Dr. Cichoke tells a story about a stroke patient in Portland, Oregon, who was treated with these enzymes. "They had given up on him. But as a last-ditch effort, nine hours after the stroke, they began to give him urokinase. Not only did he regain consciousness, he also regained the ability to move his arms and his legs. After six weeks of rehabilitation therapy he went home."

Dr. Cichoke cites a 1999 article in *The New York Times* that stated, "Enzymes offer hope for reducing devastation from strokes." Currently, Dr. Cichoke notes, the Cleveland Clinic in Cleveland, Ohio, is using prourokinase to fight strokes. He stresses the importance of proteolytic enzymes as well as antioxidant enzymes. "I suggest taking 200 micrograms of antioxidant enzymes three times a day between meals and eight to ten tablets of combination enzymes three times a day, also between meals. If you take bromelain, take four to six tablets of approximately 230 to 250 milligrams every day.

"I know this can be fairly expensive," he goes on, "but how much does health mean to you? In 1960, medical services were 5 percent of our gross national product; by 1990, this figure was over 12 percent. We eat too much fat and too many refined carbohydrates, we smoke too much, we get virtually no exercise, and we overeat. For this reason, exercising, having a positive mental attitude, and eating fresh fruits are all very important. And enzyme supplementation is critical."

CHAPTER 33

THYROID
DISEASE

T hyroid disease is about fifteen or twenty times more prevalent in women than in men. About 1.5 million women are being treated for it in the United States, compared to only about 100,000 men. Thyroid disease is at once a hot-button issue and one of the most misunderstood illnesses facing us today. To cite just one example of the importance of thyroid disease: 70 percent of women with infertility and miscarriage have hypothyroidism.

IMPORTANCE OF THE THYROID

The thyroid gland is an important component of the immune system. Dr. Stephen Langer, who practices preventive medicine in Berkeley, California, explains that the thyroid gland is a small, butterfly-shaped organ at the base of the neck that releases about a teaspoon of hormone a year, which affects the metabolism and acts as a cellular carburetor for every cell in the body—from our hair follicles down to our toenails. The thyroid can be implicated in just about any condition.

Dr. Langer says, "If a person's metabolism is hypo-functioning, every-thing is going to be slow. In a book I wrote called *Solve the Riddle of Illness*, I explain why upward of 40 percent of the population may have subclinical hypothyroidism and not detect it by the traditional blood chemistry work that is done at their general practitioner's office. The symptoms of low thyroid include weakness, dry, coarse skin, slow speech, coarse hair, hair loss, weight gain, difficulty breathing, problems with menstruation, nervous-ness, heart palpitations, brittle nails, and severe chronic fatigue and de-pression. If you have a patient with a constellation of symptoms like that, they're going to be sick and tired of feeling sick and tired. Plus they're going to feel depressed all the time because they're going from one doctor to another, sometimes with two or three or four pages worth of complaints, and the doctors tell them it's all in their head, or that they should go home and learn to live with it."

Dr. Hyla Cass, a holistic psychiatrist, emphasizes the importance of thyroid inflammation, or thyroiditis, as a root cause of a variety of emotional and physical problems. She also describes the difficulty today of establishing the diagnosis of thyroid disorder in the face of continuing skepticism from conventional physicians. According to Dr. Cass, "When the thyroid isn't working properly, the immune system is impaired, and this sets up a vicious cycle. You have a person whose immune system is depleted and who is anxious; they're told by regular doctors that the problem is all in their head, that there's nothing physically wrong with them. So then they feel worse."

HYPOTHYROIDISM

Symptoms

Dr. Mark Lader is the supervisor of nutritional services at the Natural Wellness Center in New York. He's been in practice for more than ten years and is coauthor of *The Encyclopedia of Women's Health: Herbal and Nutritional Health.* He takes an historical look at hypothyroidism.

Dr. Lader says, "A milestone in the study of the disease was the publication of Broda Barnes's *Hypothyroidism: The Unsuspected Illness.* Back in 1976 when she wrote the book, so many of the symptoms that so many people were experiencing—ones that appeared to have no obvious cause—were called hypothyroidism. Some of those symptoms were tiredness, sluggishness, lethargy, weakness, slow speech, dry, coarse skin, bumpy skin on the back of the arm, intolerance of cold, puffy face or hands, loss of the outer third of the eyebrow, cramping, infertility, absence of period, excessive menstrual bleeding, loss of appetite, thinning of hair on the scalp, face, or genitals, swelling of the neck, gaining weight easily, and abdominal swelling. There are so many symptoms of hypothyroidism that are related to dysfunctions in so many organ systems of the body."

Broda Barnes was convinced that as many as 40 percent of Americans were affected by some form of hypothyroidism. But the effects of hypothyroidism go even beyond the multiple symptoms recognized by Broda Barnes. According to an article in the online magazine *Alternative Medicine* (www.alternativemedicine.com), hypothyroidism can also aggravate many female problems, including miscarriage, fibrocystic breast disease, ovarian fibroids, cystic ovaries, endometriosis, PMS, and menopausal symptoms. All of these, the article asserts, can be caused or aggravated by hypothyroidism.

Although the exact cause-and-effect connection is not worked out, it is known that hypothyroidism is linked to hormonal imbalances, particularly an excess of estrogen over the other female hormone, progesterone. Normally, a woman's ratio of progesterone to estrogen is ten to one. If she has too much estrogen, this is bad for the thyroid, since estrogen inhibits thyroid production while progesterone promotes it. The connection between thyroid production and female hormones indicates that a disruption in one sphere will affect the other.

Causes

Dr. Lader believes that nutritional deficiencies and stress are the two major keys to hypothyroidism. He says that although iodine deficiency or excess has been fully documented as a causal factor, it is not significant in the United States because most of the salt consumed here is iodized.

Micronutrient deficiencies are important. Some of the major nutrients involved in thyroid metabolism are selenium, glutathione, and zinc, which are known to be required for proper conversion of T4 into T3, the form of thyroid hormone that is active in the tissues. Dr. Lader says that we also should examine protein, fat, and carbohydrate consumption to really get an idea of what's happening with the thyroid gland. With hypothyroidism, as with so many other chronic illnesses, excess carbohydrate intake can be a major contributing factor. Too much carbohydrate can push blood sugar high and stimulate cortisol production, leading to hypoglycemia, and this increases thyroid production.

Dr. Lader also notes that suboptimal intake of calories, especially in women, may contribute to hypothyroidism. Diets high in caffeine may also adversely affect thyroid function. In addition, Dr. Lader notes, "Food allergies affect our thyroid glands, and that is why we see so many people with allergies who commonly have other systemic endocrine problems in their bodies. You also have to stop and look at chemical and medical toxicity. People whose cholesterol rises year after year may have hypothyroidism."

The gut is another place where problems can start. Our bodies detoxify and eliminate thyroid hormones through the gut, where certain enzymes in a healthy intestine help to break apart the soluble thyroid hormones so that we can reabsorb them through our intestines. Many people have had a lot of antibiotic therapy, and poor diet or intestinal problems have led to imbalances in microflora. This imbalance decreases the body's ability to reuptake active thyroid hormone. It's very important to establish a healthy environment in the intestines in order to maintain normal levels of thyroid hormones.

"We also have to look at the liver," Dr. Lader continues, "which is probably the most abused, overworked, and stressed organ in the body. Our liver is exposed to a number of toxins, which we have to make soluble so that we can excrete them out of our bodies. The same enzymes that break down many environmental toxins also break down thyroid chemicals. If our livers are overworked due to exposure to toxins, and those enzymes speed up, we are also going to be moving lots of thyroid hormone out of the body. This is really the X factor in thyroid illness."

Dr. Lader says that many drugs that people take also interfere with thyroid function. These include antidepressants and interferon, which is taken to treat hepatitis C but can affect thyroid function.

Testing

In conventional medicine, hypothyroidism is diagnosed by serum testing of the hormones thyroxine (T4), triiodothyronine (T3), and thyrotropin or thyroid-stimulating hormone (TSH). The textbook explanation is that low T4 and T3 levels along with high TSH indicate hypothyroidism. Dr. Lader comments, "On the face of it, hypothyroidism seems to be a real simple illness. The symptoms and blood values seem to correlate very well to a hypothyroid case, and then when we give levothyroxin, the symptoms seem to go away."

However, these tests are not as accurate as they might seem. An *Alternative Medicine* article points out that "most of the standard thyroid tests (for T3, T4, and TSH levels) often fail to pinpoint an underfunctioning thyroid, leading physicians to make erroneous diagnoses." The article goes on to say that doctors diagnose by symptoms, even while they remain unaware of the medical cause. So a patient with depression gets Prozac; one with weight gain is prescribed a weight loss drug; and one who is continually tired is said to suffer from chronic fatigue syndrome and gets no treatment.

In Dr. Lader's opinion, the standard blood tests do little to pinpoint the actual cause of the thyroid problem. Instead, he looks at the patient's overall environment to locate key problem sectors. The first step is ascertaining the patient's body temperature.

"For my own diagnosis, I ask the women about their symptoms and also use something called a basal temperature test, which is a very simple way to learn if the body is running cold. [Basal body temperature is a person's resting temperature upon waking up in the morning.] We ask the woman to use an oral thermometer. She shakes it down before she goes to sleep at night. First thing upon arising in the morning, she puts it under her armpit for about seven minutes.

"The temperature should be above 97.8. If it's below that level, many doctors will say that is diagnostic for hypothyroidism. However, we must remember that some people have a lower body temperature than others. They tend to run a little cool but don't have the hypothyroid symptoms. Some people's underarm temperature doesn't even rise after they have a significant improvement in their symptoms."

Dr. Lader looks at the whole body and a person's whole environment. In his experience, most of the symptoms that people with hypothyroidism come in with are lethargy, weakness, dryness, and cold intolerance. By studying both the temperature and the patient's whole history, he is able to assess the patient's condition.

Conventional Treatment

Conventional treatment relies on prescription drugs. According to Dr. Lader, on the surface, it would seem reasonable to treat the symptoms of hypothyroidism with synthroid or Armour thyroid, (the natural form of thyroid), or levothyroxin. These drugs make the symptoms disappear in a high percentage of cases. "But," he asks, "are we really getting to the true causes of the problem?" He cautions that there are certain drawbacks to these medicines.

Dr. Lader explains: "We know that in conventional treatment the patient will be on the medication for her whole life. Natural doctors believe we don't need to medicate people that long. Moreover, the increasingly larger doses these people are getting over the course of a lifetime cause more and more adverse symptoms."

If we look at the big picture, according to Dr. Lader, we see it's important to treat the whole body. "One of the true hallmarks of an alternative, natural practitioner is that she or he believes that eliminating symptoms is not really enough to determine if a successful therapy has been carried out." He adds, "Probably most readers realize that we have a medical tradition in this country of relegating hypothyroidism to the idiopathic trash heap. *Idiopathic* is a term used when traditional medicine does not know what the cause is. In my opinion, though, it means we are not asking the right questions. Saying that this problem has unknown causes or ones that cannot be addressed nutritionally is really a cop-out. At the same time, many doctors just whip out the hormone replacement therapy prescription pad in order to treat the symptoms while ignoring the cause. To me this is sad, a sad commentary on our whole health care system in this country."

Dr. Lader notes that there are many different agents in our environment that decrease thyroid function, ranging from stress to food. And, he says, treating environmentally induced hypothyroidism by using hormones or drugs is an excuse for those who are not willing to do the right work to get people well. He argues that to treat hypothyroidism, "We have to use a natural approach to make the body stronger and healthier. To really give optimal treatment for hypothyroidism, we have to treat the ultimate cause of the illness. So we will have to deal with diet, nutrition, and all the environmental factors that can affect our thyroid gland."

Alternative Treatment

"The first thing I like to have my patients do is take the underarm temperature test," says Dr. Lader. "Women who are menstruating need to do it on Day 2, Day 3, and Day 4 of their blood flow. Remember, if the temperature's 97.8 or below, they might have hypothyroidism.

"The next step is to keep a seven-day diary, which records foods eaten, stress, symptoms, and physical conditions. This diary can sometimes convert what appears to be a very difficult case into one that's obvious by giving you an idea of what is really happening in the body."

Next he concentrates on developing a healthier lifestyle. This includes eating right. "One thing I urge my patients to try to avoid is the *Brassica* family foods—cabbage, broccoli, cauliflower." He acknowledges that these foods have many health benefits, but says that some people are eating way too many of them, especially if they are exhibiting thyroid symptoms. Stress management is also important. One of the major problems of hypothyroidism, as noted, is inadequate conversion of inactive thyroid (thyroxine) into active thyroid (triiodothyronine). Stress elevates cortisol, which inhibits this conversion process. Heavy activity, exercise, and different stress-reduction methods are needed. One also has to take a good, high-quality multiple vitamin and eat a healthy, balanced diet.

Another aspect of treatment is nutritional supplementation. The creation of a supplement program has to be handled carefully, Dr. Lader explains. "It comes down to the fact that every hypothyroid patient is different and requires a different approach. Supplemental programs need to be customized so that they address all the factors that have been ascertained during the diagnosis and workup. In general, we have to make sure people are taking in adequate amounts of selenium, glutathione, and zinc."

Dr. Lader concludes, "People who are suffering from hypothyroidism should view the disease as a chance to make some positive changes in their lifestyle, especially in terms of stress and toxicity."

THYROIDITIS

Over the past fifteen years or so, it has become apparent that some people with thyroid conditions have normal thyroid hormone levels and are suffering from another condition, known as Hashimoto's disease, or autoimmune thyroiditis.

Causes

What triggers an autoimmune response? Dr. Langer explains: "Imagine autoimmune thyroiditis to be like rheumatoid arthritis of the thyroid gland. A person can have rheumatoid arthritis, which is an autoimmune condition where the body puts out antibodies to the joints. Frequently people with rheumatoid arthritis can experience long periods of remission. When they are under a great deal of stress, the body puts out antibodies to the joints and all their joints swell up. A similar thing happens with thyroiditis; if a person gets stressed out for any reason whatsoever, the body can start pumping out antibodies to the thyroid gland. The thyroid becomes acutely inflamed, and thyroid hormone, which under normal circumstances would not be released, starts escaping. It's almost like pumping speed into your system."

Clinical Experience

Dr. Langer notes, "There is a very precise blood test that any doctor can order called the autoimmune thyroid antibody test, and most of the people who I suspect have thyroid conditions and have normal thyroid hormone levels will have an elevation in their antithyroid antibodies. If they have an elevated antithyroid antibody level, they have the symptoms that go along with low thyroid, which can be any one of 125 symptoms that we enumerate in *Solve the Riddle of Illness*."

Like hypothyroidism, thyroiditis can cause a number of psychological symptoms. Dr. Langer explains: "With thyroiditis people get anxiety attacks and panic attacks for no apparent reason. They could be sitting and reading a book. All of a sudden they will develop a cascade of heart palpitations and fearfulness.

"I've had a number of patients who have been rushed, almost on a monthly basis, to the emergency room to be worked up by cardiologists because their heart was pounding over 200 beats a minute. Cardiologists would do EKGs and echocardiograms and then tell them to go see a psychiatrist. The psychiatrist would work them up, not find anything, and then put them on an antidepressant or a tranquilizer, and actually make the condition worse. When you have an undiscovered organic basis for a psychological problem, being put on psychotropic medication is like sitting on a thumbtack and being put on pain pills for the rest of your life. It has about the same effect. It wears the system down, and as a result the patient's condition not only does not improve but will in fact deteriorate, because the underlying cause is not being treated."

A large number of Dr. Hyla Cass's patients also have thyroiditis. "I really can't emphasize the importance of this problem enough," she says, "because thyroiditis often accompanies the mixed infection syndrome, which can consist of any combination of the following: parasites, candidiasis, and the viral syndromes, including Epstein-Barr virus and cytomegalovirus. Psychological components include depression, anxiety, and even panic attacks.

"To treat thyroiditis, I've done nutritional consults on people who were under the care of other physicians. When I suggested that they had thyroiditis and that it was to be treated with low doses of thyroid hormones, I was met with skepticism from the other doctors.

"When people have these long-standing chronic conditions, they can become extremely depressed. They feel like they can't go on anymore, particularly when their body has been so racked by the continuing illness. Also, some of the mixed infection of thyroiditis and the parasites or other viruses can actually affect the brain directly. Thyroiditis and its accompanying infections affect the central nervous system along with every other organ of the body. So people come in extremely depressed, both as a reaction to their prolonged illness and as a primary symptom of the illness, and this is usually totally overlooked. That's why it's crucial to do a good medical workup on a patient whose disorder may at first appear purely psychological in origin."

"There is one more connection to be drawn between depression and thyroid dysfunction," Dr. Langer adds. "Poor libido. One of the classic symptoms of depression is a loss of interest in sex. Those people who in the past were sexually active but who all of a sudden or gradually started to lose interest in sex will be diagnosed as being depressed right away. Men come into my office by the score—many of them young—who have potency problems, and they can't figure it out because they have no apparent organic illness. As a result, they get performance anxiety, and if that continues long enough, they wind up getting severely depressed. But I have found that if you go to the root cause of their depression, very often it's the thyroid that's malfunctioning.

"If a person develops an acute depression that leads to a sexual dysfunction—which it frequently does—a doctor would be remiss if he or she didn't look for an imbalance in the thyroid. Patients have got to start taking their health destinies into their own hands and demanding that doctors do thyroid testing and look for autoimmune thyroid disorders and nutritional imbalances, which are frequently the underlying causes of sexual dysfunction and depression."

Alternative Therapies

"The question for holistic clinicians to ask themselves, regarding each individual patient is where they're going to intervene," Dr. Langer says. "Different physicians will intervene at different places, depending upon their background and interests. I try, to the best of my ability, to get to the root cause of what's going on. If I am having difficulty figuring out the cause, then

I try to intervene at a point in a person's imbalance that will cause the least disruption to their lifestyle and give them the best results for the least amount of money in the quickest period of time. Frequently, that turns out to be treating with small doses of thyroid and altering eating habits. In my clinical experience, I have found that with the thyroid and nutritional support, very often a person will get better. The thyroid is not a lifetime treatment and can be removed after the person's condition has been stabilized. Thyroid treatment is inexpensive, works rapidly, and when done properly is absolutely nontoxic."

Dr. Allan Spreen, a general practitioner who specializes in nutrition-based medicine, reminds us that while thyroid supplementation is an important modality, it is not fail-safe. "I'd love to say that correcting thyroid function is a panacea. While it doesn't work 100 percent of the time, if a patient comes in complaining of fatigue and depression that is linked with the physical findings of foods not digesting well, and cold extremities, then an underactive thyroid may be the root cause. People come and say, 'Oh, my husband says, "Don't touch me with your feet at night because they're just ice cold."' These are the same people who are comfortable in a room when everybody else is boiling and who are freezing in a room when everybody else is comfortable. Their thinking seems to have slowed down. They just don't seem to be able to concentrate like they used to, and they don't remember lists the way they used to.

"In this kind of a situation, once I find that their blood levels of thyroid are normal, I go back to the old school of Broda Barnes, who, forty or fifty years ago, did axillary temperature testing. I ask my patients to keep a record of their early-morning basal body temperature. If their basal metabolic rate based on early-morning body temperatures is really low, then I consider them to be candidates for thyroid supplementation. In axillary testing, Broda Barnes talked about temperature ranges between 97.8 and 98.2 degrees Fahrenheit, which is lower than the 98.6 people think of as normal. But the axillary temperature is taken in the armpit first thing in the morning, using a mercury thermometer that stays there for ten minutes before they get up. If their temperature is, much of the time, down in the 96.8, 96.7, 96.5 range, I at least consider the possibility that the person needs low doses of natural thyroid, which is still available.

"Thyroid is a prescription drug. Some doctors who use this type of testing use synthetic thyroid. I prefer to prescribe natural thyroid in very low doses. If a person responds—either their temperature rises or their symptoms lift— then I retest them to see if their blood levels of thyroid have changed. Many times a person with this profile of symptoms who takes thyroid begins to feel better, but their blood tests remain unchanged, including levels of thyroid stimulating hormone (TSH) and actual thyroid hormone. This means that the blood testing has missed the diagnosis, and yet the person feels well with the increased, but undetectable, dose of thyroid hormone."

PATIENT STORIES

I came to be treated by Dr. Spreen only after first following the conventional route in medical treatment. In 1988, I was in my fifth year of infertility treatments, had taken multiple infertility drugs, and wound up severely depressed, which caused me to lose thirty-five pounds in two months. I couldn't sleep, I had panic attacks, the whole horrible group of symptoms associated with depression. The doctors put me on the conventional Xanax treatment for three years before I met Dr. Spreen, who was helping me with some other related medical problems. I had hair loss, skin problems, nail-biting problems. I had aches all over my body, especially in my legs. Dr. Spreen got me on a vitamin regimen, which made me feel somewhat better.

Then Dr. Spreen put me on very low doses of thyroid and immediately—within two to three weeks—all the problems I just mentioned were gone. Now, I had had thyroid checks three times during the whole time when I was being treated for infertility, and the blood tests had always come up negative. But I knew that in my family there were thyroid problems. There are at least six members of my family I can think of who have thyroid disorders, but mine just never showed up on my tests. After taking these very low doses of thyroid, my skin problem cleared up, I stopped biting my nails, and my legs stopped aching. The mild depression I was still suffering from all of a sudden in August vanished. I felt great. I slept like a normal person again. I had energy. People started commenting on how I seemed to be like my old self again. It was like getting a new lease on life!

I feel rather fed up with the original doctors I went to see. They treated me like I was a hysterical woman who needed to get a grip on things. I have never told them about my recovery using alternative methods because I don't think they'd be receptive to it.

—Jenny

I had hives, some kind of an allergic response, about five years ago and it progressed to the point where I had hives on my vocal cords. It was a pretty serious allergic reaction, for which I was first treated with antihistamines. Later, I was treated with prednisone. When small doses of prednisone given every other day didn't help, my doctor began increasing the dosage until I was taking 70 milligrams every day. After about six weeks I started declining physically from taking this tremendous dose. I gained about fifty pounds. I had conjunctivitis in both of my eyes. I had open sores.

I was so weak I was almost bedridden. I did find another doctor who slowly weaned me off of the prednisone. But when it was all over, my immune system had been damaged. I had a lot of viral illnesses that are usually associated with chronic fatigue syndrome. I could scarcely get out of bed, and I couldn't lose all the weight I had gained. So I went from doctor to doctor. I was living in the Midwest at the time, and many of these doctors said, "Your metabolic system has been altered by prednisone. Too bad, but you will never lose that weight. And prednisone can damage the immune system. Too bad, but your immune system has been damaged." No one could offer me any help at all.

I first went to Dr. Atkins in New York and he was a lot of help. It was through Dr. Atkins and his association with Dr. Huggins that I learned about dental amalgams, because when your immune system is depleted, you are much more susceptible to any kind of toxins, including mercury leaching from mercury amalgam fillings. It was causing me a great deal of trouble and I did have those removed.

Then I moved to California and I had heard, previous to my moving, about Dr. Slagle and her work with depression. In fact, I referred friends to her, friends I had made in California, and they had these miraculous cures from depression after two weeks of taking B-complex vitamins and amino acids. But I didn't think of going to her myself for quite a while because I thought of her as someone who only treated depression. In fact, like many alternative physicians, she treats the whole person. She had worked with fatigue a lot, and she first tested me thoroughly and found that my thyroid and, in fact, my whole endocrine system, was not functioning properly, most likely as a result of prednisone. She picked up subtleties in the test that other doctors ignored. She has the philosophy that a body should be healthy and whole. She doesn't need gross parameters of unusual test results to say something is wrong here. So she was able to discover that I had a rather unusual problem in my thyroid and she was able to treat it.

When I began seeing her, I still had very limited energy. Even though Dr. Atkins had helped me lose weight so I looked normal, I still didn't feel normal. In one day, I could either go to the grocery store or go to a doctor's appointment. That was all I could do. The remainder of the day I had to rest. I went to Dr. Slagle and after she began treating my thyroid, I had a leap of improvement. I regained my energy. She also gave me amino acids, which heightened my mood. Even though I hadn't thought I was depressed—and I still don't think I was—generally the amino acids made me feel healthier. And while I don't have the energy of a lot of people around me, I can pretty much function normally, which is a miracle. It has been a five-year struggle and I'm finally living practically a normal life.

Here's what I have learned from my experience: You simply cannot go to a traditional physician and carelessly allow that doctor to treat your symptoms with drugs. Traditional physicians tend not to look at the whole person, but to give drugs to ameliorate the symptoms, or to treat individual problems without regard to what that treatment does to the rest of the body. I learned to use tremendous caution when entrusting my body to someone. If you're going to trust your body to someone, you should know a lot about the physician. You should know whether the physician treats the whole person and sees you as more than an allergy or a gallbladder.

—Helen

I recently saw a young woman who came in depressed, tired, unable to get up in the morning, and feeling overwhelmed by her work responsibilities. Her history revealed that she was often cold, especially in her hands and feet (she even wore socks to bed), had thinning hair, dry skin, constipation, and was losing the outer part of her eyebrows. I suspected an imbalance in her thyroid. When I asked about thyroid disease, she said that it had been suspected before, but her tests had been normal. I checked her thyroid hormones, including thyroid antibody levels.

Often despite "normal" blood tests, there is an underactive thyroid. Dr. Broda Barnes's technique of monitoring thyroid function through body temperature is used by many alternative practitioners. Although this patient's thyroid hormone blood levels were normal, she did, in fact, have antithyroid antibodies, confirming a diagnosis of Hashimoto's thyroiditis. This is an autoimmune disease, treatable with thyroid hormone, antioxidants, and adrenal support. Her signs were those of hypothyroidism, indicating that the circulating hormone was being rendered ineffective. With Hashimoto's thyroiditis, there are often also intermittent signs of hyperthyroidism, or overactive thyroid, such as irritability or heart palpitations.

I prescribed thyroid hormone from natural animal sources, and asked her to monitor her body temperature so that I could adjust the dosage. She asked whether this supplementation would suppress her own thyroid function, and whether she would be taking it for the rest of her life. The answer was no on both counts. The treatment actually supported her own gland, allowing it to heal. Within ten days of starting the program she was feeling alive again.

—Dr. Hyla Cass

CHAPTER 34

URINARY INCONTINENCE

CAUSES

Eighty-five percent of the thirteen million people who are incontinent are women. This is because urinary incontinence is related to childbirth and menopause. Gynecologist Vicki Hufnagel explains, "In many cases, women are given episiotomies after delivery, without proper closure. Since muscles are not put back together correctly, the whole area is unable to provide support." Dr. Hufnagel adds that during menopause, urinary incontinence occurs when a woman is not making enough estrogen. Too little estrogen enters the vaginal tissue, causing the area to become thin, inelastic, and weak.

Urinary incontinence can also be the result of brain and spinal cord lesions, trauma, multiple sclerosis, and allergies.

There are many causes of transient incontinence. Some common ones are infection, strophic urethritis or vaginitis, certain medications (sedatives, hypnotics, diuretics, anticholinergics, alpha-adrenergic agonists or antagonists, and calcium-channel blockers), psychological disorders (especially depression), endocrine disorders, hyperglycemia, restricted mobility, and stool impaction.

Smoking has been found to be the cause of 28 percent of cases of urinary incontinence in women. Smoking increases the odds of both stress and motor urinary incontinence, and with increased daily and lifetime cigarette consumption, the odds for genuine stress incontinence rise. A study of six hundred women showed that genuine stress incontinence was twice as common for both former and current smokers as for nonsmokers.

SYMPTOMS

Urinary incontinence is a partial or total loss of control over one's bladder and urinary sphincter muscles. Sometimes, incontinence is accompanied by a feeling of urgency. This is usually the result of a person's inability to empty the bladder completely. Coughing and other stressors can set off urinary incontinence. Overflow can occur when bladder capacity is small.

CLINICAL EXPERIENCE

Women with urinary incontinence are often advised to get bladder surgery, even hysterectomies. But this drastic approach may be completely unnecessary, according to Dr. Hufnagel, who says that women need to be educated about more conservative treatments for this common problem.

Outpatient Surgery and Hormone Replacement

Women need to repair their failed episiotomy, or to receive hormones, Dr. Hufnagel explains. Often, they simply need outpatient surgery to put the muscles and tissues back the way they should have been restored at the time of delivery.

Regarding menopause, Dr. Hufnagel adds, "We can treat this locally, without surgery, by simply putting hormones into the vagina. One or two months later, we see normal, healthy tissue."

Electrical Stimulation

This treatment became popular in Europe after it was learned that high voltages of electricity to the vaginal area caused muscles to contract. However, the effects were short-lived, and the technique was not without problems. Voltages had to be applied constantly, which sometimes resulted in tissue burning and nerve damage.

In the United States, electrical stimulation is being performed with lower voltages and a pulsing sequence of one second on and one second off to prevent muscle fatigue. The objective is to strengthen the urethral muscles and the puborectalis muscle, which control the opening and closing of the bladder muscles. This form of electrical stimulation, combined with pelvic floor exercises, has produced favorable results in trial studies. It allows for a retraining, toning, and strengthening of muscles so that a patient can regain continence. One electrical product that looks promising is called Cystotron, put out by a company called Biosonics.

Homeopathic Remedies

Dana Ullman suggests in an article posted on HealthWorld Online (www.healthy.net) that homeopathic medicines can help prevent involuntary urination. He advises consulting a homeopathic practitioner who can individualize the treatment and work on strengthening the overall immune system, rather than just treating the bladder symptoms.

But there are homeopathic medicines that you can use on your own. One new, inexpensive homeopathic medicine he recommends is EnurAid, which is nontoxic and nonaddictive. Other homeopathic remedies that he recommends are listed below. Ullman recommends that someone who has not used homeopathic remedies before should start all the remedies suggested at the sixth potency and take the medication three or four times a day. If there is no improvement after taking a medication for a week, a different homeopathic remedy should be tried.

ARNICA (LEOPARD'S BANE)—Arnica is good for involuntary urination after surgery.

BELLADONNA (DEADLY NIGHTSHADE)—Belladonna is helpful for people who dribble urine and who sometimes have a burning sensation when they urinate.

CAUSTICUM—Causticum may help if involuntary urination gets worse in the winter and better in the summer. Often people with these symptoms lose urine when they cough or sneeze.

EQUISETUM (SCOURING RUSH)—Equisetum is a general remedy for anyone who loses urine or is a bedwetter, with no apparent cause.

FERRUM PHOS (IRON PHOSPHATE)—Ferrum phos works best for people who tend to lose urine during the day. Often people with this symptom have the strongest urge to urinate when standing; lying down lessens the urge.

KREOSOTUM (BEECHWOOD)—Kreosotum is recommended for people who cannot control sudden urges to urinate. Ullman says that these people tend to wet their bed during the first part of the night, and may dream that they are urinating.

CHAPTER 35

URINARY TRACT INFECTIONS AND INFLAMMATIONS

U rinary tract infections and inflammations are quite common, accounting for approximately six million office visits per year in the United States. Dr. Jennifer Brett, a naturopathic physician from Stratford, Connecticut, says only 60 percent of people with symptoms of urinary tract infections have true infections; the other 40 percent have inflammations. Three types of infections and inflammations that Dr. Brett commonly sees are true urinary tract infections, urinary tract inflammations, and interstitial cystitis, a more distressing form of inflammation that can last for months or even years.

CAUSES

The cause of urinary tract inflammations is unknown, but some doctors believe they may be caused by viruses, food allergies, candida in the colon, hormonal changes, new sexual partners, or vigorous sexual activity. Interstitial cystitis may result from infection by candida or allergic reactions to foods and additives. "These irritants inflame the pelvis and bladder, and the body responds by increasing blood flow to the area," Dr. Brett explains. "Pelvic congestion causes further irritation and pressure on the bladder. Again, the body responds by sending more blood. This becomes a vicious cycle."

Dr. David L. Hoffman, in an article posted on the HealthWorld Online website (www.healthy.net), adds that microcrystals of calcium phosphate in the urine may cause mechanical irritation to the bladder walls, resulting in inflammation.

High-Risk Groups

Dr. David Kaufman, a specialist in women's urological problems, says that there are basically four types of women at high risk: "The most common patients are young, sexually active females. Another large group at risk are postmenopausal women. In fact, 8 to 10 percent of all women over sixty will get a bladder infection at some point. We also see a lot of patients who are hospitalized. The risk of bladder infection increases about 5 percent per day for every day that a catheter is in place. For this reason, medical doctors try to get catheters out as quickly as possible. The last high-risk group are patients with neurological problems. An example would be multiple sclerosis; patients with MS do not completely empty their bladders."

Dr. Kaufman says, "Many sexually active women get cystitis as a result of intercourse because the bacteria that normally live in the vaginal vault area get pushed up into the urethra. A woman's urethra is only about an inch and a half long, while in men it is much longer. In females, it doesn't take too much for bacteria to migrate from the outside of the urethra to the inside of the bladder. That's why we see so many more young women than men with bladder infections.

"It is very important for women to know that their partners are not giving them infections. The bacteria are already in the vaginal area and simply get pushed into the bladder during intercourse."

Dr. Hoffman mentions several other risk factors. One is being diabetic or eating a lot of sugars. Another is use of products such as douches, feminine deodorants, antibacterial soaps, and certain contraceptive creams or jellies that irritate vaginal tissue, making it vulnerable to infection. Using a diaphragm can also irritate the urethra. Excess use of antibiotics will promote growth of bacteria resistant to those drugs, which can make cystitis more likely. Finally, he says, eating foods containing pesticides can cause some types of interstitial cystitis.

Hormonal Imbalance

Dr. Kaufman says there are many reasons that not all sexually active women get bladder infections. "One of the more interesting ones has to do with the woman's hormonal balance. We know that there are estrogen and progesterone receptors on the lining cells of the urethra. In some women bacteria sticks to these receptors, a condition that is related to hormone levels. Imagine bacteria as little organisms with Velcro hooks. Picture the lining cells of the urethra with the opposite kind of hooks. Bacteria hook on to the Velcro on the receptor sites. In most women, the urinary stream washes away most bacteria. But in women who have specific hormonal environments, the bacteria are not expelled that easily. These are the women we see in our office with recurrent bladder infections."

Dr. Kaufman adds that postmenopausal women tend to get urinary tract infections for this reason as well. Their low estrogen levels cause their urethral linings to be "stickier" for bacteria. "One way to treat that is simply to insert low-dosage estrogen cream into the vaginal vault, about once a week," he advises. "Many women are on estrogen pills, but that does not have the same protective influence on the urinary tract as does estrogen cream."

Weakened Immunity

Dr. Linda Wharton, a naturopathic physician and acupuncturist from New Zealand and author of *Natural Woman Health: A Guide to Healthy Living for Women of All Ages*, says recurrent bladder infections reflect a state of lowered immunity and weakened vitality: "Remember that cystitis is an infection. As with all infections, individuals with lowered nutritional status, poor cellular health, and lowered immunity are much more susceptible to infection. Women don't always develop acute cystitis each time a stray bacterium finds its way into the bladder. Often, women play host to these potentially problem-causing bacteria for weeks or months or even a lifetime without ever experiencing acute symptoms. It is only when the health of the whole body is reduced that an explosion of this bacterial population takes place. This may occur, for example, when a woman goes through a period of great stress, such as a divorce or the death of a loved one."

Structural Problems

Dr. Wharton adds that other causes of cystitis are often overlooked: "Pelvic floor muscles can weaken as a result of pregnancy and childbirth. When these muscles are weakened, the bladder may prolapse and bulge forward into the wall of the vagina. If the back part of the bladder droops below the neck of the bladder, it becomes virtually impossible to empty the bladder properly. This leaves an almost permanent reservoir of urine in the bladder. In time, the stagnant urine becomes a haven for bacteria to multiply, should they be present." Dr. Wharton also says that a prolapsed transverse colon— due to childbirth, age, abdominal fat, poor posture, or spinal problems—can eventually cause bladder problems.

Over time the prolapsed transverse colon—which lies across the abdomen, sags, compressing the organs beneath it, including the bladder. Blood flow is impeded, and the oxygen-starved bladder becomes ripe for infection. She adds, "This same downgrading of tissue health can occur as a direct result of a chronic back problem. All the pelvic organs receive nervous impulses from the spine, and a chronic lower back problem can interfere with those nervous impulses from the spinal cord." Dr. Wharton advises women with chronic back problems to see an osteopath or chiropractor.

Constipation

Dr. Wharton says, "Waste materials are excreted from our bodies through several different channels. The bowels excrete in the form of feces; the lungs gets rid of toxins in the form of carbon dioxide; the skin eliminates toxins as perspiration; and the kidney and bladder pass toxins out in the form of urine. If any one of these waste disposal systems is functioning inadequately, it places an excessive load on the others. If you only manage a half-hearted bowel movement every two or three days, you are placing undue stress on your kidneys and bladder, as accumulated toxins are passed out this way instead. In a sense, then, there is actually a direct link between chronic constipation and repeated urinary tract infections."

SYMPTOMS

Typical symptoms of urinary tract infections and inflammations are frequent urination, a sensation that the bladder is never quite empty, and a burning sensation upon urination. Often women get up at night to urinate. There may be cramps, and the urine may be dark and foul-smelling. In severe cases, there may be blood in the urine as well.

CLINICAL EXPERIENCE

Diagnosis

A diagnosis of cystitis is usually made by collecting a midstream urine sample and testing for the presence of bacteria. If the problem stems from an inflammation, no pathogenic bacteria will be found in the urine, nor will bacteria be found on a vaginal culture.

Conventional Treatment

The usual treatment for cystitis is a course of antibiotics, and standard therapy for chronic cystitis generally consists of repeated rounds of the same therapy.

In the long term, this practice may actually exacerbate the condition rather than cure it. It is well known that broad-spectrum antibiotics are indiscriminate killers that destroy colonies of friendly gut bacteria along with problem-causing organisms. Once the delicate balance of the normal gastrointestinal microflora has been disrupted, less desirable organisms proliferate, virtually unchecked. These include *Escherichia coli,* the prime cause of cystitis, and candida overgrowth, a suspected cause of inflammations.

Dr. Kaufman says that antibiotics should be a last-ditch effort, used only when various holistic protocols fail to achieve results. Even then, mild medicines should be used: "What of women who do all the right things, and still come back with bladder infections? In these cases, we need to turn to more traditional medical approaches. The gold standard for treating patients who do everything right and still get infections is a very gentle, bacteriostatic antibiotic. A bacteriostatic antibiotic does not kill the bacteria, but limits bacterial growth. It is gentler on the system, and generally does not cause yeast infections or gastrointestinal problems. I am not big on taking antibiotics, but this is a better alternative than constant infections."

Dr. Brett reports that radical therapies are sometimes used for persistent cases. "Treatments I have read about in recent medical journals include surgery to cut nerves to reduce irritation to the bladder, hormonal therapy, and even antidepressive medications to help women sleep better, even though this doesn't get at the root cause of the problem."

Naturopathic Treatments

DIET

It is important to drink plenty of pure water, about one 8-ounce glass each hour. "If you are in agony and you don't know what to do, start drinking water and don't stop," advises Dr. Wharton. "Stay away from tea, coffee, soft drinks, and alcohol, but drink plenty of water."

Cranberry, either in the form of unsweetened juice or capsules, changes the pH of the urine, making it more acidic and less hospitable to bacteria. Cranberries also contain powerful antibacterial substances. In fact, studies reveal that as little as 15 ounces of cranberry juice results in an 80 percent inhibition of bacterial growth. Bacteria lose the ability to cling to the bladder wall and must exit the system along with urine. Other research indicates that cranberry juice combined with vitamin C acidifies the urine further. The effect is therefore much greater when both are taken together.

Other drinks useful for temporarily acidifying the urine include lemon juice and water, buttermilk, and 2 teaspoons of apple cider vinegar stirred into a glass of water. Drink any of these substances three or four times a day.

During an acute attack of cystitis, the diet can be temporarily changed to further acidify the urine. Dr. Wharton warns that this is recommended only for short periods of time, during an acute infection: "Eat plenty of acidic foods, such as grains, nuts, seeds, fish, dairy products, meat and bread, and cut back on fruit and vegetables."

VITAMIN C

Any time the body is fighting an infection, it tolerates large amounts of C, sometimes as much as 10,000 to 15,000 milligrams orally each day (and even more intravenously). For cystitis, or for any infection, take vitamin C to bowel tolerance. (Bowel tolerance is where the stool becomes quite loose, almost to the point of diarrhea.) Vitamin C should be taken every two to three hours since it is water-soluble, which means that it is rapidly excreted from the body. According to Dr. Hoffman, recent studies indicate that ascorbic acid irritates the bladder. For this reason it is best to take vitamin C in the buffered form of calcium ascorbate. Aspartate also irritates the bladder, so avoid vitamins that contain it.

Dr. Wharton says that vitamin C fights infections in several ways: "Vitamin C concentrates in very high levels in the urine and exerts a direct bactericidal effect. It also supports systemic immune system function by helping to activate neutrophils, the white blood cells most involved in the front line defense against infection. It also works to stimulate the production of lymphocytes, which are important for coordinating immune function at the cellular level."

VITAMIN A

In addition to vitamin C, think about vitamin A. An easy way of supplementing with this vitamin is to use halibut or cod liver oil capsules, up to 25,000 IU a day, during acute phases of infection. Vitamin A helps protect the mucous membrane lining of the bladder and urethra from irritation during infection. It also improves antibody response and white blood cell function. Just a word of warning here: if you are pregnant, do not use such high doses of vitamin A, as they have been associated with birth defects. Beta carotene, with which the body can make vitamin A as it is needed, is a safer alternative.

ZINC

Zinc is essential for increasing white blood cell activity in response to infection. For acute cystitis, approximately 50 milligrams elemental zinc is needed daily.

HERBS

The classes of herbs used to treat cystitis include antiseptic herbs, demulcents, and diuretics. Antiseptic herbs for bladder infections include uva-ursi, buchu, goldenseal, juniper berries, and garlic. "Think garlic whenever you have any type of infection, including cystitis," says Dr. Wharton. Demulcents soothe inflamed mucous membranes inside the bladder and urethra, and include marsh mallow root, juniper berry, and corn silk. Diuretic herbs stimulate the production and excretion of urine, which helps to wash out bacteria. Common diuretics are parsley and goldenrod.

Dr. Wharton recommends the following old naturopathic herbal remedies for treating burning urine: "Mix together equal parts of fennel, burdock, and slippery elm. Steep a teaspoon of this mixture in a cup of boiled water for about twenty minutes. Have one cup before each meal, and one before bed."

She also recommends flaxseed tea or a combination of uva-ursi and buchu: "For either tea, use 1 teaspoon of the dried herbs to a cup of boiling water. Again, let it steep for fifteen to twenty minutes. Then drink one cup, three or four times a day. The results more than compensate for the awful taste."

Dr. Hoffman recommends the following formula for cystitis: Combine two parts corn silk, two parts uva-ursi, and one part buchu. Take 5 milliliters of this tincture three times a day. At the same time, drink an infusion of yarrow, another antiseptic herb, throughout the day.

Dr. Tori Hudson, a naturopath in Portland, Oregon, in her column for *Prevention* magazine recommends the following combination of herbs, either as capsules or in tinctures: pipsissewa, uva-ursi, echinacea or goldenseal, and buchu. For two days, take two capsules or 20 to 30 drops every two hours. For the next seven days, take the capsules or tincture three times daily.

Dr. Joseph Pizzorno adds this bit of advice: "After sexual intercourse, women should wipe the opening to the urethra with a dilute solution of Betadine or a strong solution of goldenseal tea to wash away any bacteria that may have been forced up into the urethra."

OTHER THERAPIES

Homeopathy

Judyth Reichenberg-Ullman and Robert Ullman, naturopathic and homeopathic doctors in Edmonds, Washington, in an article posted on the Health-World Online website (www.healthy.net), recommend Cantharis (Spanish fly), a frequently used remedy in cases in which extreme pain in the bladder occurs very suddenly and there is blood in the urine. Staphysagria (stavesacre) is the remedy to use when a bladder infection has developed after having sex ("honeymoon cystitis"). When cystitis is associated with pain in the kidney area, especially on the right side, they suggest Berberis aquifolium (Oregon grape).

Hydrotherapy

Hydrotherapy is another traditional naturopathic method for helping people overcome the discomforts of cystitis. Sitz baths or hot compresses stimulate blood circulation and remove toxins from the pelvic area. Dr. Wharton explains how this is done: "You can use a hot compress by dipping a small hand towel into a basin of water, as hot as you can possibly tolerate it. Wring out the water and quickly apply the cloth to the area just above the pubic bone.

As the cloth cools, repeat the process. In total, apply the compress eight or nine times. Repeat this process two to three times throughout the day. It actually feels wonderful and gives quite a bit of local relief to the symptoms.

"Alternatively, you can try making a sitz bath. Fill a small tub with water, once again, as hot as you can bear it. Add 6 drops bergamot oil, and sit in the bath so that water actually covers your pelvis and lower abdomen. Stay there for around half an hour. As the water cools, keep replenishing with fresh, hot water to keep the water up to a hot, even temperature. Just a word of warning: If you have a problem with a weak heart or high blood pressure, hot sitz baths aren't really for you. You are better off just using a local compress."

Acupuncture

Dr. Wharton reports impressive results in the treatment of chronic cystitis with acupuncture when it is accompanied by lifestyle and dietary changes: "Usually an acute attack of cystitis responds to two to four acupuncture sessions, spaced two or three days apart. Chronic cystitis sufferers often benefit from an extended course of acupuncture treatment to prevent the recurrence of their problem."

Aromatherapy

Essential oils can enhance any treatment program, according to aromatherapist Ann Berwick. To help clear up a urinary tract infection, 18 to 20 drops of juniper and cedarwood can be added to 1 ounce of lotion and massaged into the lower abdomen. Also, 6 to 8 drops of juniper, bergamot, or sandlewood can be added to a sitz bath or full bath.

A Psychological Perspective

Judyth Reichenberg-Ullman and Robert Ullman caution further that it's important not only to rest but to pay attention to whatever message your body is giving you with this bladder infection, in order to avoid recurrences. Therefore, consider what might be its underlying cause. They add that breathing into the pain and relaxing can be remarkably effective: "We had one patient who cured a bladder infection solely through visualization and meditation."

URINARY TRACT INFLAMMATIONS

For urinary inflammation not caused by bacteria, Dr. Brett says it is important to avoid foods that encourage the growth of candida, such as wheat, simple sugars, white flour, pastries, candies, alcohol, aged cheeses, vinegar, and even fruit. Avoid known food allergens. It is a good idea to get a test to determine if there are any other foods in the diet that are acting as irritants.

As with bacterial infections, you should drink one 8-ounce glass of water every hour. It is also a good idea to drink a glass of water and to urinate immediately after sexual intercourse. This tends to reduce the bladder irritation that sexual intercourse may cause.

Clothing is important too. Avoid tight-fitting pants, nylon underwear, and pantyhose. They encourage the growth of candida in the vaginal tract, which irritates the bladder and urethra.

Vitamins and herbs may also be useful. For vitamins, take 2,000 to 6,000 milligrams of buffered vitamin C and 100 to 200 milligrams of vitamin B6. Also take four to six capsules of evening primrose oil. Herbs that soothe the bladder include althea or marsh mallow, corn silk, slippery elm, and goldenrod. Finally, as with bacterial infections, the homeopathic remedy Cantharis (Spanish fly) is often effective in reducing bladder and urethra irritations.

INTERSTITIAL CYSTITIS

"The basic way to treat interstitial cystitis," says Dr. Brett, "is to remove congestion from the pelvis." The therapies she suggests in cases of interstial cystitis are listed below. "If you follow these basic guidelines," says Dr. Brett, "within three to four weeks, you are likely to notice that your ability to sleep through the night is improved and that your cramping and pain during the day is significantly lessened."

Tests

It is a good idea to be tested for food allergies to see if some food is causing an antibody-antigen reaction and irritating the bladder. It is also important to test for candida in the colon because candida can cause irritations and antibody reactions that irritate the bladder. Next, check to see that the hormones are in balance. If they are not, use vitamin B6, evening primrose oil, and herbs to restore hormonal balance.

Exercise

The two types of exercise that help in cases of interstitial cystitis are aerobic exercise and inversion exercise. Doing aerobic exercise every day helps to remove blood congestion from the pelvis. *Aerobic* means anything that gets the blood moving, such as walking briskly, jogging, swimming, and bicycling.

Specific exercises for moving the blood involve turning upside down. In yoga, this is accomplished with the headstand or shoulderstand. It can also be achieved by lying on the back, raising the legs up, and performing cycling rotations with the legs. If there is a back or neck problem, however, a simple solution is to use a slant board, which can be made simply with an old door or a couple of one-by-four boards. One end can be placed on the couch, and the other end on the floor. Once it is stable, the person lies upside down, that is, with the head near the floor and the feet near the couch. The blood is automatically pulled out of the pelvis by gravity, and moved into the chest and head. Remaining too long can cause dizziness; five or ten minutes works for most people.

Herbs

The soothing herbs previously mentioned are useful here as well: marsh mallow, corn silk, slippery elm, and goldenrod.

Diet

A low-acid diet decreases irritations. High-acid foods to omit are red meat, dairy, shellfish, and citrus fruits. The diet should include whole grains, beans, and vegetables. Essential fatty acids, such as those found in flaxseed oil, evening primrose oil, and fish oils, can help reduce inflammation. In interstitial cystitis, they are key for reversing the cycle of irritation and blood congestion.

Prevention

Long-term preventive changes obviously make a lot more sense than simply dealing with each acute infection as it arises. Here are some simple personal-hygiene measures to reduce the likelihood of reinfection:

After a bowel movement, wipe from front to back, away from the vagina.

Encourage your partner to wash thoroughly before any sexual contact.

Avoid the transfer of bacteria from the anus to the vagina during lovemaking.

During a period, change pads and tampons frequently.

Do not wear tight-fitting jeans or nylon pantyhose or pants. Cotton pants and stockings with garters allow more airflow and ventilation.

Make a habit of drinking lots of water. Aim for seven to eight glasses each day. This keeps the urine dilute so that bacterial proliferation is less likely. It also prompts frequent urination, which washes out problematic bacteria. Reduce the intake of coffee and tea.

Make a habit of emptying your bladder frequently. Research shows that women who ignore their urge to urinate for long periods of time are much more likely to develop cystitis. The motto here is:

When you need to go, go right away. Also urinate after sexual intercourse. This will help to wash out any of the bacteria that may have been pushed up into the urethra.

Try not to urinate before sex so that more bacteria is pushed out after sex. A glass of water right before intercourse will further increase the volume of liquid in the bladder for the washout of bacteria later on.

If infections are an ongoing problem, try this: Take a detachable shower head, or use a bidet, and direct a stream of water into the vaginal area before sex. This will dilute the bacteria and decrease their numbers so that fewer bacteria get pushed up into the bladder during intercourse.

Avoid chemical irritation to the urethra by staying away from perfumed or colored personal hygiene products. Diaphragms and birth control pills, as a means of contraception, often promote urinary tract infections and should not be used by women who tend to get the condition. Condoms or a properly fitted cervical cap are better.

See a registered osteopath or chiropractor if you think you may have a spinal problem that can be contributing to your recurring cystitis.

Dr. Hudson suggests drinking one glass of cranberry juice (or the equivalent in capsules) and taking vitamin C every day to reduce the frequency of recurrent attacks of cystitis by creating an acidic environment in which bacteria cannot easily grow.

"Remember that your bladder health reflects your overall health," says Dr. Wharton, "so take a good look at your lifestyle. Ask yourself, "Do I eat a nutritious, balanced diet? Do I get enough relaxation and sleep? Am I under stress?" Maybe you drink too much coffee or alcohol or smoke or use recreational drugs. If your lifestyle is unhealthy, your body will be too."

Asian Perspective

Dr. Brett explains that traditional Chinese medicine views cystitis as the end result of an accumulation of damp and heat in the bladder: "Often there is a weak flow of *chi* (energy) in the kidney and the spleen meridians. Weakness of spleen energy leads to the formation of damp in the body, which, in turn causes a stagnation of energy. As in nature, whenever anything builds up, there is friction. A stagnation of *chi* eventually leads to the development of heat, what we in the West interpret as cystitis.

"Spleen *chi* is easily disrupted through dietary indiscretion. Spleen *chi* can be damaged by any of the following: overeating; drinking with meals; overconsumption of damp-forming foods, such as dairy products, chilled foods or drinks, and raw fruits and vegetables; and eating greasy foods, such as takeout foods.

"What you do with your mind actually affects spleen energy as well. An overuse of the mind, particularly through chronic anxiety and worry, or through many years of overstudying, also tends to deplete spleen energy.

"When the cooling *yin* energy of the kidneys is weakened, cystitis becomes much more likely as well. Kidney *yin* is consumed naturally as we age, but it can also be prematurely diminished as a result of lifestyle. The long-term overwork, stress, and exhaustion that form a part of many American lives these days, along with an overconsumption of alcohol and too much sex, all deplete the vital kidney energy." Acupuncture, combined with lifestyle changes, can help to balance energy and eliminate cystitis.

VAGINAL INFLAMMATION AND INFECTION

CAUSES

According to Amanda McQuade Crawford, a medical herbalist and author of *Herbal Remedies for Women*, "There are many causes of vaginitis, which simply means an inflamed vagina. There's not always an infection. Many women use the term to refer to any number of situations where there's an irritation of the vagina. When it is caused by bacteria, it's called bacterial vaginosis. So we are talking about a number of different conditions.

"Though vaginitis isn't always caused by an infection, there are various microbes that commonly cause it. One of the microbes most commonly involved in nonspecific vaginitis is *Gardnerella vaginalis*, a bacterium that doesn't like oxygen. When men have *Gardnerella*, they don't show many signs or symptoms, so it may unsuspectingly pass to a female partner."

Some other common causes of vaginitis are candida (a yeast), *Trichomonas vaginalis*, a parasite, and a number of sexually transmitted diseases, such as gonorrhea, genital warts, and herpes. When an infecting agent is not the cause of vaginitis, it may simply be caused by a hormonal imbalance.

Vaginitis can occur at many stages of a woman's life; for example, it is common when a woman's body adjusts to a lower level of estrogen at menopause. Vaginitis can be aggravated by stress, nutritional imbalance, a foreign object such as a diaphragm or a tampon, and problems that originate in the vulva, which can lead to a vaginal irritation.

Crawford points out, "Vaginitis is not a punishment. It is the body's way of signaling an irritation of the most tender gateway to the interior that leads all the way up to our heart, and of our relationship to the person we love and let into our body."

SYMPTOMS

One common vaginal symptom is a discharge, which can be of different types and colors. These differences can help determine the necessary approach for healing.

If the discharge is clear and has a normal smell, it may well be due to ovulation and does not require treatment.

If the color is a milky white, and the discharge has a creamy texture but smells normal, this can also be a sign of ovulation.

If the discharge is white but sticky, it might be simply postovulation or an effect of taking the birth control pill.

When the discharge is brown and watery or sticky but has a normal odor, it can be spotting from the end of the menstrual period or, occasionally, spotting in between periods. If that is the case, it might be a good idea to consult a licensed practitioner to see why this is occurring.

When the discharge is watery and white, with almost a buttermilk quality, and smells fishy or foul—and especially when there's itching or other symptoms, such as fever—then you may have a case of BV (bacterial vaginosis), possibly from *Gardnerella,* which requires treatment.

Sometimes the discharge is white and flecked, like curds, smells a bit like beer or rising bread dough with a yeasty smell, and is accompanied by itching. This could be from a yeast infection, which also requires treatment with antifungal, antiyeast herbs or other remedies.

When the discharge is yellow and frothy, sometimes with dots of red, has a very foul odor, and is itchy, it may be from *Trichomonas.* See a medical practitioner to ensure that the infection is adequately treated, because this can be persistent.

Crawford notes, "Be careful if the discharge is yellow to green, and there's a heavy, thick mucous discharge, with or without a bad odor, that may be accompanied by other symptoms, such as abdominal cramps or pains, painful urination, and a fever. It could be evidence of PID [pelvic inflammatory disease] or possibly gonorrhea. Even if there's no discharge, it still might be gonorrhea if the other symptoms are present. So go to a medical practitioner for a clear diagnosis."

CLINICAL EXPERIENCE

Treatment

In treating vaginitis, some very simple herbs can be used, such as the soothing, anti-inflammatory calendula flowers. Crawford also likes licorice root, which can be used as a douche externally. Another herb that is quite good is plantain (sometimes called ribwort). These should be used with an astringent herb. They will help pull the inflamed vaginal tissues together so that the natural forces of your body can fight off whatever the infection or inflammation might be.

Crawford details, "An astringent herb which I use internally is anemone pulsatilla, or pasqueflower. Take 3 ounces of that and combine it with 1 ounce of licorice root and 2 ounces of plantain. Mix those together. Over 1 ounce of the mixture, pour a pint of boiling water. Let that stand, then take a teacup full of this tea, strained, three times a day. Alternatively, a woman can take extracts or tinctures of these herbs. The relative amounts would be the same. Take a teaspoon, diluted in 1 cup of water, three times a day."

Treat vaginitis for one or two weeks, then stop treatment and see if the condition is gone. "If there is a more deep-seated infection that doesn't resolve in that time period," Crawford says, "then I usually add 2 ounces of echinacea root to the other ingredients. Steep an ounce and use it in the same way as you did the previous tea, three to four times a day for at least ten days. If that doesn't clear things up, it is necessary to reassess."

"There's always nutritional advice that goes along with herbal treatments," Crawford adds. "Avoid sugar, including honey, maple syrup on your pancakes, or fruit juice–sweetened cookies, even if they are from the health food store. Lots of sugar is not going to help a woman fight off an infection."

VAGINAL YEAST (CANDIDIASIS)

Carol Dalton is a nurse practitioner who helped found the clinic Wellspring for Women. She explains that yeast infections are actually a general gathering of bacteria, a multiplicity of them, not just one organism. "Many of these organisms live normally within the vagina. If they are in the right balance and there are small amounts of them, they really don't cause any problem. But if they get out of hand and if the partner has a lot of bacteria as well, then it can really start to cause a lot of inflammation, itching, redness, and a foul-smelling discharge. Then it is obviously a problem."

She adds that just as we can be around someone who has a cold but not catch the cold if our immune system is good, a woman can come into contact with yeast but will not necessarily begin to grow it herself if her cells and immune system are healthy. On the other hand, if her immune system is depressed, she will pick it up and it will turn into a raging infection very easily.

Causes

A vaginal yeast infection has multiple causes, according to Dalton. She notes that the type of birth control you use will influence whether you can be infected. You may get the yeast infection from a partner, "if you are sexually active and particularly sexually active without any barrier protection or any spermicide—spermicide helps to kill off all of these things. So it may be passed more easily to women who are using the Pill or the IUD, for example, and not using female or male condoms or a diaphragm. They will be at higher risk, because everything that comes into contact with the genital area can pass way up into the vaginal canal. That's one of the reasons we are seeing more of this and have been for the last fifteen or twenty years: women are using more different kinds of birth control than we used to have. Women are tired of using the older methods, so they have switched to hormone injections (Depo-Provera), IUDs, and oral contraceptives, and those methods don't really offer any protection against yeast infections."

Dr. William Crook, author of *The Yeast Connection and Women*, says that taking antibiotics can lead to yeast overgrowth and that women are especially susceptible. "The yeast we're talking about normally live in the body of every man, woman, and child. When you are healthy, there are no problems, but when you take a lot of antibiotic drugs, you begin to get complications. Antibiotics knock out the normal, friendly bacteria. As a result the yeast overgrows, and a woman may get a vaginal yeast infection, a child may develop thrush or diaper rash, and a man or woman may get bloating, constipation, and digestive symptoms.

"But that's not the major problem. This yeast puts out toxins that weaken the immune system. It so disturbs the interior membrane of the intestinal tract that you absorb food allergens that would normally be excreted. People truly become sick all over."

"There are several reasons why a woman is more susceptible to yeast infections than a man," says Dr. Crook. "Since her genitalia are internal, yeast is able to grow on the warm interior membranes of the body. The little tube going from the urinary bladder to the outside is only an inch and a half long in a woman, whereas in a man it is many inches long. This allows the bacteria to get up into the woman's bladder much more easily. Women have fifty times more urinary tract infections than men, and they are given antibiotic drugs as treatment. Birth control pills further promote yeast growth. So does pregnancy. And teenage girls with a few pimples on their face are much more likely to run to the dermatologist and get tetracycline, an antibiotic that makes yeast grow."

Nutritionist Gracia Perlstein adds these causes to the list: "Some women are susceptible at the end of each month's menstrual flow. There are low estrogen levels present at menopause, and also pregnancy, when the rate of infection can be as high as 20 percent toward the end. Also women who have diabetes have an increased risk.

"Stress is another factor. Many people have two or three jobs. They are running around, eating on the run, not really paying attention to their diet. When people do that, they also tend to overdo sweets and processed foods, which weaken their immunity and set up a perfect environment for the candida overgrowth."

Complementary physician Dr. Robert Sorge says Candida is the result of drug pollution. In addition to antibiotic overuse, mentioned earlier, he adds, "The most likely candidate for overgrowth is a person who has been on steroids, hormone medication, cortisone, the entire gamut of prescriptions and over-the-counter drugs, especially ulcer medications such as Tagamet and Zantac, and oral contraceptives. As far as I'm concerned, the sugar and junk food diet that most people have is also a drug."

Symptoms

Classical symptoms of a yeast infection are itching, redness, irritation, and a cottage cheese–like curdly white discharge. Symptoms are not always obvious, but a gynecologist can often confirm whether or not a yeast infection exists by looking at a smear under the microscope or creating a culture to see if yeast colonies form.

Clearing up immediate symptoms is relatively simple. Many over-the-counter preparations, including homeopathic remedies, exist for that purpose. The trick, according to Dr. Marjorie Ordene, a holistic gynecologist from Brooklyn, New York, is to treat the overall yeast syndrome, not just the local infection.

"Often the vaginal itching will be the impetus for the person to come to the doctor, but it is not the only problem they have. Unless the whole person is treated, the yeast is bound to recur." Dr. Ordene breaks down symptoms of a yeast syndrome into five categories:

GENERAL SYMPTOMS—Low energy and fatigue, brain fog, depression, headaches, muscle and joint paints, memory loss, extreme sensitivity to chemicals, recurrent urinary infections, light-headedness

DIGESTIVE SYMPTOMS—Gas, bloating, intermittent constipation and diarrhea, indigestion, intestinal cramps

RESPIRATORY SYMPTOMS—Chronic postnasal drip, frequent coughs, sore throats, colds, asthma, allergies

SKIN PROBLEMS—Eczema, itching, rashes, fungal infections

HORMONAL PROBLEMS—Menstrual irregularities, menstrual cramps, premenstrual syndrome, mood swings, problems with the endocrine glands, hypothyroidism, hypoglycemia or diabetes

As already noted, the infection is more likely to take hold if a woman has a less than healthy immune system. "If the person who gets a yeast infection has a weak immune system, then the yeast, which comes out in the stool, can creep up. It grows like little tree branches, into the perineum and vaginal area. If the pH is off, it can cause an infection in that area," Dalton says.

Clinical Experience

DIAGNOSIS

Since the intestines serve as a reservoir for much of the yeast, a stool study may reveal an overgrowth. Excess yeast here indicates that yeast is present in other parts of the body, including the vagina, and is causing recurrent yeast infections.

A simple skin test may reveal a yeast allergy as well. Red or itchy skin indicates a problem. Often the results are seen quickly, within ten to fifteen minutes, although sometimes there is a delayed reaction or none at all.

These tests are not always reliable, according to Dr. Crook. "Although we physicians generally like to have a test that can say you do or do not have a particular condition, such as a chest X ray to see whether your heart is enlarged, there is not presently a single, simple laboratory test that can say whether you do or do not have a yeast-related problem. If a woman has a vaginal infection, a lab study of the secretion may help identify the yeast. Sometimes a culture may. But they are not 100 percent accurate. They may not be more than 50 percent accurate. There are studies done on stools because yeast grows there, but those are not reliable either. The best we can do is to suspect it, and then to note the response of a person to a sugar-free special diet, and oral antiyeast medication, both prescription and nonprescription."

ALTERNATIVE THERAPIES

Yeast-Free Diet

A yeast-free diet is both diagnostic and therapeutic. If a woman feels better when following the diet, this indicates a yeast sensitivity. The diet should be observed for several weeks at a minimum, and may be followed indefinitely. Some people feel much better and choose to eat this way permanently. Foods can be added back gradually, however, to see their effect. If symptoms recur, the reintroduced food should be avoided.

There are two basic principles to follow on a yeast-free diet:

AVOID SWEETS—The relationship between sugar and yeast was seen in a study performed at St. Jude Hospital in Memphis, Tennessee, where mice who were fed sugar had two hundred times greater yeast concentration than mice who were not. Yeast feeds on sugar, causing many symptoms, especially digestive problems such as gas and bloating. Avoiding sugar entails more than just not adding granulated sugar to cereal or tea; it means checking labels and staying away from corn syrup, maltose, artificial sweeteners, fructose, cornstarch, sodas, and lactose, a milk sugar found in dairy products.

AVOID FOODS CONTAINING YEASTS AND MOLDS—These include baked foods such as breads, muffins, cakes, cookies, and other refined carbohydrates, commercial fruit juices, tomato sauce (unless homemade with fresh tomatoes), foods containing vinegar, pickled foods, smoked foods, alcohol, fermented foods, smoked meats, dried fruits, mushrooms (except for shiitake), pistachio nuts, and peanuts. Leftovers may be moldy as well.

What you can eat are healthful foods that do not contain yeasts and molds. Included are whole grains, such as brown rice, millet, amaranth, quinoa, and barley, as well as fresh vegetables. Lots of steamed green vegetables are particularly beneficial because they are abundant in purifying chlorophyll. Also allowed are sea vegetables; whole wheat matzo; sourdough rye bread; popcorn; tortillas; tofu; miso; plain yogurt; lean meats; fresh fish; organically fed, free-range poultry; and eggs from free-range chickens. Organic extra-virgin olive oil, when used sparingly, can inhibit yeast overgrowth, according to recent studies. Raw garlic or lightly cooked garlic helps get rid of candida in the intestines.

Supplements

Sometimes diet alone is not enough. After all, yeast has been in the body for years. The following supplements provide additional needed help:

FLORA—The flora found in Lactobacillus acidophilus and bifida bacteria can be taken in powder form or as sugar-free yogurt. The effectiveness of flora was noted in a New York Medical School study of women with recurrent vaginal yeast infections. Those eating sugar-free yogurt had fewer infections than those who did not. Flora repopulate the intestinal tract with good bacteria, which in turn crowd out the yeast. The effects of flora are temporary, so the powder or yogurt should be consumed on a daily basis.

ANTIFUNGAL, ANTIYEAST AGENTS—Over-the-counter preparations, such as citrus seed extract, kyolic garlic, caprylic acid, pau d'arco, and berberine, may be helpful. Sometimes prescription agents such as nystatin are needed. These remedies get rid of excess yeast only. Since they are not absorbed into the blood, they are safe to take, even during pregnancy and while nursing.

HOMEOPATHIC CANDIDA—Helps desensitize the body to yeast.

GARLIC SUPPOSITORIES—Simple insertion of a clove of garlic into the vagina has a powerful healing effect. *The New Our Bodies, Ourselves* suggests that the clove should be peeled but not nicked, and then wrapped in gauze before inserting.

A strong body is better able to rebalance its health. In addition to supplements that target yeast infections specifically, the following nutrients provide overall nutritional support:

MULTIVITAMIN/MINERAL SUPPLEMENT—Formulas containing zinc, magnesium, yeast-free vitamins, trace minerals, and essential fatty acids boost immune function and help prevent recurrent yeast infections.

CHLOROPHYLL—Cleanses the intestines and purifies the blood.

ESSENTIAL FATTY ACIDS—3,000 mg of evening primrose, borage, or black-currant seed oil daily in three divided doses, or one tablespoon of organic flaxseed oil. (Never cook flaxseed oil, and keep refrigerated.)

VITAMIN C—3,000–5,000 mg daily in three divided doses helps fight infections.

B COMPLEX—50–100 mg with each meal combats stress.

Herbs

The following Asian and Western herbs can help alleviate yeast problems:

DIGESTIVE HARMONY AND HERBASTATIN—Digestive Harmony is a combination of bitter herbs that work together to cleanse the digestive tract and other internal organs of yeast infections. Herbastatin gets rid of yeast caused by phlegm.

YU DAI WAN—This Chinese remedy helps to eliminate creamy discharges.

KU SHEN—Used as a wash to clean the vagina.

BLACK WALNUT TINCTURE—Thirty drops three times daily, added to water before meals.

PAU D'ARCO—This herb has wonderful immune-enhancing and antifungal properties. As a tea, take three to four cups daily.

SUMMA—This is another good herbal tea for helping the immune system. Also helpful are goldenseal, bearberry, Oregon grape, German chamomile, aloe vera, rosemary, ginger, alfalfa, red clover, and fennel.

Colon Therapy

"My battle with candida lasted a long time," says colon therapist Tovah Finman-Nahman. "I tried everything, including a strict diet, antifungals, and vitamin C drips. But I never got it under control until I started doing colonics. Then I saw quick results. The gas and bloating went away, and my chronic fatigue amazingly disappeared. I have seen similar results with a lot of people who come to see me. I can't stress how good colonics are."

What makes colon therapy such an effective treatment? First, it creates a clean internal environment. "We want a good environment so that flora can grow and flourish. That is paramount when we have candida overgrowth," says Finman-Nahman. Second, colonics calm an irritated colon: "Herbs can be added to the water, such as pau d'arco, which has antifungal properties. Yellow dock can also be added to soothe any inflammation. Fennel can be used to dissipate gas and eliminate the bloating that a lot of people with candida tend to get. Aloe vera gel is absolutely wonderful. It is very soothing to an inflamed colon. And of course, it can be taken orally in the form of aloe vera juice.

"In conjunction with colonics, psyllium can be taken orally. This moisturizes impacted fecal material in the congested colon, which further aids cleaning.

"People ask, 'How many colonics should I get?' That depends on the individual. The more the merrier. For a healthy person I recommend at least ten in a series, and then a maintenance program. Sometimes, it can take as long as six months to get candida under control because it is a very hearty bacteria. When yeast is at the point of being candidiasis, it can grow through the colon walls and run rampant. The more we cleanse, the better our chance of getting it under control and regaining health."

Aromatherapy

Tea tree oil is scientifically shown to be antifungal, antiyeast, and antiviral. One tablespoon of the oil added to a pint of water, and used in a douche, helps eliminate yeast infections. Follow this by placing acidophilus tablets or capsules into the vagina to reestablish proper vaginal bacteria.

Lifestyle Factors

Nutritionist Gracia Perlstein notes the following important habits for minimizing the incidence of vaginal infections:

Wear underpants with a cotton crotch so that air can circulate.

Avoid pantyhose or any tight-fitting clothing for the same reason.

Develop good toilet habits of always wiping from front to back.
This keeps anal bacteria from entering the vagina.

Avoid feminine hygiene sprays and powders, which can cause irritation.
Douching is not necessary; a healthy vagina is naturally clean.

Keep stress under control. Take a few deep breaths. Go for a brisk walk
in the open air. Do something to alleviate the stress that builds up.

Homeopathy

Since homeopathy treatments are chosen according to symptoms, deciding on a remedy depends on the quality of the discharge and the sensations, according to Dr. Ken Korins. Here he offers some of the major remedies for vaginal yeast infections:

PULSATILLA—This remedy is often indicated in vaginitis. The woman has a thick, yellowish-to-green discharge. Sometimes the consistency is milky or creamy. Mentally, she is often moody, gentle, and weepy, and craves sympathy.

SILICA—The main symptom is an itching of the vulva and vagina. It is sensitive to touch. The discharge tends to be thin, and sometimes curdly.

KREOSOTUM—The person has violent symptoms. Discharges are excoriating, burning is profuse, and there is a foul odor, as well as violent itching and a burning and swelling of the labia. Discharge tends to be yellow and may actually have a watery, bloody consistency.

HEPAR SULPH—Symptoms are similar to Silica, but more chronic. The vagina itches, particularly after sexual intercourse, and often has an odor similar to that of old cheese. Both Hepar sulph and Silica can be used to treat sores or cysts, particularly Bartholin's cysts.

KALI BICHROMIUM—Here discharges tend to be thick, green, and sometimes jellylike.

ALUMINA—Discharge is thick and transparent.

NITRIC ACID—Helps when there are sores or ulcers on the vaginal mucosa. The sensation tends to be a sharp, sticking pain. Discharges are brown. Often, there is a stain on underwear that leaves a yellow perimeter.
MERCURIUS—The discharges are excoriating but greenish and bloody. There is a sensation of rawness.

MEDORRHINUM—Discharge is thick and acrid, with a sensation way up in the uterus.

Wellspring for Women Treatment

The holistic program at the Wellspring for Women clinic treats chronic cases of yeast infection. As Carol Dalton points out, the conventional treatment for yeast is to prescribe antifungal medications. "If a woman went to a more traditional medical care facility, that would be the first choice. It would be an antifungal of some sort in either a vaginal or an oral preparation.

"The problem with this approach is that you are not really addressing why this problem develops in the first place; why there is an unhealthy environment that allows this organism to grow. By prescribing these drugs, you are actually adding to the imbalance in the environment. This makes it even more likely that the person is going to pick it up again or that she will develop a yeast infection, because you have killed off her normal bacteria and allowed yeast to overgrow there. Often that starts a cycle of bacteria, then yeast, sometimes even developing into bladder infection because the whole area gets so inflamed."

Dalton notes that she often sees patients who have had chronic infections for a long time. "What we try to do is establish what their general immune system looks like. Then we try to help them systemically to get that into balance.

"We look at their diet, their lifestyle, their stress factors, their supplements, all those things, and try to help them create a healthier, better balance. For example, if the woman was low on protein in her diet and eating a lot of sugar and carbs, then we might recommend a lower-carb, lower-sugar diet so that we are not feeding the yeast.

"If the woman is not doing any kind of supplementation, we would tend to recommend things to raise the immune system and to help balance the flora in the vagina. We might suggest B-complex vitamins, zinc, beta carotene, vitamin C, all of those things that seem to help the immune system in general."

Dalton also uses natural suppositories to treat the yeast, as well as oral antifungal remedies including garlic. This is a traditional treatment. "I've even had patients who were told to tie some dental floss onto a clove of garlic or to thread it through a garlic clove and insert the clove in the vagina. It is very antifungal, so it probably does work.

"There are many ways to treat this, but the basic premise when you have developed a chronic problem should be to look at the whole body."

Describing the difference between acute versus chronic yeast infections, Dalton says, "If somebody gets a onetime infection, then perhaps she has a new partner and is having more sex than usual. In that case I would recommend she get some over-the-counter Monistat cream or use a little antifungal vaginal gel for a few days, to get rid of it. However, if it's an ongoing problem, we try to look more at the whole person and why she is having infections over and over again."

For chronic yeast problems, Dalton looks at the digestive system, because there is likely a yeast imbalance in the digestive system. That means the woman is getting more vaginal contamination than average. "Often you'll see symptoms such as gas, bloating, constipation or diarrhea, and rectal itching."

In chronic cases, it is important to determine what strain of yeast is present. At Wellspring for Women, Dalton says, "We do tests through our local lab or, more often than not, through Great Smokies Lab in North Carolina. The patient gets a kit from the clinic and takes a stool sample, and it's sent to North Carolina to be analyzed. With chronic yeast, the problem is that over time the yeast will mutate into a form that becomes resistant to most, if not all, of the medications typically used to treat yeast. The lab not only cultures but also tests the strain or strains that are found for sensitivities to medications and natural treatments. We have sometimes found yeast that has become resistant to garlic, for example. Though garlic in general is considered a great antifungal, there are some yeast strains that have mutated into a form in which garlic doesn't bother them at all—in fact, they probably thrive on it. And the same is true for resistance to various types of medication.

"So for chronic problems, we not only look a little deeper into the person's situation—into her lifestyle and habits—but we try to identify the exact organism we are dealing with and what that organism is sensitive to, so that we can help the person get rid of it completely."

PATIENT STORY

I had a patient who had a chronic yeast infection for about twelve years. It developed out of chronic bladder infections. She was given so many antibiotics that they ended by killing off the normal bacteria in the gut, which allowed the yeast to overgrow. Eventually that developed into vaginal yeast infections. We worked on it systemically. We tested to find out what organism she had and what it was sensitive to. We looked at her diet and her stress levels, which were high. After medication as well as natural treatments, we thought we'd gotten rid of it.

"Recently she had to be on antibiotics for twelve weeks for an abscessed tooth, so we wanted to check her. We found that she was fine. She had gone three months on antibiotics and there was no sign of yeast at all. We felt that she was really clear of it, since, being on the antibiotics that long, any average woman would have gotten a yeast infection. She was able to avoid it. So that was a very good sign that she was clear.

—Carol Dalton

TRICHOMONAS

Trichomonas is another vaginal infection, caused by a one-celled protozoan called *Trichomonas vaginalis*. Trichomonas, says herbalist Amanda McQuade

Crawford, "is usually sexually transmitted. It's a parasite, not a virus or a bacterium, and is not to be confused with trichinosis, the infestation of worms that can result from eating uncooked pork."

Symptoms

Trichomonas causes an inflammation of a woman's vaginal lining. The symptoms, says Crawford, are intense vaginal itching, irritation, and discharge. These symptoms are worse than similar symptoms that appear with bacterial vaginitis or yeast infections. The thin vaginal discharge trichomonas produces is yellow or green, and occasionally gray, and has a bubbly or frothy appearance. This discharge produces a burning sensation; a raw feeling; and a characteristic bad, fishy smell. Sexual intercourse is painful.

Trichomonas is a very serious condition, and it is important to know how it is distinct from other vaginal infections. Some general medical symptoms are also present; fever, chills, nausea, and fatigue. It can mimic a bladder infection (cystitis). The organisms that cause trichomonas can sit in the tissues of the vagina or the urethra, or hidden away deep in some of the glands inside the vagina, which makes it difficult to treat with natural remedies. When the infection goes on, you need to consult a licensed health care practitioner.

Treatment

In herbal treatment, Crawford indicates, "We try to eliminate the parasite by optimizing natural immune system defenses and work on preventing a recurrence at the same time. This means eliminating risk factors, particularly unsafe sex. The woman's sex partners may need to be tested to see if they require treatment. If they test positive, they need to be tested until they are shown to be negative. It's not enough just to have the symptoms go away. The herbal treatment requires consistency and should be done for at least two months before a retest to see if the parasite has disappeared."

One of the best herbal treatments is cassia bark. Others are myrrh and barberry root. These herbs together are often used to kill off the parasite causing the infection. Tonics promoting long-term immune system health also offer benefits. Two herbs used for this purpose are reishi, a Chinese mushroom, and astragalus root. Astragalus has often been used to boost immunity, especially with long-term infections.

Crawford cautions, "The herbs that are strong enough to kill the organism are ones that taste particularly bad. I say that so that women will know, when they are treating themselves for this, that it is not something like a beverage herbal tea. To take it will require some rigor and some willingness to gulp the things down." You can also take these herbs in capsule form. It can take as long as two months to eliminate the infection.

To make a capsule, combine 4 ounces cassia with 3 ounces barberry root. Add to that 3 ounces reishi mushrooms and 2 ounces astragalus. These herbs can be mixed together and put into capsules at home very easily. It's also very affordable.

If you don't want to take them as powdered herbs in capsules, you can take them in extracts and tinctures. The proportions would be the same, and the dose would be 1 teaspoon in 1 cup of water with meals four times a day for six to eight months.

Alternatively, you can take the herbs separately, although if you do, after three weeks you might encounter a little stomach distress. In that case, dilute them with even more water and be sure to take them with meals so that there is some food in your stomach. This will slow down the speed with which the herbs get into your bloodstream but will not neutralize their effects.

Don't forget that what you eat can also help the body heal. For trichomonas there is no one specific food that will make the difference. Crawford's recommendations are to decrease excess sugar and refined carbohydrates. Eat low-protein, high-quality whole foods with at least four to five servings a day of fresh fruits and vegetables in season. She says you must keep in mind that "We are eating foods that will nourish our whole being, not just the fruits or plants that will kill off parasites, because that won't get to the root of the whole problem."

Dalton also recommends certain supplements. She cites "good research on using fairly high doses of zinc, C, and beta carotene, which seem to systemically help the body throw off trichomonas."

Crawford uses douches in her treatment. One douche formula is cassia bark combined with equal amounts of licorice root bark to soothe the irritated, raw vaginal lining. Simmer 1 ounce of each on low heat for about fifteen minutes, then strain and use the tea as a douche.

A douche Dalton recommends contains aloe, vinegar, and tea tree oil. This is a drawing solution that helps get rid of the infection.

Crawford warns, "The thing to remember about douching is that it has some short-term benefits but also some long-term drawbacks. It should not be done every day, but only to relieve symptoms. At the same time, you must undergo a long-term treatment, such as taking the capsules, to deal with the root of the problem."

After six or eight weeks on the herbal treatment, get tested to see if the parasite has been eliminated. If it is still present, use the herbal treatment for an additional two weeks.

Crawford also notes that there's a need to counter the effect of the stronger herbal remedies. "If you are going to continue taking fairly strong herbs to kill off a small living organism, it's necessary to take some other herbs to help you counteract the negative side effects of these strong herbs. One of these counteracting herbs would be milk thistle. Take it as a standard extract, or in one of the many proprietary forms that are now in the marketplace. The dose would be 300 or 400 milligrams a day." Milk thistle can help the body develop long-term immunity as well as cope with the other herbs being used to treat the infection.

PATIENT STORY

Trichomonas is generally treated with a drug called Flagyl. In traditional medicine, it's thought that Flagyl or other antiparasitic drugs are the only way to treat this. About twenty years ago I had a patient who had a resistant case of trichomonas. She had been in the university hospital in Denver and they had given her intravenous Flagyl. Still they had not been able to get rid of the trichomonas. We used the douche solution and oral supplements to boost her immune system, and, lo and behold, in about three weeks, the trichomonas was gone and never recurred. So the natural treatments really can work if people are willing to put forward the effort. Obviously, it's easier in many cases to take a pill or two a day than to do all of this regime. However, it helps the body be healthier in general.

—Carol Dalton

BACTERIAL VAGINOSIS

Bacterial vaginosis (BV) is caused by *Gardnerella*, a gram-negative bacterium that hates oxygen. An alternative treatment that has been used at women's health clinics across America is to mix 1 cup of distilled or sterilized water and 1 tablespoon of a 3 percent solution of hydrogen peroxide. Douche with this mixture once a day for a week. Then repeat every three days, for an additional two weeks. The hydrogen peroxide and distilled water increase oxygen in the vaginal canal and tissues, which is antagonistic to the *Gardnerella*. This douche is a noninvasive, effective way to treat the problem. If it doesn't work within a week to ten days, consult a licensed health practitioner for other kinds of help that might be appropriate.

Plants containing phytochemicals with antibacterial/antifungal activity, in order of potency, include:

Coptis chinensis (Chinese goldthread)
Coptis sp. (generic goldthread)
Mangifera indica (mango)

Coptis japonica (huang lia)
Hydrastis canadensis (goldenseal)
Hamamelis virginiana (witch hazel)
Phyllanthus emblica (emblic)
Punica granatum (pomegranate)
Quercus infectoria (aleppo oak)
Berberis vulgaris (barberry)
Phellodendron amurense (huang po)
Argemone mexicana (prickly poppy)
Fragaria sp. (strawberry)
Rheum rhaponticum (rhubarb)
Glycine max (soybean)

CHAPTER 37

VARICOSE
VEINS

V aricose veins, a common condition in women that usually affects the lower extremities, is the result of damaged valves in the veins. Normally, these tiny valves ensure that the blood flowing through the veins will return fully to the heart. But when these valves are injured, and do not open and close properly, some of the blood runs backward in the veins, pools, and finally engorges the vessels. Varicose veins are large, contorted, unsightly, and sometimes even painful.

CAUSES

Three mechanisms help return blood to the heart, says Dr. Leon Chaitow, a naturopath, osteopath, and acupuncturist from England, in an article on the HealthWorld Online website (www.healthy.net): the action of muscles through which veins run, the pulsation of arteries that run alongside veins, and the movement of the diaphragm during breathing. Thus, he says, poor breathing function and lack of exercise, as well as various mechanical stresses, such as those resulting from occupations that require long periods of standing, will make venous return less efficient. Other factors that can increase the chance of developing varicose veins are inadequate fiber, vitamins C and E, and bioflavonoids in the diet; increased pressure in the pelvis, as from chronic constipation; and use of birth control pills.

Another cause of varicose veins, says Dr. Chaitow, is thrombophlebitis, a condition in which the veins are obstructed due to clot formation or an aggregation of platelets and fibrin, which restricts blood flow, causing inflammation and damage to the veins.

Herbalist David L. Hoffman lists several other reasons why the walls of the veins receive inadequate support, resulting in varicose veins:

OBESITY—A buildup of fatty tissue in the legs results in inadequate support for veins.

GENETIC PREDISPOSITION—In about 40 percent of cases, there seems to be an inherited tendency to varicosity.

AGE—Over time the connective tissue that supports the veins degenerates, and a decrease in exercise worsens the problem.

TIGHT CLOTHING—Tight clothing constricts and weakens tissue.

PREGNANCY—Pregnancy creates intrapelvic pressure, which interferes with venous return.

SYMPTOMS

According to Dr. Chaitow, the earliest symptom is feeling leg fatigue more often than usual. Other standard symptoms are an ache and heavy feeling in the legs, itching in the skin over the veins, and swelling, sometimes of the entire leg. The skin is discolored, and sometimes an eczema develops, with a breakdown of the skin that may lead to ulcers.

CLINICAL EXPERIENCE

Standard procedures for treating varicose veins include elevating the legs, wearing elastic stockings, and, in severe cases, surgery.

Many types of support stockings are available, but it is best to buy them at a pharmacy or surgical supply store, where they will be better quality. If you have a severe problem with varicose veins, you might look into custom-made surgical support stockings. In this country, two companies, Jobst and Sigvaris, make them. If you can't afford support stockings, sometimes an Ace bandage will give you the support you need. Wrap a 3- or 4-inch bandage around the leg where the varicosity is a problem. This may require wrapping your legs from the toes to the groin if the problem is severe.

With early intervention, the following natural remedies have a high rate of effectiveness.

Nutrients and Herbs

Certain foods and supplements may strengthen the integrity of the vein wall. These include dark-skinned fruits and berries, such as blueberries, cherries, and purple grapes. Vitamin C with bioflavonoids, especially quercetin or bilberry, improves elasticity, so that blood can return more effectively to the heart.

Dr. Chaitow also recommends vitamin E, in a daily dose of 500 to 800 IU, which is thought to help develop other channels of circulation, thus relieving the pressure in the veins. Vitamin E can also be applied directly to leg ulcers. Selenium, which works together with vitamin E, should also be taken daily in a dose of 50 micrograms. Essential fatty acids in the form of 500 milligrams of evening primrose oil and four to six capsules of EPA (eicosapentaenoic acid) a day will help decrease the likelihood of inflammation and lower the viscosity of the blood. Finally, he says, it is essential to consume enough fiber to keep the bowels functioning well so that no straining occurs.

Astringent herbs, such as horse chestnut, witch hazel, gotu kola, and butcher's broom, are good to take, although the first two should not be used when pregnant or lactating. Naturopathic physicians often recommend 1,000 milligrams of butcher's broom, two to three times daily, for pregnant women in their third trimester who are troubled by varicose veins or hemorrhoids.

David Hoffman adds that prickly ash and ginkgo can be used to stimulate circulation; hawthorn, yarrow, horse chestnut to tone the veins; comfrey to soothe irritation and heal wounds. He offers the following lotion, which can be used as necessary to relieve irritation:

8 parts distilled witch hazel
1 part horse chestnut tincture
1 part comfrey tincture
Rose water, if desired

Another factor to consider is dietary support for the liver. This is because a congested liver backs up venous circulation and places additional pressure on the veins, which can then damage valves. Foods such as beets and artichokes and herbs such as milk thistle and dandelion can improve liver circulation. At the same time, it is important to refrain from substances known to cause liver damage, such as drugs, alcohol, and other harsh chemicals.

Exercise

The main way to help relieve varicose veins is to do what you can to keep your blood flow moving, in spite of the fact that the veins are not doing their job properly. Helping the blood flow counteracts some of the problems caused by the damaged valves. Daily exercise is key. It is also important for keeping weight down. Excess weight creates stress on the body. Maintaining one's optimal weight lessens stress on the body, which, in turn, decreases the chance of damaging the valves in the veins. In addition, exercise improves overall circulation in the arteries and veins. Dr. Chaitow suggests exercises that involve contracting the leg muscles, circling the ankles, and upside-down bicycling movements.

Of particular benefit are maneuvers that take pressure off the legs. It is helpful to sit with your feet and legs elevated, waist-level or higher, whenever you can. This allows gravity to help the blood flow back to your heart. Inverted postures in yoga or even just lying on a slant board with the legs elevated for a few minutes a day are beneficial. You can also raise the foot of your bed by 6 to 12 inches. Medical magnets can be placed over the feet for added healing power. Maneuvers that take weight off the feet are particularly important for people who work in occupations in which they are constantly on their feet.

Another form of exercise to consider is qi gong, which strengthens the veins' ability to pump blood back to the heart.

Chelation Therapy

Chelation therapy flushes toxins out of the blood. Many people know that chelation therapy improves arterial integrity, but few realize that it can aid venous circulation as well, thereby helping varicose veins. Chelation therapy also helps to overcome liver congestion and thrombophlebitis, two conditions that put women at risk for varicose veins. (See chapter 1 for a more in-depth discussion of chelation therapy.)

Additional Suggestions

Dr. Tori Hudson, a naturopath in Portland, Oregon, offers the following tips in her column in *Prevention* magazine:

Eat a high-fiber diet.

Avoid standing for long periods and lifting heavy objects.

Use supplements: Every day take 1,000 mg of vitamin C; 1,000 mg of bioflavonoids; 150 mg of pycnogenols; and 400 IU of vitamin E.

Dr. Chaitow adds a few more suggestions:

Instead of standing still, shift from one leg to the other, or walk gently back and forth.

Don't cross your legs when you sit.

Take warm, not hot, baths, and end by splashing cold water on the legs.

Take regular sitz baths, alternating between hot and cold, but finish with cold; this stimulates circulation.

Alexander technique and osteopathic manipulation both improve body mechanics and thereby aid circulation. (For more information on the Alexander technique, see chapter 28.)

Garlic is excellent for thinning the blood; Dr. Chaitow recommends two or three capsules or raw cloves a day.

CHAPTER 38

SELECTING AN ALTERNATIVE HEALTH PRACTITIONER

A lternative health practitioners can help define the weak links in your body's structure and function and then direct you toward optimal personal care. There are many different approaches, but some general guidelines are worth mentioning here

YOUR RIGHTS AS A PATIENT

A good alternative medical practitioner will perform at least these three basic types of analysis before prescribing any treatment plan: (a) Take a detailed medical history; (b) perform a physical examination that goes beyond conventional methodologies; and (c) study carefully the results of appropriate laboratory tests taken at the time of the history taking and the physical examination.

In addition, you have the right to expect that the practitioner include in his or her repertory, some or all of the following:

As many noninvasive diagnostic techniques as possible.

An awareness of the potential diagnostic value of even very minor signs and symptoms in the prevention of major dysfunction.

A preference for noninvasive over invasive techniques; for example, substances will be administered orally rather than intravenously (except when a condition calls for the more direct route).

A recognition of the importance of strengthening the body's resistive capacities and an interest, wherever possible, in attempting to repair any malfunctioning organ or gland.

A tendency, whenever possible, to treat the primary weak link first if more than one has been discovered. (For example, if the stomach is producing insufficient hydrochloric acid, resulting in the malabsorption of calcium, among other substances, the resulting calcium deficiency could lead to osteoarthritis, periodontal disease, or skin problems; by treating the hydrochloric acid insufficiency, the physician would be treating the primary weak link.)

An approach that treats the person as a whole person, not just a collection of ailing parts.

The demonstrated ability to listen carefully and to skillfully classify any relevant symptoms to arrive at the best possible diagnosis.

An orientation toward optimal health and sensitivity to dysfunctions that signal an imbalance in the individual.

Familiarity with a combination of approaches to help the person regain balance. (For example, in addition to orthodox treatments, the physician's recommendations may include advice about stress reduction and lifestyle changes to reduce or eliminate causative factors in the environment.)

A willingness to refer the individual, when the condition warrants, to other medical practitioners whose specialized knowledge in a given area may be necessary to provide the most valuable restorative program.

A demonstrated awareness of the importance of the individual's own attitudes toward health and disease, and a willingness to communicate openly with the individual.

YOUR ROLE AS A PATIENT

Your alternative health practitioner should expect you to be an active, committed participant in the process, not a passive, disinterested patient who accepts everything the doctor recommends.

One form of this active participation may be the questions you ask with a view to getting the important information you need to help in your contributions to the healing process. Some examples are:

What, specifically, is being treated?

How do you know that that's the problem?
What are some realistic goals in my situation?

What is the time frame?

Does every individual with this condition get exactly the same tests and treatments?

What are my weak links?

Are these tests and this treatment relevant to my body and my condition?

THE IMPORTANCE OF COMMONPLACE SYMPTOMS

Many people are living with symptoms that, because they are mild and do not constitute a full-blown disease state, are accepted, needlessly, as being an inevitable consequence of getting older. In fact, such people are often told by their conventional physicians, "Nothing is wrong with you. Everything is normal." And yet, the symptoms may be early warnings that something is out of balance. Gas in the lower bowel (flatulence), belching, heaviness in the stomach, heartburn, and bloating, for example, may all be indicators of a malfunctioning digestive system, depending on their frequency and severity. These conditions are not normal in a healthy state, and they are often correctable.

Similarly, many of the symptoms that accompany delayed allergic reactions (the masked, cyclical allergies) are widely accepted as normal, and therefore to be tolerated for no better reason than "that's the way it is." The failure to recognize a connection between these symptoms and allergies may be due to the fact that they do not appear for upward of thirty hours after the ingestion of the offending food or chemical substance. Typical symptoms are headache, irritability, anxiety, sudden changes of mood, and excessive fatigue, as well as unexplained body aches and pains. These symptoms may not be severe enough to be labeled disease states, so the underlying cause is repeatedly overlooked or denied by traditional practitioners. Even when the disorders are recognized, their true significance may still be missed by those who try to reverse the symptoms without addressing the underlying causes for their appearance.

Thus frequent colds, recurring infections, and fatigue are all part of the warning mechanisms used by the body to signal a malfunctioning immune system. But they are rarely recognized as such. The phenomenal sales of cold remedies, for example, reflect how little attention is paid to strengthening the immune system—an approach that would far more effectively reduce the incidence of these and other disorders.

TYPES OF THERAPIES

It has never been my policy to make specific recommendations, to suggest to a person that a specific practitioner is the best doctor to see. The quality of a doctor's health care may depend on both the physician and the patient, as well as on their mutual compatibility. This is not something I, or anyone else, can predict in advance. But I still feel that people should be given some direction. So, what I have done here is supplied a directional guide. Below are descriptions of the therapies described in this book. Where applicable, I have listed organizations to contact for referrals or more information.

Acupressure

Acupressure, also known as shiatsu, is based on the principle that a vital energy, called *qi (chi),* flows through the body. The primary cause of pain is an imbalance in this energy. The goal of the healer is to balance the client's energy so that pain and discomfort do not manifest or, if they do appear, will be relieved.

The practitioner concentrates on certain pressure points that have metaphoric names that tell us something of what they do or how they are to be worked with. He or she uses thumbs, fingers, palms, forearms, elbows, and even knees to apply pressure to specified points in the body to modulate the flow of energy. During a treatment, the client lies on the floor on a comfortable padded surface, such as a futon, fully clothed or undressed to her level of comfort. What the client feels is pressure, which can be gentle or deeper at the places where the practitioner is working. As the pressure continues, the patient will generally feel relaxed and energized at the same time.

Acupressure is good for treating a variety of different pains. It is especially beneficial in combating chronic pain in the back, neck, or shoulders, but it has also proved effective in treating whiplash, herniated disk, and nerve problems, such as Bell's palsy.

Contact:
ACUPRESSURE INSTITUTE
(800) 442-2232
info@acupressure.com

Acupuncture

Acupuncture sees pain as derived from blocked energy or *qi* (*chi*). In treating this blockage, the practitioner has to determine whether it stems from an overabundance or a deficiency in energy, so the treatment can be adjusted depending on whether it is necessary to strengthen or decrease *qi*. To accomplish this, the acupuncturist will work to open blocked energy pathways, so that healing energy can go directly to the point in the body where it is needed, thereby stimulating the body's natural healing capacities.

The acupuncturist first records the patient's medical history in the manner of a conventional doctor. Then, with the patient lying down or seated, depending on the area to be treated, fine-gauge, stainless steel needles are inserted into significant points and meridians (channels through which *qi* flows) to exert different physiological effects on the body and induce both relaxation and energization. The patient will remain in this position from twenty to thirty minutes, though an appointment with an acupuncturist may last up to an hour, since part of the time will be spent consulting about the employment of other traditional and herbal treatments that might be recommended. Bodywork and massage might also be included in the session.

According to Abigail Rist-Podrecca, a registered nurse, acupuncture works by "dilating the blood vessels, so that the vessels can open. You get more circulation, more of the nutrients, more oxygen flowing through the meridians."

Practitioners attend three- to four-year postgraduate-type programs. Schools are accredited for master's degree programs through the National Accreditation Commission of Schools and Colleges of Acupuncture and Oriental Medicine. A certification examination is offered through the National Certification Commission for Acupuncture and Oriental Medicine. A minimum of 1,300 hours of training is required to sit for this exam. Medical doctors and dentists rarely require specialized training to perform acupuncture, although training is available through the American Academy of Medical Acupuncturists.

Contact:
AMERICAN ACADEMY OF MEDICAL ACUPUNCTURE
(323) 937-5514
www.medicalacupuncture.org

AMERICAN ASSOCIATION OF ORIENTAL MEDICINE
(888) 500-7999
www.aaom.org

NATIONAL ACUPUNCTURE AND ORIENTAL MEDICINE ALLIANCE
(253) 851-6896
www.acuall.org

Alexander Technique

Alexander technique is based on the concept that all of us know how to move comfortably as children but lose that natural flexibility over time. The teacher acts to help the student recapture this freedom and lightness of movement. Practitioners see themselves as teachers, and their sessions not as therapy but as teaching.

Each session is an experiential process in which the teacher guides the student with hands-on training to help her learn a new way of moving, by means of the teacher's hands stimulating the student's nervous system.

This technique can help mothers, for example, learn how to bend over and lift children in a new way that avoids stress on the back.

There are ten affiliated societies for teachers of Alexander technique worldwide. Teacher certification requires 1,600 practical hours over a three-year period.

Contact:
AMERICAN SOCIETY OF THE ALEXANDER TECHNIQUE
(800) 473-0620
www.alexandertech.org

Applied Kinesiology

This discipline is related to Chinese acupuncture. Practitioners use it to determine which foods and herbs are best assimilated by the individual, in order to develop a healing diet and supplementation program that is finely calibrated to the person's own biology.

The patient extends her arm at shoulder level while holding a food or supplement in the other hand, and the practitioner pushes down on the extended arm. If the substance is appropriate for her, the arm will be strong and harder to force down. If the substance is not good for her, the arm will be weak. This is because the body can feel the value of the substance. Using various techniques, kinesiologists can study these reactions more precisely to determine proper individual diet.

Contact:
INTERNATIONAL COLLEGE OF APPLIED KINESIOLOGY
(913) 384-5336
www.icakusa.com

Aromatherapy

Aromatherapy depends on the therapeutic powers of essential oils. These oils are commonly used in skin and body care products in the United States, but their medicinal properties have long been accepted in other countries, particularly France, where, in many instances, their antimicrobial properties make them acceptable replacements for drug therapy. Pure essential oils can be used to cure cold and canker sores, calm the emotions, diminish joint swelling, clear the nasal passages and lungs, balance hormones, and for many other applications.

Contact:
NATIONAL ASSOCIATION FOR HOLISTIC AROMATHERAPY
www.naha.org

Ayurveda

Ayurveda means "the science of life." It is a system of medicine widely used in India for the past four thousand years. Ayurveda believes that balance is the key to perfect health. It basically determines which of three body-mind types a person belongs to and, based on that type, helps people choose the type of foods he or she should eat as well as the best type of exercise. For more information, read *Perfect Health and Ageless Body, Timeless Mind* by Deepak Chopra.

Contact:
THE AYURVEDIC INSTITUTE
(505) 291-9698
www.ayurveda.com

MAHARISHI AYURVED PRODUCTS INTERNATIONAL
(800) 255-8332
www.mapi.com

Bach Flower Remedies

The Bach flower remedies were developed by Dr. Edward Bach during the 1930s. They consist of thirty-eight plant extracts that are used to treat physical and emotional problems. The extracts used in each case are selected according to the individual patient's personality. For instance, for a person who is critical and intolerant of others, the suggested remedy derives from the beech tree. For some with an unhealthy fear of the unknown, a remedy derived from the aspen would be prescribed. Bach flower remedies are said to have positive effects on the psychological and emotional stresses that underlie many illnesses.

Contact:
THE BACH FLOWER ESSENCES INTERNATIONAL EDUCATION PROGRAM
(800) 334-0843
www.nelsonbach.com

ELLON USA
644 Merrick Road
Lynbrook, NY 11563
(516) 593-2206

FLOWER ESSENCE SOCIETY
(800) 736-9222
www.floweressence.org

Biofeedback

Biofeedback is a technique that teaches a person to consciously regulate normally involuntary bodily processes, such as heartbeats, brain waves, blood pressure, and muscle tension. The bodily process, such as heart rate, may be monitored by electronic equipment or by natural observation, such as holding a finger against an artery. With practice, the patient learns to slow down the heart rate, relax tension, and so on. Biofeedback is helpful for conditions such as migraine, tension headache, digestive upset, and other disorders that are aggravated by stress.

Practitioner certification is recommended but not required. Practitioners are certified through the Biofeedback Certification Institute of America.

Contact:
ASSOCIATION FOR APPLIED PSYCHOPHYSIOLOGY AND BIOFEEDBACK
(303) 422-8436
www.aapb.org

BIOFEEDBACK CERTIFICATION INSTITUTE OF AMERICA
(303) 420-2902
www.bcia.org

Body Rolling

Body Rolling, a form of bodywork developed by Yamuna Zake, uses a 6- to 10-inch ball in a series of routines designed to elongate muscles and increase blood flow in all parts of the body. As the body weight presses into the ball, the ball applies pressure onto bone and creates traction that allows the entire length of a muscle to release. Body Rolling is useful for relieving pain and tension in many parts of the body.

YAMUNA ZAKE
(888) 226-9616
www.bodylogic.com

Chelation Therapy

Chelation therapy flushes toxins out of the blood. A synthetic amino acid, EDTA, is administered to the patient through an intravenous drip. The EDTA moves through the blood vessels and attaches itself to heavy metals in the blood such as mercury and lead, holding on to these substances until they are washed out of the body in the urine. Chelation therapy is being used increasingly to treat heart disease as well as other illnesses. Protocols for the intravenous administration of EDTA are set by the American College for the Advancement of Medicine (ACAM) and require a prior medical examination.

Contact:
AMERICAN COLLEGE FOR ADVANCEMENT IN MEDICINE
(800) 532-3688
www.acam.org

Chiropractic

Chiropractic treatment involves the manual manipulation of vertebrae that have become misaligned, exerting pressure on nerves and blocking the flow of energy to various organs. The manipulation is called an adjustment. It involves the chiropractor's gentle and painless application of direct pressure to the spine and joints. The chiropractor may squeeze or twist the torso, pull or twist the limbs, or wrench the head or back. In this manner she or he is readjusting the spinal column to restore the normal relationship of one vertebra to another. This eliminates the body's energy blocks.

Chiropractic is effective in dealing with pain and as a preventive measure because it relieves nerve pressure as the spine is properly adjusted.

While chiropractic is still far from being accepted as a part of standard health care, it attracts more patients now than ever before and is more accepted than ever before by the mainstream medical community. There are now about twenty chiropractic colleges nationwide, and chiropractors can get licensed in all fifty states. Some liberal arts colleges offer undergraduate degrees in chiropractic, and some facilities at member hospitals of the American Hospital Association have been opened to chiropractors.

Contact:
AMERICAN CHIROPRACTIC ASSOCIATION
(703) 276-8800
www.acatoday.com

INTERNATIONAL CHIROPRACTORS ASSOCIATION
(800) 423-4690
www.chiropractic.org

Colon Therapy

Colon cleansing refers to washing out the colon in order to remove toxic buildups. First the colon is irrigated with warm water, washing out encrustations and old fecal matter. Next, healing substances to reduce inflammation and strengthen the colon wall are infused.

Contact:
AMERICAN ASSOCIATION OF NATUROPATHIC PHYSICIANS
(877) 969-2267
www.naturopathic.org

INTERNATIONAL ASSOCIATION FOR COLON HYDROTHERAPY
(210) 366-2888
www.i-act.org

Craniosacral Therapy

The sacral region is that at the bottom of the spine. Between that region and the head there should be maintained a balanced relation for the health of the organism. If a restriction is experienced at that point, pain will be felt and other problems may arise.

In craniosacral therapy, the practitioner places her or his hands on the patient's body in such a way as to bring the cranium and sacrum back into alignment and to reestablish a natural rhythm between them. Treatment usually centers on the head or lower back, although it may be done on many different parts of the body.

Contact:
INTERNATIONAL ASSOCIATION OF HEALTHCARE PRACTITIONERS
(800) 311-9204
www.iahp.com

Detoxification Therapy

A person whose health is compromised, or on a diet that is too high in fats, processed proteins, and refined foods, has a reduced capacity to rid the body of toxins. When this happens, the toxins accumulate.

Frances Taylor, coauthor of *The Whole Way to Natural Detoxification*, explains: "As we journey through life the way most people do, we become overloaded with the toxins that absorb in the body. Unless we do something to get rid of these things, our bodies become overloaded and our health suffers. We develop symptoms such as headaches, digestive problems, sluggishness, after-meals fatigue. Many health benefits can be obtained by simply detoxifying the body."

Among the methods of detoxification are diet, nutritional supplementation, chelation therapy, colon cleansing, detox baths, exercise, deep breathing, and bodywork.

Contact:
AMERICAN ASSOCIATION OF NATUROPATHIC PHYSICIANS
(877) 969-2267
www.naturopathic.org
AMERICAN COLLEGE FOR ADVANCEMENT IN MEDICINE
(800) 532-3688
www.acam.org

AMERICAN ASSOCIATION FOR HEALTH FREEDOM
(800) 230-APMA
www.apma.net

Enzyme Therapy

Enzyme therapy uses enzymes to cure illness and enhance life. South American Indians used papaya as a healing agent, and medieval Europeans used the milky juice of plants of the spurge family for medical reasons. Today, many practitioners advocate enzyme supplementation to enable vitamins and other supplements, as well as food, to be properly absorbed.

There are many different types of enzyme therapy. One example is that which relies on the Wolfe and Benitez formulas, which combine animal and vegetable enzymes. The preparations are said to be powerful weapons against bacteria and other invasive microorganisms. Many naturopaths and chiropractors use enzyme therapy.

Contact:
DR. HOWARD F. LOOMIS
(800) 662-2630
www.loomisenzymes.com

VITAL PRODUX
44 Mine Road
Stafford VA 22554
(540) 286-2400
www.vitalprodux.com

Feldenkrais

Feldenkrais is a practice that helps eliminate poor movement habits and relieve chronic tensions. It uses very gentle movements that the student does herself, guided by the instructor, while lying on the floor. Alternatively the student lies on a massage table and the teacher uses a hands-on approach, taking the student through gentle movements to enable the student to let go of a chronic holding pattern.

The goal is to learn to differentiate between parts of the body that are relaxed and parts that are still tense. Thus the nervous system learns a new way of functioning.

Contact:
FELDENKRAIS GUILD
(800) 775-2118
www.feldenkrais.com

Guided Imagery

Guided imagery can be practiced either by an individual with a therapist or in a group setting. In the individual setting, the practitioner helps the client elicit her own mental images, which she then interacts with, perhaps in dialogue. For example, if the client is ill, she may call up images of the distressed part of her body and encourage it to heal through an imagistic interaction.

In a group, a facilitator helps the participants concentrate on building certain images whose healing power they can tap into. In this setting, the participant has the added benefit of being able to discuss the process with another participant afterward so as to further affirm and enrich the healing process.

Contact:

ACADEMY FOR GUIDED IMAGERY
(800) 726-2070
www.interactiveimagery.com

INTERNATIONAL ASSOCIATION OF INTERACTIVE IMAGERY
www.iaii.org

AMERICAN HOLISTIC MEDICAL ASSOCIATION
(703) 556-9728
www.holisticmedicine.org

AMERICAN HOLISTIC NURSES ASSOCIATION
(800) 278-AHNA
www.ahna.org

Hellerwork

Hellerwork is a bodywork technique derived from Rolfing (see below). Both modalities work to improve body structure with deep tissue work, but Hellerwork, unlike Rolfing, is not painful. The practice has three components. In the first, hands-on part, the practitioner finds a misalignment in the body and works with the client to release it.

The second part is movement education. The practitioner analyzes the patient's posture and movements, then offers more relaxed and stressless ways to move. The third component is body-mind dialogue, whose purpose is to identify emotional patterns that underlie dysfunctional movement patterns.

Contact:

HELLERWORK INTERNATIONAL
(800) 392-3900
www.hellerwork.com

Herbal Medicine

American interest in herbal medicine has exploded in recent years. Not long ago, we had to seek out an herbalist or visit a health food store to obtain herbal formulas. Today supplements are being manufactured by mainstream drug and vitamin companies, and can be found on store shelves everywhere. The National Institutes of Health has even established an office to maintain a database and fund research into herbals. It may seem as if herbal medicine is a new field. In actuality, herbs have been used for healing for as far back as we can trace the existence of humans.

Herbs can play a vital role in our day-to-day lives by stimulating our immune systems. Many people find that their health seems to be sapped by recurring or chronic colds and viruses. Synthetic drugs, far from being a solution, seem merely to encourage new, more resistant strains of bacteria and viruses. People with more serious immune problems, such as AIDS and cancer, can help their systems to fight back as much as possible by using herbs to stimulate a healthy immune system.

In addition to fresh herbs and dried herbs, there are several other forms in which herbal medicines can be taken. *Infusions* and *decoctions*, two of the simpler forms, are both made with boiling water. *Tinctures* are made by macerating herbs in a mixture of water and alcohol for at least 2 weeks. *Ointments*, which are useful for treating some skin conditions, can be made with herbs and oils.

Contact:

AMERICAN HERBALISTS GUILD
(770) 751-6021
www.americanherbalistsguild.com

HERB RESEARCH FOUNDATION
(800) 748-2617
www.herbs.org

AMERICAN ASSOCIATION OF NATUROPATHIC PHYSICIANS
(877) 969-2267
www.naturopathic.org

Homeopathy

Homeopathy is based on the Law of Similars, the principle that what causes illness can also cure it. If a person has a head cold, you would give the person a substance that would cause cold symptoms in a healthy person, but in a sick person it helps to cure them. Homeopathy is limited in scope at this time in the United States, although one hundred years ago it was the prevailing form of medicine—until allopathic medicine, and the American Medical Association in particular, launched an intensive drive against it, which culminated in its being virtually banned in this country.

Recently, there has been a renewed interest in homeopathy, and growing numbers of physicians are using its principles. Homeopathy is particularly effective in the treatment of fevers, bacterial infections, toxicity, and the cumulative effects of alcohol, drugs, tobacco, caffeine, or sugar. It is not recommended for cancer, AIDS, or heart disease.

Contact:
HOMEOPATHIC ACADEMY OF NATUROPATHIC PHYSICIANS
www.healthy.net/hanp

NATIONAL CENTER FOR HOMEOPATHY
(703) 548-7790
www.homeopathic.org

Hydrotherapy

Hydrotherapy is a traditional naturopathic method that uses hot and/or cold water to treat a range of ailments, including urinary tract inflammations, fibrocystic breast disease, migraine headaches, and infertility. For urinary tract inflammations, for example, sitz baths or hot compresses can be used to stimulate blood circulation and remove toxins from the pelvic area. For migraines, there are many inventive forms of hydrotherapy that involve applying cold to the head and heat to the feet.

Contact:
AMERICAN ASSOCIATION OF NATUROPATHIC PHYSICIANS
(877) 969-2267
www.naturopathic.org

Massage Therapy

Massage therapy is used to treat a variety of ailments, including muscle spasm and pain, soreness, swelling and inflammation, temporomandibular joint syndrome, whiplash, headaches, and stress. It helps to release tension and enhance relaxation. It can help in detoxification. Some states require massage therapists to be licensed, others do not. Many massage therapists perform a variety of bodywork techniques.

Contact:
AMERICAN MASSAGE THERAPY ASSOCIATION
(888) 843-2682
www.amtamassage.org

Midwifery

Midwives help women give birth, providing care and advice during pregnancy and after a baby is born. They may also provide general gynecologic care. Midwives work in homes, clinics, birthing centers, and hospitals. Midwifery views pregnancy as a natural, normal, and individual process in which medical intervention should be as minimal as possible. Most midwives only accept women who are likely to have a normal delivery and are not considered at high risk for complications.

Certified nurse-midwives (CNMs) are registered nurses who have been trained in midwifery and certified by the American College of Nurse-Midwives. Some states require nurse-midwives to have a special license. Other states allow them to practice under their nursing license. Most CNMs have back-up doctors at hospitals.

Lay midwives have no formal training in midwifery. A few states license lay midwives.

Contact:
AMERICAN COLLEGE OF NURSE MIDWIVES
(202) 728-9860
www.acnm.org

Natural Hygiene

Natural hygiene is the practice of creating optimal conditions for the body and its constituent cells, tissues, and organs to pursue and sustain health. This means environmental purity of air, food, and water; a balanced primordial diet based on natural foods; and stress reduction and management. It precludes the use of most drugs, since they are antithetical to a modality that perceives illness to be due to inappropriate nutrition and toxic accumulations (drugs are usually toxic substances). Finally, it means a symbiotic relationship of all humankind and harmony with God and nature.

Contact:
AMERICAN ASSOCIATION OF NATUROPATHIC PHYSICIANS
(877) 969-2267
www.naturopathic.org

Naturopathy

Naturopathic physicians can treat most conditions. They are not, however, allowed to perform major surgery (although they can perform minor surgery). Their very extensive background is centered in the botanical sciences, including the use of herbs and tinctures with a wide variety of natural immune-stimulating properties. Becoming a doctor of naturopathic medicine requires four years of graduate-level study in the medical sciences. The accrediting agency is the Council on Naturopathic Medical Education (CNME).

The naturopath practices a natural form of health care whose traditions precede the advent of modern medicine. In this the naturopath resembles the traditional Tibetan physician, who must be able to identify nearly one thousand different healing herbs, mineral sources, and animal sources. The naturopath has years of extensive study in the healing potential of such substances. He or she is also able to understand muscular and skeletal bodily adjustment. Naturopaths use a much broader basis for diagnosis than do conventional allopathic physicians.

Contact:

AMERICAN ASSOCIATION OF NATUROPATHIC PHYSICIANS
(877) 969-2267
www.naturopathic.org

AMERICAN PREVENTIVE MEDICAL ASSOCIATION
(800) 230-APMA
www.apma.net

AMERICAN NATUROPATHIC MEDICAL ASSOCIATION
(702) 897-7053
www.anma.com

Orthomolecular Medicine

Orthomolecular medicine is an alternative approach to mental and physical health whose goal is to identify and treat the root cause of disease. The objective is to balance and rebuild the whole body, not merely to mask or suppress symptoms. To do this, orthomolecular physicians try to establish equilibrium among the essential nutrients that may be lacking, present in excess, or are being poorly absorbed. Orthomolecular physicians are conventionally trained medical doctors who feel that such an imbalance is often responsible for psychiatric as well as physical disorders.

The physician looks at diet, glandular function, glucose metabolism, and a host of other biochemical factors that may play a role in the patient's mental health. Imbalances in the body are corrected through judicious use of vitamins, minerals, amino acids, and other naturally occurring nutrients. Orthomolecular physicians frequently use a very high-dose vitamin regimen.

Contact:

INTERNATIONAL SOCIETY FOR ORTHOMOLECULAR MEDICINE
(416) 733-2117
www.orthomed.org

Polarity Therapy

Polarity therapy is based on the belief that any stagnation or stopping of the natural flow of energy in the human body is the underlying cause of disease. The naturally occurring positive and negative energy fields of the body are in a polarity relationship with each other. However, when the energy is blocked, it turns neutral, and the surrounding tissues stagnate and become painful.

Practitioners use light forms of touch, gentle manipulation, and techniques such as rocking to restore the flow of energy, relieving stress and pain and encouraging healing.

Polarity therapy is particularly useful for depression, anxiety, fatigue, headaches, fibromyalgia, and other conditions involving emotional blockages. Standards of practice and a code of ethics are established by the American Polarity Therapy Association.

Contact:

AMERICAN POLARITY THERAPY ASSOCIATION
(303) 545-2080
www.polaritytherapy.org

Qi Gong

The Chinese phrase qi gong means "air" (considered the vital essence) and "work." This traditional Asian practice utilizes aerobic exercise, meditation, relaxation techniques, and isometrics to control the vital energy of the body in the most efficient way. Like many Chinese practices, it emphasizes the unity of mind, spirit, and world.

The central practice is a combination of breathing, movement, and shallow meditation, in which the person is aware of what is going on but in a tranquil state in which positive images flow quietly through a relaxing mind. Once the person is in this state, the flow of the *qi* through the body is stimulated. This unobstructed flow will heal sickness or increase an existing sense of wellness.

Contact:

QI GONG INSTITUTE OF EAST WEST ACADEMY OF HEALING ARTS
(415) 788-2227

AMERICAN COLLEGE OF TRADITIONAL CHINESE MEDICINE
(415) 282-7600
www.actcm.org

Reflexology

Reflexology is based on the principle that people have reflex areas in their feet that correspond to every part of the body. The locations of the reflex points on the foot correspond to the way the organs and glands are distributed within the body. Massaging these specific areas on the feet thus helps to improve the functioning of particular organs and glands.

For example, the toes reflect the head area, the ball of the foot represents the chest area, and so on. The practitioner presses his or her fingers into the foot, using a variety of techniques, to massage and relax ill or stressed parts of the body.

Contact:
REFLEXOLOGY ASSOCIATION OF AMERICA
(702) 871-9522
www.reflexology-usa.org

Reiki

Reiki is a type of massage therapy or bodywork in which pressure-point techniques are used to move energy through the body in order to create balance and harmony. The practice, Japanese in origin, teaches the student to attain an attunement with the universal energy.

Whereas many Asian techniques involve learning a discipline to guide the flow of energy, in Reiki the student attains attunement from a Reiki Master, who transmits it during a ritual process. This single attunement can never be lost, although with further attunements one can move to a higher spiritual level. There are schools of Reiki with three levels or "degrees" of proficiency.

Contact:
INTERNATIONAL ASSOCIATION OF REIKI PROFESSIONALS
(781) 729-3530
www.iarp.org

Rolfing

According to practitioners of Rolfing, pain is caused by chronic shortenings in the tissue. Correction of the pain can be accomplished by soft-tissue manipulation. This manipulation creates order in the body so that the client stands tall and free of restriction.

Rolfing is generally performed in a series of ten sessions, designed to address all the shortenings in the structure systematically. Each session works in a different area. The basic goal of Rolfing is not pain relief per se; still it has been found useful for TMJ, frozen shoulder, carpal tunnel syndrome, tennis elbow, chronic hip problems, sciatica, cervical neuropathies, and knee, foot, and ankle problems.

The Rolf Institute of Structural Integration certifies Rolfers.

Contact:
ROLF INSTITUTE OF STRUCTURAL INTEGRATION
(800) 530-8875
www.rolf.org

Therapeutic Touch

Therapeutic Touch represents a reinvigoration of the old process of the laying on of hands, whereby the subtle touch of a healer on the patient's body will infuse her with positive energy. This therapy was originally developed by nurses and emphasizes the nurturing aspect of the practitioner.

A key ingredient of the practice is compassion for the patient being touched. Unlike most of the therapies reviewed here, this technique requires minimal training, which is why it is widely practiced by both professional medical practitioners and laypeople.

Nurse Healers Professional Associates is responsible for guidelines and curricula for teaching practitioners. There is no certification program. Therapeutic Touch can be practiced by nurses after a twelve-hour or minimum six-hour program.

Contact:
NURSE HEALERS PROFESSIONAL ASSOCIATES
(801) 273-3399
www.therapeutic-touch.org

Traditional Chinese Medicine

Traditional Chinese medicine is based on ancient Taoist philosophy, which treats the whole person. The philosophy is that body and mind are one; there is no separation between the two. When qi, or universal energy, flows freely through the meridians, a person is healthy, but when qi is blocked or disrupted, the person develops pain or illness.

Practitioners begin by examining the patient to identify patterns of disharmony. They then prescribe herbal remedies based on these patterns.

Contact:
AMERICAN COLLEGE OF TRADITIONAL CHINESE MEDICINE
(415) 282-7600
www.actcm.org

Trager Technique

According to the theory behind Trager technique, pain is caused when someone frequently tightens her muscles in movement and posture. To correct this, the practitioner uses gentle motions to increase the patient's pleasure in the quality of her tissues and decrease the restriction and sense of holding. Gentleness is important, so that no message is sent to the body telling it that pain is on the way or that causes the patient to tighten up.

The movement reaches into the central nervous system to convey the sensations of pleasure, lengthening, softening, and opening to the tissues and joints. This practice is used to relieve lower back, neck, and upper back pain; sciatica; migraines; TMJ disorders; carpal tunnel syndrome and other repetitive stress disorders.

The Trager Institute offers information, training, and certification in the Trager approach.

Contact:
TRAGER INSTITUTE
(216) 896-9383
www.trager.com

Yoga

Yoga is a system of mental and physical exercise. It combines physical postures, breathing exercises, and meditation. Studies have shown that yoga can help improve overall health and prevent and/or manage many conditions and diseases. Among other things, it has been proven to reduce stress, improve metabolism, enhance blood flow, aid digestion, and manage menstrual problems. Various forms of yoga have become popular in the United States and Europe.

Contact:
INTERNATIONAL ASSOCIATION OF YOGA THERAPISTS
(415) 928-9898
www.iayt.org

RESOURCE GUIDE

Below you will find contact information for many of the alternative health practitioners whose work and/or wisdom are profiled in this book.

DR. MAJID ALI
The Institute of Integrative Medicine
95 East Main Street
Denville NJ 07834
(201) 586-4111

NINA ANDERSON
P.O. Box 36
E. Canaan CT 06024
(860) 824-5301

DR. RICHARD ASH
Center for Complementary Medicine
New York NY 10021
(212) 758-3200

DR. ROBERT ATKINS
Atkins Center for
Complementary Medicine
152 East 55th Street
New York NY 10022
(888) ATKINS-8

DR. ERIC BRAVERMAN
212 Commons Way, Building 2
Princeton NJ 08540
(609) 921-1842
(800) 224-7105

JEANETTE BREEN
Baldwin Midwifery Service
660 Merrick Road
Baldwin NY 11510
(516) 223-1251

DR. JENNIFER BRETT
998 Nichols Avenue
Stratford CT 06497
(203) 377-1525

SUSAN BUCCI
86 Coppersmith Road
Levittown NY 11756
(516) 731-4648

DR. CHRISTOPHER CALAPAI
18 E. 53rd Street, 3rd floor
New York NY 10022
(212) 838-9100
or
1900 Hempstead Turnpike
East Meadow NY 11554
(516) 794-0404

DR. HYLA CASS
1608 Michael Lane
Pacific Palisades CA 90272
(310) 459-9866

DR. ROBERT CATHCART
127 2nd Street
Los Altos CA 94022
(415) 949-2822

ROBERTA CERTNER
677 West End Avenue
New York NY 10025
(212) 865-7505

DR. JANE CICCHETTI
Five Element Center
115 Route 46W
Mountain Lake NJ 07046
(201) 402-8510

DR. ANTHONY CICHOKE
P.O. Box 92094
Portland OR 97292

DR. WILLIAM CROOK
International Health Foundation
Jackson TN 38303
(901) 423-5400

DR. PAUL CUTLER
652 Elmwood Avenue
Niagara Falls NY 14301
(716) 284-5140

DR. MARTIN DAYTON
18600 Collins
N. Miami Beach FL 33160
(305) 931-8484

DR. MARTIN FELDMAN
132 East 76th Street
New York NY 10021
(212) 744-4413

TOVAH FINMAN-NAHMAN
Lifeline Hygienics
Rye NY 10580
(914) 921-5433

DAVID FROME
165 West 91st Street
New York NY 10024
(212) 724-6677

DR. HERBERT GOLDFARB
29 The Crescent
Montclair NJ 07042
(201) 744-7470

DR. WILLIAM J. GOLDWAG
7499 Cerritos Avenue
Stanton CA 90680
(714) 827-5180

DR. PAT GORMAN
5 East 17th Street
New York NY 10003
(212) 620-0506

DR. JANE GUILTINAN
1307 North 45th Street
Seattle WA 98103
(206) 632-0354

DR. ELSON HAAS
25 Mitchell Boulevard
San Rafael CA 94903
(415) 472-2343

LETHA HADADY
310 West 21st Street
New York NY 10021
(212) 807-1006

DR. JESSE HANLEY
22917 Pacific Coast Highway
Malibu CA 90265
(310) 456-9393

DR. BRUCE HEDENDAL
301 Crawford Boulevard, Suite 206
Boca Raton FL 33432
(407) 391-4600

DR. ROGER HIRSCH
9730 Wilshire Boulevard, Suite 105
Beverly Hills CA 90212
(800) 967-3898

DR. TORI HUDSON
2067 Northwest Lovejoy
Portland OR 97209
(503) 222-2322

DR. VICKI HUFNAGEL
Women's International
FRS Surgical Center
Juarez Baja California
(323) 650-6182

DR. HAL A. HUGGINS
P.O. Box 49145
Colorado Springs CO 80949
(866) 948-4638

DR. MICHAEL JANSON
2557 Massachusetts Avenue
Cambridge MA 02140
(617) 661-6225

KIM JESSOR
229 Berkeley Place
Brooklyn NY 11217
(212) 925-1169

DR. DAVID KAUFMAN
210 Central Park South
New York NY 10019
(212) 969-9540

DR. KEN KORINS
200 W. 57th Street
New York NY 10019
(212) 246-5122

JANE KOSMINSKY
41 West 70th Street
New York NY 10023
(212) 724-9755

SUSAN LACINA
The Healing Center
175 West 72nd Street
New York NY 10023
(212) 439-4781

DR. STEPHEN LANGER
3031 Telegraph Avenue
Berkeley CA 94705
(510) 548-7384

DR. MICHAEL LESSER
2340 Parker Street
Berkeley CA 94704
(510) 845-0700

DR. WARREN LEVIN
18 East 53rd Street
New York NY 10022
(212) 838-4926

DR. SHARI LIEBERMAN
New York NY
(212) 929-3152

DR. GENNARO LOCURCIOAS
610 3rd Avenue
Elizabeth NJ 07202
(908) 351-1333

DR. JAY LOMBARD
1180 Morris Park Avenue
Bronx NY 10461
(212) 863-8465

SUSANA LOMBARDI
We Care Health Center
18000 Long Canyon Road
Desert Hot Springs CA 92241
(800) 888-2523

DR. NANCY LONSDORF
Maharishi Ayurveda Center
4910 Massachusetts Avenue
Washington DC 20016
(202) 244-2700
(800) THE-VEDA

DR. MARSHALL MANDELL
3 Brush Street
Norwalk CT 06850
(203) 838-4706

DR. JOHN MCDOUGALL
McDougall Wellness Center
Santa Rosa CA 95402
(800) 570-1654

DR. LANCE MORRIS
1601 North Tucson Boulevard
Suite 37
Tucson AZ 85716
(520) 322-8122

DR. LINDA OJEDA
c/o P.O. Box 2914
Alameda CA 94501
(800) 266-5592

DR. MARY E. OLSEN
42 High Street
Huntington NY 11743
(516) 427-3724

SHARON OLSON
20-61 32nd Street
Astoria NY 11105
(718) 726-3817

DR. MARJORIE ORDENE
2515 Avenue M
Brooklyn NY 11210
(718) 258-7882

DR. DEAN ORNISH
Preventive Medicine
Research Institute
900 Bridgeway
Sausalito CA 94965
(415) 332-2525

DR. ANTHONY PENEPENT
Great Neck NY 11022
(212) 239-9582

DOLORES PERRI
315 West 70th Street
New York NY 10023
(212) 787-2404

DR. JOHN PITTMAN
Carolina Center for Alternative
and Nutritional Medicine
4505 Fair Meadow Lane
Raleigh NC 27607
(919) 571-4391

DR. JOSEPH PIZZORNO
Bastyr University
Kenmore WA 98028
(425) 823-1300

DR. MITCHELL PROFFMAN
144-02 69th Avenue
Flushing NY 11367
(718) 268-9080

DR. STEPHANIE ODINOV PUKIT
20 W. 20th Street, Suite 1002
New York NY 10011
(212) 206-8100

DR. DORIS RAPP
1421 Colvin Boulevard
Buffalo NY 14223
(716) 875-0398
or
8179 E Del Cuarzo
Scottsdale AZ 85258
(480) 905-9195

DR. JUDYTH REICHENBERG-ULLMAN
131 3rd Avenue
Edmonds WA 98020
(425) 774-5599

ABIGAIL RIST-PODRECCA
130 West 57th Street
New York NY 10016
(212) 957-5266

DR. HOWARD ROBINS
200 West 57th Street
New York NY 10019
(212) 581-0101

DR. MICHAEL SCHACHTER
Schachter Center for
Complementary Medicine
Suffern NY 10901
(845) 368-4700

BARBARA SEAMAN
110 West End Avenue, #5D
New York NY 10023
(212) 580-1838

SHERRILL SELLMAN
13707 East 31st Place
Tulsa OK 74134
(918) 437-1058

DR. CHARLES SIMONE
123 Franklin Corner Road
Suite 108
Lawrenceville NJ 08648
(609) 896-2646

DR. CARL SIMONTON
Simonton Cancer Center
Pacific Palisades CA 90272
(310) 459-4994

DR. PRISCILLA SLAGLE
16542 Ventura Boulevard
Encino CA 91436
(310) 826-0175

DR. DAVID STEENBLOCK
Health Restoration Center
Mission Viejo CA 92691
(800) 300-1063

DR. JANICE STEFANACCI
6801 Jericho Turnpike
Syosset NY 11791
(516) 496-7766

DR. WALT STOLL
267 Yorkshire Court
Gurnee IL 60031
(606) 233-4273

SARAH SUATONI
731 Greenwich Street
New York NY 10014
(212) 966-9005

ROGER TOLLE
292 West 93rd Street
New York NY 10025
(212) 787-5167

DANA ULLMAN
2124 Kittredge Street
Berkeley CA 94704

DR. ROBERT ULLMAN
131 3rd Avenue
Edmonds WA 98020
(425) 774-5599

DR. ELIZABETH VILET
P.O. Box 64507
Tucson AZ 85728
(800) 509-1688

NILSA VERGARA
7609 34th Avenue
Jackson Heights NY 11372
(718) 651-2260

DR. MICHAEL WALD
Advanced Medical of Mount Kisco
Mount Kisco NY 10549
(914) 241-7030

DR. ALLAN WARSHOWSKY
2001 Marcus Avenue
New Hyde Park NY 11042
(516) 488-2877

DR. JULIAN WHITAKER
Whitaker Wellness Institute
Newport Beach CA
(949) 851-1550

DR. JONATHAN WRIGHT
515 West Harrison Street
Kent WA 98032

DR. RAY WUNDERLICH
1152 94th Avenue North
St. Petersburg FL 33702
(813) 822-3612

DR. YUAN YANG
The Healing Center
175 West 72nd Street
New York NY 10023
(212) 501-7521

DR. JOSE YARYURA-TOBIAS
935 Northern Boulevard
Great Neck NY 10021
(516) 487-7116

DR. JANET ZAND
1441 West Smith Road
Ferndale WA 98248
(800) 232-4005

INDEX

ABC drops, 246
abortion aftercare, 479–80
Abraham, Dahlia, 57–58, 59, 60
abuse and depression, 366
acetyl-l-carnitine, 373
aconite, 74, 474
activity disorders, 192
acupressure, 407–8, 428–29, 469–70, 560
acupuncture, 560–61
    for addiction, 390
    for AIDS, 50–51
    for arthritis, 72
    for back pain, 428
    for chronic fatigue syndrome, 159–60
    for depression, 376
    for fibroids, 137
    for infertility, 327, 328–29
    for lupus, 335
    for migraines, 403
    for osteoporosis, 455
    for pain management, 428
    pressure points for digestive
        disorders, 179–80
    for urinary tract problems, 532, 536
acyclovir (Zovirax), 310
adaptogens, 248
    See also herbs

addiction, 387–97
    to alcohol, 388, 390, 391–93
    to caffeine, 388, 393–94
    and depression, 397
    detoxification, 387–89
    to food, 389, 390, 395–96
    hypnotherapy, 389–91
    to nicotine, 388, 389, 390
    to sugar, 388, 394–95
addictive allergic reaction, 274–75
adrenal function, 14–15, 19, 418
adrenaline, 13
Aesoph, Laurie, 89–92
age spots, 262, 263
Agho, Peter, 67
aging, 11–38
    of brain, 32–38
    causes, 12–14
    clinical experience, 14–31
    symptoms, 14
AIDS, 39–55
    alternative treatments, 45–55
    causes, 40–43
    clinical experience, 43–45
    and human papilloma virus (HPV), 501
    survivor portraits, 55
    in women, 40

air purifiers, 229

air quality, indoor, 229, 230–31

alcohol
addiction, 197, 388, 390, 391–93
and breast cancer, 112
and hormonal imbalance, 316
and infertility, 325

Alcoholics Anonymous, 392–93

Alexander technique, 430, 470, 556, 561–62

Ali, Majid, 150, 151, 153, 154–55, 155, 160–61

allergies, 150, 249, 399–400, 559

allergy shots, 279

aloe vera, 242–43, 353

alpha lipoic acid, 201

alternative health practitioner selection, 557–76
patient rights, 557–58
patient role, 558–59
symptom importance, 559
therapy types, 559–76

alternative health therapy concepts, 54–55

alumina, 546

aluminum, 226, 227, 445–46

Alzheimer's disease, 444–48
alternative therapies, 446–48
causes, 445–46
conventional treatment, 446
signs and symptoms, 444–45

amenorrhea, 355–59

American College of Gynecologists and Obstetricians (ACOG), 470–71

American Diabetes Association (ADA), 167, 267

American ginseng, 311
See also ginseng

American Heart Association, 290, 291, 295

amino acids, 372–73, 382–83
See also gluthathione; l-glutamine; phenylalanine; tryptophan; tyrosine

anabolic processes, 52, 78

Anderson, Nina, 26–27

anemia, 57–62

causes, 57–59
clinical experience, 59–61
diagnosis, 59
and fibroids, 135
patient story, 61–62
and stomach acid, 177–78
symptoms, 59

angelica, 257

angina pectoris, 288

animal proteins, 316

anorexia nervosa, 191, 193, 196, 197–98
See also eating disorders

Anshen bu nao pien, 299

antiaging diet, 15–16

antibiotics
and depression, 365
and immune system, 247
for sexually transmitted diseases, 495, 497, 499
and urinary tract problems, 528–29
and yeast infections, 540, 548–49

antidepressants, 156, 196–97, 369–70

antifungal, antiyeast agents, 543

antifungal medicine, 547, 548

antihistamines, 463

antioxidants, 17–18, 280, 294

anxiety disorders, 378–84
causes, 378–81
clinical experiences, 381–84

anxiolytics (antianxiety agents), 253–54

aphrodisiacs, 255–57, 328

apis, 312

apis mellifera, 87–88

appendicitis, 186–87
See also pressure diseases

applied kinesiology, 278, 403, 562

Aricept, 446

Arms, Suzanne, 457, 458, 474–75, 481

arnica, 245, 406, 474, 478, 523

aromatherapy, 562
for AIDS, 51
for herpes, 313
for menopause, 348
for menstrual cramps, 355
for osteoporosis, 453
for pregnancy, 471–72
for sexual dysfunction, 493–94

for urinary tract problems, 532
for vaginal yeast infections, 545
arsenicum, 255, 312–13, 375, 473
arthritis, 63–94
    alternative treatments, 67–73
    arthritis cure, 75–77
    and atherosclerosis, 92–94
    causes, 65
    defined, 63–65
    diagnosis, 75
    and environmental allergies, 81–85
    and food allergies, 285
    gout, 73–74
    Holistic Balanced Treatment, 77–81
    homeopathy, 85–89
    nutrition, 89–92
    patient stories, 79–81, 83–85
    traditional medicine, 65–67
    types, 64–65
    See also lupus
Ash, Richard, 18–19
Asian medicine. *See* Chinese medicine
aspirin, 66, 75, 80, 365, 463
assisted reproductive technology (ART),
    323–24
astragalus, 48, 118, 439
Atacama, Jeie, 304
atherosclerosis, 92–94, 300–301
Atkins, Robert, 116–17, 121–22, 163–64,
    168, 203, 254, 385, 386, 517, 518
Atkins diet, 204
Auerbach, K. G., 475–76
Aurigemma, Anthony, 209, 213–14
aurum metallicum (gold), 375, 479
aurum muriaticum, 138
autoimmune thyroiditis, 508, 512–15
Ayurveda, 61–62, 161, 348–49, 563
AZT, 43–45

Bach, Edward, 563
Bach flower remedies, 563
back pain, 423–24, 428
    See also pain management
bacteria identification, 249
bacterial vaginosis, 551–52
Baker, Jeanine Parvati, 462
Baltimore, David, 41

baoxin wan, 299
Barnard, Neal, 425–26
Barnes, Broda, 295, 508, 515, 518
Bar-Shalom, Ruth, 123, 124, 125, 355–56,
    357–58, 359
basements, 224–25
bathrooms, 227
baths
    detox, 238–39
    for insomnia, 255
    sitz, 329–30, 359, 532, 556
B complex. *See* vitamin B complex
beans, 241
bedrooms, 216–17, 228–29
beechwood, 523
beet juice, 23
behavioral therapy, 386, 387
    See also psychotherapy
belladonna (deadly nightshade), 74,
    346–47, 487, 523
bellis perennis, 473
Beltz, Richard, 43
Benson, Herbert, 302
Berwick, Ann, 348, 453, 471–72, 493–94,
    532
beta carotene, 17, 46–47, 258, 416
    See also vitamin A
Bialy, Harvey, 41–42
Bic, Zuzana, 249–51
Billings method, 95–97
biochemical factors in depression,
    364–65
biofeedback, 404–5, 564
bioflavinoids, 18, 19–20
biological clock, 13
biomechanics, 76
bipolar disorder, 364, 369, 373
birth control, 95–105
    fertility awareness, 95–97
    methods, 97–105
        birth control pills, 101–4
        cervical cap, 98–99
        diaphragm, 99–101
        female condom, 98
        male condom, 97–98
        Norplant, 104
        sterilization, 105

vaginal contraceptive film, 101
birth control pills, 101–4
    and anemia, 59
    and carpal tunnel syndrome, 417
    and depression, 365
    and hormonal imbalance, 316
    and infertility, 322–23, 329
birth defects, 325
Biting Insect (remedy), 244
bittersweet, 312
Black, Dean, 42, 45, 147–48
black currant seed oil, 118
black ointment, 245
black walnut tincture, 544
bladder infections. See urinary tract
        infections and inflammations
Blank, Arnold, 71–72
Block, Neil, 151, 155–56
blood-type diet, 204
blood vessels, broken, 264
blueberry extract, 19
Body Rolling, 422, 455, 564
bodywork, 428–32
    See also Alexander technique;
        craniosacral therapy; magnet
        therapy; Rolfing; shiatsu; Trager
        technique
bojemni slimming tea, 299
borage oil, 118
boron, 35, 70, 344
bovista, 486
Bradshaw, John, 152
brain aging, 32–38
    Brain Electronic Activity Map
        (BEAM), 36–37
    and brain function, 32–33
    chelation therapy, 38
    diet and nutrition, 33–34
    electrostimulation, 38
    exercise, 37
    mental stimulation and stress
        management, 37–38
    other nutrients, 35–36
    Reiki, 38
    supplements, 34–35
Brain Electronic Activity Map (BEAM),
    36–37

brain reflex, 410
bras and breast disease, 109–10
Braverman, Eric, 19, 32, 36–37, 38, 290
breast cancer, 107–22
    alternative treatment, 116–21
    causes, 107–12
    clinical experience, 112–16
    and estrogen, 345
    patient stories, 121–22
    symptoms, 112
    See also fibrocystic breast disease;
        lymphedema
Breast Cancer Prevention Trial, 113–14
breast-feeding, 474–76
breathing exercises, 28
Breen, Jeanette, 459, 474
Breiner, Mark, 269, 270
Brett, Jennifer, 404, 525, 529, 532–36
Brill, Gerri, 408–11
British Migraine Association, 402
bromelain, 74, 438
brown spots, 262, 263
Brownstein, Art, 423–24, 433
bryonia, 74, 87, 348, 473
Bucci, Luke, 68, 70
Bucci, Susan, 30–31
bugleweed, 296
Buhner, Steven Harrod, 242–43
bulimia nervosa, 191, 193, 195, 196,
        197–98
    See also eating disorders
burns, 242–43
Burton, Lawrence, 120
B vitamin complex. See vitamin B
        complex

cabbage juice, 23
caffeine, 316, 325
caffeine addiction, 388, 393–94
Calapai, Christopher, 12, 14–15, 45–46,
        50, 51–52
calcarea phosphorica, 456
calcium
    for aging, 20
    for Alzheimer's disease, 446
    for anxiety, 383
    for arthritis, 69

for dental health, 267
for digestive disorders, 177
for estrogen replacement therapy, 451
for menopause, 344
for osteoporosis, 450–51, 455
for pregnancy, 466
for repetitive strain injuries, 415
for temporomandibular joint (TMJ) dysfunction, 422
calendula, 245, 474
califilum, 474
candida, 220
capsaicin, 425–26
capsicum, 22
carbo vegetabilis, 473
cardiomyopathy, 17
carnivora (Venus flytrap), 118
carpal tunnel syndrome, 414, 417–20
    alternative treatments, 419–20
    causes, 417–19
    conventional treatment, 419
    See also repetitive strain injuries
Carpenter, Karen, 194
carpeting, 223, 228
carrot juice, 23
carrots, 463–64
cars, 223
cartilage growth factors, 416
    See also chondroitin; glucosamine
Cass, Hyla, 196–97, 508, 513–14, 518–19
castor oil packs, 124, 359
catabolic processes, 52, 78
Cathcart, Robert, 47
cat's claw, 118
causticum, 523
cayenne, 296–97, 361
celery juice, 23
Certner, Roberta, 346
cervical cancer, 139–40, 499–500
cervical cap, 98–99
cervical dysplasia, 129–32, 140, 500, 501
cervical subluxation, upper, 400, 403
Chaitow, Leon, 553, 554, 555, 556
Chalker, Rebecca, 98–99, 491–92
chamomile, 254
chamomilla, 355

chelation therapy
    for aging, 24–25
    for arthritis, 93–94
    for brain aging, 38
    defined, 564–65
    for diabetes, 170
    for environmental illness, 221
    for heart disease, 300–301
    for varicose veins, 556
chemicals
    and environmental illness, 218
    for gardening, 224
    toxic, 226, 227, 231, 234
    in the workplace, 419
cherries, 74
chest muscles stretch (yoga), 454–55
china, 347
Chinese medicine
    defined, 575
    for endometriosis, 212
    for hair health, 271
    for heart disease, 297–300
    for infertility, 327–29
    for interstitial cystitis, 535–36
    for menopause, 346
    for sexual dysfunction, 494
    and tongue, 266
chiropractic, 565
    for arthritis, 71
    for migraines, 403
    for pain management, 427–28
    for temporomandibular joint (TMJ) dysfunction, 421–22
chlamydia, 322–23, 496–98, 498, 499
chlorophyll, 136, 544
Cho, Y. K., 49
chondroitin, 63, 70, 75–76, 91–92, 94, 416
Chopra, Deepak, 349, 563
Christie, Huw, 44
chromium, 20, 201
chromium picolinate, 169, 294
chronic disease and food allergies, 280–81
chronic fatigue syndrome, 147–61
    about, 147–48
    causes, 148–52

clinical experience, 154–61
symptoms, 152–53
chuan xiong, 137
Cicchetti, Jane, 477–79
Cichoke, Anthony, 504–5
cigarettes. *See* smoking
cimicifuga, 355, 474, 478, 488
circumcision, 481
Claire, Thomas, 428–29
clay compress, 359
Clement, John, 120
Cleveland Clinic, 505
clinical ecology, 81–82
clove, 298
cobalamin (vitamin B12), 21, 58, 296, 438, 447–48
cobra (yoga pose), 126, 454
Coca Pulse test, 278
cocculus, 473, 479
cod liver oil, 68–69, 220
coenzyme 1, 21
coenzyme Q10
for aging, 20, 34
for eating disorders, 202
for heart disease, 294–95
for repetitive strain injuries, 416
for temporomandibular joint (TMJ) dysfunction, 423
coffea cruda, 255
coffee, 424, 425–26
See also caffeine
coffee enemas, 142–43
cognitive therapy, 196
See also psychotherapy
colchicum, 74
colds, 246–49
homeopathic remedies, 246
and immune system, 246–48
natural remedies, 248–49
cold sores, 307, 308, 309, 312, 313
See also herpes
Coley's toxins, 143–44
colocynthis, 354, 487
colon
irritation, 177
natural therapies, 181
therapy, 25–26, 545, 565–66

color therapy, 408
common cold. *See* colds
compression bandaging, 127
congestive heart failure, 288
conium maculatum, 125
constipation, 175, 176, 186, 528
consumer advocacy groups for infertility, 331
Cooksley, Valerie, 313
corn silk tea, 353
corrective vaginal surgery (episiotomy), 476
cortex cinnamomi, 328
Corticoid, 456
cortisol, 38, 365
cortisone, 13
cosmetic laser surgery, 262–66
cosmetics, 216, 227
Costin, Carolyn, 191–93, 194–95, 196, 197–98
Cousins, Norman, 433
cranberry, 529, 535
cranial faults, 400, 402–3
cranioelectrical stimulation (CES) device, 38
craniosacral therapy, 421–22, 431, 566
cravings (food and alcohol), 197
Crawford, Amanda McQuade, 132, 496–98, 537, 538–39, 549–51
Crook, William, 540, 542
cryptococcois, 243
Cutler, Paul, 291, 293, 294, 300, 303
cuts, salve for, 245
cyclic food allergy, 274
cystitis, interstitial. *See* interstitial cystitis

D'Adano, Peter, 67
Dalkon Shield, 498
Dalton, Carol, 495, 497, 498, 499–501, 539–40, 542, 547–49, 551
danazol, 209
dandelion, 118, 124, 353, 467–68
dan shen wan, 298
Davis, Ronald M., 335
Dayton, Martin, 24–25
deadly nightshade, 74, 346–47, 487, 523
dehydration, 15–16

dementia, 440, 441, 445
    See also Alzheimer's disease
dental care, 266–70
dental fillings, 13, 150, 267–69, 517
deprenyl, 36
depression, 363–78
    and addiction, 397
    alternative therapies, 370–78
    causes, 364–68
    diagnosis, 368–69
    and eating disorders, 195
    major, 363
    manic, 364, 369, 373
    postpartum, 477–79
    traditional treatments, 369–70
    types, 363–64
Derosis, Helen, 378–79, 381
detox bath, 238–39
detoxification
    for addiction, 387–89
    for aging, 22–31
    for carpal tunnel syndrome, 419
    by drinking water, 238
    of environment, 221–31
    for environmental illness, 221
    at home, 238–42
    of liver, 488
    for reproductive system cancers, 142
    therapy, 566–67
devil's claw, 74
DHEA
    and aging, 18–19, 22
    and Alzheimer's disease, 447, 448
    for menopause, 345
    and osteoporosis, 452
diabetes, 163–73
    and carpal tunnel syndrome, 418
    causes, 163–65
    clinical experience, 165–70
    gestational diabetes, 171–73
    monitoring and preventing, 170–71
    symptoms, 165
    types, 164–65
Diabetes Control and Complications
        Trial (DCCT), 166
diaphragm (birth control), 99–101
diarrhea, 175, 176

diary-writing, 255
diet, 237
    for amenorrhea, 357
    for anemia, 60
    for anxiety, 382–83
    for arthritis, 67–68, 76–77
    for breast cancer, 111–12, 115–16,
        117, 139
    for carpal tunnel syndrome, 418–19
    for chronic fatigue syndrome, 158–59
    for dental health, 266–67
    for depression, 370–71
    for diabetes, 166–67, 168
    for endometriosis, 214
    for fibrocystic breast disease, 123
    for fibroids, 135–36
    general, 239–41
    for gestational diabetes, 171–72
    for hair health, 270–71
    for headaches, 250
    for heart disease, 291–93
    for hormonal imbalance, 357
    for hypothyroidism, 509–10, 512
    for immune system, 247–48
    for infertility, 325–26
    for interstitial cystitis, 534
    for lupus, 335–36
    for menopause, 342–43
    for menstrual cramps, 352–53
    for migraines, 406
    for multiple sclerosis, 436–37
    for osteoporosis, 450–51
    for pain management, 424–26
    for pregnancy, 459, 465–66
    for repetitive strain injuries, 414–15
    for toxic shock syndrome, 361
    for ulcers, 190
    for urinary tract problems, 529
    for vaginal problems, 539
    for vaginal yeast infections, 542–43,
        547
    for varicose veins, 554–55, 556
diets and eating disorders, 191–92,
        202–5
di Fabio, Anthony, 333, 334, 335
digestion and anxiety, 380–81
digestive aids, 20

digestive disorders, 175–90
  causes, 175–77
  clinical experience, 178–81
  and endometriosis, 210–11
  and food allergies, 275
  food allergy and digestion, 181–83
  gastritis, 183–84
  lactose intolerance, 183
  pressure diseases, 184–87
  symptoms, 177–78, 559
  ulcers, 187–90
Digestive Harmony (herbal remedy),
    299, 544
diuretics, 463
diverticulitis, 184–85
  See also pressure diseases
DMAE, 34
dong quai, 328, 358, 494
Donnelly, Patrick, 50
Dorsman, Jerry, 395–96
douching, 132, 497–98, 545, 550–52
Douillard, John, 378
dowager's hump, 453–54
downward-facing dog (yoga), 454
drug addiction, 390
drug use and chronic fatigue syndrome,
    151
dulcamara (bittersweet), 312
Dushkin, Ron, 433
dust, 228
dysmenorhea. See menstrual cramps and
    irregular menstruation
dysthymia, 363

E. coli infections, 243
Eades, Michael, 203
earaches, 246
ear infections, 220
eating disorders, 191–205
  causes, 191–94
  clinical experience, 194–202
  and diets, 191–92, 202–5
echinacea, 158, 243, 311, 439
EDTA, 18, 24, 300, 564
eicosapentaenoic acid, 485
Elavil, 370
electrical stimulation, 38, 522

electromagnetic pollution, 36–37, 150
  See also pollution
Eli Lilly (firm), 489–90
elimination diet, 279
elimination testing, 278
Ellner, Michael, 389–91
endocrine system, 33
endometrial cancer, 140–41
endometriosis, 207–14
  alternative therapies, 210–14
  causes, 207–8
  conventional therapy, 209–10
  diagnosis, 209, 212
  patient story, 214
  symptoms, 208–9
endorphins, 364
enemas, 142–43, 405
EnurAid, 523
environmental allergies, 81–85, 402
environmental factors
  and chronic fatigue syndrome, 150
  and depression, 366
  and environmental illness, 216–17
  and Parkinson's disease, 441
environmental illness, 215–35
  causes, 216–17
  detoxifying the body, 221
  detoxifying the environment, 221–31
  diagnosis, 218–19
  patient story, 231–35
  symptoms, 218
  treatment clues, 219–21
environmental medicine, 81–82
enzymes
  for aging, 26–27
  for breast cancer, 119
  for chronic fatigue syndrome, 156–57
  for diabetes, 169
  for multiple sclerosis, 438
  for stroke, 504–5
enzyme therapy, 567
ephedra, 438
episiotomies, 476, 492, 521, 522
Epsom salts, 239
Epstein, Paul, 152, 160, 161
Epstein-Barr (EB) virus, 148–49, 307
  See also herpes

equisetum (scouring rush), 523
er jow, 136
essential fatty acids
    for aging, 20–21, 34
    for arthritis, 68
    for breast cancer, 111
    for eating disorders, 201
    for endometriosis, 212
    for immune system, 280
    for menopause, 344
    for skin care, 260
    for vaginal yeast infections, 544
    See also omega-3 fatty acids; omega-6
        fatty acids
essiac, 118
estonia, 243
estradiol, 77–78, 337–38
    See also estrogen
estriol, 345
estrogen
    and Alzheimer's disease, 447
    and breast cancer, 107–8, 345
    and environmental illness, 217
    and hormonal imbalance, 315,
        317–18, 319
    and menopause, 337–38
    and migraines, 400
    and osteoporosis, 450
    and ovarian cancer, 341
    triple, 345
    See also hormonal imbalance
estrogen dominance, 108, 325, 326
estrogen replacement therapy, 451
    See also hormone replacement
        therapy (HRT)
estrone, 337–38
evening primrose oil, 118, 299, 353,
        437–38
    See also omega-6 fatty acids
exercise(s)
    for aging, 27–28
    for arthritis, 76, 79
    for brain aging, 37
    for breast cancer, 119
    breathing, 28
    for depression, 376–77
    for diabetes, 168–69

    for eating disorders, 202
    for fibroids, 135–36
    and free radical damage, 28
    for gestational diabetes, 172–73
    for headaches, 250
    for heart disease, 293
    for hormonal imbalance, 316
    for interstitial cystitis, 533–34
    for menopause, 348
    for migraines, 405
    for multiple sclerosis, 439–40
    for osteoporosis, 452–53, 455
    for pregnancy, 470–71
    for premenstrual syndrome, 485
    strengthening, 28
    for varicose veins, 555–56

facial herpes. *See* cold sores
Farnsworth, Norman, 48–49
fasting, 23, 239–40, 336
fasting test, 278
fathers and eating disorders, 192–93
fatty acids. *See* essential fatty acids;
        omega-3 fatty acids; omega-6 fatty
        acids
feldenkrais, 567
Feldman, Martin, 11–12, 44, 152, 153,
        155, 179–81, 188–90
female condom, 98
female reconstructive surgery (FRS),
        134, 210
ferrum phos (iron phosphate), 523
fertility awareness, 95–97
fever blisters. *See* cold sores
feverfew, 404, 405
fiber, 326
fibrocystic breast disease, 110, 122–26
    See also breast cancer
fibroids and uterine bleeding, 132–38
    alternative therapies, 134–38
    conventional approach, 133–34
    symptoms, 133
fibromyalgia, 86–87, 318, 401
fillings, dental, 13, 150, 267–69, 517
Finman-Nahman, Tovah, 545
fish pose (yoga), 125–26
fixed food allergy, 274

Flagyl, 551
Fleckenstein, Al, 301
flora, 543
Floradix with iron, 358
fluorescent lighting, 231
fluoride, 269–70
folic acid, 58, 74, 296
folliculinum, 487
food addiction, 196–98, 389, 390, 395–96
food allergies, 239–40, 273–85
    alternative treatments, 279–85
    and arthritis, 81–85, 285
    and carpal tunnel syndrome, 418
    causes, 275–77
    and chronic disease, 280–81
    and diabetes, 169
    and digestion, 181–83
    and eating disorders, 197
    and environmental illness, 232–33
    and headaches, 281–82
    and mental health, 281
    and migraines, 402
    and multiple sclerosis, 436–37
    and obesity, 284–85
    and prostaglandins, 352
    and tension fatigue syndrome, 282–84
    testing, 277–79
    types, 274–75
    and ulcers, 189
Food and Drug Administration, 372–73, 386
food cravings, 198–99, 396
food rotation, 182–83, 239, 278–79
foot-and-toe boogie, 409
formaldehyde, 222–23, 234
formulas. See recipes and formulas
fo-ti, 21
Fox, Michael J., 440, 441
frankincense, 298
free radicals
    and aging, 12, 16
    and breast cancer, 117, 119
    and cancer, 111
    and dementia, 445
    and diet, 247
    and enzyme therapy, 504–5
    and exercise, 28

and smoking, 12
freon, 225
Friedman, Richard, 301–3
Frome, David, 430–31
Fuhrman, Joel, 336
Furman, Joel, 202–5

Gadol, Elmira, 268
Galante, Michele, 150, 151, 159, 377–78
Gallo, Robert, 39, 40
gamma linolenic acid (GLA), 316, 319, 344, 485
garages, 223–24
Gard, Zane, 221
gardenia, 353, 358
garlic
    for aging, 22
    for AIDS, 48, 243
    as antibiotic, 243
    for heart disease, 297
    and immune system, 243, 280
    for vaginal yeast infections, 544, 547, 548
    for varicose veins, 556
Garson, Barbara, 413–14
gas stoves, 225, 285
gastritis, 183–84
gelsemium, 474
genital herpes, 307, 309, 312
genital warts, 499, 501–2
Gentile, Andrew, 148–49, 151–52, 154
gestational diabetes, 171–73
    See also pregnancy
ginger, 361, 468
ginger tea, 358
ginko biloba, 22, 34, 297, 404, 448
ginseng, 22, 48–49, 157, 298, 311, 361
Gittelman, Ann Louise, 342–43
Gladstar, Rosemary, 254
GLA (gamma linolenic acid), 316, 319, 344, 485
Glenville, Marilyn, 325–26
glonoine, 347
glucocorticoids, 77–78
glucosamine, 63, 70, 72, 75–76, 91–92, 416
glucose tolerance test, 379

glutamine, 392
gluthathione
    for aging, 17, 20
    for AIDS, 46
    for multiple sclerosis, 438, 439, 442, 443
glycemic index, 171–72, 200–201
glycyrrhizin, 158
Gofman, John, 110–11
gold, 66, 85, 375, 479
goldenbook, 298
goldenseal, 243, 311, 439, 464
Goldfarb, Herbert, 133–34
Goldwag, William J., 366, 370–71, 376–77
gonadotropin-releasing hormone compounds, 209–10
gonorrhea, 495–96, 538
Gordon, Yehudi, 325–26
Gorman, Pat, 58–59, 351, 355, 356, 358
gotu kola, 22, 255
gout, 64–65, 73–74, 90
    See also arthritis
grains, 240
grapeseed extract, 18
Greenboro, William, 27–28
green tea, 20, 299, 353
Griffin, Judy, 136
GST (glutathione S-transferases) enzyme system, 143
guan xin su he wan, 298
guided imagery, 433, 568
    See also imagery
Guiltinan, Jane, 342, 449, 451
gunpowder 6x, 245

Haas, Elson, 14, 18, 22, 387–89, 391–92, 393–95
Hadaday, Letha, 70–71, 115, 122, 124, 157–58, 297–300, 352, 484, 485–86
Hahnemann, Samuel, 354
hair care, 270–72
hair removal, 264
hangovers, 245, 251–52
Hanley, Jesse, 104, 483, 484, 488
han lian cao (warrior's grass), 137
Harkness, Carla, 321, 323–24, 331
har shar woo, 494

Hashimoto's disease, 508, 512–15
hawthorn, 22, 202, 297, 361
Hazlehurst, G., 44
headaches, 244, 249–51, 281–82
    See also migraines
healing, promotion of, 245
Healing Center of New York City, 18
heart disease, 287–306
    causes, 287–88
    complementary approach, 290–306
    conventional treatment, 289–90
    symptoms, 288
heat and pregnancy, 462–63
heating systems, 223, 230
Hedendal, Bruce, 341
Heimowitz, Colette, 200–202
Helicobacter pylori bacteria, 181, 187, 188–89, 303
Hellerwork, 212–13, 568
    See also Rolfing
hemorrhoids, 185–86, 245
    See also pressure diseases
Hepar sulph, 546
herba epimeti, 328
herbal antibiotics, 242–43
herbal medicine, 569
herbal ointment, 261
herbal skin cleanser, 262
herbal sleep pillow, 253, 254
herbal teas, 23, 25, 261, 405–6
Herbastatin, 544
herbs
    for age spots, 262
    for aging, 21–22
    for AIDS, 47–49
    for anemia, 60–61
    with antibacterial/antifungal activity, 552
    for anxiety, 383
    for arthritis, 70–71
    for breast cancer, 117–18
    for cervical dysplasia, 132
    for chronic fatigue syndrome, 157–58
    cycle for taking, 439
    for depression, 374
    for diabetes, 170
    for endometriosis, 212

for fibrocystic breast disease, 124
for fibroids for uterine bleeding,
    136–37
for gestational diabetes, 173
for heart disease, 296–97
for herpes, 311
for hormonal imbalance, 319–20
for immunity, 248
for infertility, 328
for insomnia, 252–54
for interstitial cystitis, 534
for lupus, 334
for menopause, 345–46
for menstrual problems, 353–54, 358
for migraines, 405–6
for miscarriage, 462, 463–64
for multiple sclerosis, 439
for osteoporosis, 452
for pregnancy, 463–64, 466–68
for premenstrual syndrome, 485–86,
    488
for repetitive strain injuries, 416–17
for sexual dysfunction, 494
for sexually transmitted diseases, 496,
    497–98, 501–2
for skin care, 260–62
for toxic shock syndrome, 360–61
for trichomonas, 549–51
for urinary tract problems, 530–31
for vaginal problems, 538–39
for vaginal yeast infections, 544–45
for varicose veins, 555
herpes, 307–13
    causes, 308–9
    clinical experience, 310–13
    symptoms, 309
herpes simplex virus 1 (HSV-1).
    See cold sores
herpes simplex virus 2 (HSV-2), 307,
    309, 312
herpes zoster, 307, 309, 312–13
    See also herpes
hiatus hernia, 186
    See also pressure diseases
high-fiber diet, 92–93
high-protein, low-carbohydrate diet, 202–4
high-protein diet, 182

Hildebrand, Gar, 141–45
Hinton, Howard, 268
Hippocrates, 25
Hirsch, Roger, 212, 327–29
histamine, 493
Hoffer, Abram, 367–68, 392
Hoffman, David L., 525, 526, 530, 531,
    553–54, 555555
Holistic Balanced Treatment (HBT),
    77–81
holistic medicine, 55
home births, 457, 458
homeopathic candida, 543
homeopathy
    for amenorrhea, 359
    for arthritis, 85–88
    for chronic fatigue syndrome, 159
    defined, 569–70
    for depression, 375–76
    dosages, 88–89
    for endometriosis, 213–14
    for everyday health, 243–46
    for fibrocystic breast disease, 125
    for fibroids and uterine bleeding,
        137–38
    for fibromyalgia, 86–87
    for heart disease, 303–4
    for herpes, 312–13
    for insomnia, 254–55
    for menopause, 346–48
    for menstrual problems, 347, 354–55
    for migraines, 406–7
    for osteoporosis, 456
    for postpartum depression, 477–79
    for pregnancy, 472–74
    for premenstrual syndrome, 486–88
    for repetitive strain injuries, 417
    for urinary incontinence, 523
    for urinary tract problems, 531
    for vaginal dryness and thinning,
        347–48
    for vaginal yeast infections, 546–47
honey, 170, 243
honeybee venom, 87–88
hops, 253
hormonal imbalance, 315–20
    causes, 315–17

and chronic fatigue syndrome, 151
clinical experience, 318–20
and hypothyroidism, 509
and infertility, 322, 325
and massage, 469
and menorrhagia, 357
and migraines, 402
and premenstrual syndrome (PMS), 483
symptoms, 317–18
tests, 318
and urinary tract problems, 526–27
hormone replacement therapy (HRT)
and Alzheimer's disease, 448
and carpal tunnel syndrome, 417
dangers, 339–41
and heart disease, 289–90
and urinary incontinence, 522
See also estrogen replacement therapy
hormones, 18–19, 209, 400, 451–52
hot compresses, 531–32
See also hydrotherapy
hot flashes, 346–47
houseplants, 229, 402
HPV (human papilloma virus), 129, 130, 499–501
Hudson, Tori, 60, 115, 129–31, 134, 211, 492–93, 531, 535, 556
Hufnagel, Vicki, 134, 210, 356, 357, 476, 492, 521, 522
Huggins, Hal A., 13, 517
human herpes virus 6 (HHV-6), 149
human immunodeficiency virus (HIV)
and acupuncture, 50
and AIDS, 39, 40–42
and alternative health therapy, 54
and AZT, 44
herbal treatments, 49
and human papilloma virus (HPV), 501
and ozone, 53
See also AIDS
human papilloma virus (HPV), 129, 130, 499–501
humor in pain management, 433
hunger, 199
Hydergine, 35, 36

hydrastinum muriaticum, 138
hydrogenated oil, 216
hydrotherapy, 125, 405, 531–32, 570
See also hot compresses; sitz bath
hyperbaric oxygen, 143
hypericin A, 34–35, 447
hypericum perforatum (St. John's wort), 49, 313, 374
hypertension, 287–88, 289
hypnotherapy, 389–91
hypoglycemia, 379
hypothyroidism, 12–13, 507, 508–12
hysterectomy, 133–34, 476
hysteroscopic surgery, 134

ignatia, 375, 477–78, 487
ileocecal valve, 176, 181
imagery, 160–61
See also guided imagery
immune system
boosters, 247–48, 280
"busters," 246–47
symptoms of problems, 559
and urinary tract problems, 527
and vaginal yeast infections, 539
Immuno-Augmentative Therapy (IAT), 120, 132
indoor pollution, 229, 230–31
See also pollution
infections, 220, 245, 530
infertility, 321–31
causes, 322–23
clinical experience, 323–31
and gonorrhea, 495
and hypothyroidism, 507
insect bite prevention, 244
insomnia, 252–55
conventional treatment, 252
and DHEA, 18
herbal remedies, 252–54
homeopathy, 254–55
nutrition and supplements, 254
other natural therapies, 255
Institute for Traditional Medicine, 47–48
insulin, 164, 165–66
insulin resistance, 200–201
interstitial cystitis, 533–36

intrauterine device (IUD), 498
intravenous therapies, for lupus, 335
iodine, 123–24, 259
ipecac, 137
iron, 24, 57–58, 177–78
iron phosphate, 523
IUD (intrauterine device), 498

jalapeño peppers, 425–26
Jameson, Timothy, 414–17
Jamison, Richard, 389
Janson, Michael, 287–88, 289, 292, 293,
    294, 296, 484, 488, 493
Jariwalla, Raxit, 47
Jessor, Kim, 470
joint disease, 12
    See also arthritis; osteoarthritis
Joseph, Jim, 431
juice fasting, 23
    See also fasting
juices, 16, 23, 240

kali bichromium, 546
kali carbonicum, 473–74, 478
Kane, Emily, 405–8, 428
Kaplan, Charles A., 431
Kaslow, Andrew, 285
Kaufman, David, 213, 526–27, 529
Keeper (rubber cup), 361
Keep Fit, Reduce Fat (herbal remedy),
    299
Kennedy, David, 269
Keuneke, Robin, 111, 118
Khalsa, Dharma Singh, 32–33, 33–35,
    37–38
kidney function, 494
kitchen, 225–27
Kleinman, Deborah, 420–22
Korins, Ken, 137, 303–4, 346–48, 354–55,
    456, 486–87, 546–47
Kosminsky, Jane, 430
kreosotum (beechwood), 523
Kresse, James, 119–20, 126, 127
ku shen, 544

lacaninum, 486
lachesis, 346, 406, 486

Lacina, Susan, 460–61, 468–69
lactase, 183
lactose intolerance, 183
Lader, Mark, 508, 509–12
Langer, Stephen, 507–8, 513, 514–15
laparoscopic surgery, 105, 134, 209
large intestine. *See* colon
l-arginine, 294
Lark, Susan M., 211–12
Lauritsen, John, 44
lavender, 405
laxatives, 463
l-carnitine, 20, 294
l-cysteine, 20
lecithin, 295
ledum, 74
legumes, 241
Lehrer, Danise, 271
lemon balm, 253, 256–57, 311
leopard's bane, 245, 406, 474, 478, 523
Lesser, Michael, 379, 382, 384
Levin, Warren, 67, 70
Lewy body disease, 445
l-glutamine, 392
licorice, 49, 243, 311
Lieberman, Shari, 150, 155, 158
Liefman, Robert, 77–81
lifestyle
    and AIDS, 50
    and infertility, 325–26
    and lymphedema, 127–28
    and urinary tract problems, 534–35
    and vaginal yeast infections, 545–46
light, 229–30
lighting, 231
liquid zinc. *See* zinc
Liv.52, 251
liver, 181, 488, 510
liver spots, 262, 263
Locurcioas, Gennaro, 375–76
Lombard, Jay, 441, 442–43, 446–47
Lombardi, Susana, 22–23, 28, 30
Lonsdorf, Nancy, 161
Lotson, Anita, 25–26
Lucidril, 35, 36
lung press (reflexology), 409
Lupron, 134

lupus, 333–36
  causes, 333
  clinical experience, 334–36
  symptoms, 333–34
  See also arthritis
lutaigou, 328
lymphatic cleansing, 28
lymphatic drainage, 109–10
lymphedema, 109–10, 126–28
  See also breast cancer
lysine, 310, 311

MacEoin, Beth, 137
magnesia phosphorica, 354, 487
magnesium
  for aging, 21
  for Alzheimer's disease, 446
  for anxiety, 383
  for arthritis, 70
  for depression, 366–67
  for diabetes, 169
  for eating disorders, 201–2
  for fibromyalgia, 401
  for heart disease, 295
  for menstrual cramps, 353
  for migraines, 401, 403, 404
  for premenstrual syndrome, 484
  for repetitive strain injuries, 415–16
  for temporomandibular joint (TMJ)
    dysfunction, 422
magnet therapy, 30–31, 72, 431–32, 556
malabsorption syndrome, 17, 177–78,
    179, 188
malaria, 243
male condom, 97–98
Mandell, Marshall, 81–85, 217, 285
manganese, 202, 416
manganum, 347
manual lymphatic drainage (MLD),
    119–20, 127
mao dong qing, 300
Marcus, William, 269–70
massage, 255, 468–69, 570
  See also manual lymphatic drainage
    (MLD)
Masters and Johnson model of sexual
    response, 491–92

Maver, Robert, 42
maxEPA, 295
McBride, Molly, 73
McCreary, Bill, 43
McDougall, John, 290
medications
  and depression, 365, 369
  for diabetes, 165–66
  and migraines, 401, 403–4
  and yeast infections, 541
medicine cabinet, natural, 242–46
meditation, 302–3, 377–78, 390
medorrhinum, 547
melatonin, 31, 34
menopause, 337–49
  causes, 337–38
  clinical experience, 339–49
  misconceptions, 339
  natural therapies, 341–42
  symptoms, 338–39
menorrhagia, 356–59
menstrual cramps and irregular
    menstruation, 351–61
  amenorrhea and menorrhagia,
    355–59
  causes, 351–52
  clinical experience, 352–55
  homeopathy, 347, 354–55
  and infertility, 322
  toxic shock syndrome, 359–61
menstrual sponges, 361
mental health, 281
  See also addiction; anxiety disorders;
    depression; obsessive-compulsive
    disorders; psychotherapy
mercurius, 547
mercury in silver amalgam fillings, 13,
    150, 267–69, 517
meridian imbalance, 400, 403
Mertz, David, 43
metabolism, 52–53, 150, 379
Michaels, Gina, 335
microwave ovens, 225
midwifery, 457, 459–60, 571
migraines, 399–411
  causes, 399–401
  clinical experience, 401–11

and food allergies, 281–82
symptoms, 401
See also headaches
mildew, 226
milk thistle, 22
Millar, Heather, 215–16, 217, 218–19, 231–35
Millen, Barbara, 453–55
Mills, Dian Shepperson, 208, 210–11
mind-body connection, 120–21, 433
minerals, 151, 259–60, 343–44
See also supplements; *specific minerals*
mint, 118
miscarriage, 321, 325, 461–62, 463–64, 507
See also infertility
miso, 240
mistletoe, 297
mold, 224–25, 226
molybdenum, 21
monoamine oxidase inhibitors, 253
morning sickness, 472–73
Morris, Lance, 13, 17, 28
mothballs, 229
mothers and eating disorders, 192
motherwort, 297
mouthwash, 269, 270, 313
MS. *See* multiple sclerosis (MS)
mucokehl, 170
mucus observation, 95–97
multiple sclerosis (MS), 435–40
causes, 436
clinical experience, 436–40
musculoskeletal injuries, 413–33
pain management, 423–33
repetitive strain injuries, 413–20
temporomandibular joint (TMJ) dysfunction, 420–23
myelin basic protein, 437
myoma coagulation, 134
myomectomy, 133

n-acetyl-cysteine (NAC), 438–39
Nader, Ralph, 216
NADH, 21
Nair, Muraleedharan, 74
National Osteoporosis Foundation, 450

natrum muriaticum, 312, 348, 359, 406–7, 477
natural childbirth, 457, 458–59
natural family planning, 95–97
natural hygiene, 214, 330–31, 571
natural killer cell, 246
naturopathy
for cervical dysplasia, 131
defined, 571–72
for endometriosis, 211
for infertility, 329–30
key tenet, 152
for osteoporosis, 450–52
for urinary tract problems, 529–31
for uterine bleeding, 136
Navajo society, 27
neighborhoods and environmental illness, 219
nervous system disorders. *See* Alzheimer's disease; multiple sclerosis (MS); Parkinson's disease
neurotransmitters, 364
neutralizing-dose therapy, 279–80
New York Medical School, 543
niacin (vitamin B3), 21, 295, 371, 404
Nickel, Nancy, 256–57
nicotine addiction, 388, 389, 390
See also smoking
nitric acid, 348, 546
noise pollution, 225–26, 231
See also pollution
nonsteroidal anti-inflammatory drugs (NSAIDs), 66, 75, 91, 325
norepinephrine, 364
Norman, Laura, 349, 489
Norplant, 104
NSAIDs (nonsteroidal anti-inflammatory drugs), 66, 75, 91, 325
Null, Gary, 391
nutrition
for addiction, 391
for AIDS, 45–50
for alcohol addiction, 391–92
for arthritis, 89–92
for chronic fatigue syndrome, 150
for eating disorders, 194
for herpes, 310–11

for hormonal imbalance, 319
for infertility, 323
for insomnia, 254
for reproductive system cancers,
141–42
nux vomica, 245, 255, 407, 473, 488

obesity, 191, 193, 284–85, 317
See also eating disorders
obsessive-compulsive disorders, 384–87
alternative therapies, 385–87
causes, 384–85
conventional treatment, 385
symptoms, 385
Odinov Pukit, Stephanie, 472–74
Ojeda, Lybda, 339
Olsen, Mary, 399–404
Olson, Sharon, 313
omega-3 fatty acids, 260, 280, 373,
437–38
See also essential fatty acids
omega-6 fatty acids, 260, 437–38
See also essential fatty acids
one-month, one-year law, 58–59
Ordene, Marjorie, 137, 324, 351–52, 477,
479, 541
Ornish, Dean, 168, 290–91
orthomolecular medicine, 572
osteoarthritis, 12, 64, 69–70, 177
See also arthritis
osteoporosis, 449–56
causes, 449–50
clinical experience, 450–56
diagnosis, 450
and hormone replacement therapy,
341
Ostrom, Neenyah, 149, 150
ovarian cancer, 138–39, 341
ovulation, 324
oxygen therapy, 53–54, 219, 439
ozone therapy, 53–54

Page, Linda, 360–62, 496, 498, 501–2
pain management, 423–33
back pain, 423–24
for carpal tunnel syndrome, 419
diet and nutrition, 424–27

for endometriosis, 209, 210, 214
mind-body connection, 433
physical therapies, 427–32
pancreatic enzymes, 176, 177
pantothenic acid, 423
papain, 438
Pap smears, 129, 130, 139, 140, 141,
499–500
parathyroid, 456
Parkinson's disease, 440–43
alternative approaches, 442–43
causes, 441
conventional treatment, 442
passionflower, 253
patient rights, 557–58
patient role, 558–59
pau d'arco, 544
Peat, Ray, 12–13, 292, 295, 330
Peel Report, 458
Pelton, Ross, 32, 33, 34, 35, 36
pelvic inflammatory disease (PID),
329–30, 495, 496, 497, 498–99, 538
Penepent, Anthony, 136, 214, 330–31,
352–53, 357
peppermint oil, 124, 244
perimenopause, 337–38
See also menopause
Perlstein, Gracia, 135–36, 158–59,
464–66, 540–41, 545–46
peroneal massage, 469
Perri, Dolores, 316–17, 319
personal hygiene for urinary tract
problems, 534–35
pesticides and infertility, 325
PET (positron emission tomography)
scan, 37
PET (progesterone, estrogen, and
testosterone), 19
petroleum, 312, 473
phenylalanine, 382
philodendron, 353
Philpott, William, 171
phosphates, 316
phosphatidyl choline, 448
phosphatidyl serine, 34, 374
phospholipids, 52
phosphoric acid, 478

phosphorus, 69–70, 138, 312, 347, 407

photodamage, 262, 263

physical therapy, 72–73, 422

Physicians for Complementary
    Medicine, 67

phytochemicals, 49–50

phytoestrogens, 326

phytolacca, 125

Picozzi, Michele, 307, 308, 309, 311

Pierce, Robert, 50

piracetam, 35–36

Pittman, John, 53–54

pituitary insufficiency, 329

Pizzorno, Joseph, 28, 136, 329–30, 531

plant protein, 203–4

plants, house, 229, 402

plastics, 218

Plumley, P., 42–43

Podell, Richard, 222

polarity therapy, 573

pollution, 217
    electromagnetic, 36–37, 150
    indoor, 229, 230–31
    noise, 225–26, 231

polyphosphates, 316

poo wah, 136

postpartum depression, 477–79

potassium, 169

prednisone, 78, 91, 516–17

pregnancy, 457–81
    abortion aftercare, 479–80
    and anemia, 58–59
    breast-feeding, 474–76
    circumcision, 481
    corrective vaginal surgery, 476
    midwifery, 457, 459–60
    miscarriage, 321, 325, 461–62,
        463–64, 507
    natural childbirth, 457, 458–59
    postpartum depression, 477–79
    stages, 460–61
    things to avoid, 462–64
    See also gestational diabetes

pregnenolone, 345

premenstrual dysphoric disorder
    (PMDD), 489–90

premenstrual syndrome (PMS), 483–90

causes, 483
    clinical experience, 484–89
    herbs, 358
    premenstrual dysphoric disorder
        (PMDD), 489–90
    symptoms, 483

pressure diseases, 184–87

Price, Erika, 312–13

Price, Weston, 266

Priestley, Joan, 46

Proffman, Mitchell, 27–28, 71

progesterone, 315–16, 318
    and menopause, 338, 344–45
    for menorrhagia, 357
    for osteoporosis, 451–52
    for postpartum depression, 479
    for premenstrual syndrome, 488
    See also hormonal imbalance

progestin, 340, 344

prolapsed transverse colon, 527

prolapsed uterus, 476

prostaglandins, 352

proteolytic enzymes, 416

Prozac, 489–90

psoralens, 261–62

psychotherapy, 194–95, 384, 386, 387

public speaking, 390–91

pulsatilla
    for amenorrhea, 359
    for menstrual cramps, 354
    for migraines, 407
    for postpartum depression, 478
    for pregnancy, 472, 473
    for premenstrual syndrome, 487
    for vaginal yeast infections, 546

Pure Cream Cleanser, 262

pyridoxine (vitamin B6), 251, 386–87,
    479, 484

qi (chi) manipulation, 304

qi gong, 556, 573

Rachlin, Steven, 117

Randolph, Theron, 81

Rapp, Doris, 366

recipes and formulas
    for age spots, 262

bath, 239
douche, 132, 498, 545, 550, 551–52
gotu kava tea, 256
herbal drink for amenorrhea, 358
herbal ointment, 261
herbal tea, 261, 405–6
hops tea, 253
juiced garlic, 243
kava kava tea, 256
lemon balm tea, 253, 256–57
for menstrual cramps, 352
mouthwash, 313
passionflower tea, 253
for premenstrual syndrome, 486
to prevent miscarriage, 462
Pure Cream Cleanser, 262
red raspberry tonic, 466–67
salad, 370–71
for skin care, 260–62
skullcap tea, 253
soup, immune-enhancing, 159
stinging nettle tonic, 467
tea for vaginal problems, 539
for trichomonas, 550
for urinary tract problems, 531
vaginal ointments, 498
for varicose veins, 555
reconstructive therapy for arthritis,
    71–72
red cabbage extract, 19
red raspberry tonic, 466–67
refeeding, 196
reflexology
    and AIDS, 51
    defined, 574
    for menopause, 349
    for migraines, 408–11
    for premenstrual syndrome, 489
refrigerators, 225–26
Reichenberg-Ullman, Judyth, 254–55,
    531, 532
Reid, Susanna, 138–41, 171–73, 479–80
Reiki, 29–30, 38, 574
reishi mushroom, 253
relaxation response, 302–3, 377–78, 390
repetitive strain injuries, 413–20
    carpal tunnel syndrome, 414, 417–20

clinical experience, 414–17
    symptoms, 414
reproductive system cancers, 138–46
    combination treatments, 141–45
    patient story, 145–46
    types, 138–41
rescue remedy, 244
Resolve (consumer advocacy group), 331
restorative foods, 89–90
Revici, Emmanuel, 52–53
Rezulin, 166
rheumatoid arthritis, 64, 90, 513
    See also arthritis
rhus tox, 86–87, 407
Ribner, Rich, 68
Rist-Podrecca, Abigail, 51, 133, 136–37,
    159–60, 450, 455, 494, 561
RNA, 21
roach sprays, 226
Robins, Howard, 18, 68, 452, 453
Rolfing, 212, 430–31, 574–75
    See also Hellerwork
romania, 494
rosemary, 118
Ross, Gary, 125–26
rotary diversified diet, 182–83, 239,
    278–79
Rothblatt, Henry, 78

sabina, 137, 347
sacro-occipital technique, 421–22
Sahelian, Ray, 246–47
salad recipe, 370–71
salivary IgA, 18–19
SAMe (S-adenosyl-l-methionine), 373
Sarnoff, Debra, 262–66
sarsaparilla, 353
saunas, 30
Sawaf, Talha, 325–26
Schachter, Michael, 107–9, 116, 119,
    219–21, 268
Schauss, Alexander, 193–94, 195, 373–74
schizandra, 299
Schneider, Eric, 160
Scolastico, Ron, 304–6
scouring rush, 523
sea algae, 21

Seaman, Barbara, 322–23
Sears, Barry, 203
seasonal affective disorder, 229–30
sea sponges, 361
sea vegetables, 240–41
secale, 137, 347
sedatives, 253–54
selenium, 17, 416, 438
self-healing, 161
Sellman, Sherrill, 102–3, 112–13, 115,
    289–90, 315–16, 318, 320, 337–39,
    339, 340, 341, 344–45, 489–90
sepia
  for depression, 375–76
  for fibrocystic breast disease, 125
  for menopause, 347–48
  for migraines, 407
  for postpartum depression, 477
  for pregnancy, 472, 473
  for premenstrual syndrome, 487
Seraphim, 489–90
serotonin, 364, 385, 386, 387
sexual dysfunction, 491–94
  causes, 491–93
  clinical experience, 493–94
sexually transmitted diseases (STDs),
    495–502
  chlamydia, 496–98
  and condoms, 97–98
  genital warts, 499, 501–2
  gonorrhea, 495–96, 538
  human papilloma virus (PMV),
    499–501
  pelvic inflammatory disease (PID),
    329–30, 495, 496, 497, 498–99, 538
SGOT enzymes, 179
shiatsu, 407–8, 428–29, 469–70, 560
shina, 137
shingles, 307, 309, 312–13
shoulder and neck reflex, 410
shoulder stand, 125
Siberian ginseng, 298, 311
  See also ginseng
sick building syndrome, 222–23
silica, 407, 546
silicon, 259–60
silicone breast implants, 217

Silverman, Stephen M., 216–17
Simone, Charles, 111, 112, 116
Simonton, Carl, 120–21
simple stretch for chest muscles (yoga),
    454–55
Singer, Sidney Ross, 109–10
sitz bath, 329–30, 359, 532, 556
  See also hydrotherapy
skin brushing, 30
skin care, 257–66
  cosmetic laser surgery, 262–66
  essential fatty acids, 260
  herbal formulas, 260–62
  minerals, 259–60
  vitamins, 257–59
skin resurfacing, 263, 264–65
skullcap, 253, 257
Slagle, Priscilla, 364–65, 369, 372–73,
    517–18
sleep and immune system, 149, 246
  See also insomnia
slivers, 245
smell, sense of, 233
Smith, Lendon, 366–67
smoking
  and cancer, 112
  and depression, 367–68
  and free radicals, 12
  and hormonal imbalance, 316
  and immune system, 246
  and infertility, 325
  and nicotine addiction, 388, 389, 390
  and urinary incontinence, 521
social support and pregnancy, 459–60
soft drinks, 69–70
Soileau, John, 123, 124, 125, 355–56,
    357–58, 359
Sorge, Robert, 132–33, 541
soup, immune-enhancing, 159
spermicide, 99–101
spine reflex, 410
splinters, 245
Spreen, Allan, 382–83, 515–16
sprouts, 240
St. John's wort, 49, 313, 374
staphylococcus bacteria, 242–43
Stay, Flora Para, 267

Steenblock, David, 69–70, 92–94, 287, 289, 300–301
Stefanacci, Janice, 339, 491
sterilization, 105
stinging nettle tonic, 467
Stoll, Walt, 380–81
stomachache, 181, 244, 245
stomach acid, 176, 177–78, 180, 189–90
strengthening exercises, 28
streptococcal bacteria, 243
stress
    and arthritis, 65
    and depression, 365
    and environmental illness, 220–21
    and food allergies, 276
    and headaches, 250
    homeopathic remedies, 244
    and hormonal imbalance, 317
    and immune system, 246
    and infertility, 327
    management, 28, 280, 301–3, 355, 384, 424
    and migraines, 401, 404
    and temporomandibular joint (TMJ) dysfunction, 420–21
stressor foods, 90–91
stroke, 503–5
    causes, 503
    clinical experience, 504–5
    symptoms, 503
Suatoni, Sarah, 212–13
subluxation, upper cervical, 400, 403
sugar
    addiction, 388, 394–95
    and hormonal imbalance, 317
    and pain management, 425–26
    and vaginal problems, 539, 542–43
sulfur, 260
summa, 544
sunscreen, 261–62
sun spots, 262, 263
superoxide dismutase (SOD), 18
Super Slow (weight-training program), 28
supplements
    for addiction, 397
    for aging, 16–22

for Alzheimer's disease, 447–48
for amenorrhea and menorrhagia, 357
for anemia, 60
for arthritis, 68–70
for breast cancer, 116
for chronic fatigue syndrome, 155–56
for depression, 373–74
for detoxification, 241–42
for diabetes, 169
for digestive disorders, 181
for eating disorders, 195
for endometriosis, 211–12
for environmental illness, 219–20
for fibrocystic breast disease, 123–24
for fibroids, 135–36
for hair health, 271–72
for heart disease, 294–96
for hormonal imbalance, 319
for human papilloma virus (HPV), 500–501
for hypothyroidism, 512
for infertility, 327
for insomnia, 254
for lupus, 334–35
for menopause, 344–45
for menstrual cramps, 353
for migraines, 402
for multiple sclerosis, 437–39
for pain management, 426–27
for pregnancy, 466
for premenstrual syndrome, 484–85
for repetitive strain injuries, 415–16
for sexual dysfunction, 493
for temporomandibular joint (TMJ) dysfunction, 422–23
for urinary tract problems, 530
for vaginal yeast infections, 543–44, 547
for varicose veins, 555, 556
support stockings, 554
suppositories, 544, 547, 548
surgery, carpal tunnel syndrome, 419
Swank, Roy, 437
symptoms, importance of, 559
systemic lupus erythematosis.
    See lupus

tai chi, 160
tamoxifen, 112–15, 138, 140
tampons, 360, 361
Taromaro Indians, 28
tarragon, 311
tattoo removal, 263–64
Tatz, Shmuel, 72
taurine, 295
Taylor, Frances, 238–42, 566
tea tree oil, 244, 545
Teich, Morton, 70
Temin, Howard, 41
temporomandibular joint (TMJ)
        dysfunction, 420–23
    causes, 420–21
    clinical experience, 421–23
    symptoms, 421
tension fatigue syndrome, 282–84
testosterone, 77–78, 493
Tew, Marjorie, 458
Theodosakis, Jason, 64, 75–77
Therapeutic Touch, 575
therapy types, 559–76
thiamine (vitamin B1), 296, 447
thuja occidentalis, 407
thymus extract, 21
thymus gland, 13
thyroid disease, 507–19
    hypothyroidism, 12–13, 507, 508–12
    patient stories, 516–19
    thyroid importance, 507–8
    thyroiditis, 508, 512–15
thyroid disorders, 318, 330, 418
thyroiditis, 508, 512–15
thyroid supplements, 295, 515, 516, 519
Tienchi ginseng, 298
    See also ginseng
Tirtha, Sada Shiva, 61
tobacco. See smoking
Tolle, Roger, 430
tongue as indicator of health, 266
toothpaste, 269, 270
Tourles, Stephanie, 257–62
toxic home syndrome, 36–37
toxic shock syndrome (TSS), 359–61
toxic thinking, 391
Trager technique, 429–30, 576

tranquilizers, 365, 369
transcutaneous electrical stimulation
        (TENS) unit, 38
trans-fats, 111
trauma ointment, 245
trichomonas, 549–51
trigger foods, 199–200
trillium, 138
tryptophan, 254, 372–73, 382, 386
tuberculosis, 243
turmeric, 118
tyrosine, 21, 202, 372–73, 382

ulcers, 187–90
    alternative treatment, 188–90
    diabetic, 170
    diagnosis, 188
    and food allergies, 189
    traditional treatment, 187–88
Ullman, Dana, 85–89, 487–88, 523
Ullman, Robert, 254–55, 531, 532
Ulrich, Gail, 247–49
upper cervical subluxation, 400, 403
urinary incontinence, 521–23
    causes, 521
    clinical experience, 522–23
    symptoms, 522
urinary tract infections and
        inflammations, 525–36
    causes, 525–28
    clinical experience, 528–32
    and diaphragm method of birth
        control, 101
    interstitial cystitis, 533–36
    symptoms, 528
    urinary tract inflammations, 532–33

vacticime drops, 245
vaginal contraceptive film (VCF), 101
vaginal dryness and thinning, 347–48
vaginal inflammation and infection,
        537–52
    bacterial vaginosis, 551–52
    causes, 537
    clinical experience, 538–39
    symptoms, 538
    trichomonas, 549–51

vaginal yeast (candidiasis), 539–49
vaginal ointments, 498
vaginal yeast (candidiasis), 539–49
   alternative therapies, 542–48
   causes, 539–41
   clinical experience, 542
   patient story, 548–49
   symptoms, 541–42
valerian, 253, 353
vanadium, 201
vanadyl sulfate, 169
varicose veins, 553–56
   causes, 553–54
   clinical experience, 554–56
   symptoms, 554
vegetable juices, 240
ventilation, 230–31
Venus flytrap, 118
Vergara, Nilsa, 29–30
Vesselago, Michael, 152–53
viburnum, 354
vincristine, 35
viral infection and chronic fatigue
   syndrome, 148–49
Virtue, Doreen, 198–200
virus identification, 249
vitamin A
   for aging, 17
   for arthritis, 68–69
   for endometriosis, 211
   for pregnancy, 463
   for sexually transmitted diseases, 501
   for skin care, 258
   for urinary tract problems, 530
vitamin B complex
   for depression, 371
   for endometriosis, 212
   for menopause, 343–44
   for repetitive strain injuries, 415
   for skin care, 258
   for temporomandibular joint (TMJ)
     dysfunction, 422–23
   for vaginal yeast infections, 544
vitamin B1 (thiamine), 296, 447
vitamin B3 (niacin), 21, 295, 371, 404
vitamin B6 (pyridoxine), 251, 386–87,
   479, 484

vitamin B12 (cobalamin), 21, 58, 296,
   438, 447–48
vitamin C
   for aging, 17–18
   for AIDS, 47
   for arthritis, 69, 72
   for colds, 248–49
   for detoxification, 241
   for endometriosis, 212
   for genital warts, 501
   for gout, 74
   for heart disease, 296
   for infections, 530
   for repetitive strain injuries, 415
   for skin care, 258
   for urinary tract problems, 530
   for vaginal yeast infections, 544
vitamin D, 258–59, 344, 463
vitamin E
   for aging, 17, 34
   for AIDS, 47
   for arthritis, 69
   for eating disorders, 201
   for endometriosis, 212
   for heart disease, 296
   for menopause, 343
   for pregnancy, 463
   for premenstrual syndrome, 485
   for repetitive strain injuries, 416
   for skin care, 259
vitamins
   for chronic fatigue syndrome, 151
   for menopause, 343–44
   for pregnancy, 463
   for skin care, 257–59
   See also supplements; *specific vitamins*
vitral syndromes, 220
Vleit, Elizabeth, 317–18

Wald, Michael, 435–40, 440, 445–46,
   447–48
Wald, Robin, 322, 325, 326, 327
Walker, Lynn Page, 244–46
warrior poses (yoga), 454
Warshowsky, Allan, 480, 495–96, 502
warts, genital, 499, 501–2
water

and aging, 15–16
for detoxification, 238
and environmental illness, 216, 226–27
and headaches, 250
during pregnancy, 466
for urinary tract problems, 529
Weed, Susun, 452, 462–64, 466–68
weight-training programs, 28
Wellspring for Women, 547–49
Wharton, Linda, 527–28, 529, 530–31, 531–32
Whitaker, Julian, 290, 293
Whiting, Steven, 156–57, 310–11, 383
wild yam, 19, 22, 297
Willard, Terry, 253–54
willow, 405
Women's Precious (herb formulation), 358
Women's Rhythm (herb formulation), 358
workplace and environmental illness, 218–19, 230–31
wormwood, 328
wound healing, 245
Wright, Jonathan, 334–35
Wunderlich, Ray, 65, 417–20

xenoestrogens, 108–9, 325, 326
xiao yao wan, 118, 124, 299, 353
X rays and breast cancer, 110–11

yam, 19, 22, 297
Yang, Yuan, 72
yans shen jia jiao wan, 298–99
Yaryura-Tobias, José, 196, 384–87
yeast-free diet, 542–43
yeast infections. See vaginal yeast (candidiasis)
yoga
for arthritis, 73
defined, 576
for depression, 377–78
for fibrocystic breast disease, 125–26
for osteoporosis, 453–55
yu dai wan, 544
yunnan pai yao, 354

Zake, Yamuna, 422, 455, 564
Zamm, Alfred, 222
Zand, Janet, 60–61, 319–20, 485
Zeines, Victor, 266
Zhang, Quingcai, 48
zinc
for aging, 17, 35
for Alzheimer's disease, 448
and children, 249
for colds, 248–49
for depression, 373–74
for diabetes, 169
for eating disorders, 193–94, 195, 201
for menopause, 343
for repetitive strain injuries, 416
for skin care, 260
for urinary tract problems, 530
zone walking, 409–10
Zovirax, 310